Anabolic Steroids in Sport and Exercise

Second Edition

Charles E. Yesalis, MPH, ScD
The Pennsylvania State University
Editor

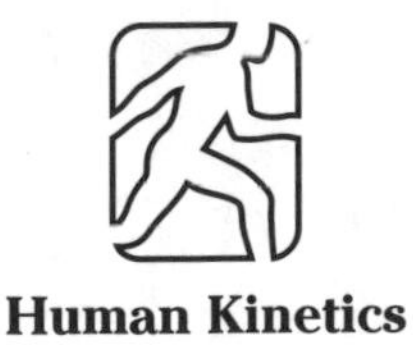

Human Kinetics

Library of Congress Cataloging-in-Publication Data

Anabolic steroids in sport and exercise/Charles E. Yesalis, editor.
-- 2nd ed.
p. cm.
Includes bibliographical references and index.
ISBN 0-88011-786-9
1. Anabolic steroids--Health aspects. 2. Doping in sports.
I. Yesalis, Charles.
RC1230.A522 2000
362.29'088'796--dc21 99-38353
CIP

ISBN 0-88011-786-9

Permission notices for material reprinted in this book from other sources can be found on pages xvii–xviii.

Acquisitions Editor: Loarn D. Robertson PhD; **Developmental Editor:** Joanna Hatzopoulos; **Assistant Editor:** Susan C. Hagan; **Copyeditor:** John Mulvihill; **Proofreader:** Sarah Wiseman; **Indexer:** Robert Howerton; **Permission Manager:** Heather Munson; **Graphic Designer:** Fred Starbird; **Graphic Artist:** Dawn Sills; **Photo Editor:** Clark Brooks; **Cover Designer:** Jack W. Davis; **Illustrator:** Kristin King; **Printer:** Versa Press; **Binder:** Dekker & Sons

Printed in the United States of America 10 9 8 7 6 5 4 3 2 1

Human Kinetics
Web site: http://www.humankinetics.com/

United States: Human Kinetics, P.O. Box 5076, Champaign, IL 61825-5076
1-800-747-4457
e-mail: humank@hkusa.com

Canada: Human Kinetics, 475 Devonshire Road Unit 100, Windsor, ON N8Y 2L5
1-800-465-7301 (in Canada only)
e-mail: humank@hkcanada.com

Europe: Human Kinetics, P.O. Box IW14, Leeds LS16 6TR, United Kingdom
+44 (0)113-278 1708
e-mail: humank@hkeurope.com

Australia: Human Kinetics, 57A Price Avenue, Lower Mitcham, South Australia 5062
(08) 82771555
e-mail: liahka@senet.com.au

New Zealand: Human Kinetics, P.O. Box 105-231, Auckland Central
09-523-3462
e-mail: humank@hknewz.com

This book is dedicated in memory of:

Philip Bonnet, M.D., my mentor, teacher, and friend. He taught me the value of logic and clarity in one's work and thoughts.

Charles Kochakian, PhD., a true pioneer in endocrinology. His monumental contributions in anabolic-androgenic steroid research spanned more than a half century.

My father, Charles Yesalis, a great athlete, a warrior, and a patriot. He taught me to speak the truth regardless of the consequences.

For a great many years I have believed that the weakness of old men depended on two causes—a natural series of organic changes and the gradually diminishing action of the spermatic glands.

E.C. Brown-Séquard
Lancet, 1889 (**2**)

The use of artificial means [to improve performance] has long been considered wholly incompatible with the spirit of sport and has therefore been condemned. Nevertheless, we all know that this rule is continually being broken, and that sportive competitions are often more a matter of doping than of training. It is highly regrettable that those who are in charge of supervising sport seem to lack the energy for the campaign against this evil, and that a lax, and fateful, attitude is spreading. Nor are the physicians without blame for this state of affairs, in part on account of their ignorance, and in part because they are prescribing strong drugs for the purpose of doping which are not available to athletes without prescriptions.

O. Riesser
"Über Doping und Dopingmittel" in
Leibesübungen und körperliche Erziehung, 1933
Found in John M. Hoberman, Mortal Engines, *1992*

Lie #1: Anabolic steroids do not enhance athletic performance.
Lie #2: Steroids will kill you.
Lie #3: You can get the same results without steroids, you just have to work longer and harder.

Dan Duchaine
Underground Steroid Handbook II, 1989

My definition of cheating is doing something nobody else is doing.

Charlie Francis
Former coach of Ben Johnson
Sports Illustrated, *December 17, 1990*

That evening I spied two of the G.D.R.'s female throwers on their way to the cafeteria for dinner. They were gotten up in frilly dresses with matching purses, and were perched on improbably flimsy high heels. In between the dresses and the shoes, one was reminded of why these women were here: their calves were like tree trunks, their Achilles tendons like bridge cables. A childhood memory flashed before me: the dancing hippos from *Fantasia.*

Charlie Francis
Speed Trap, *1990*

"It is absolutely rampant right now," says one American League front-office executive, who talked only on the condition his name would not be used. "But baseball doesn't care. The Players Association doesn't care. The owners don't care."

Steroids have completely changed the game. Guys try to cover it up by saying they're using creatine (a muscle-enhancer). Or they're just lifting weights now. Come on. It's a completely different look. I can pick out a kid using creatine from a kid on 'roids.

Go ahead and get pictures of guys when they were 22 years old, and look at them now. Look at their faces. Look at the size of their heads now. That's not creatine.

Ken Rosenthal
Regular writer for MSNBC on the Internet, and columnist for the Baltimore Sun
Steroids: Baseball's Darkest Secret, August 25, 1998

By 2000, unless we are testing blood, we haven't got a chance.

Professor David Cowan, head of the International Olympic Committee (IOC) accredited laboratory in London, fears certain drugs are being used by athletes with the knowledge they cannot be detected by existing testing methods involving urine analyses.
Dublin, Ireland, November 9, 1998

People who get caught are either badly managed or have very stupid doctors.

Anonymous British sportsman

Far and away the most frequently occurring side effect of using steroids is that you become a liar.

Anonymous bodybuilder
Peter Hildreth, OP/ED London Times, August 23, 1999

Anabolic steroid's biggest side effect is loss of memory because no one can remember taking them.

Anonymous All-Pro Lineman

Contents

Preface

> ***No one is guilty of steroid use except the other guy, the other team or the other school—what a laugh.***
>
> Charles Yesalis, Sr. (1915–1999)
> Chicago Golden Gloves Team 1934
> University of Illinois Basketball and Track 1935–36

In 1992, I began the preface by stating, "The use of performance-enhancing drugs by athletes, most notably anabolic steroids, is likely the greatest problem facing sport today. Hardly a week goes by that another revelation of drug use by high school, collegiate, professional, or Olympic-level athletes is not highlighted in the news." Today this assertion still rings true. In a recent investigative report on drug use in sport conducted by *Sports Illustrated* (Bamberger and Yaeger, 1997), the authors stated:

> *the use of steroids—and other, more exotic substances, such as human growth hormone (hGH)—has spread to almost every sport, from major league baseball to college basketball to high school football. It is the dirty and universal secret of sports, amateur and pro, as the millenium draws near . . . Dozens of athletes, coaches, administrators and steroid traffickers interviewed by SI say that the Atlanta Olympics, like other Games of the last half century, was a carnival of sub-rosa experiments in the use of performance-enhancing drugs.*

In 1998 in the United States, Olympic gold medalists and world record holders Randy Barnes (shot-putter) and Dennis Mitchell (sprinter) have been suspended by the International Amateur Athletic Federation (IAAF) for positive drug tests (Patrick, 1998). The Tour de France cycling race, a world-class event, was "transformed from a triumphant test of man and machine into a scandal-sodden drug debacle" (Ruibal, 1998). Team physicians, trainers, and cyclists have detailed an epidemic of drug use in professional cycling. This has all taken place despite the presence of a so-called rigorous, state-of-the-art drug testing program—the same program used by the world's major sport federations, including the International Olympic Committee, the National Football League, and the National Collegiate Athletic Association. Drug scandals seem to go on and on, and doping is not confined to humans. Livestock shows at state fairs, where large cash prizes are awarded, have increasingly employed drug testing in the wake of episodes of cheating where drugs were used to make the animals appear larger or more muscular ("State Fair Weighing," 1996). There have even been accusations of doping in auto racing—not of the drivers, but tires! It has been alleged that some teams have used chemicals to illegally treat tires to increase traction (Newberry, 1998). It is rumored that some of these chemicals are undetectable.

It is also increasingly obvious that performance-enhancing drug use is not just confined to professional and Olympic athletes. There is a growing body of evidence that high school and even junior high students are using anabolic steroids during the physically and emotionally vulnerable period when hormonal cycles are changing. In fact, since the publication of the first edition of this book in 1993, anabolic steroid use among adolescents has increased significantly. Moreover, in the United States today there are approximately 375,000 adolescent males and 175,000 adolescent females who have used anabolic steroids at least once in their lives. The American Academy of Pediatrics (1997) concluded the following:

> *To our knowledge, no study has identified an adolescent population without the temptation and risks of anabolic steroid use. Furthermore, no study has been published showing a decrease in the prevalence of anabolic steroid use over time.*

In addition, the level of anabolic steroid use among adolescents in other developed nations appears remarkably similar to that observed in the United States. Unfortunately, anabolic steroid use at the professional and Olympic levels is still poorly documented and veiled in secrecy.

Given the magnitude of this problem, it is important that physicians, athletic trainers, nurses, physical therapists, and other medical professionals who treat and counsel athletes have a thorough knowledge of performance-enhancing drugs.

For some time there has been a lack of trust and communication between members of the athletic community and the scientific and medical communities regarding anabolic steroids and other drugs. This, in part, is a function of a poor understanding by clinicians and researchers of the motivations of athletes, and vice versa. The medical community has lost much credibility as a result of repeated denials that anabolic steroids significantly enhance performance (American College of Sports Medicine [ASCM], 1977; Ryan, 1981; Elashoff, Jacknow, Shain, & Braunstein, 1991). For the past three decades, some physicians and scientists have dogmatically reported that any weight an athlete gains while taking steroids is mainly the result of fluid retention and that any strength gain is largely psychological (a placebo effect). Since the first edition, further research has been conducted on the efficacy and mechanisms of action of anabolic steroids, which will hopefully help put this issue to rest. Along the same line, some members of the sports medicine community have, with the best of intentions, adopted an overly aggressive educational strategy and have used strong, but often unfounded, pronouncements regarding the adverse health effects of anabolic steroids. Athletes, on the other hand, simply have not witnessed longtime steroid users "dropping like flies." This credibility gap has been exacerbated by the apparent contradiction between these warnings of dire health consequences and new clinical applications of these drugs, such as the 10-center worldwide trial sponsored by the World Health Organization to test the efficacy of anabolic steroids as a male contraceptive (World Health Organization Task Force, 1996) as well as multicenter trials to assess the effects of testosterone supplementation in older men ("Testosterone Replacement Therapy," 1996). To help close this gap, our book seeks to provide the reader with a comprehensive, accurate, and objective discussion of anabolic steroid use in sport.

Since the first edition, our knowledge of effects of anabolic steroids has continued to expand. While the long-term health effects of anabolic steroids remain unclear, the acute or short-term health effects are more clearly understood, especially those related to heart and cerebrovascular disease. A pattern of association between endogenous testosterone levels and aggressive behavior in humans has been increasingly established. On the other hand, a number of clinical studies using moderate doses of exogenous testosterone have failed to note any demonstrable effect on behavior. However, the picture is still clouded by case reports and several other studies that show affective and psychotic syndromes—some of violent proportions—among individuals using high doses of anabolic steroids.

During the past five years, a prevention program targeted at anabolic steroid use among male high school students has been developed. By all appearances, it works! Nonetheless, given the increase in anabolic steroid use among female adolescents, more work needs to be done.

The contributors to this text have spent a number of years researching anabolic steroids. They have backgrounds in various areas of science, clinical medicine, and law as well as journalism. Many of the authors also have actively assisted the federal government and state governments as well as national sport federations in dealing with drug use in athletics. The authors have collaborated on this book to attempt to answer, at least in part, the following questions about anabolic steroids.

- What are anabolic steroids?
- Who uses anabolic steroids?
- Do anabolic steroids enhance physical capacities?
- How do anabolic steroids work?
- How do anabolic steroids affect physical and psychological health?
- What alternatives do we have as a society in dealing with this problem?

To best answer these questions, this book is divided into three parts. Part I, "History and Incidence of Use," contains four chapters that explain the chemical development of anabolic steroids and trace the progression of anabolic steroid use by athletes. Physical and psychological effects of these drugs, as well as approaches to assessment and treatment, are discussed in part II, "Effects, Dependence, and Treatment Issues." The contributors to part III, "Drug Testing and Societal Alternatives," explain the origins, history, and problems of testing for anabolic steroids and pose some thought-provoking solutions to anabolic steroid use.

By providing our perspectives on these issues, we trust that this text will help clinicians and health educators better provide potential or current users of anabolic steroids with the best information available with which to make informed judgments. Furthermore, we hope that this book will give health professionals a better understanding of anabolic steroid use in sport and will help them solve this societal problem.

References

American Academy of Pediatrics. (1997). Adolescents and anabolic steroids. *Pediatrics, 99*, 904–908.

American College of Sports Medicine. (1977). Position statement on the use and abuse of anabolic-androgenic steroids in sports. *Medicine and Science in Sports and Exercise, 9,* 11–13.

Bamberger, M., & Yaeger, D. (1997, April 14). Over the edge. *Sports Illustrated, 86*(15), 60–70.

Elashoff, J., Jacknow, A., Shain, S., & Braunstein, G. (1991). Effects of anabolic-androgenic steroids on muscular strength. *Annals of Internal Medicine, 115*, 387–393.

Newberry, P. (1998, September 2). Gordon: Roush owes Rainbow Warriors an apology over tire flap. *Centre Daily Times,* (State College, PA) p. 1B.

Patrick, D. (1998, July 28). Positive drug tests sideline Olympic pair. *USA Today*, p. 1c.

Ruibal, S. (1998, July 30). Cyclists' drug protest wipes out Tour stage. *USA Today,* p. 1c.

Ryan, A. (1981). Anabolic steroids are fool's gold. *Federation Proceedings, 40,* 2682–2688.

State fair weighing more livestock testing. (1996, 23 January). *News-Gazette,* (Champaign, IL) p. B6.

Testosterone replacement therapy: May improve life for aging males. (1996, February). *Endocrine News, 21*(1), 1–7.

World Health Organization Task Force on Methods for the Regulation of Male Fertility. (1996). Contraceptive efficacy of testosterone-induced azoospermia and oligozoospermia in normal men. *Fertility and Sterility, 65*, 821–829.

The State of the Game

I woke up this morning after a night of killing pain.
I went to the practice field to deal with it again.
My coach, he tells me, "Fight hard and be a man!"
But with his chalk board theories we all wonder if he can?
So knock 'em down, block 'em hard and strive to win the fight.
I wonder why they're so concerned, is it economic plight?
The battle in the trenches, won and lost, and who does realize
But the gladiator in its midst whose soul in anguish cries.
What keeps him in the arena but those fine and great ideals,
But it's become just a business, what matter how he feels.
The battle fought, the game is won, and victor duly glorified.
But the sad fact, businessman, is the sporting soul has died.
In the end in retrospect what's glorified and gained
But the almighty dollar, not the spirit of the game.

Steve Courson
Pittsburgh Steelers 1977–1983
Tampa Bay Buccaneers 1984–1985

Credits

Chapter 1 Portions of this chapter are reprinted from "The Evolution From 'The Male Hormone' to Anabolic-Androgenic Steroids" by C.D. Kochakian, 1988, *Alabama Journal of Medical Sciences* 25 (1): 96–102. Reprinted by permission of the University of Alabama School of Medicine. The journal article is an abbreviated version of the November 1986 History of Medicine Seminar from the Reynolds Historical Library Lecture Series. The complete lecture was recorded on videotape and is available with the original manuscript from the Reynolds Library, University of Alabama at Birmingham. The lecture was also presented at the Panel on Steroid Abuse, National Institute of Drug Abuse, March 1989 (Kochakian, 1990a) and an abbreviated version has been published in *Trends in Biochemical Sciences* 1986, 11: 399–400.

Figure 1.1 Reprinted, by permission, from L.V. Domm, 1927, "New Experiments on Ovariotomy and the Problem of Sex Inversion in the Fowl," Journal of Experimental Zoology 48 (1): 151. Copyright © 1927. Reprinted by permission of Wiley-Liss, a division of John Wiley and Sons, Inc.

Figures 1.2 and 1.3 Reprinted, by permission, from L.F. Fieser and M. Fieser, 1959, *Steroids* (New York: Reinhold), 505, 514. Copyright ©1959 by Reinhold Publishing Corporation.

Figure 1.5 Reprinted, by permission, from C.D. Kochakian and C. Tillotson, 1957, "Influence of Several C-19 Steroids on the Growth of Individual Muscles of the Guinea Pig," *Endocrinology* 60: 607–618.

Table 1.2 Reprinted, by permission, from A. Arnold, G.O. Potts, and A.L. Beyler, 1963, "Evaluation of the Protein Anabolic Properties of Certain Orally Active Anabolic Agents Based on Nitrogen Balance Studies in Rats," *Endocrinology* 72: 408–417.

Table 1.3 Reprinted, by permission, from G.W. Liddle and H.A. Burke, Jr., 1960, "Anabolic Steroids in Clinical Medicine," *Helvetica Medica Acta* 27:14.

Table 1.4 Reprinted, by permission, from A.A. Albanese, 1963, "Newer Methodology in the Clinical Investigation of Anabolic Steroids, " *Journal of New Drugs* 5:208–224.

Chapter 3 Portions of this chapter are reprinted, by permission, from C.E. Yesalis, W.E. Buckley, W.A. Anderson, M.Q. Wang, J.A. Norwig, G. Ott, J.C. Puffer, and R.H. Strauss, 1990, "Athletes' Projections of Anabolic

Steroid Use," *Clinical Sports Medicine* 2: 155–171, and from C.E. Yesalis, J.E. Wright, and J.A. Lombardo, 1989, "Anabolic-Androgenic Steroids: A Synthesis of Existing Data and Recommendations for Future Research," *Clinical Sports Medicine* 1: 109–134.

Table 3.7 Reprinted, by permission, from C.E. Yesalis, W.E. Buckley, W.A. Anderson, M.Q. Wang, J.A. Norwig, G. Ott, J.C. Puffer, and R.H. Strauss, 1990, "Athletes' Projections of Anabolic Steroid Use," *Clinical Sports Medicine* 2: 168.

Chapter 8 This chapter is adapted, by permission, from M.S. Bahrke, C.E. Yesalis, and J.E. Wright, 1990, "Psychological and Behavioural Effects of Endogenous Testosterone Levels and Anabolic-Androgenic Steroids Among Males: A Review," *Sports Medicine* 10 (5): 303–337.

Tables 9.1 and 9.2 are reprinted, by permission, from K.J. Brower, F.C. Blow, J.P. Young, and E.M. Hill, 1991, "Symptoms and Correlates of Anabolic-Androgenic Steroid Dependence," *British Journal of Addiction* 86: 763.

Chapter 10 Portions of this chapter, including figure 10.1, are reprinted, by permission, from K.J. Brower, 1997, Withdrawal From Anabolic Steroids. In C.W. Bardin (Ed.), *Current Therapy in Endocrinology and Metabolism*, 6th ed. (St. Louis: Mosby), 338–343.

Chapter 14 Portions of this chapter are from "Winning and Performance-Enhancing Drugs—Our Dual Addiction" by C.E. Yesalis, 1990, *The Physician and Sportsmedicine, 18*(3), 161–163, 167. Published by McGraw-Hill. Copyright © 1990 by McGraw-Hill, Inc. Adapted by permission of McGraw-Hill, Inc.

Introduction

The pill, capsule, vial and needle have become fixtures of the locker room as athletes increasingly turn to drugs in the hope of improving performances. This trend . . . poses a major threat to U.S. sport even though the Establishment either ignores or hushes up the issue.

Bill Gilbert
Sports Illustrated, June–July 1969

This introduction will provide the reader with a foundation for the discussion of anabolic steroids as well as develop a conceptual framework in which to place the chapters that follow. The introduction will define the term *anabolic-androgenic steroids* and will examine the reasons and methods for the use of steroids in sport and exercise. The use of drugs in sport as well as our societal concern for and knowledge of this issue will be placed in a historical context, and the underlying philosophical basis for our concern will be discussed.

Definition of Terms

Anabolic-androgenic steroids are synthetic derivatives of testosterone (see chapter 1). *Testosterone,* the natural male hormone that is produced primarily by the testes in men, is responsible for the *androgenic* (masculinizing) and *anabolic* (tissue-building) effects noted during male adolescence and adulthood. *Androgenic effects* are those that relate to the growth of the male reproductive tract or to the development of secondary sexual characteristics in men. In the pubertal male, these are increases in the length and diameter of the penis, development of the prostate and scrotum, and the appearance of the pubic, axillary, and facial hair. *Anabolic effects* are the changes that occur in the somatic and nonreproductive tract tissue; these include an acceleration of linear growth that appears before bony epiphyseal closure, enlargement of the larynx, thickening of the vocal cords, development of libido and sexual potentia, and an increase in muscle bulk and strength as well as a decrease in body fat.

Why and How Athletes Use Anabolic Steroids

The goals of individuals who use anabolic steroids depend on the activities in which they participate. Bodybuilders desire more lean mass and less body fat (Klein, 1993; Fussell, 1991). Weightlifters, both power and Olympic, desire to lift the maximum amount of weight possible. Field athletes want to put the shot or throw the hammer, discus, or javelin farther than competitors or record holders. Swimmers and runners hope to perform their frequent, high-intensity, long-duration workouts without physical breakdown (Francis, 1990). Football players want to increase their lean body mass and strength so that they can be successful at the high school, college, or professional level. Another group of users of anabolic steroids simply wants to look good, which currently for many means big and muscular. In addition, there are others, such as fashion models, film actors/actresses, rock and roll band members, and dancers (exotic, ballet, and others), who, although they do not necessarily strive to be big, nonetheless want to be lean and muscular ("ripped," "cut," "defined," "buffed"). There also appears to be a segment of the population—for example, bouncers, police officers, and soldiers—who use steroids to, in their mind, improve their job performance.

Anabolic steroids have traditionally been taken in cycles, which are episodes of use lasting 6 to 12 weeks or more (Gallaway, 1997; Phillips, 1990). However, there are athletes, such as some powerlifters, who use the drugs on a relatively continuous basis and increase their doses at certain times of the year—for example, to prepare for a competition (Duchaine, 1989). Often, athletes will take more than one steroid at a time; this is referred to as "stacking." The purported rationale for stacking is that it allows the user to activate more receptor sites than if only one steroid is used, or that the user can achieve a synergistic effect with certain combinations of steroids (Duchaine, 1989; Hatfield, 1982; Phillips, 1990). In order to avoid plateauing (developing a tolerance to a particular anabolic steroid), some users stagger their drugs and will take the steroids in an overlapping pattern or will stop taking one drug and start another—though this does not necessarily mean that only one drug is taken at a time (Duchaine, 1989; Hatfield, 1982; Phillips, 1990). Often steroid users will pyramid their dosing patterns such that they move from low daily doses at the beginning of the cycle to higher doses and then taper their doses down toward the end of the cycle (Wright, 1982). In addition, the athlete may use a number of other drugs concurrently with anabolic steroids to further enhance physical capacities or to counteract the common side effects of steroids. These drugs include stimulants, diuretics, antiestrogens, human chorionic gonadotropin (HCG), human growth hormone (hGH), anti-acneiform medications, as well as anti-inflammatories (Di Pasquale, 1984). Moreover, some anabolic steroid users will take other illegal drugs such as marijuana to relax after an intense workout. They also tend to use so-called natural food supplements, such as creatine, DHEA, androstenedione, megavitamins, caffeine, protein, amino acids, ginseng, and bee pollen (Phillips, 1995). This polypharmacy is termed an array (Duchaine, 1989).

Athletes primarily use the oral and intramuscular forms of anabolic steroids, and needle sharing to inject steroids has been reported, especially among adolescents (Durant, Rickert, Ashworth, Newman, & Slavens, 1993; Korkia & Stimson, 1993). More recently, some elite athletes have begun using testosterone via transdermal patches, sublingual tablets, dermatological gels, and nasal sprays (Catlin, Hatton, & Starcevic, 1997; Franke & Berendonk, 1997) as possible means of circumventing drug tests (see chapter 13).

The dose of anabolic steroids depends on the sport as well as the particular needs of the athlete. Endurance athletes use steroids primarily for their alleged catabolism-blocking effects (Yesalis, Wright, & Lombardo, 1989) and employ doses at or slightly below physiologic replacement levels—that is, about 7 mg/d (Yen & Jaffee, 1978). (Because the bioequivalence of various forms and types of anabolic steroids has not been established, the estimates of dosages used by athletes relative to physiologic replacement levels are approximate.) Although sprinters desire similar results, the strength and power requirements of their activity result in doses that are approximately one and one-half to more than double the replacement levels (Francis, 1990). Participants in the traditional strength sports, seeking to "bulk up," have generally used amounts that exceed physiologic levels by 10 to 100 times, or more (Kerr, 1982; Wright, 1982). Dosing patterns will also vary among athletes within a particular sport based on each athlete's training goals and response to the drugs and the biological activity of different anabolic steroids (Di Pasquale, 1984; Kerr, 1982; Kochakian, 1990; Wright, 1982). Women, regardless of sport, are thought to generally use lower doses of anabolic steroids than males.

Sources of Anabolic Steroids

The majority of individuals who use anabolic steroids to enhance athletic performance and physical appearance obtain the drugs from the black market (Tolliver, 1998). Black-market steroids come from three sources:

1. those manufactured legally and illegally in other countries and smuggled into the United States;

2. those manufactured in this country by licensed pharmaceutical companies and diverted into the black market by the producer, distributor, pharmacist, veterinarian, or physician; and
3. those produced by clandestine laboratories.

There are two types of clandestinely produced anabolic steroids:

1. counterfeit products sold as steroids but containing no active anabolic agents; and
2. counterfeit preparations containing an anabolic steroid, but of a different type or dose than is indicated on the package.

International smuggling is the predominant source of illicit anabolic steroids in the United States, followed by illegally diverted and clandestinely manufactured anabolic steroids (Tolliver, 1998).

Of international sources, the Baja California area of Mexico is particularly important. The steroids are manufactured in Mexico City and shipped to pharmacies in the Baja region (Kenney, 1994). Traffickers come from the United States, purchase prescriptions at the pharmacies and fill them in unlimited quantities, and then smuggle the steroids across the border. Other international sources of supply for the U.S. black market include Russia, Poland, Hungary, Spain, Italy, Greece, Canada, and the Netherlands (Tolliver, 1998).

Because some of these black-market drugs are counterfeit and do not contain any anabolic steroid or contain an anabolic steroid other than that indicated on the package, the actual types and doses taken by illicit users are difficult to determine (USDHHS, 1991; Walters et al., 1990). Moreover, some of the drugs taken are intended for veterinary use (Duchaine, 1989), so the equivalent human doses are unknown. It is estimated that 10 to 15% of illicit steroid users obtain these drugs by prescription (Kenney, 1994).

Drug Use Is Not New

The use of drugs to enhance physical performance has been a feature of athletic competition since the beginning of recorded history (Prokop, 1970; Strauss & Curry, 1987). The legendary Berserkers of Norse mythology used bufotenin for stimulating effects, whereas West Africans used *Cola acuminita* and *Cola nitida* for running competitions since ancient times (Prokop, 1970; Bøje, 1939). The ancient Greeks ate hallucinogenic mushrooms as well as sesame seeds to enhance performance, and the gladiators in the Roman Colosseum used stimulants to overcome fatigue and injury (Wadler & Hainline, 1989). For centuries South American Indians have chewed coca leaves to increase endurance (Bøje, 1939; Karpovich, 1941).

During the 19th century, performance-enhancing drug use among athletes was commonplace. Swimmers, distance runners, sprinters, and cyclists used drugs such as caffeine, alcohol, nitroglycerine, digitalis, cocaine, strychnine, ether, opium, and heroin to get an edge on their opponents (Bøje, 1939; Hoberman, 1992; Prokop, 1970). Indeed, the first fatality attributed to a performance-enhancing drug was that of an English cyclist who overdosed on tri-methyl during a race between Bordeaux and Paris in 1886 (Prokop, 1970). In 1939, in a paper entitled "Doping," Bøje stated,

> *There can be no doubt that stimulants are to-day widely used by athletes participating in competitions; the record-breaking craze and the desire to satisfy an exacting public play a more and more prominent role, and take higher rank than the health of the competitors itself. (p. 439)*

Today, athletes employ a wide variety of drugs other than anabolic steroids to enhance performance; these include human growth hormone (hGH), IGF-1, erythropoietin, thyroid hormone, insulin, human chorionic gonadotropin (HCG), gonadotropin-releasing hormone (GnRH), clenbuterol, L-dopa, clonidine, DHEA, ephedrine, gamma hydroxy butyrate (GHB), and amphetamines. Currently over 100 substances are banned by the International Olympic Committee, including over 17 individual anabolic steroids and related compounds (International Olympic Committee, 1995).

Concerns Over Drug Use

Prokop (1970) wrote that by the early 1930s the word "doping" had already been incorporated into our language, and not only had the medical aspects of drug use in sport been discussed but the moral and ethical aspects as well. In 1924, a German physician, Dr. Willner, wrote,

> *At competitions we want to measure physical performances, not test the effects of drugs. . . . In my view, there is nothing more reprehensible than using pharmacological substances in an attempt to improve one's performances in competition with others who bring to the sporting encounter only that fitness that they have achieved through training. (Hoberman, 1992)*

In the same year, the German Association of Physicians for the Promotion of Physical Culture condemned doping on both medical and ethical grounds. Bøje (1939) wrote that in regard to doping "the ethical and medical aspects are so intermingled that the problem as a whole becomes most confused" (p. 440).

The most obvious reason we are concerned about anabolic steroid use in sport is that it is cheating—the use of these drugs violates the rules of virtually every sport federation (Wadler & Hainline, 1989). A more important question, however, is, Why have sport federations outlawed the use of these drugs?

Our concern over drug use in sport is generally founded on one or more of the following moral and ethical issues:

- The athlete may suffer physical or psychological harm as a result of drug use (Brown, 1984; Karpovich, 1941; Murray, 1983; Olivier, 1996; Simon, 1984).
- The use of drugs by one athlete may coerce another athlete to use drugs to maintain parity (Murray, 1983; Olivier, 1996; Simon, 1984).
- The use of drugs in sport is unnatural in that any resulting success is due to external factors (Murray, 1983).
- The athlete who uses drugs has an unfair advantage over athletes who do not use them (Gardner, 1989).

Although on its surface each argument has an intuitive appeal, each holds inconsistencies.

Physical Harm

Although protecting the health of participants by banning drugs is admirable, one must keep in mind that a number of sports, such as boxing, football, and auto racing, pose an inherent and significant physical threat to participants. Due to the fervor of competition as well as the intensity, frequency, and duration of training, it is also difficult to imagine an elite athlete in any sport who has not experienced some level of sport-related injury. Moreover, the argument of protecting adult steroid users from harm is viewed by some sport libertarians as a paternalistic intrusion on personal liberties (Olivier, 1996). On the other hand, by banning steroid use, harm to nonusers in contact sports could possibly be reduced by minimizing inappropriate aggression on the part of steroid users, as well as minimizing the strength and size differentials of participants.

The rationale of banning drugs to protect the health of athletes assumes that performance-enhancing drugs are harmful under all circumstances. In the case of anabolic steroids, this assumption does not appear to hold. Anabolic steroids are approved for use in certain medical conditions (see chapter 1) at doses that approximate those currently used by a number of strength, sprint, and endurance athletes. The use of anabolic steroids in clinical trials to evaluate their effect as a contraceptive, as hormone replacement in aging males, and in studies to assess their impact on strength and muscle mass, supports the argument that some anabolic steroids can be used safely at moderate to supraphysiologic doses, at least in the short term (Hoberman & Yesalis, 1995; Bhasin et al., 1996; World Health Organization Task Force, 1990, 1996). In fact, based on current knowledge, one could argue, epidemiologically, that the rate of death or permanent disability among participants in "violent" sports, including boxing, football, and auto racing, far exceeds that observed among steroid users. The physical and psychological health effects of anabolic steroids will be discussed at length in chapters 6 through 8.

Coercion of Athletes

Some have argued that at the elite level of certain sports—namely weightlifting, field events in track, bodybuilding, and perhaps the line positions in football—an athlete either uses steroids or will not be able to compete effectively (*Proper and Improper Use of Drugs,* 1973; *Steroids in Amateur and Professional Sports,* 1989; Dubin, 1990; Francis, 1990; Wade, 1972; Yesalis, Herrick, Buckley, Friedl, Brannon, & Wright, 1988). If this is true, potential competitors are coerced into using these drugs or "resign themselves to either accepting a competitive disadvantage or leaving the endeavor entirely" (Murray, 1983, p. 27). Strength training with heavy weights, a basic requirement of most strength and power sports, is itself a significant health risk that many athletes are pressured to endure. Although these circumstances are unfortunate, the final decision to use steroids, strength train, or participate in the sport still lies with the athlete. However, Olivier (1996) notes,

> *in professional sports one's future may depend on winning. At this level, sports is one's means of employment, and the greater the incentive to succeed, the greater the temptation to use any method available to achieve that end. The pressure may thus be greater than some mere primeval satisfaction of the will-to-win.*

Nevertheless, these ethical dilemmas are not peculiar to sport. If a scientist wishes to do laboratory research on virulent strains of viruses or bacteria, he or she must accept certain risks; the only way to completely avoid such risks is to not participate in this type of research.

Success Due to External Factors

Ideally, superior performance in sport should be a function of factors internal to the athlete, such as genetic endowment, intelligence, motivation, courage, and dedication. Thus, it is argued that drugs, in this instance anabolic steroids, are an external factor and therefore unnatural (Simon, 1984). Anabolic steroids are, however, a derivative of a hormone that is endogenous to the human body; athletes who use steroids are supplementing what is already there. Moreover, is there a difference between athletes' use of anabolic steroids and their use of vitamins, aspirin, amino acids, creatine, or corticosteroids, all of which are allowed by most sport governing bodies? The use of fiberglass poles, synthetic track surfaces, lifting suits, and high-tech tennis rackets raises similar questions of unnaturalness.

Unfair Advantage

The contention that anabolic steroids grant the user an unfair advantage is interesting in that the use of these drugs was banned at least nine years before the sports medicine community acknowledged that steroids could enhance performance (American College of Sports Medicine, 1977, 1984; Wadler & Hainline, 1989). There is little or no doubt, however, among athletes that the use of steroids offers a competitive edge (see chapter 5)—but so do differences in genetic endowment. Athletes who have access to elite coaches, the most sophisticated equipment, the latest training techniques, and the most knowledgeable sport scientists also have significant advantages over those without access to such luxuries. Perhaps as Gardner (1989) pointed out,

> *What renders a substance-gained advantage unacceptable, and what we may be ultimately objecting to, is not that an advantage is gained over other athletes but that one is gained over the sport itself—either its intended purpose or its conceived obstacles. (p. 68)*

Once again the distinctions are unclear. Although corked bats, high-pressure golf balls, and swim fins are not allowed in their respective sports, fiberglass poles, ultralight racing bicycles, and compound bows are.

Moral and Philosophical Concerns

In summary, none of the traditional ethical arguments for banning the use of anabolic steroids in sport is without limitations. Perhaps the most compelling argument against steroid (or any drug) use in sport is that it is morally wrong because it reduces sport to competition between biochemical machines: "it dehumanizes by not respecting the status of athletes as persons" (Fraleigh, 1985, p. 25). When high jumpers take anabolic steroids and other performance-enhancing drugs, the competition is not decided by who has best developed his or her skill but whose body has taken the most effective drugs at the proper time at the most productive dosage.

Simon (1984) concluded the following:

> *It is of course true that the choice to develop one's capacity through drugs is a choice a person might make. Doesn't respect for persons require that we respect the choice to use performance enhancers as much as any other? The difficulty, I suggest, is the effect that such a choice has on the process of athletic competition itself. The use of performance-enhancing drugs in sports restricts the area in which we can be respected as persons. Although individual athletes certainly can make such a choice, there is a justification inherent in the nature of good competition for prohibiting participation by those who make such a decision. Accordingly, the use of performance-enhancing drugs should be prohibited in the name of the value of respect for persons itself. (p. 13)*

Sport should be a quest for personal excellence through competition, as well as a source of fun, enjoyment, and camaraderie. Drugs are unnecessary to achieve these ends. If the primary objective of participation in sport, however, is to achieve victory over an opponent, the use of drugs to achieve that end becomes an increasingly rational behavior.

Has Steroid Use Been a Secret?

Some might think that until recently the dimensions of the problem of steroid use in sport were the privileged information of a few insiders. This is not true. In 1969, *Sports Illustrated* (Gilbert, 1969a–c) published a three-part series on drug use that named athletes and sports and detailed the magnitude of the issue; between 1971 and 1972 *Science* and the *New York Times Magazine* published similar articles (Wade, 1972; Scott, 1971). As a result of these and like revelations, the United States Senate Committee on the Judiciary held hearings in 1973 on drug use in sports (*Proper and Improper Use of Drugs,* 1973); no new laws resulted and public interest in this issue dwindled.

With the possible exception of a few comments made in the news media during the 1970s, such as comments related to the masculine appearances of some Eastern European Communist bloc female athletes, little public attention was given to the use of performance-enhancing drugs until the 1983 Pan American Games in Caracas, Venezuela. During these games, international attention was focused on 19 athletes (two from the United States) who tested positive for anabolic steroids and on a number of U.S. athletes who returned home prior to competition—in the minds of many, to avoid detection and sanctions. Three years later Brian Bosworth and 25 other college football players were suspended from postseason competition for anabolic steroid use. Once again, public interest appeared to subside, and it was not until the fall of 1988 that the issue was thrust once more into the spotlight when Ben Johnson was stripped of his gold medal at the Seoul Olympics. Since that time, the media, governments, and sport federations have given significant attention to assessing the magnitude of the problem and identifying solutions.

Why has it taken several decades to develop a sustained level of public and sport federation interest as well as government scrutiny? For one thing, the fact that high school students have been using anabolic steroids has been given wide public exposure only since the late 1980s (Buckley, Yesalis, Friedl, Anderson, Streit, & Wright, 1988). Ironically, our society was confronted with the news of adolescent steroid use only one month after the Ben Johnson incident—and all of this took place during a period of heightened concern over illicit drug use, especially among young people. The negative image of drug use and its potential deleterious effect on the marketing of collegiate, Olympic, and professional sport might explain, in part, the apparent lack of motivation of many sport officials in dealing with this problem during the prior 30 years. Another possible reason for this lack of motivation is that anabolic steroids and other drugs work well! Drugs can assist greatly in achieving "superhuman" bodies and performances—both of which dramatically enhance the interest of fans and, therefore, the financial viability of sport.

Conclusion

In the past several thousand years, humans have tried numerous substances to enhance their performance. Anabolic steroids and a rapidly growing list of other drugs are merely the 20th century's contribution to this practice. Long before a world sports figure was stripped of his medal at the Seoul Olympics, concerned voices—most often unheeded—warned of the problem of drug use and other excesses in sport. Their concerns about drug use included the well-being of the athlete, coercion to cheat, unfair advantage, and excellence achieved through artificial means. In the end, however, the main effect of drug use in sport is to degrade athletic competition to a battle of biochemical machines.

References

American College of Sports Medicine. (1977). Position statement on the use and abuse of anabolic-androgenic steroids in sports. *Medicine and Science in Sports and Exercise, 9,* 11–13.

American College of Sports Medicine. (1984). Position stand on the use of anabolic-androgenic steroids in sports. *Sports Medicine Bulletin, 19,* 13–18.

Bhasin, S., Storer, T., Berman, N., Callegari, C., Clevenger, B., Phillips, J., Bunnell, T.J., Tricker, R., Shirazi, A., & Casaburi, R. (1996). The effects of supraphysiologic doses of testosterone on muscle size and strength in normal men. *New England Journal of Medicine, 335*, 1–7.

Bøje, O. (1939). Doping. *Bulletin of the Health Organization of the League of Nations, 8,* 439–469.

Brown, W.M. (1984). Paternalism, drugs, and the nature of sports. *Journal of Philosophy of Sport, XI,* 14–22.

Buckley, W.E., Yesalis, C.E., Friedl, K.E., Anderson, W., Streit, A., & Wright, J. (1988). Estimated prevalence of anabolic steroid use among male high school seniors. *Journal of the American Medical Association, 260*, 3441–3445.

Catlin, D., Hatton, C., & Starcevic, S. (1997). Issues in detecting abuse of xenobiotic anabolic steroids and testosterone by analysis of athletes' urine. *Clinical Chemistry, 43*, 1280–1288.

Di Pasquale, M.G. (1984). *Drug use and detection in amateur sports.* Warkworth, ON: M.G.D. Press.

Dubin, C. (1990). *Commission of inquiry into the use of drugs and banned practices intended to increase athletic performance* (Catalog No. CP32-56/1990E, ISBN 0-660-13610-4). Ottawa, ON: Canadian Government Publishing Centre.

Duchaine, D. (1989). *Underground steroid handbook II.* Venice, CA: HLR Technical Books.

DuRant, R., Rickert, V., Ashworth, C., Newman, C., & Slavens, G. (1993). Use of multiple drugs among adolescents who use anabolic steroids. *New England Journal of Medicine, 328*, 922–926.

Fraleigh, W.P. (1985). Performance-enhancing drugs in sport: The ethical issue. *Journal of the Philosophy of Sport, XI,* 23–29.

Francis, C. (1990). *Speed trap*. New York: St. Martin's Press.

Franke, W., & Berendonk, B. (1997). Hormonal doping and androgenization of athletes: A secret program of the German Democratic Republic government. *Clinical Chemistry, 43*, 1262–1279.

Fussell, S.W. (1991). *Muscle: Confessions of an unlikely bodybuilder.* New York: Avon Books.

Gallaway, S. (1997). *The steroid bible*. Golden, CO: Mile High.

Gardner, R. (1989). On performance-enhancing substances and the unfair advantage argument. *Journal of the Philosophy of Sport, XVI,* 59–83.

Gilbert, B. (1969a, June 23). Drugs in sport: Part 1. Problems in a turned-on world. *Sports Illustrated,* 64–72.

Gilbert, B. (1969b, June 30). Drugs in sport: Part 2. Something extra on the ball. *Sports Illustrated,* 30–42.

Gilbert, B. (1969c, July 7). Drugs in sport: Part 3. High time to make some rules. *Sports Illustrated,* 30–35.

Hatfield, F. (1982). *Anabolic steroids: What kind and how many.* Venice, CA: Fitness System.

Hoberman, J. (1992). The early development of sports medicine in Germany. In J. Berryman & R. Park (Eds.), *Sport and exercise science: Essays in the history of sports medicine.* Champaign, IL: University of Illinois Press.

Hoberman, J., & Yesalis, C. (1995). The history of synthetic testosterone. *Scientific American, 272*(2), 60–65.

International Olympic Committee. (1995). *International Olympic committee medical code.* Lausanne, Switzerland: IOC. ISBN 92-9149-003-2.

Karpovich, P.V. (1941). Ergogenic aids in work and sports. *Research Quarterly, 12*(Suppl.), 432–450.

Kenney, J. (1994). Extent and nature of illicit trafficking in anabolic steroids. In *Report of the International Conference on the Abuse and Trafficking of Anabolic Steroids* (pp. 34–35). Washington, DC: United States Drug Enforcement Administration Conference Report.

Kerr, R. (1982). *The practical use of anabolic steroids with athletes.* San Gabriel, CA: Kerr.

Klein, A. (1993). *Little big men: Bodybuilding subculture and gender construction.* Albany, NY: State University of New York Press.

Kochakian, C.D. (1990). History of anabolic-androgenic steroids. In G. Linn & L. Erinoff (Eds.), *Anabolic steroid abuse* (NIDA Research Monograph No. 102). Rockville, MD: National Institute on Drug Abuse.

Korkia, P., & Stimson, G. (1993). *Anabolic steroid use in Great Britain: An exploratory investigation.* London, England: Centre for Research on Drugs and Health Behaviour.

Meikle, A., Arver, S., Dobs, A., Sanders, S., Rajaram, L., & Mazer, N. (1996). The pharmacokinetics and metabolism of a permeation-enhanced testosterone transdermal system in hypogonadal men: Influence of application site—a clinical research center study. *Journal of Clinical Endocrinology and Metabolism, 81,* 1832–1840.

Murray, T.H. (1983). The coercive power of drugs in sports. *The Hastings Center Report, 13*(24), 24–30.

Olivier, S. (1996). Drugs in sport: Justifying paternalism on the grounds of harm. *American Journal of Sports Medicine, 24*(6), S43–S45.

Phillips, B. (1995). *1996 supplement review.* Golden, CO: Mile High.

Phillips, W. (1990). *Anabolic reference guide.* 5th ed. Golden, CO: Mile High.

Prokop, L. (1970). The struggle against doping and its history. *Journal of Sports Medicine and Physical Fitness, 10*(1), 45–48.

Proper and improper use of drugs by athletes: Hearings before the Subcommittee to Investigate Juvenile Delinquency, of the Committee on the Judiciary, U.S. Senate. 93d Cong., 1st Sess. (1973, June 18, July 12, 13).

Scott, J. (1971, October 17). It's not how you play the game, but what pill you take. *New York Times Magazine.*

Simon, R.L. (1984). Good competition and drug-enhanced performance. *Journal of the Philosophy of Sport, XI,* 6–13.

Steroids in amateur and professional sports. The medical and social costs of steroid abuse: Hearings before the Committee on the Judiciary, U.S Senate. 101st Cong., 1st Sess. (1989, April 3, May 9).

Strauss, R.H., & Curry, T.J. (1987). Magic, science and drugs. In R.H. Strauss (Ed.), *Drugs and performance in sports* (pp. 3–9). Philadelphia: Saunders.

Tolliver, J. (1998, February 9–14). *Anabolic steroid black-market in the United States.* Paper presented at Drugs and Athletes: A Multidisciplinary Symposium. Meeting of the American Academy of Forensic Sciences, San Francisco.

U.S. Department of Health and Human Services, Public Health Service. (1991, January). *Interagency Task Force on Anabolic Steroids.* Washington, DC: Author.

Wade, N. (1972). Anabolic steroids: Doctors denounce them, but athletes aren't listening. *Science, 176,* 1399–1403.

Wadler, G., & Hainline, B. (1989). *Drugs and the athlete.* Philadelphia: Davis.

Walters, M., Ayers, R., & Brown, D. (1990). Analysis of illegally distributed anabolic steroid products by liquid chromotography with identity confirmation by mass spectrometry or infrared spectrophotometry. *Journal of the Association of Official Analytic Chemists, 73,* 904–926.

World Health Organization Task Force on Methods for the Regulation of Male Fertility. (1990). Contraceptive efficacy of testosterone-induced azoospermia in normal men. *Lancet, 336,* 955–959.

World Health Organization Task Force on Methods for the Regulation of Male Fertility. (1996). Contraceptive efficacy of testosterone-induced azoospermia and oligozoospermia in normal men. *Fertility and Sterility, 65,* 821–829.

Wright, J. (1982). *Anabolic steroids and sport II.* Natick, MA: Sports Science Consultants.

Yen, S., & Jaffe, R. (1978). *Reproductive endocrinology.* Philadelphia: Saunders.

Yesalis, C.E., Herrick, R.T., Buckley, W.E., Friedl, K.E., Brannon, D., & Wright, J.E. (1988). Self-reported use of anabolic-androgenic steroids by elite power lifters. *The Physician and Sportsmedicine, 16,* 91–100.

Yesalis, C.E., Wright, J.E., & Lombardo, J.A. (1989). Anabolic-androgenic steroids: A synthesis of existing data and recommendations for future research. *Clinical Sports Medicine, 1,* 109–134.

PART I

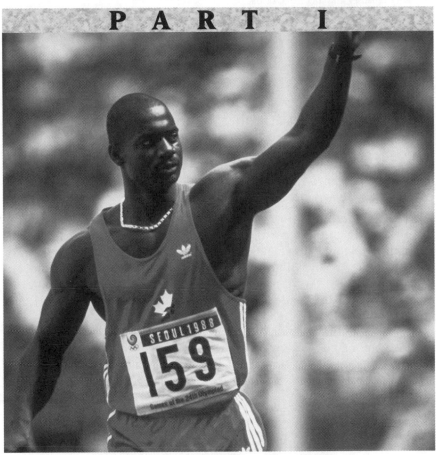

© Photo Run

History and Incidence of Use

The chapters in part I lay the groundwork for the study of anabolic steroids. You will gain a detailed knowledge of the history of anabolic steroids and their use, and also become aware of the current level of use among students at the secondary school level and the methodological problems associated with researching anabolic steroid use.

In **Chapter 1,** the authors provide a historical perspective and definition of anabolic steroids. They discuss the loss of secondary male sex characteristics by castration, the family of male hormones termed *androgens,* the discovery of the male hormone testosterone, the discovery of the anabolic activity of testosterone, and the attempt to modify the testosterone molecule, resulting in anabolic-androgenic steroids. They also describe therapeutic and veterinary applications of anabolic steroids.

Whereas chapter 1 deals with the history of the development of anabolic steroids, **chapter 2** details the history of anabolic steroid *use,* especially use in sport and exercise settings. The authors describe the history of use among several categories of athletes, from Olympic level to high school. Of particular interest are the factors that influenced spread from one class of athlete to another.

In **chapter 3,** the authors critique methods of assessing the level of steroid use, inlcuding investigative journalism, government investigations, drug testing, and scientific surveys. They also review the results of systematic surveys of anabolic steroid use given to adolescent and adult populations. They provide information gained from both of these assessment measures and discuss the methodological problems in these processes.

The data mentioned in chapter 3 suggesting widespread anabolic steroid use among adolescents prompted the groundbreaking ATLAS prevention program. In addition a detailed analysis of prevention and intervention programs, including drug testing, is provided.

CHAPTER

1

Anabolic-Androgenic Steroids: A Historical Perspective and Definition

Charles D. Kochakian, PhD, and Charles E. Yesalis, ScD

The more we understand how past discoveries have been made, the better we are able to plan for future discoveries.

W.I.B. Beveridge
Frontiers in Comparative Medicine, 1972

Portions of this chapter are reprinted from *Alabama Journal of Medical Sciences* 1988; see credits page for more information.

In this chapter we will discuss the historical development and definition of anabolic steroids. We will also discuss the loss of the secondary male sex characteristics in fowl and men by castration, the discovery of the male hormone testosterone (the endocrine function of the testis), the family of male hormones termed androgens, the discovery of the anabolic activity of testosterone (the synthesis of new tissue), and the attempt to modify the testosterone molecule to produce a steroid with strong anabolic activity and no or very weak androgenic activity. These modified steroids became popularized as anabolic steroids, but they contain sufficient androgenic activity to produce virilization and have been classified along with testosterone as anabolic-androgenic steroids. Testosterone, in the form of several potent esters, and many of the modified steroids have been explored therapeutically in humans and in animals, with surprising results; this research has explored the abilities of these drugs to correct a variety of conditions of protein deficiency and more recently to increase musculature and performance by athletes, race horses, and dogs.

Endocrine Function of the Testis

The scientific community did not recognize the endocrine function of the testis until almost one hundred years after the initial demonstration by Berthold in 1849. Berthold's experiments and interpretation of the results clearly anticipated the fundamentals of endocrinology; 56 years later Starling (1905) named the blood-borne factors *hormones* (which means "to excite or arouse").

In this section we will describe the initiation and evolution of the concept that the testis produces a chemical substance that is secreted into the bloodstream and carried to the target tissues—for example, the comb and wattles of the rooster and the accessory sex organs of the rat—to effect their growth and maintenance.

Castration and Secondary Male Characteristics

It has been known for centuries that castration of the male results in the loss of not only fertility but also the secondary male sex characteristics (Hoskins, 1941; Spencer, 1946). The Neolithic peoples of Asia Minor practiced castration as early as 4000 B.C. to domesticate animals for work and meat production (Spencer, 1946).

The practice of castration of humans probably originated in Babylonia about 2000 B.C., originally as a punitive measure (e.g., for adultery), and traveled to India by 1500 B.C., to Egypt by 1200 B.C., to China by 1122 B.C., and to neighboring countries (Spencer, 1946). The practice flourished in the early days of the Eastern Roman Empire and was used by the early Christian Church for its priesthood and to retain the soprano voices of choirboys. Castration was forbidden at the Church Council of Nicea in A.D.

325. However, as late as the early 20th century, religious cults (e.g., the Skoptz) continued the practice (Spencer, 1946). The Greeks and later the Romans did not accept the concept of castration, probably because of their emphases on physical culture and the Olympic games (Spencer, 1946).

Early Primitive Attempts to Reverse Effects of Castration

Primitive people commonly ate organs of animals and even of humans to improve or cure the dysfunction of their respective organs. As early as 140 B.C., Sucruta of India advocated the ingestion of testis tissue for the cure of impotence (Newerla, 1943). The endocrine function of the testis was speculated upon by Arataeus in about A.D. 150 and more vigorously by de Bordeu in 1775. They proposed that each organ of the body produces a substance that is secreted into the blood to regulate bodily function. Although this concept touched on the now-recognized function of the endocrine glands, it was mere speculation based on casual observation. However, early scientists made some progress in the knowledge of the anatomy and physiology of the testis. Aristotle (300 B.C.) clearly described the effect of castration on the bird (capon). Furthermore, in the first half of the 19th century, scientists recognized that the ductless glands are closely allied with the vascular system (Newerla, 1943).

In 1889, a respected French physician, Brown-Sequard, reported that aqueous extracts of animal testes injected into other animals (e.g., dogs) and even into himself produced improvements in general health, muscular strength, appetite, regulation of the intestinal tract, and mental faculties. Ironically, these uncontrolled studies and bold claims stimulated an increase in clinical endocrinology. Numerous similar reports soon followed and continued until the early 1920s. Surgeons developed lucrative practices by transplanting testes from animals (e.g., monkeys), and internists administered injections of aqueous and glycerol extracts of animal testes to humans. It seemed that the fountain of youth had been discovered. But serious experimentation in reproduction, initiated in the 1920s (Parkes, 1966, 1985), caused scientists to become concerned with the blatant claims of rejuvenation. An international committee that was appointed to investigate concluded that claims of rejuvenation as a result of testis transplantation or injection of testicular extracts were unfounded (Parkes, 1985, 1988). The practice disappeared as scientists learned how to produce active extracts and then isolated, characterized, and synthesized the active substance.

Discovery of the Endocrine Function of the Testis

In spite of the early speculations, the general consensus as late as the middle of the 19th century was that the changes after castration were mediated through the nervous system. The first inkling of the real regulation of these changes was provided in 1849 by Berthold, professor of medicine at Göttingen. In a simple and elegantly designed experiment with only six roosters, he demonstrated that the well-known regression of the comb and wattles (see figure 1.1) and changes in behavior, all of which occurred after castration, were prevented by the transplantation of the testis in the abdominal cavity. The transplants developed new blood supplies and maintained the roosters in the normal manner. Berthold correctly deduced that because the transplanted testis no longer had its nerve connections, it produced something that was secreted into the bloodstream and transported to the target tissues to regulate their growth and maintenance.

In the subsequent 60 years, Berthold's results were questioned. Others who attempted to repeat the transplantation experiments were unsuccessful, except for Lode (1891, 1895), who did confirm Berthold's experiment but whose results were ignored. Pezard in 1911 successfully repeated the effects of castration in roosters and in 1912 fragmented the removed testes and deposited the fragments in the abdominal cavities of the castrated roosters (capons). The size of the combs and wattles of the capons were maintained.

Preparation of Active Extracts of Testis and Male Urine: Male Hormone

In the early 1920s, interest in the development of the male reproductive tract was accelerated. Many studies of laboratory rodents were conducted, and extracts of the testis were prepared that reversed the effects of castration (Moore, 1939). Regeneration—of the regressed accessory sex organ of the castrated rat (Moore, 1939; Moore & Gallagher, 1930), and the seminal vesicles of the castrated mouse (Voss, 1930)—was suggested as a method of assay.

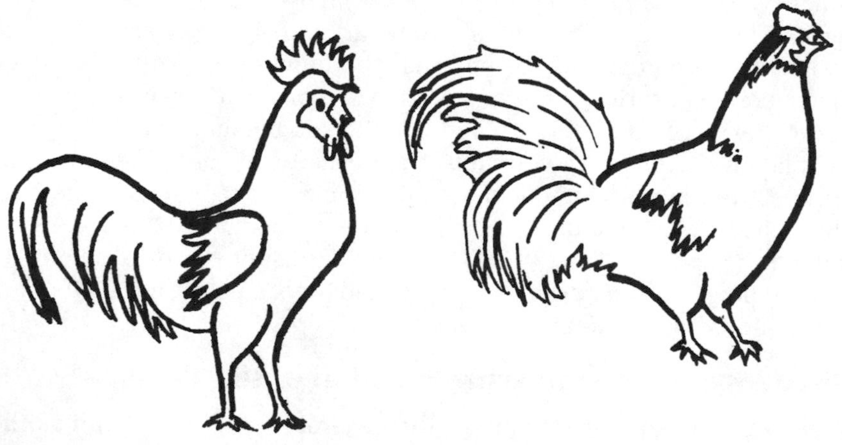

Figure 1.1 Effect of castration on the comb and wattles of the brown leghorn rooster.

Reprinted from *Journal of Experimental Zoology* 1927; see also Moore 1939.

In 1927, McGee reported that an alcohol extract of bull testicles stimulated the growth of the capon comb. Gallagher and Koch (1930) developed the stimulation of growth of the capon comb into a quantitative procedure and improved the extraction procedure to produce a highly purified and very active preparation (Gallagher & Koch, 1934b).

In the meantime, in 1926 Pezard and Caridroit transplanted two fragments of the comb of a normal rooster to its back through an incision in the skin and found that the fragments were maintained (i.e., they did not regress). Another rooster was castrated, and 1 week later two fragments of the comb were transplanted to its back; both the comb in situ and the transplanted fragments exhibited the usual postcastration regression. The researchers deduced, as had Berthold, that the active principal was in the blood and that it acted directly on the comb. On the basis of this observation, Funk and Harrow in 1929 assumed that the active substance should be cleared by the kidney and appear in the urine. The researchers found that a crude concentrate of alcohol-treated male urine stimulated the growth of the capon comb. Acidification of the urine, followed by chloroform extraction, provided an oily active concentrate (Funk, Harrow, & Lejwa, 1930). Further purification and an increase in yield were effected by stronger acidification prior to chloroform extraction, followed by hydrolysis of the extract with sodium hydroxide solution (Funk & Harrow, 1930), which removed many impurities and also estrogens. Other investigators (Freud, deJongh, Laqueur, & Munch, 1930; Loewe & Voss, 1930) almost simultaneously developed similar extraction procedures. Thus, relatively simple methods for the assay and production of highly active concentrates of what was designated the "male hormone" became available.

Androgens: Multiplicity of Male Hormones

Androsterone, a substance with the ability to stimulate the growth of the capon comb, was isolated from human male urine and synthesized from cholesterol. This event was quickly followed by the isolation, synthesis, and chemical characterization of the biologically active principal in bull testes, testosterone, which was biologically more active and chemically slightly different from androsterone. The isolation of other chemically related and biologically active compounds from human male urine suggested that testosterone was metabolized in the body to several other related steroids. Appraisal of the testosterone molecule indicates that testosterone has the potential to be oxidized or reduced to approximately 600 related steroids. These steroids have been given the general name of androgens (*andro* = "male"; *gen* = "to produce").

Isolation and Characterization of Androsterone

Butenandt (1931) succeeded in isolating 15 mg of a pure substance (Butenandt & Tscherning, 1934a) from an extract of 15,000 L of policemen's urine. Analysis of the urinary product (Butenandt & Tscherning, 1934b) indicated a hydroxyl and a ketone attached to a polycyclic nucleus like that of cholesterol; the researchers named this substance androsterone (*andro* = "male"; *ster* = "sterol"; *one* = "ketone").

The final elucidation of the ring structure of cholesterol was in the process of being accomplished (see Fieser & Fieser, 1959). In the meantime, Ruzicka (1973) had become intrigued by the possible polycyclic structure of androsterone. Ruzicka, Goldberg, Meyer, Brunigger, and Eichenburg (1934) oxidized cholesterol and obtained the anticipated ketone. The free compound possessed only one-seventh of the comb-growth-stimulating property of androsterone and was assumed to be a stereoisomer of androsterone. Ruzicka's group then immediately proceeded to convert cholesterol to androsterone and its three possible isomers (figure 1.2). Thus, the chemical structure of androsterone and its relationship to cholesterol were established.

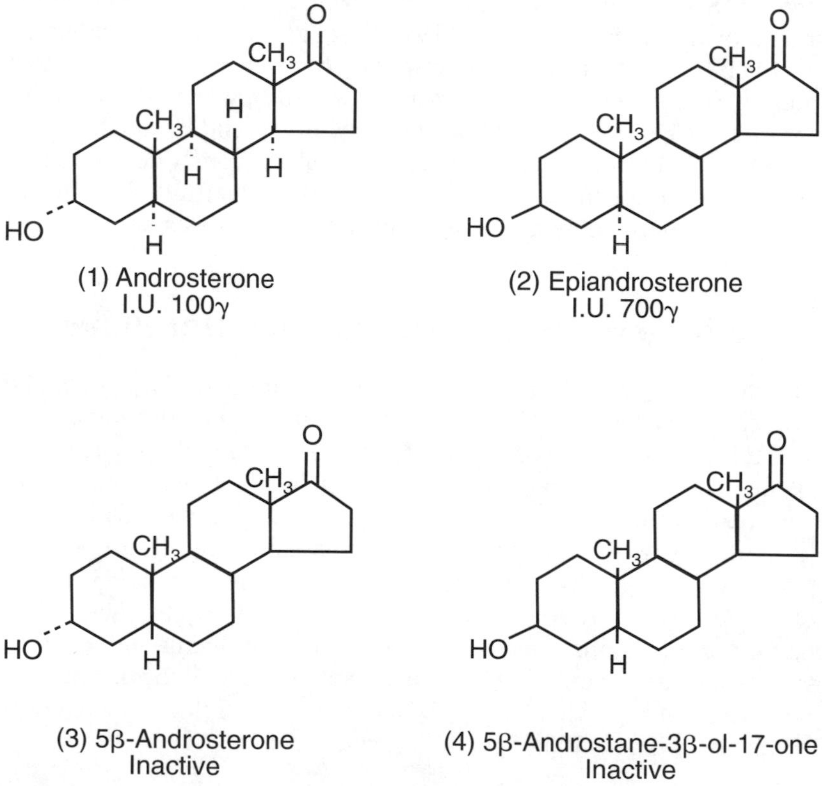

(1) Androsterone
I.U. 100γ

(2) Epiandrosterone
I.U. 700γ

(3) 5β-Androsterone
Inactive

(4) 5β-Androstane-3β-ol-17-one
Inactive

Figure 1.2 Androsterone and its three isomers.
Reprinted from Fieser & Fieser 1959; see also Ruzicka et al. 1934.

Synthesis, Isolation, and Characterization of Testosterone

The biological and chemical properties of the newly synthesized androsterone were compared with those of the testis extract; the testis extract was found to be more active in the stimulation of growth of the seminal vesicles and prostate of the castrated rat and mouse (Freud et al., 1930), and it was labile to hot alkali (Gallagher & Koch, 1934a). The alkaline lability, based on studies with progesterone, suggested the presence of an α,β-unsaturated ketone in the testis product (see Fieser & Fieser, 1959; Tausk, 1984). Both Ruzicka and Wettstein (1935a) and Butenandt and Kudszus (1935) immediately (in July 1935) reported the synthesis of androsterone from cholesterol. The compound possessed the chemical lability of the testis extract and showed a substantial increase in biological activity, but it was not as biologically active as the testis extract. In August, Butenandt and Hanisch (1935) and Ruzicka and Wettstein (1935b) quickly converted the ketone at position 17 to a hydroxyl (figure 1.3). This compound proved to have both the chemical and biological properties of the partially purified bull testis extract.

In May 1935, David of Laqueur's group in Amsterdam reported the isolation of a crystalline compound from bull testes (10 mg of 100 kg) that had the chemical and biological properties of the compound newly synthesized by the Butenandt and Ruzicka groups, and named it testosterone. Shortly thereafter, the Amsterdam group (David, Dingemanse, Freud, & Laqueur, 1935) reported that the chemical structure of their compound was identical with that of the recently synthesized compound.

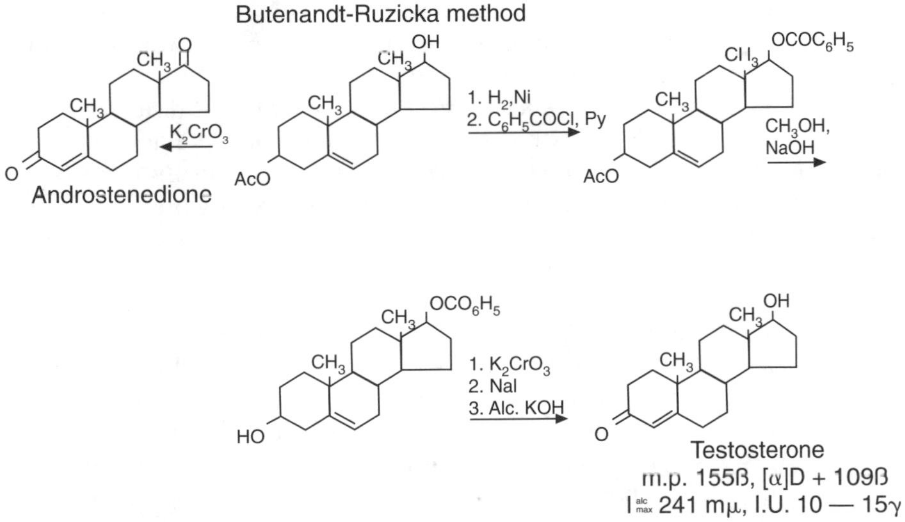

Figure 1.3 Synthesis of androstenedione and testosterone from cholesterol via dehydroepiandrosterone.

Reprinted from Fieser & Fieser 1959.

Family of Related C_{19}-Steroids

It was becoming apparent that the body produces more than one compound with male hormonelike activity. Butenandt and Dannenbaum (1934) already had isolated dehydroandrosterone and a second compound from the male urine extract, an artifact (chlorodehydroandrosterone) of dehydroandrosterone formed during the hydrochloric acid hydrolysis of the urine. Furthermore, they indicated that there probably were several more related compounds present in the urine, which was amply confirmed over the subsequent years (Dorfman & Ungar, 1965). Thus, a family of compounds had been discovered, which was soon given the generic name *androgens*.

Testosterone has the potential to be converted by tissue enzymes to 27 compounds (Kochakian, 1959, 1990b). The polycyclic nucleus of each compound has nine potential sites for α- or β-hydroxylation and also potential hydroxylation of the angular methyls at C_{18} and C_{19}. Thus it is possible for the tissues to produce at least another 540 compounds (Kochakian, 1990a, 1990b). Moreover, the unsaturated steroids may be converted to estrogens. Many of these compounds are already recognized (Kochakian, 1959; Kochakian & Arimasa, 1976).

In 1935, Ruzicka, Goldberg, and Rosenberg (see Fieser & Fieser, 1959) reported that the substitution of a methyl for the 17α-hydrogen yielded a highly effective oral compound, 17α-methyltestosterone, which was immediately accepted for clinical use. Testosterone in the early studies (Foss, 1939) appeared to be completely ineffective by oral administration, but later studies of mice (Kochakian, 1952) and humans (Johnsen, Bennett, & Jensen, 1974) demonstrated that testosterone was active by mouth if administered in sufficient quantity.

It was observed early (see Kochakian, 1938) that the addition of fatty acids or impurities from extracts enhanced the biological activity of a parenterally administered oil solution of testosterone. These studies (see Kochakian, 1938) suggested that esters of testosterone would prove effective. The acetates of testosterone and related compounds already were available; they had been prepared to establish the presence of hydroxyl in the molecule. On bioassay, the acetate of testosterone proved to be more effective and also to provide a more prolonged activity. The propionate was even more effective (see Kochakian, 1938) and became the standard compound for parenteral administration. The further prolongation of activity with the propionate prompted the synthesis of several other esters with even greater extension of activity that correlated with the length of the carbon chain of the carboxylic acid. The prolongation of biological activity has been extended as long as four months after the single injection of testosterone-trans-4n-butylcyclohexyl-carboxylate (Weinbauer, Marshall, & Nieschlag, 1986).

The introduction and recognition of 5α-dihydrotestosterone, 5α-dihydro-19-nortestosterone, and 19-nortestosterone as effective agents were followed by the preparation of esters of these steroids. The esters are hydrolyzed by blood and/or tissue esterases to release the steroid for biological action.

Anabolic Activity

The discovery that testosterone stimulates the synthesis of new tissue opened many potential new uses for this steroid. Kochakian found that a male hormonelike extract from male urine stimulated a strong positive nitrogen balance in castrated dogs. As soon as androstenedione and testosterone were synthesized from cholesterol, these steroids were found also to produce a strong positive nitrogen effect in the castrated dogs. Shortly thereafter, testosterone propionate became commercially available and proved to produce an identical effect in eunuchoid men.

Nitrogen Balance in Dog and Man

The demonstration of male hormonelike activity in male urine stimulated many biological studies. Murlin, the discoverer of glucagon, was prompted to investigate whether this material also was responsible for the difference in basal metabolic rate (BMR) between males and females. He assigned two medical students in 1931 to conduct a pilot study as their class project. They found that an extract of medical student urine (similar to extracts studied by Funk, Harrow, & Lejwa, 1930) increased the BMR of a castrated dog. In the fall of 1933, I (CDK) was appointed as a graduate assistant (Kochakian, 1984) to confirm and extend this exciting observation. In spite of repeated experiments on a similar extract at several dose levels, I was unable to confirm the increase in BMR. Thereupon, Murlin suggested the investigation of protein metabolism, a suggestion probably prompted by his earlier (1911) studies on nitrogen balance in pregnant dogs. The urine extract produced an immediate and strongly positive nitrogen balance in two castrated dogs. The results were reported in 1935 (Kochakian, 1935; Kochakian & Murlin, 1935) at the same time that androsterone, androstenedione, and testosterone were being characterized and synthesized. The experiments were immediately repeated with androstenedione (Kochakian & Murlin, 1936), which I (CDK) synthesized from cholesterol by the method of the Butenandt and Ruzicka groups (see figure 1.3), and with testosterone and testosterone acetate (Kochakian, 1937), which had become commercially available. The results obtained were identical with those of the urinary extract. Shortly thereafter, Kenyon, Sandiford, Bryan, Knowlton, and Koch (1938) reported identical results in eunuchoid men with the commercially available testosterone propionate. In addition to the retained nitrogen, the other elements (Na^+, K^+, $C1^+$, H_2O, PO_4^{-3}) for the synthesis of new tissue were retained by the subjects in proportionate amounts.

The experiments involving the castrated dogs and the eunuchoid men clearly indicated that the secretion of the testis (testosterone) not only regulated the development of the secondary male characteristics and the accessory sex organs but also had a general anabolic effect. Subsequent experiments in rats, mice, guinea pigs, and hamsters demonstrated that testosterone influenced the synthesis of new tissue in practically every organ of the body. Thus testosterone is a general anabolic agent (Kochakian, 1975, 1976b).

Nitrogen Balance in Rats

Nitrogen balance studies in dogs proved to be too expensive and time consuming. Therefore, these studies were extended to rats as one phase in the delineation of the nature and mechanism of the action of testosterone. The comparison of available natural androgens demonstrated testosterone propionate to be the most active; androsterone showed only a trace of activity (Kochakian, 1950, 1964). Testosterone was more active than androsterone but less active than testosterone propionate. The esterification enhanced and prolonged the activity. The various steroids produced a log/dose response.

An unexpected effect on the positive nitrogen balance and a simultaneous increase in body weight was revealed. Prolongation of the injections after 7 to 10 days resulted in a gradual return of the positive nitrogen balance to equilibrium and a cessation of the increase in body weight, followed by a gradual decrease to the initial level. This "wearing-off" effect could be reversed by increasing the dose of the steroid.

An identical pattern of response was reproduced with testosterone propionate in the normal male rat, the normal and ovariectomized female rat, the normal and castrated hypophysectomized male rat, the castrated-adrenalectomized rat, the surgically and thiouracil hypothyroid male rat, and the alloxan-diabetic rat (and the depancreatized dog). This indicated that the protein-synthesizing activity of testosterone and related steroids was not mediated through any of the other endocrine glands.

Partial Dissociation of Anabolic Activity From Androgenic Activity

The potential therapeutic usefulness of the protein-synthesizing property of testosterone in patients who exhibited a decrease in the formation of tissue was immediately recognized. The use of testosterone in such patients, however, was always accompanied with the virilizing effect, especially evident in women and children. The first indication that it might be possible to avoid this effect surfaced in experimentation on castrated mice, in comparing the differential effect of a number of natural steroids on the kidney weight as representative of the anabolic activity and on the prostates and seminal vesicles as representative of the androgenic activity. In general, the reduction of the polar groups of testosterone resulted in a decrease in androgenic activity without decreasing the weight of the kidney. A similar relationship was obtained in comparing the response of the sensitive muscles of the castrated male guinea pig. A comparison of the response of the levator ani muscle with that of the prostate or seminal vesicles of the castrated rat was suggested as a simple and inexpensive screening assay to find a chemically modified testosterone that would have no or weak androgenic activity but have retained or enhanced activity of the muscle. Many modifications of testosterone were synthesized and exploited in clinical use as anabolic steroids. Unfortunately, the dissociation was never sufficient to prevent the residual virilizing activity from occurring.

Renotrophic/Androgenic Activity in Mice and Rats

The potential therapeutic value of the anabolic activity of testosterone and its commercial availability stimulated many investigations of diverse anabolic-deficient conditions (Landau, 1976; Reifenstein, 1942), including intensive studies in women with breast cancer. The clinical use, however, was always accompanied by virilization, especially evident in women and children. A possible answer to this problem appeared imminent (Kochakian, 1942). As one aspect of my (CDK) program to elucidate the nature and mechanism of the anabolic action, I decided to compare the abilities of a number of steroids to stimulate growth in the sensitive mouse kidney (anabolic effect) (Kochakian, 1977; Pfeiffer, Emmel, & Gardner, 1940; Selye, 1939) with their abilities to stimulate growth in the seminal vesicles and prostate (androgenic effect).

These studies indicated for the first time a possible separation of the stimulation of growth in two target tissues through a modification of the testosterone molecule. Reduction in the A-ring decreased the androgenic activity without significantly changing the renotrophic activity. The opposite effect was produced by oxidation of the 17-hydroxyl (Kochakian, 1944, 1946). I (CDK) noted a similar response in the castrated rat (Kochakian, 1964). An even more striking dichotomous effect was produced by the oral administration of the mono-oxygenated steroid, 17α-methyl-5α-androstan-17β-ol (Kochakian, 1952). In 1961 another steroid without a 3-ketone (17α-ethylestrenol) demonstrated a favorable dissociation between its effect on the weight of the levator ani muscle and that of the prostate of the rat (see Potts, Arnold, & Beyler, 1976).

Myotrophic/Androgenic Activity in Guinea Pigs

Papanicolaou and Falk (1938) had reported that the temporal and the masseter muscles of the guinea pig were much larger in the male than in the female and that castration of the male resulted in female-sized muscles. Administration of testosterone propionate restored the weight of the muscles in the castrated male and increased muscle weights of the female. I (CDK) confirmed a decrease in temporal muscle weight of the castrated male guinea pig and a growth-stimulating effect of testosterone propionate on the temporal muscle of the normal female and the castrated male guinea pig (table 1.1) (Kochakian, Humm, & Bartlett, 1948). The increase in weight of the muscle was due to hypertrophy. The diameter of the cross section of the muscle fibers was much greater in the normal adult guinea pig than in the castrated guinea pig (figure 1.4). The diameter of the muscles of the treated guinea pigs was identical with that of the normal guinea pigs and is not shown. Furthermore, the total DNA, which is indicative of the number of cells, was not changed by castration or testosterone propionate treatment (Kochakian, Hill, & Harrison, 1964).

A comparison of the effectiveness of several steroids revealed that 5α-androstane-3α, 17β-diol produced a partial dichotomy between the growth of the muscle and the accessory sex organs. The study was then extended (Kochakian, 1975; Kochakian & Tillotson, 1957) to include 47 other muscles to determine the general nature of the response. The increase in size of the different muscles differed not only for the several steroids but also for the individual muscles. The sensitivity of the muscles to the steroids was greatest in the head and neck region and gradually diminished from head to hindquarters (figure 1.5). Of further interest was the effect of 5α-dihydrotestosterone (5α-DHT). It was more active than testosterone in its androgenic effect and even more active in the myotrophic effect.

Table 1.1 Comparison of Temporal Muscle Weight (g) of Adult Guinea Pigs and of the Effect of Testosterone Propionate

Male			Female	
Normal	Castrated*	Castrated** plus TP	Normal	Normal** plus TP
2.08	0.98	1.80	0.54	1.01

*Castration was at approximately 400 g body weight.

**Testosterone propionate (TP) was implanted subcutaneously as two ±15 mg cylindrical pellets at the time of castration. The pellets were recovered at autopsy (54 days after castration), cleaned, dried, and weighed. The amount absorbed was 340 μg/day for the castrated males and 390 μg/day for the normal females.

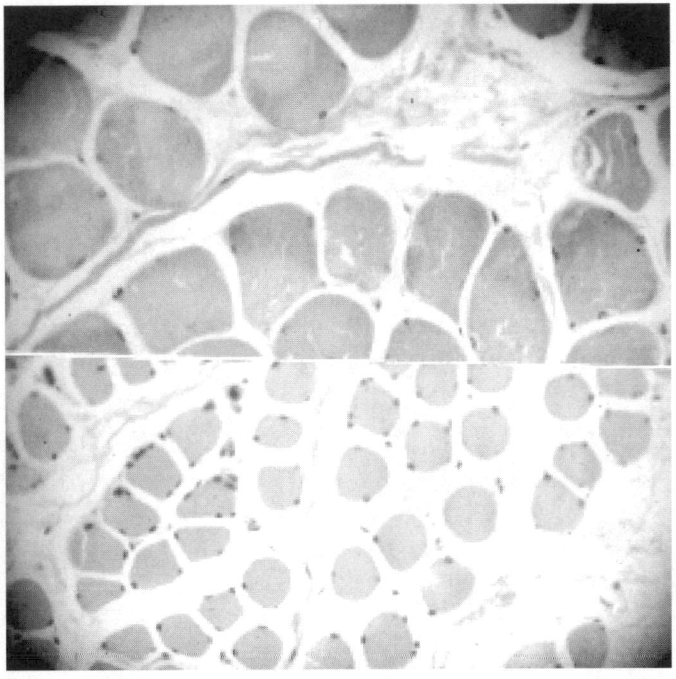

Figure 1.4 A comparison of the diameter of the fibers in the temporal muscle of the normal and castrated guinea pig.
Reprinted from Kochakian 1990a.

Rat: Skeletal Muscles

Castration of young rats (36 to 40 days of age) slightly decreased the rate of body growth and proportionately decreased the weight of practically all of the skeletal muscles (Kochakian, Tillotson, & Endahl, 1956). Our preliminary unpublished experiments with the injection of testosterone propionate and methyltestosterone did not produce any remarkable disproportionate increase in any of the many skeletal muscles, but suggested a small increase in several of the muscles. Thompson, Boxhon, King, and Allen (1989) reported that the injection of trenbolone acetate (17β-acetoxy-3-oxo-estra-4,9,11-triene) at 80 μg per 100 g body weight per day for 14 days (initial body weight was 63 to 124 g) increased the rate of growth of female rats with no acceleration of the growth of the gastrocnemius, anterior tibialis, and peroneus complex muscles but a small increase in the growth of the semimembranosus muscle. The DNA of all of the muscles was increased.

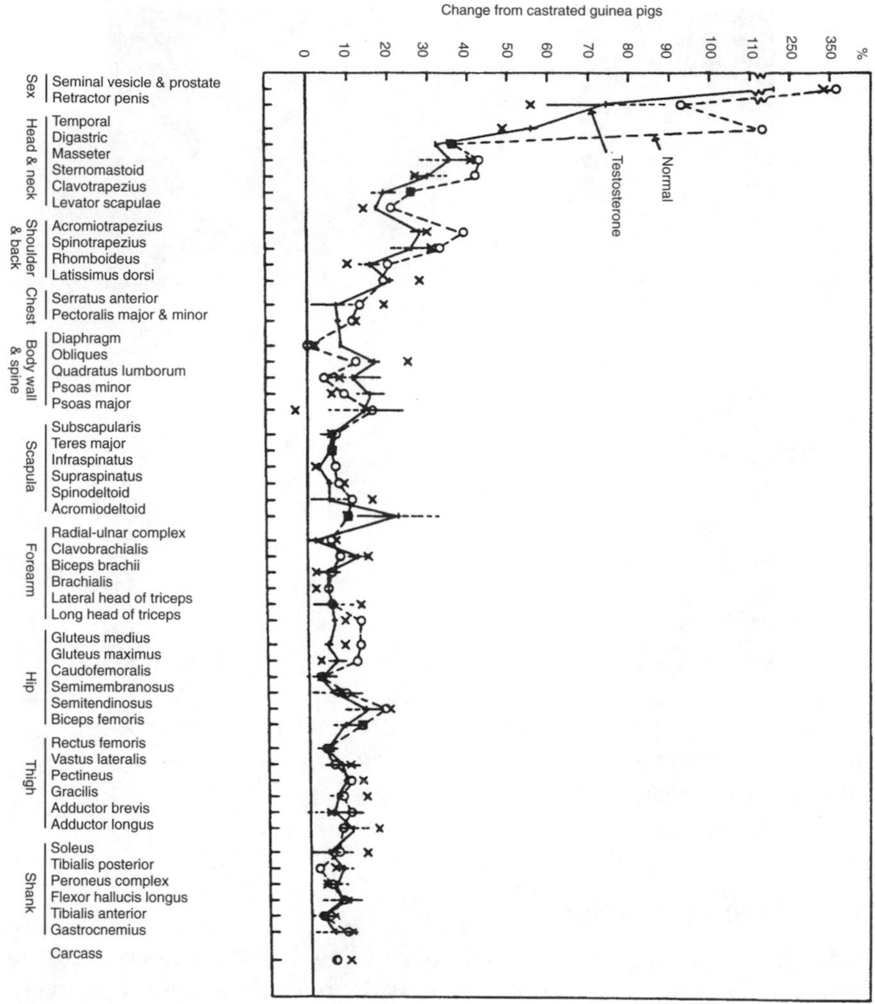

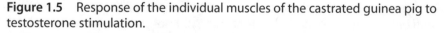

Figure 1.5 Response of the individual muscles of the castrated guinea pig to testosterone stimulation.

Reprinted from *Endocrinology* 1957.

Anabolic Steroids

Although a group of synthetically modified testosterone steroids have been popularized as anabolic steroids, there is no such thing as a pure anabolic steroid. All of the modified steroids still retain sufficient virilizing activity to make them objectionable as therapeutic agents, especially in children and women. Furthermore, researchers have presumed but never demonstrated that the response of the levator ani (dorsal bulbocavernosus) muscle is representative of the responses of the skeletal muscles. This muscle is in fact one of the perineal complex muscles that are located in the pelvic cavity.

Levator Ani

Hershberger, Shipley, and Meyer (1953) used the suggestion of Eisenberg and Gordan (1950) to develop a quantitative assay procedure and found that 19-nortestosterone stimulated a greater response in the levator ani muscle than in the accessory sex organs of the castrated rat. The authors presumed that the changes in weight of this muscle were representative of the skeletal muscles and designated its response to the steroids as anabolic, but this has not been proven (see sections on the muscles of guinea pigs and rats [Kochakian, 1976a pp. 14–16]. The protein of the skeletal muscles of the rat represents approximately 60% of the protein of the body (Kochakian & Webster, 1958). The levator ani muscle proved to be the sex-linked dorsal bulbocavernosus muscle (Hayes, 1968; also see Nimni & Geiger, 1957), but the assay because of its simplicity, inexpensiveness, and use of the common laboratory animal was widely accepted as a screening procedure (Overbeek, 1966; Overbeek, Delver, & deVisser, 1961).

Syntheses of many modifications of the natural compounds rapidly followed. Some of the more active steroids have been examined by nitrogen balance studies in castrated rats (table 1.2; Potts, Arnold, & Beyler, 1976), in monkeys (Stucki, Forbes, Northam, & Clark, 1960), and in humans (Albanese, 1965; Kochakian, 1975; Liddle & Burke, 1960; tables 1.3 and 1.4). The partial dissociation of the effect of some of the more active modified steroids on levator ani muscle from their effect on the prostate of the rat is presented in table 1.2 (Arnold, Potts, & Beyler, 1963). Potts, Arnold, and Beyler (1976) critically reviewed these and many other modified steroids. The researchers performed the assay for the muscle and the prostate (androgenic) on the same animals and studied the effect on nitrogen retention on a separate set of rats. The data clearly demonstrate the enhancement of nitrogen retention, as much as 10-fold, and a decrease in but not an elimination of the effect on the weight of the prostate by the modified steroids as compared with methyltestosterone. The effect of methyltestosterone on nitrogen retention is less than 20% of the effect of parenterally administered testosterone propionate (Kochakian, 1950; Potts, Arnold, & Beyler, 1976). These promising results prompted comparative nitrogen balance studies in humans, with several of the active oral steroids. Although many of the steroids demonstrated a marked enhancement when compared with methyltestosterone (table 1.3; Liddle & Burke, 1960) and testosterone propionate (table 1.4; Albanese, 1965), the differences are greatly diminished if compared with the more effective parenterally administered testosterone propionate or the other esters of testosterone. Orally administered testosterone is barely effective (see p. 10).

Table 1.2 Summary of Nitrogen-Retaining, Myotrophic, and Androgenic Activities of Several Orally Active Steroids Relative to Methyltestosterone

	Anabolic activity		Activity ratio		
Steroid	**Nitrogen retention**	**Levator ani**	**Androgenic activity**	**Nitrogen retention**	**Levator ani**
Methyltestosterone	1.0	1.0	1.0	1.0	1.0
Methandrostenolone	1.2		0.35	3.4	
(Δ^1-17α-methyltestosterone)	10		—	—	
		2.1	0.6		3.5
		2.3	—		—
		0.9	0.45	—	2.0
Oxymetholone	1.75		0.2	8.75	
	3		—	—	
		1.5	0.3		5.0
Norethandrolone	3.9		0.19	20	
(17α-Ethyl-19-nortestosterone)	2		—	—	
		2	(0.19)		(10.5)
		5.6			
		0.7	0.2		3.5
		1.0	0.34		3.1
Methylandrostanol-isoxazole	9.7		0.24	4.0	
		2	0.24		8.3
Stanozolol	10.0		0.33	3.0	
		2	0.33		6
		3.2	0.3		10.6

From *Endocrinology* 1963.

Table 1.3 Comparison of the Nitrogen-Retaining Activity of Orally Administered Steroids in Humans

Steroid	Relative activity
17α-methyltestosterone	1
17α-Ethyl-19-nortestosterone	2
9α-Fluoro-11β-hydroxy-17α-methyltestosterone (Halotestin)	3
2-Hydroxy-methylene-5α-dihydro-17α-methyltestosterone (Oxymetholone)	3
Oxandrolone	6
Δ^1-17α-methyltestosterone (Methandrostenolone; Methandienone)	10

Reprinted from *Helvetic Medica Acta* 1960.

Table 1.4 Comparison of Steroid Protein Anabolic Index (SPAI) of Some Newer Oral Steroids in Convalescent Adults

Steroid	Number of assays	Dosage mg/day	Average SPAI
Testosterone propionate	12	10–25	+6
19-Nortestosterone	14	25–75	+9
Norethandrolone (17α-ethyl-19-nortestosterone)	10	30–60	+8
Oxandrolone	27	10–20	+20
4-Hydroxy-17α-methyltestosterone	14	15–45	+11
Methandrostenolone (Δ^1-17α-methyltestosterone)	16	5–30	+16
Stanozolol	10	6–12	+29
17β-Hydroxy-17α-methylandrost-4-ene-(3.20)-pyrazol	9	15–25	+30
Norbolethone [(dl)-13-Ethyl-17b-hydroxy-18, 19-dinor-17α-pregn-4-en-3-one]	6	7.5–10	+34

$$\text{Steroid protein anabolic index} = \frac{\text{NBSP}}{\text{NISP}} - \frac{\text{NBCP}}{\text{NICP}} \times 100$$

NBSP = nitrogen balance in steroid period; NISP = nitrogen intake in steroid period; NBCP = nitrogen balance in control period; NICP = nitrogen intake in control period.

Reprinted from Albanese 1965.

The failure of the levator ani assay to reveal a steroid with an increased effect on the levator ani muscle and no or minimal effect on the accessory sex organs of the rat might indicate that the selection of this muscle as representative of the anabolic action of testosterone was a poor choice (Kochakian, 1975). The translation to clinical usage of the apparent favorable differential effect has been disappointing (i.e., the dissociation effect is not sufficient; Edgren, 1963).

Although at present the dissociation of anabolic activity from androgenic activity seems to be an impossible dream, we may be encouraged by the fact that several natural and synthetically modified steroid hormones have exhibited sufficient dissociation of specific biological activities to be exploited for beneficial therapeutic use (see Kochakian, 1990a, 1990b).

Anabolic-Androgenic Steroids

The synthetically modified steroids became known as anabolic steroids, but none of them exhibited a complete separation of anabolic from androgenic activity. They are now being more correctly recognized as anabolic-androgenic steroids (Kochakian, 1976a).

Although the new designation is more descriptive of the two better known effects of these compounds, it is not all-inclusive. Testosterone directly or indirectly through its metabolites influences the development and function of practically every organ in the body (Kochakian, 1959). The tissues influenced by testosterone can be classified into at least four categories:

- *Complete influence*—The accessory sex organs and the sex-linked muscles (e.g., bulbocavernosus in rats and mice and retractor penis in the guinea pig) are decreased after castration to vestigial organs by the loss of cells and atrophy of the residual cells, and are increased to at least double normal size in castrated and also normal animals by testosterone administration.
- *Supplementary influence*—The kidney, liver, heart, skeletal muscles, bone, bone marrow, salivary and orbital glands, urinary bladder, skin, sebaceous glands, larynx, and body hair are partially regressed after castration without an apparent loss in the number of cells and are restored to normal or greater size by testosterone administration.
- *Reverse influence*—Castration results in an increase in the size of the thymus, spleen, adrenals, and lymph glands. Testosterone administration decreases the thymus to a vestigial organ but only partially decreases the size of the spleen, adrenals, and lymph glands. Testosterone also causes a loss of scalp hair (male baldness).

• *Structural and functional changes in specific cells*—The dendritic length and size of motoneurons in the lumbar region of the male rat are reduced by castration and restored by testosterone administration (Breedlove, 1984, 1985; Kurz, Sengelaub, & Arnold, 1986). These neural units are involved in the mediation of the effect of steroids on the bulbocavernosus muscles.

The ability of specific cells in the brain to accumulate and metabolize testosterone is less in the castrated male and the female rat and is enhanced by testosterone administration. These changes and the resulting metabolites of testosterone are correlated with behavior (Balthazart & Schumacher, 1985).

Secretion of luteinizing hormone (LH) and follicle-stimulating hormone (FSH) by the anterior pituitary is enhanced after castration and decreased by testosterone administration.

The degrees of responses of the tissues in the complete influence category are characteristic and are the same for all species, but those in the other categories vary greatly among the different animal species and in some instances even among strains of the same species (Kochakian, 1975). Furthermore, parallel changes are not produced in these tissues by the many anabolic-androgenic steroids. Some of the lesser-studied responsive tissues (e.g., epithelial cells of the gastrointestinal tract) have not been included in the classification.

Many of the tissues in cell culture have shown diverse positive responses after the addition of physiological quantities and inhibition after excessive quantities of testosterone or other anabolic-androgenic steroids.

Therapeutic and Other Applications

Many of the synthetic modified sex steroids are of the orally active 17α-alkylated type (figure 1.6) and are more active than methyltestosterone (tables 1.3 and 1.4). These steroids have been popularized as anabolic steroids. Testosterone and 5α-dihydrotestosterone and their esters and Halotestin and methyltestosterone are considered androgens. The so-called anabolic steroids, however, still retain sufficient virilizing activity to be undesirable if given to women or adolescents, but not adult men (Edgren, 1963), whereas the so-called androgens have potent anabolic activity (nitrogen retention), which is accentuated by esterification and is accompanied by a small decrease in androgenic activity. Methyltestosterone is much less active than parenterally administered testosterone and even less active than parenterally administered testosterone esters (Kochakian, 1976b). More recently, transdermal preparations of testosterone have become increasingly popular as a delivery modality because they avoid the inconvenience and discomfort

Oral

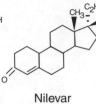

Methyltestosterone Nilevar Dianabol Ethylestrenol

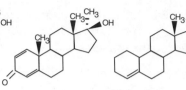

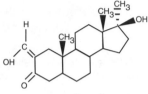

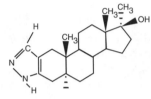

Anadrol Winstrol Anavar

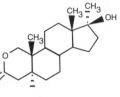

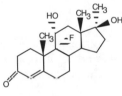

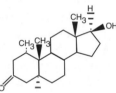

Halotestin Mesterolone Danazol

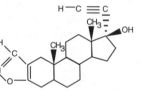

Parenteral

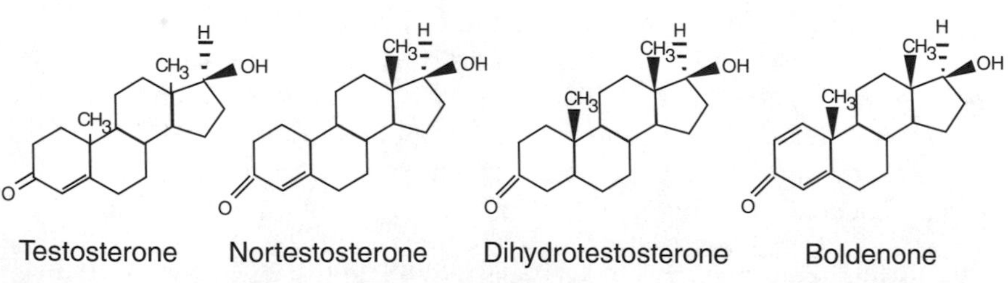

Figure 1.6 Some of the more common oral and parenteral anabolic-androgenic steroids and their familiar trivial or trade names.

of injections (*Drug Facts and Comparisons,* 1997). Initially, transdermal application of testosterone was limited to scrotal skin (Cunningham, Cordero, & Thornby, 1989), but more patient-friendly, enhanced transdermal patches are now available to effectively deliver physiological amounts of testosterone across nonscrotal skin (Mazer et al., 1992; Meikle et al., 1992). Testosterone buccalate and injectable, long-acting microcapsules of testosterone are also being examined as potential delivery modalities (Bagatell & Bremner, 1996).

Many of the modified steroids are prepared for oral use. Figure 1.6 shows the chemical modifications produced in each molecule of the more commonly used compounds. The possible undesirable effects on the liver, however, have discouraged the use of these preparations. On the other hand, the natural hormone testosterone and also 19-nortestosterone have been widely used parenterally as esters, which have been synthesized to produce efficient and long-lasting effects by a decrease in their rate of absorption. The most useful have been the propionate, $(\text{-}\overset{\text{O}}{\overset{\|}{\text{C}}}\text{-CH}_2\text{CH}_3)$, cypionate $(\text{-}\overset{\text{O}}{\overset{\|}{\text{C}}}\text{-CH}_2\text{-CH}_2\text{-}$⬠$)$, enanthate $(\text{-}\overset{\text{O}}{\overset{\|}{\text{C}}}\text{-(CH}_2)_5\text{-CH}_3)$, and undecanoate $(\text{-}\overset{\text{O}}{\overset{\|}{\text{C}}}\text{-(CH}_2)_9\text{-CH}_3)$ of testosterone and the decanoate $(\text{-}\overset{\text{O}}{\overset{\|}{\text{C}}}\text{-(CH}_2)_8\text{-CH}_3)$, and phenpropionate $(\text{-}\overset{\text{O}}{\overset{\|}{\text{C}}}\text{-CH}_2\text{-CH}_2\text{-}$⬡$)$ of nortestosterone.

Overbeek (1966) and Arnold, Potts, and Beyler (1976) have listed the manufacturers, the structure, and the systemic, generic, and trivial names of many of the anabolic-androgenic steroids (also see chapter 13; American Hospital Formulary Service, 1996; American Medical Association [AMA], 1994, 1990; *Drug Facts and Comparisons,* 1997).

Anabolic steroids have been used in a variety of clinical conditions (Bagatell & Bremner, 1996; Kopera, 1976, 1985; Tenover, 1997; World Health Organization, 1996) and in sports (Dubin, 1990; Ryan, 1976; Voy, 1990; Wade, 1972; Wright, 1980).

The AMA (1990) is uncertain about the beneficial value of these steroids as adjunct therapy for conditions of protein deficiency (such as chronic debilitating diseases) and for patients convalescing from severe infections, surgery, burns, trauma, irradiation, and cytotoxic drug therapy. The AMA acknowledges, however, that these steroids induce a sense of well-being, stimulate the appetite, induce protein synthesis, and may be helpful in terminal patients.

In the past, anabolic steroids, such as nandrolone decanoate, were used to treat anemia associated with chronic renal failure. However, their use for this condition has been supplanted, for the most part, by recombinant erythropoietin (Bagatell & Bremner, 1996).

From the 1930s to the late 1970s, anabolic steroids were used to successfully treat depression, melancholia, and involutional psychoses (Bahrke, Yesalis, & Wright, 1990). It is unclear why the use of anabolic steroids to treat certain psychiatric disorders diminished over time. However, this change is presumably due to reports of adverse interactions of anabolic steroids with other antidepressive agents, mixed results in clinical investigations employing androgens for treatment of depression, and the development of other, more efficacious, drugs whose mode of action is to modulate selected neurotransmitter systems (Green, Mooney, Posener, & Schildkraut, 1995; Rubin, 1981; Wilson, Prange, & Lara, 1974).

Hypogonadism

Anabolic steroids are given in physiological doses as replacement therapy to males with hypogonadism to induce or maintain secondary sexual characteristics, sexual behavior, and muscle development (Bagatell & Bremner, 1996). Because of the potential hepatotoxicity of oral steroids, primary hypogonadism as well as hypogonadotropic hypogonadism is generally treated with the injectable, long-lasting esters of testosterone (testosterone enanthate or cypionate) or with transdermal patches (American Hospital Formulary Service, 1996; AMA, 1994; Bagatell & Bremner, 1996; *Drug Facts and Comparisons,* 1997).

Delayed Puberty

Constitutional delay of puberty in boys age 15 or older has been treated with physiological doses of testosterone esters administered for 6 months. Thereafter, puberty continues because endogenous production of androgens begins. Because anabolic steroids may adversely affect epiphyseal centers, bone age needs to be monitored (AMA, 1994; Bagatell & Bremner, 1996).

Impotence and Male Climacteric Symptoms

In hypogonadal men, anabolic steroid therapy (testosterone and methyltestosterone) therapy can restore libido and potency (AMA, 1994). Androgen therapy in men with normal serum testosterone is ineffective.

Hereditary Angioedema

Anabolic steroids are used prophylactically for hereditary angioedema. To minimize virilizing effects, especially with women, anabolic steroids with low androgenic activity (e.g., danazol and stanozolol) are used (AMA, 1994; Bagatell & Bremner, 1996).

Metastatic Breast Cancer

Anabolic steroids have been used in the treatment of estrogen receptor-positive metastatic breast cancer in postmenopausal women.

Fluoxymesterone and nandrolone phenpropionate have been preferred in place of the testosterone esters because they are less virilizing (AMA, 1994; *Drug Facts and Comparisons,* 1997). However, today the antiestrogen tamoxifen is the primary therapy for these patients.

Postpartum Breast Pain and Engorgement

Methyltestosterone, fluoxymesterone, and testosterone propionate have been used for the prevention of postpartum breast pain and engorgement, although there is no satisfactory evidence that these drugs prevent or suppress lactation (American Hospital Formulary Service, 1996).

Endometriosis

Danazol is a common treatment for the signs and symptoms of endometriosis (AMA, 1994). When therapy is stopped, recurrence is common. In addition, while danazol is a weak anabolic steroid, many women will experience masculinization and an altered lipid profile (Bagatell & Bremner, 1996; chapter 7).

HIV/AIDS

Anabolic steroids appear to be increasingly used in the treatment of HIV illness. Case reports of HIV/AIDS patients treated with a variety of oral and injectable anabolic steroids indicate increases in appetite, strength, lean body mass, libido, and an improved sense of well-being in these patients (Berger, Pall, & Winfield, 1993; Hengge, Baumann, Maleba, Brockmeyer, & Goos, 1996; Jekot & Purdy, 1993; Rabkin, Rabkin, & Wagner, 1995; Wagner, 1998).

Contraception

A series of multinational evaluations of the contraceptive efficacy of testosterone esters (primarily cypionate and enanthate) has been conducted during the past 20 years. These studies have demonstrated spermatogenic suppression to severe oligozoospermia and resulted in sustained, reversible, effective contraception with minimal side effects (Waites & Farley, 1996; World Health Organization, 1996).

Aging Males

It appears that testosterone esters are being used increasingly to counteract age-associated decrease in serum testosterone concentrations in healthy adult men. Preliminary results indicate that testosterone supplementation therapy may help restore muscle strength and mass as well as bone mass in older men (Tenover, 1997). Other results, although less clear, suggest potential positive effects on mood, libido, and cognition.

Veterinary Applications

The anabolic-androgenic steroids are widely used in veterinary medicine (Dakin, 1966; Scoggins, 1980) based on studies of humans and experimental animals. However, scientific reports on veterinary use are scarce (Dennis, 1990). The available reports and anecdotes indicate improvements in nitrogen retention, weight gain, appetite, stamina, and general vigor, and report beneficial results as adjunct therapy for certain anemias; immunomediated thrombocytopenia; catabolism associated with illness, surgery, or trauma; overwork; old age; and glucocorticoid-related debilitation (Ettinger, 1986; McDonald, 1982). Improvements of coat hair and of attitude are also reported.

Trenbolone and testosterone propionate are used in pellet form in cattle to increase the rate of weight gain and improve feed efficiency (Veterinary Medicine Publishing Group, 1995).

Stanozolol (Winstrol V) and boldenone (Equipoise) are approved for horses (Dennis, 1990; FDA, 1991; Veterinary Medicine Publishing Group, 1995). Stanozolol is also approved for use in small animals (cats, dogs), especially older animals, to improve appetite and increase strength and vitality. But many other steroids, especially oxymetholone (Adroyd, Anadrol) and testosterone enanthate, are commonly prescribed (Ettinger, 1986). Mibolerone (Cheque Drops) is effective for estrus prevention in adult female dogs (Veterinary Medicine Publishing Group, 1995).

The effectiveness and dose of the steroid depend on the metabolic status of the horse. The beneficial effect is barely perceptible in the normal (especially growing) horse and shows decreasing efficacy from gelding to mare to stallion. Excessive doses produce adverse symptoms similar to those in the human.

Steroids also are used frequently in performance horses and racing horses to alleviate the stale and sour attitude (Blanchard, 1985; Dawson & Gertson, 1981; Genovese, 1981); 17β-hydroxy-17α-methylandrosta-1,4-dien-3-one (methandienone) and boldenone undecylenate improved the performances of race horses (Genovese, 1981). This use has prompted the development of methods to detect these steroids and their metabolites in equine urine (Edlund, Bowers, Herrion, & Covey, 1989).

Summary

Androsterone and testosterone were shown to stimulate growth and maintenance in not only the secondary sex organs of the rooster and mammals but also in practically every organ in the body. Attempts were made to modify the testosterone molecule to provide a molecule with strong anabolic activity but no or weak androgenic activity; a partial separation was accomplished in many compounds, but the separation was not sufficient to prevent virilization in therapeutic use. Testosterone esters and some of the modified compounds have proven useful in treating diverse types of protein deficiency in both human and veterinary medicine. New clinical applications, including contraception and supplementation therapy in older males, are being evaluated. The muscle-building effect of anabolic-androgenic steroids has caused them to be widely used by bodybuilders and athletes.

References

Albanese, A.A. (1965). Newer methodology in the clinical investigation of anabolic steroids. *Journal of New Drugs, 5,* 208–224.

American Hospital Formulary Service. (1996). *Drug information*. Bethesda, MD: American Society of Health-System Pharmacists.

American Medical Association, Council on Scientific Affairs. (1990). Medical and non-medical use of anabolic-androgenic steroids. *Journal of the American Medical Association, 264,* 2923–2927.

American Medical Association. (1994). *Drug evaluations.* Chicago: Author.

Arnold, A., Potts, G.O., & Beyler, A.L. (1963). Evaluation of the protein anabolic properties of certain orally active anabolic agents based on nitrogen balance studies in rats. *Endocrinology, 72,* 408–417.

Arnold, A., Potts, G.O., & Beyler, A.L. (1976). Structures, systematic, trivial, generic, and trade names of protein anabolic steroids. In C.D. Kochakian (Ed.), *Handbook of experimental pharmacology: Vol. 43. Anabolic-androgenic steroids* (pp. 627–636). Berlin: Springer-Verlag.

Bagatell, C., & Bremner, W. (1996). Androgens in men—uses and abuses. *New England Journal of Medicine, 334,* 707–714.

Bahrke, M., Yesalis, C., & Wright, J. (1990). Psychological and behavioural effects of endogenous testosterone and anabolic-androgenic steroids: An update. *Sports Medicine, 22,* 367–390.

Balthazart, J., & Schumacher, M. (1985). Role of testosterone metabolism in the activities of sexual behavior in birds. In R. Gilles & J. Balthazart (Eds.), *Current comparative approaches, neurobiology* (pp. 121–140). Berlin: Springer-Verlag.

Berger, J., Pall, L., and Winfield, D. (1993). Effect of anabolic steroids on HIV-related wasting myopathy. *Southern Medical Journal, 86,* 865–866.

Berthold, A.A. (1849). Transplantation des Hoden [Transplantation of testis]. *Archives Anatomic Physiologie Wissenschaftliche Medizin, 16,* 42–46.

Blanchard, T.L. (1985). Some effects of anabolic steroids—specially on stallions. *Compendium, 7,* S372–378.

Breedlove, M.S. (1984). Steroid influences on the development and function of a neuromuscular system. In G.J. DeVries, J.P.C. DeBruin, H.B.M. Uylings, & M.A. Corner (Eds.), *Progress in brain research: Vol. 61. Sex differences in the brain* (pp. 147–167). Amsterdam: Elsevier Science.

Breedlove, M.S. (1985). Hormonal control of the anatomical specificity of motoneuron-to-muscular innervation in rats. *Science, 227,* 1357–1359.

Brown-Sequard, E.C. (1889). The effects produced in man by subcutaneous injections of a liquid obtained from the testicles of animals. *Lancet, 2,* 105–107.

Butenandt, A. (1931). Über die chemische Untersuchung der Sexualhormon [The chemical research of sex hormones]. *Zeitschrift Angewandte Chemie, 44,* 905–908.

Butenandt, A., & Dannenbaum, H. (1934). Über Androsteron, und Kristallisietes männliches Sexualhormon III. Isolierung eines neuen, physiological unwirksamen Sterinderivatives aus Männerharn, seine Verknupfung mit Dehydro-Androsteron und Androsterons, ein Beitrag zur Konstitution des Androsterons [Androsterone, a crystalline male sex hormone III. Isolation of a new, physiologically inactive steroid derivative from male urine, its relationship with dehydroandrosterone and androsterone, a contribution to the constitution of androsterone]. *Zeitschrift Physiologische Chemie, 229,* 192–208.

Butenandt, A., & Hanisch, G. (1935). Über die Umwandlung des Dehydroandrosterons in Androstenol-(17)-one-(3) (Testosterone); um Weg zur Darstellung des Testosterons auf Cholesterin (Vorlauf Mitteilung) [The conversion of dehydroandrosterone into androstenol-(17)-one-3 (testosterone); a method for the production of testosterone from cholesterol (preliminary communication)]. *Berichte Deutsche Chemie Gesellschaft, 68,* 1859–1862.

Butenandt, A., & Kudszus, H. (1935). Über Androstendion, einen hochwirksamen mannlichen Pragungstoff [Androstenedione, a highly active male synthetic compound]. *Zeitschrift Physiologische Chemie, 237,* 75–88.

Butenandt, A., & Tscherning, K. (1934a). Über Androsteron, ein Krystallisiertes männliches Sexualhormon I. Isolierung und Reindarstellung aus Männerharn [Androsterone, a crystalline male sex hormone I. Isolation and purification from urine]. *Zeitschrift Physiologische Chemie, 229,* 167–184.

Butenandt, A., & Tscherning, K. (1934b). Über Androsteron ein Krystallisiertes Sexualhormon II. Seine Chemische Characterisierung [Androsterone, a crystalline sex hormone II. Its chemical characterization]. *Zeitschrift Physiologische Chemie, 229,* 185–191.

Cunningham, G., Cordero, E., & Thornby, J. (1989). Testosterone replacement with transdermal therapeutic systems: Physiological serum testosterone and elevated dihydrotestosterone levels. *Journal of the American Medical Association, 261,* 2525–2530.

Dakin, P.W. (1966). The use and misuse of hormones in veterinary medicine: Some recent developments in steroid therapy. *Veterinary Record, 78*(17) (P. Suppl. 1), IV–VII.

David, K. (1935). Über des Testosteron, des Kristallisierte männliches Hormon des Steerentestes [Testosterone, the crystalline male hormone from bulls' testes]. *Acta Brevia Neerland Physiologie, Pharmacologie, Microbiologie, 5,* 85–86, 108.

David, K., Dingemanse, E., Freud, J., & Laqueur, E. (1935). Über Kristallinisches männliches Hormon aus Hoden (Testosteron) wirksamer als aus Harn oder Cholesterin Bereitetes, Androsteron [Crystalline male hormone from testes (testosterone) more active than androsterone preparations from urine or cholesterol]. *Zeitschrift Physiologische Chemie, 233,* 281–293.

Dawson, H.A., & Gertson, K.E. (1981). Boldenone undecylenate: The way we see it. In R.L. Genovese (Ed.), *The symposium on anabolic steroids in equine medicine.* Princeton, NJ: E.R. Squibb & Sons, Animal Health Division.

Dennis, J.S. (1990). Anabolic steroids: Their potential in small animals. *The Compendium, 12,* 1403–1410.

Dorfman, R.I., & Ungar, R. (1965). *Metabolism of steroid hormones.* New York: Academic Press.

Drug facts and comparisons. (1997). St. Louis: Wolters Kluwer.

Dubin, C. (1990). Commission of inquiry into the use of drugs and banned practices intended to increase athletic performance (Catalogue No. CP32-56/1990E, ISBN 0-660-13610-4). Ottawa, ON: Canadian Government Publishing Center.

Edgren, R.A. (1963). A comparative study of the anabolic and androgenic effects of various steroids. *Acta Endocrinologica, 44*(Suppl. 87), 1–24.

Edlund, B., Bowers, L., Herrion, J., & Convey, T.R. (1989). Rapid determination of methandrostenolone in equine urine by isotope dilution, liquid-chromatography-tandem mass spectrometry. *Journal of Chromatography, 497,* 49–57.

Eisenberg, E., & Gordan, G.S. (1950). The levator ani muscle as an index of myotrophic activity of steroidal hormones. *Journal of Pharmacology and Experimental Therapeutics, 99,* 39–44.

Ettinger, S.J. (1986). Diseases of blood cells, spleen, and lymph nodes. *Veterinary Internal Medicine, 2,* 1606.

Fieser, L.F., & Fieser, M. (1959). *Steroids.* New York: Reinhold.

Food and Drug Administration. (1991). Regulation to prevent abuse of anabolic steroids. *FDA Veterinarian, VI,* 3–4.

Foss, G.L. (1939). Clinical administration of androgen: Comparison of various methods. *Lancet, 1,* 562–564.

Freud, J., deJongh, S.E., Laqueur, E., & Munch, A.P. (1930). Über männliches (Sexual) Hormon [Male (sex) hormone]. *Klinische Wochenschrift, 9,* 772–774.

Funk, C., & Harrow, B. (1929). The male hormone. *Proceedings of the Society for Experimental Biology and Medicine, 26,* 325–326, 569–570.

Funk, C., & Harrow, C. (1930). The male hormone IV. *Biochemical Journal, 24,* 1678–1680.

Funk, C., Harrow, B., & Lejwa, A. (1930). The male hormone. *American Journal of Physiology, 92,* 440–449.

Gallagher, T.F., & Koch, F.C. (1930). The quantitative assay for the testicular hormone by the comb growth reaction. *Journal of Pharmacology and Experimental Therapeutics, 40,* 327–339.

Gallagher, T.F., & Koch, F.C. (1934a). Biochemical studies on the male hormone as obtained from urine. *Endocrinology, 18,* 107–112.

Gallagher, T.F., & Koch, F.C. (1934b). The testicular hormone. *Journal of Biological Chemistry, 84,* 495–500.

Genovese, R.L. (1981). Introductory notes. In R.L. Genovese (Ed.), *The symposium on anabolic steroids in equine medicine* (pp. 5–6, 42). Princeton, NJ: E.R. Squibb & Sons, Animal Health Division.

Green, A., Mooney, J., Posener, J., & Schildkraut, J. (1995). Mood disorders: Biochemical aspects. In B. Kaplan & B. Sadock (Eds.), *Comprehensive textbook of psychiatry/VI,* 6th ed. (pp. 1089–1102). Baltimore: Williams & Wilkins.

Hayes, K.J. (1968). The so-called "levator ani" of the rat. *Acta Endocrinologica, 48,* 337–347.

Hengge, U., Baumann, M., Maleba, R., Brockmeyer, N., and Goos, M. (1996). Oxymetholone promotes weight gain in patients with advanced human immunodeficiency virus (HIV-1) infection. *British Journal of Nutrition, 75,* 129–138.

Hershberger, L.D., Shipley, E.G., & Meyer, R.K. (1953). Myotrophic activity of 19-nortestosterone and other steroids determined by modified levator ani method. *Proceedings of the Society for Experimental Biology and Medicine, 83,* 175–180.

Hoskins, R.G. (1941). *Endocrinology, the glands and their functions.* New York: Norton.

Jekot, W., & Purdy, D. (1993). Treating HIV/AIDS patients with anabolic steroids. *AIDS Patient Care, 7,* 68–74.

Johnsen, S.G., Bennett, E.P., & Jensen, V.G. (1974). Therapeutic effectiveness of oral testosterone. *Lancet, 2,* 1473–1474.

Kenyon, A.T., Sandiford, I., Bryan, A.H., Knowlton, K., & Koch, F.C. (1938). The effect of testosterone propionate on nitrogen, electrolyte, water and energy metabolism in eunuchoidism. *Endocrinology, 23,* 135–153.

Kochakian, C.D. (1935). Effect of male hormone on protein metabolism of castrate dogs. *Proceedings of the Society for Experimental Biology and Medicine, 32,* 1064–1065.

Kochakian, C.D. (1937). Testosterone and testosterone acetate and the protein and energy metabolism of castrate dogs. *Endocrinology, 21,* 750–755.

Kochakian, C.D. (1938). The comparative efficacy of various androgens as determined by the rat assay method. *Endocrinology, 22,* 181–192.

Kochakian, C.D. (1942). In E.C. Reifenstein Jr. (Ed.), *Josiah Macy Jr. Foundation Conference on Bone and Wound Healing, 2,* 25–32.

Kochakian, C.D. (1944). A comparison of the renotrophic with the androgenic activity of various steroids. *American Journal of Physiology, 142,* 315–325.

Kochakian, C.D. (1946). The effect of dose and nutritive state on the renotrophic and androgenic activities of various steroids. *American Journal of Physiology, 145,* 549–556.

Kochakian, C.D. (1950). Comparison of protein anabolic property of various androgens in the castrated rat. *American Journal of Physiology, 160,* 53–61.

Kochakian, C.D. (1952). Renotrophic-androgenic properties of orally administered androgens. *Proceedings of the Society for Experimental Biology and Medicine, 80,* 386–388.

Kochakian, C.D. (1959). Mechanisms of androgen actions. *Laboratory Investigation, 8,* 538–556.

Kochakian, C.D. (1964). Protein anabolic property of androgens. *Alabama Journal of Medical Sciences, 1,* 24–37.

Kochakian, C.D. (1975). Definition of androgens and protein anabolic steroids. *Pharmacology and Therapeutics B, 1*(2), 149–177.

Kochakian, C.D. (1976a). Historical review of anabolic-androgenic steroids. In C.D. Kochakian (Ed.), *Handbook of experimental pharmacology: Vol. 43. Anabolic-androgenic steroids* (pp. 1–4). Berlin: Springer-Verlag.

Kochakian, C.D. (1976b). Metabolic effects of anabolic-androgenic steroids in experimental animals. In C.D. Kochakian (Ed.), *Handbook of experimental pharmacology: Vol. 43. Anabolic-androgenic steroids* (pp. 5–44). Berlin: Springer-Verlag.

Kochakian, C.D. (1977). Regulation of kidney growth by androgens. In M.H. Briggs & G.A. Christie (Eds.), *Advances in steroid biochemistry and pharmacology* (Vol. 6, pp. 1–34). London: Academic Press.

Kochakian, C.D. (1984). *How it was: Anabolic actions of steroids and remembrances.* Birmingham: School of Medicine, University of Alabama.

Kochakian, C.D. (1990a). History of anabolic-androgenic steroids. In G.C. Linn & L. Erinoff (Eds.), *Anabolic steroid abuse* (National Institute on Drug Abuse, Research Monograph 102, pp. 29–59). Rockville, MD: U.S. Department of Health and Human Services, Public Health Services.

Kochakian, C.D. (1990b). Metabolites of testosterone: Significance in the vital economy. *Steroids, 55,* 92–97.

Kochakian, C.D., & Arimasa, N. (1976). The metabolism in vitro of anabolic-androgenic steroids by mammalian tissues. In C.D. Kochakian (Ed.), *Handbook of experimental pharmacology: Vol. 43. Anabolic-androgenic steroids* (pp. 287–359). Berlin: Springer-Verlag.

Kochakian, C.D., Hill, J., & Harrison, D.G. (1964). Regulation of nucleic acids of muscles and accessory sex organs of guinea pigs by androgens. *Endocrinology, 74,* 635–642.

Kochakian, C.D., Humm, J.H., & Bartlett, M.N. (1948). Effect of steroids on body weight, temporal muscle and organs of the guinea pig. *American Journal of Physiology, 155,* 242–250.

Kochakian, C.D., & Murlin, J.R. (1935). The effect of male hormone on the protein and energy metabolism of castrate dogs. *Journal of Nutrition, 10,* 437–459.

Kochakian, C.D., & Murlin, J.R. (1936). The relationship of synthetic male hormone, androstenedione, to the protein and energy metabolism of castrated dogs and the protein metabolism of a normal dog. *American Journal of Physiology, 117,* 642–657.

Kochakian, C.D., & Tillotson, C. (1957). Influence of several C19-steroids on the growth of individual muscles of the guinea pig. *Endocrinology, 60,* 607–618.

Kochakian, C.D., Tillotson, C., & Endahl, G.L. (1956). Castration and the growth of muscle in the rat. *Endocrinology, 58,* 226–231.

Kochakian, C.D., & Webster, J.A. (1958). Effect of testosterone propionate on the appetite, body weight, and composition of the normal rat. *Endocrinology, 63,* 737–742.

Kopera, H. (1976). Miscellaneous uses of anabolic steroids. In C.D. Kochakian (Ed.), *Handbook of experimental pharmacology: Vol. 43. Anabolic-androgenic steroids* (pp. 535–625). Berlin: Springer-Verlag.

Kopera, H. (1985). The history of anabolic steroids and a review of clinical experiences with anabolic steroids. *Acta Endocrinologica* (Suppl. 271—*Anabolics in the '80s*), *110,* 11–18.

Kurz, E.M., Sengelaub, D.R., & Arnold, A.P. (1986). Androgens regulate dendritic length of mammalian motoneurons in adulthood. *Science, 232,* 395–398.

Landau, R.L. (1976). The metabolic effects of anabolic steroids in man. In C.D. Kochakian (Ed.), *Handbook of experimental pharmacology: Vol. 43. Anabolic-androgenic steroids* (pp. 45–72). Berlin: Springer-Verlag.

Liddle, G.W., & Burke Jr., H.A. (1960). Anabolic steroids in clinical medicine. *Helvetica Medica Acta, 27,* 505–513.

Lode, A. (1891). Zur Transplantation der Hoden bei Hahnen: [The transplantation of the testis in roosters]: Part I. *Wiener Klinische Wochenschrift, 4,* 847.

Lode, A. (1895). Zur Transplantation der Hoden bei Hahnen: [The transplantation of the testis in roosters]: Part II. *Wiener Klinische Wochenschrift, 8,* 341–346.

Loewe, S., & Voss, H.E. (1930). Der Stand der Erfassung des männlichen Sexualhormons (Androkinins) [The status of the detection of the male sex hormone (Androkinins)]. *Klinische Wochenschrift, 9,* 481–487.

Mazer, N., Heiber, W., Moellmer, J., Meikle, A., Stringham, J., Sanders, S., et al. (1992). Enhanced transdermal delivery of testosterone: A new physiological approach for androgen replacement in hypogonadal men. *Journal of Controlled Release, 19,* 347–362.

McDonald, L.E. (1982). Hormones affecting reproduction. In N.H. Booth & L.E. McDonald (Eds.), *Veterinary pharmacology and therapeutics* (pp. 534–535). Ames: Iowa State University Press.

McGee, L.C. (1927). The effect of the injection of a lipoid fraction of bull testicle in capons. *Proceedings of the Institute of Medicine* (Chicago), *6,* 252.

Meikle, A., Mazer, N., Moellmer, J., Stringham, J., Tolman, K., Sanders, S., et al. (1992). Enhanced transdermal delivery of testosterone across nonscrotal skin produces physiological concentrations of testosterone and its metabolites in hypogonadal men. *Journal of Clinical Endocrinology and Metabolism, 74,* 623–628.

Moore, C.R. (1939). Biology of the testes. In E. Allen, C.H. Danforth, & E.A. Doisy (Eds.), *Sex and internal secretions* (pp. 354–451). Baltimore: Williams & Wilkins.

Moore, C.R., & Gallagher, T.F. (1930). Threshold relationship of testis hormone indicators in mammals: The rat unit. *Journal of Pharmacology and Experimental Therapeutics, 40,* 341–349.

Murlin, J.R. (1911). Metabolism of development III. Qualitative effects of pregnancy on the protein metabolism of the dog. *American Journal of Physiology, 28,* 442–454.

Newerla, G.J. (1943). The history of the discovery and isolation of the male hormone. *New England Journal of Medicine, 228,* 39–47.

Nimni, M.E., & Geiger, E. (1957). Non-suitability of levator ani method as an index of anabolic effect of steroids. *Proceedings of the Society for Experimental Biology and Medicine, 96,* 606–610.

Overbeek, G.A. (1966). *Anabolic steroids.* Berlin: Springer-Verlag.

Overbeek, G.A., Delver, A., & deVisser, J. (1961). Pharmacological comparisons of anabolic steroids (ethylestrenol, nandrolone esters). In J.W.R. Everse & P.A. van Keep (Eds.), *Symposium on anabolic steroids. Acta Endocrinologica, 39*(Suppl. 63), 7–17.

Papanicolaou, G.N., & Falk, E.A. (1938). General muscular hypertrophy induced by androgenic hormone. *Science, 87,* 238–239.

Parkes, A.S. (1966). The rise of reproductive endocrinology, 1926–1940. *Journal of Endocrinology, 34,* xx–xxxii.

Parkes, A.S. (1985). *Off-beat biologist: The autobiography of A.S. Parkes.* Cambridge, England: The Galton Foundation.

Parkes, A.S. (1988). *Biologist at large: The autobiography of A.S. Parkes* (Vol. 2). Cambridge, England: The Galton Foundation.

Pezard, A. (1911). Sur la determination des caractères sexuels secondaire chez les gallinaces [The determination of the secondary sexual characteristics of fowl]. *Compte Rendu Academie des Sciences, 153,* 1027–1032.

Pezard, A. (1912). Sur la determination des caractères sexuels secondaire chez les gallinaces [The determination of the secondary sexual characteristics of fowl]. *Compte Rendu Academie des Sciences, 154,* 1183–1186.

Pezard, A., & Caridroit, M. (1926). Le presence de l'hormone testiculaire dans le sang du coq normal, demonstration directe fondu sur la greffe autoplastique des cretillons [The presence of the testicular hormone in the blood of the normal rooster based on the auto-transplantation of the comb]. *Compte Rendu Société des Biologie, 92,* 296–298.

Pfeiffer, C.A., Emmel, V.M., & Gardner W.U. (1940). Renal hypertrophy in mice receiving estrogen and androgen. *Yale Journal of Biology Medicine, 12,* 493–501.

Potts, G.O., Arnold, A., & Beyler, A.L. (1976). Dissociation of the androgenic and other hormonal effects of steroids. In C.D. Kochakian (Ed.), *Handbook of experimental pharmacology: Vol. 43. Anabolic-androgenic steroids* (pp. 361–406). Berlin: Springer-Verlag.

Rabkin, J., Rabkin, R., & Wagner, G. (1995). Testosterone replacement therapy in HIV illness. *General Hospital Psychiatry, 17,* 37–42.

Reifenstein, E.C., Jr. (1942). The protein anabolic activity of steroid compounds. *Josiah Macy Jr. Foundation Conference on Bone and Wound Healing, 1*(Suppl).

Rubin, R. (1981). Sex hormone dynamics in endogenous depression: A review. *International Journal of Mental Health, 10,* 43–59.

Ruzicka, L. (1973). In the borderline between bioorganic chemistry and biochemistry. *Annual Review Biochemistry, 41,* 1–20.

Ruzicka, L., Goldberg, M.W., Meyer, J., Brunigger, H., & Eichenberg, E. (1934). Zur Kenntnis der Sexualhormon II, Über die Syntheses des Testikelhormons (Androsteron) und Steroisomers desselben durch Abbau Hydrieter Sterine [Information on the sex hormones II. Concerning the synthesis of the testicle hormone (androsterone) and its stereoisomers by hydrogenation of steroids]. *Helvetica Chimica Acta, 17,* 1395–1406.

Ruzicka, L., & Wettstein, A. (1935a). Sexualhormon, trans-Dehydroandrosteron und des Androsten-3, 17-dion [Sex hormones, trans-dehydroandrosterone and androsten-3, 17-dione]. *Helvetica Chimica Acta, 18,* 986–994.

Ruzicka, L., & Wettstein, A. (1935b). Über die kristallinische Herstellung des Testikelhormons, Testosteron (Androsten-3-ol-17-ol) [The crystalline production of the testicle hormone, testosterone (Androsten-3-ol-17-ol)]. *Helvetica Chimica Acta, 18,* 1264–1275.

Ryan, A.J. (1976). Athletics. In C.D. Kochakian (Ed.), *Handbook of experimental pharmacology: Vol. 43. Anabolic-androgenic steroids* (pp. 515–534). Berlin: Springer-Verlag.

Scoggins, R.D. (1980). The anabolic steroids. *Equine Practice, 2*(1), 26–30.

Selye, H. (1939). The effect of testosterone on the kidney. *Journal of Urology, 42,* 637–641.

Spencer, R.F. (1946). The cultural aspects of eunuchism. *CIBA Symposia, 8*, 406–420.

Starling, E.H. (1905). The chemical correlation of the functions of the body. *Lancet, 1,* 339–341.

Stucki, J.C., Forbes, A.D., Northam, J.I., & Clark, J.J. (1960). An assay for anabolic steroids employing metabolic balance in the monkey: The anabolic activity of Fluoxymesterone and its keto analogue. *Endocrinology, 66,* 585–598.

Tausk, M. (1984). Androgens and anabolic steroids. In M.J. Parnham & J. Bruinvels (Eds.), *Discoveries in pharmacology* (Vol. 2, pp. 305–320). Amsterdam: Elsevier.

Tenover, L. (1997). Testosterone and the aging male. *Journal of Andrology, 18,* 103–106.

Thompson, S.H., Boxhon, L.X., King, W., & Allen, R.E. (1989). Trenbolone alters the responsiveness of skeletal muscle satellite cells to fibroblast growth factor and insulin-like growth factor-I. *Endocrinology, 24,* 2110–2117.

Veterinary Medicine Publishing Group. (1995). *Veterinary pharmaceuticals and biologicals.* Lenexa, KS: Veterinary Publishing Co.

Voss, H.E. (1930). Die Vesiculardrüsen (Samenbläsen) des Kastraten Nach Hodentransplantation [The vesicular gland (seminal vesicle) of castrates after testis transplantation]. *Pflugers Archives gesellschaft Physiologie des Menschen und der Tier, 226,* 138–147.

Voy, R. (1990). *Drugs, sport, and politics.* Champaign, IL: Leisure Press.

Wade, N. (1972). Anabolic steroids: Doctors denounce them, but athletes aren't listening. *Science, 176,* 1399–1403.

Wagner, G., & Rabkin, J. (1998). Testosterone therapy for clinical symptoms of hypogonadism in eugonadal men with AIDS. *International Journal of STD & AIDS, 9,* 41–44.

Waites, G., & Farley, T. (1996). Contraceptive efficacy of hormonal suppression of spermatogenesis. In S. Bhasin (Ed.), *Pharmacology, biology, and clinical applications of androgens* (pp. 345–353). New York: Wiley-Liss.

Weinbauer, G.F., Marshall, G.R., & Nieschlag, E. (1986). New injectable testosterone ester maintains serum testosterone of castrated monkeys in the normal range for four months. *Acta Endocrinologica, 113,* 128–132.

Wilson, I., Prange, A., and Lara, P. (1974). Methyltestosterone with imipramine in men: Conversion of depression to paranoid reaction. *American Journal of Psychiatry, 131,* 21–24.

World Health Organization Task Force on Methods for the Regulation of Male Fertility. (1996). Contraceptive efficacy of testosterone-induced azoospermia and oligozoospermia in normal men. *Fertility and Sterility, 65,* 821–829.

Wright, J.E. (1980). Steroids and athletics. *Exercise and Sports Science Review, 8,* 149–202.

CHAPTER

2

History of Anabolic Steroid Use in Sport and Exercise

Charles E. Yesalis, ScD; Stephen P. Courson; and James E. Wright, PhD

I feel sorry for Ben Johnson. All sportsmen—not all, but maybe 90%, including our own—use drugs.

Anonymous Soviet coach
New York Times, October 1988
1988 Seoul Olympics

Americans like to think the U.S. leads the "Sports without Drugs Crusade," but "the reality is that the U.S. is viewed as one of the dirtiest nations in the world," says John Ruger, past chair of the United States Olympic Committee Athletes' Advisory Council.

"Mass Deception: Today's Athlete is Getting Bigger, Stronger, Faster . . . Unnaturally"
Sport, August 1998

By 1935 the hormone testosterone had been isolated and chemically characterized, and the basic nature of its anabolic effects had been elucidated (Butenandt & Hanisch, 1935; David, Dingemanse, Freud, & Laqueur, 1935; Kochakian & Murlin, 1935). Shortly thereafter, both oral and injectable preparations were available to the medical community.

It has been rumored that some German athletes were given testosterone in preparation for the 1936 Berlin Olympics (Francis, 1990). Although the effects of other drugs on the physiology of human performance are well documented in the German medical literature, no mention of the use of testosterone as an ergogenic aid has been noted during that period (Hoberman, 1992b). Moreover, Hoberman contends,

> *It is likely that public anti-doping sentiment after 1933 was related to Nazi strictures against the self-serving, individualistic, record-breaking athlete and the abstract ideal of performance. It is also consistent with Nazi rhetoric about sportsmanship, e.g., the importance of the "noble contest" and the "chivalric" attitude of the German athlete.*

Wade (1972) has alleged that during World War II, German soldiers took steroids prior to battle to enhance aggressiveness. This assertion, although often cited, has yet to be documented, in spite of efforts to do so. Furthermore, the Nazis were opposed to organism-altering drugs in general (Hoberman, 1992a,b). There was a concerted campaign against the "poisons" alcohol and tobacco, and Nazis "were not particularly interested in the popular gland transplant techniques of that period, since their idea of race improvement was genetic" (Hoberman, 1992a,b).

Bøje, writing in the *Bulletin of the Health Organization of the League of Nations* in 1939, appears to have been the first to suggest that sex hormones, based on their physiologic actions, might enhance physical performance. At the same time, the anabolic effects of anabolic steroids were being confirmed in eunuchs and in normal men and women (Kenyon, Knowlton, Sandiford, Koch, & Lotwin, 1940; Kenyon, Sandiford, Bryan, Knowlton, & Koch, 1938). Uncontrolled studies also demonstrated improvements in strength and dynamic work capacity in eugonadal males (Simonson, Kearns, & Enzer, 1941) and otherwise healthy older males complaining of fatigue (Simonson, Kearns, & Enzer, 1944).

The first recorded case of an "athlete" using testosterone was a gelding trotter named Holloway (Kearns, Harkness, Hobson, & Smith, 1942). Prior to the implantation of testosterone pellets, this 18-year-old horse had "declined to a marked degree in his staying power and during February of 1941 in several attempts at ice racing, failed to show any of his old speed or willingness" (Kearns et al., 1942, p. 199). After the administration of testosterone and several months of training, Holloway won or placed in a number of races and established a trotting record of 2:10 at age 19.

In *The Male Hormone,* de Kruif (1945) further raised hopes and expectations for the newly synthesized anabolic steroids. He argued that these hormones had the potential to rejuvenate individuals and improve their productivity, and he assuringly reported that testosterone "caused the human body to synthesize protein [and] . . . to be able to build the very stuff of its own life" (p. 130). De Kruif went on:

> *I'll be faithful and remember to take my twenty to thirty milligrams a day of testosterone. I'm not ashamed that it's no longer made to its old degree by my own aging body. It's chemical crutches. It's borrowed manhood. It's borrowed time. But just the same, it's what makes bulls bulls (p. 226).*

With regard to athletes, de Kruif commented:

> *We know how both the St. Louis Cardinals and the St. Louis Browns have won championships supercharged by vitamins. It would be interesting to watch the productive power of an industry or a professional group (of athletes) that would try a systematic supercharge with testosterone (p. 223).*

De Kruif's pseudoscientific writings were not without effect. Combined with the significant positive observations reported from clinical studies in professional journals, it was a relatively easy extrapolation for some in the physical culture of bodybuilding to expect that additional anabolic-androgenic hormones, at that time universally assumed to exert no adverse effects when taken in therapeutic dosages, would allow development of greater than "normal" body size and strength. According to several unpublished interview reports with Wright, et al., experimental use of the new testosterone preparations began among West Coast bodybuilders in the early 1950s. Also suggestive of anabolic steroid use are physique photos of this time showing highly significant changes over relatively short periods in the muscle mass of established elite bodybuilders. Since then, bodybuilding has been and continues to be strongly and consistently linked to steroid use (Duchaine, 1982, 1989; Fussell, 1990; Klein, 1986, 1993; Nack, 1998; Phillips, 1990; Wright, 1978), as has the sport's best-known participant, Arnold Schwarzenegger (Johnston, 1974; Leigh, 1990).

The initiation of systematic use of anabolic steroids in sports has been attributed to reports of their use by successful Soviet weightlifting teams in the early 1950s. Statistical analysis of the performance of the Soviet lifters during this period is consistent with this assertion (Fair, 1988).

In 1954, at the world weightlifting championships in Vienna, Dr. John Ziegler, the U.S. team physician, reportedly was told by his Soviet counterpart that the Soviets were taking testosterone (Fair, 1993; Starr, 1981; Todd, 1987). Ziegler returned to the United States and experimented with testosterone on himself and a few weightlifters in the York Barbell Club. Dr. Ziegler was concerned, however, with the androgenic effects of testosterone, and in 1958, when the Ciba Pharmaceutical Company released Dianabol (methandrostenolone), he began experimentation with this new drug. After he described some of his results in the popular physical training periodicals of the time, and after several of the early users of anabolic steroids achieved championship status, news of the efficacy of these drugs apparently spread by word of mouth during the early 1960s to other strength-intensive sports, from field events to football.

Olympic Sports

Anabolic steroid use was apparently not a major problem at the 1960 Olympic Games in that it was probably limited to Soviet strength athletes and a few American weightlifters. By 1964, however, the secret behind the startling progress of a number of strength athletes began to leak out, and as a result steroids were soon being used extensively by athletes in all the strength sports (*Hearings Before the Subcommittee,* 1973; Gilbert, 1969a–c; Payne, 1975; Starr, 1981; Todd, 1987).

The weightlifters themselves were quickly convinced that steroids made them bigger and stronger, and they began to tout the drugs. In track and field, the throwers were early converts. By the mid-1960s most of the top-ranking throwers had tried anabolic steroids, including Randy Matson, the 1968 Olympic champion and world record holder in the shot put; Dallas Long, the 1964 Olympic shot put champion; Harold Connolly, the 1956 Olympic champion in the hammer throw; and Russ Hodge, a world record holder in the decathlon (Gilbert, 1969a–c).

By 1968, according to H. Connolly (*Hearings Before the Subcommittee,* 1973) and Francis (1990), athletes in a number of track-and-field events, including sprinters, hurdlers, and middle-distance runners, were using anabolic steroids. Dr. Tom Waddell, a U.S. decathlete, estimated that one-third of the entire U.S. track-and-field team (not just strength and field-event athletes) had used steroids at the 1968 pre-Olympic training camp (Todd, 1987). This was a time when steroid use was not banned and had become much less secretive than previously, and it was a year after the International Olympic Committee established a medical committee and banned certain drugs.

During the 1968 Olympic Games in Mexico City, athletes and coaches did not debate the morality or propriety of taking drugs; the only debate was over which drugs were more effective. Bill Toomey, gold medalist in the decathlon at the 1968 Olympics and winner of the Amateur Athletic Union's prestigious Sullivan Award, admitted he used drugs to aid his performance at the Mexico City Olympics (Scott, 1971).

Dosages used by strength athletes had increased by the late 1960s to 2 to 5 times therapeutic recommendations (for replacement therapy), and the variety of steroids used had increased as well, although it was not until this time that use of multiple drugs (stacking) and the simultaneous use of oral and injectable anabolic steroids began. From the time substances marketed as anabolic steroids were introduced, some athletes preferred them to the more androgenic preparations (such as the oral and injectable testosterones and fluoxymesterone), primarily because the anabolic steroids were marketed for their "anabolic" effects but also because of concern over what athletes considered undesirable androgenic effects (including aggression). However, steroid users who wished to maximize muscle mass and strength continued to use the more "androgenic" preparations.

By 1969, the cat was completely out of the bag. Users were praising the effects of anabolic steroids on performance (Brown & Tait, 1973), and Jon Hendershott (1969), then editor of *Track and Field News,* was nonfacetiously categorizing anabolic steroids as the "breakfast of champions." That same year a mainstream sports magazine published a three-part exposé of drug use in sports, which indicated on the basis of numerous interviews and observations that "athletes were popping more pills for more purposes than were dreamt of in anybody's philosophy—or pharmacy" (Gilbert, 1969c, p. 30).

After winning in the 1971 Pan American games in Cali, Colombia, weightlifter Ken Patera relished meeting Russian superheavyweight Vasily Alexeyev in the 1972 Olympics in Munich. Patera was quoted in the *Los Angeles Times:*

> *Last year the only difference between me and him was I couldn't afford his drug bill. Now I can. When I hit Munich I'll weigh in at about 340, or maybe 350. Then we'll see which are better, his steroids or mine (Scott, 1971).*

Prior to the 1984 Olympics, a newspaper article alleged that shot-putters and throwers of the discus, javelin, and hammer had been given information by the coordinator of a U.S. Olympic Committee's instructional program, within the year before the Olympics, to help them beat tests for anabolic steroids ("Steroid Information," 1984). Others have argued that this program was merely an educational effort to familiarize the athletes with the adverse consequences of anabolic steroid use and had nothing to do with evading drug tests. During the 1990s, not only was performance-enhancing drug use still pervasive in weightlifting and the field events (Noden, 1993; "Drugs Detected," 1995; "Out of Action," 1997; "Lifetime Drug," 1998), but anabolic steroid use was present in other Olympic sports, including hockey, swimming, cycling, skiing, volleyball, wrestling, handball, pentathlon, bobsledding, and soccer (Dubin, 1990; "We'll Take It," 1997). After a lengthy investigation of drug use in Olympic sports, Bamberger and Yaeger (1997) concluded that

> *three distinct classes of top-level athletes have emerged in many Olympic sports. One is a small group of athletes who are not using any banned performance enhancers. The second is a large, burgeoning group whose drug use goes undetected; these athletes either take drugs that aren't tested for, use tested-for drugs in amounts below the generous levels permitted by the IOC or take substances that mask the presence of the drugs in their system at testing time. The third group comprises the smattering of athletes who use banned performance enhancers and are actually caught.*

Female Athletes

The powerful masculinizing effects of anabolic steroids in females had been established prior to 1960 (Kochakian, 1976; Kruskemper, 1968). However, it is difficult to say when exactly women athletes began using anabolic steroids. It is reasonable to speculate that the Soviet female track-and-field athletes of the 1960s or perhaps even the 1950s were the first women athletes to use these drugs.

The masculine appearances of a number of female track-and-field athletes from the Eastern European Communist bloc countries in the mid-1960s led to speculation that they were either hermaphrodites or men disguised as women. In response, a chromosome test was initiated in 1967 at the European Cup (Todd, 1987). Although several athletes did indeed fail the screening over the years and several others mysteriously retired from competition prior to being tested, many of the women who initially were suspected may have been neither genetic "mistakes" nor charlatans but simply had been administered testosterone (see chapter 7).

The spread of steroid use among female athletes probably followed a pattern similar to that of males, with the strength athletes the first among women to adopt the drugs. Evidence of steroid use among female throwers from Eastern European Communist bloc countries goes back at least to the 1968 Olympic Games at Mexico City (Fikotova-Connolly, personal communication, 1991; Franke & Berendonk, 1997). By the 1972 Munich Games, it was alleged that several U.S. women participating in the field events had used anabolic steroids (*Hearings on Steroids,* 1989). Anabolic steroids continued to be used by female athletes in strength sports (Franke & Berendonk, 1997; Patrick, 1997), and based on government records, testimonials, and the results of drug tests, by the late 1970s steroid use had spread to sprinters and middle-distance runners, swimmers, rowers, and athletes in various winter sporting events as well (Berendonk & Franke, 1997; Dubin, 1990; Williams, 1989). As with men's use, women's steroid use has diffused beyond Olympic sport and has now been reported at the collegiate level in sports including basketball, volleyball, soccer, field hockey, swimming, gymnastics, lacrosse, and softball (Anderson, Albrecht, McKeag, Hough, & McGraw, 1991; "Survey Shows," 1997; Yesalis, Anderson, Buckley, & Wright, 1990; see chapter 3 in this book). In 1995, a 14-year-old female long jumper and sprinter from South Africa became the world's youngest athlete to test positive for anabolic steroid use ("Ban," 1995).

National Doping Programs

Although the existence of well-organized, nationwide sport doping programs has been rumored for decades, solid evidence has now come to light to document their reality. National doping programs transcend the all too common informal collusion of elite athletes, coaches, and rogue physicians and sport scientists to use performance-enhancing drugs. Rather they are constituted under the direction or strong support of government and sport federation officials, as well as the active collaboration of mainstream physicians and scientists.

Thanks to the courage and persistence of Werner Franke and Brigitte Berendonk (1997) we now have detailed information on the heinous activities of the German Democratic Republic (GDR) sport doping system.

Top-secret doctoral theses, scientific reports, progress reports of grants, proceedings of symposia of experts, and reports of physicians and scientists who served as unofficial collaborators for the Ministry of State Security (Stasi) reveal that, from 1966 on, hundreds of physicians and scientists, including top-ranking professors, performed doping research and administered prescription drugs as well as unapproved experimental drug preparations. Several thousand athletes were treated with androgens every year, including minors of each sex. Special emphasis was placed on administering androgens to women and adolescent girls because the practice proved to be particularly effective for sport performance.

This communist state-sponsored program was not only a highly organized assault on the rules of sport, but, more importantly, it also flagrantly violated scientific and medical ethics. Girls and boys, 14 years of age or younger, were given anabolic steroids—often without them or their parents being informed. At the time of this writing, criminal prosecutions of some of these coaches and physicians are now under way in Germany ("Athletes Live," 1997; "East German," 1998). Interestingly, the IOC has been denounced for hesitating to aggressively investigate the East German scandal. John Leonard of the World Swimming Coaches Association couched his criticism in terms of the IOC fixation on its image and money:

> *The reason the IOC needs to be cautious about this [i.e., the East German program] is because this has nothing whatsoever to do with sports. It has everything to do with the IOC's business relationships with its sponsors . . . once you start to pull on the thread of this, the entire garment of the Olympic fabric begins to come apart. . . . And what you begin to realize is the IOC itself has nothing to do with sport. It has to do with raising money and putting money in the IOC's coffers and the relationships it has with its major sponsors.*
>
> *The evidence has been there since 1989. . . . The IOC doesn't want to act on this because they don't want the full extent of doping activities revealed (Nightline, 1998).*

In addition, it is reasonable to conclude that similar organized sport doping programs existed in the Soviet Union and other Soviet-bloc countries (Gilmour, 1998; Hoberman, 1992a; Rosellini, 1992; Voy, 1991). As early as 1945, evidence exists from a Soviet government document that there were formal discussions regarding the viability of doping in sport (i.e., the use of stimulants) (Gilmour, 1998). The document shows a significant range of opinions on the matter, both pro and con. The conclusions reached in these discussions were the following: stimulants were already being used in sport, athletic trainers and coaches were involved, more research was needed to assess their effects, and variations in reaction to the drugs did not justify the risks *at that time* (Gilmour, 1998). This latter judgement may well have been reassessed when in 1948 Soviet sport established a goal of meeting or exceeding all world records. Regardless, by 1954 it appears that the Soviets employed systematic use of testosterone with their weightlifters, and thereafter use spread to other sports (Starr, 1981; Todd, 1987). While Edelman (1993) states that it is unlikely that the Soviet program was as well organized or systematic as it was in the GDR (Edelman, 1993), he nevertheless concludes that

> *officials, team doctors, and pharmacologists made drugs available to coaches who were under enormous pressure from the Party to produce winners. Facilities and assistance, especially pre-emptive testing, were provided to insure athletes could escape both detection and death (Kidd, Edelman, & Brownell, 1998).*

After the fall of communism in Europe in the late 1980s, many East German coaches sought employment elsewhere, and a number of these coaches began working in Communist China's sport programs (Fish, 1994; Hersh, 1993a; Whitten, 1994). The Chinese even established the National Research Institute, a high-performance sport science laboratory uncomfortably similar to the GDR's Research Institute for Physical Culture and Sports in Leipzig (Hoberman & Todd, 1992). Shortly thereafter, Chinese female athletes moved from a position of relative obscurity to world dominance, especially in swimming, track and field, and weightlifting. Almost immediately, accusations of doping and comparisons with the GDR spewed forth (Fish, 1993; Hersh, 1993a,b; Montville, 1994; Moore, 1993; Patrick, 1993; "Chinese Swimmers," 1994; Whitten, 1994). These accusations were supported in part by the large number of positive drug tests the Chinese experienced during this decade, including 29 track-and-field athletes and 19 swimmers (Allen, 1998). While at this time there is no compelling evidence of a centrally controlled system of drug use in China (Kidd, Edelman, & Brownell, 1998), as was the case with the GDR, there is little doubt that well-organized, systematic sports doping has taken place at the provincial level, at the very least.

Professional Football

Not long after word of the effectiveness of anabolic steroids disseminated among weightlifters and throwers in the early 1960s, football players began to incorporate these drugs into their training regimens. In 1963 the San Diego Chargers hired Alvin Roy, a Baton Rouge gym owner, as the first strength coach in professional football. Roy, previously an assistant coach for the U.S. Olympic weightlifting team, was probably already familiar with anabolic steroids, and it is alleged that he introduced the

San Diego players to Dianabol (Gilbert, 1969a–c; Mix, 1987). Some of the former Chargers say that they were not informed that the "little pink pills" placed next to their plates at the training table were anabolic steroids, and they add that there was a clear implication that players who refused to take the pills would be fined (Scott, 1971). Several years later, Roy left the Chargers to become the strength coach of the Kansas City Chiefs, who were known for their massive offensive and defensive lines during their heyday in the late 1960s. According to the accounts of physicians and players, members of the Kansas City Chiefs, Atlanta Falcons, and Cleveland Browns used anabolic steroids during the 1960s (Gilbert, 1969a–c). It is fair to assume that trades, coaching changes, and word-of-mouth interaction among football players and other strength athletes further facilitated the diffusion of steroid use in the National Football League (NFL).

From the mid-1970s to the early 1980s the Pittsburgh Steelers were said to possess one of the most sophisticated strength programs in pro football and one of the most physical styles of play. More importantly, the Steelers were a dominant force in the NFL during this period as well as in the NFL's Strongest Man competitions (1980–1982). Some of the athletes who contributed to this success used anabolic steroids (Courson, 1988, 1991). One cannot discount that this had an effect on the further spread of steroid use in the league, where strength and power are highly valued.

The testimony of former players supports the charge that steroid use escalated in the NFL from the late 1970s onward. Pat Donovan, a Dallas Cowboys offensive lineman for 9 years who retired in 1983, said, "Anabolic steroids are very, very accepted in the NFL. In my last five or six years it ran as high as 60–70% on the Cowboys on the offensive and defensive lines" (Johnson, 1985, p. 43). In the same article, the Buffalo Bills' Fred Smerlas said he thought that 40% of the players in the NFL use anabolic steroids. "On some teams between 75–90% of all athletes use steroids," said former Los Angeles Raider defensive lineman Lyle Alzado (p. 43). Other NFL players estimate steroid use as high as 90% (Johnson, 1985).

Joe Klecko, former New York Jets defensive lineman, said that anabolic steroids were commonplace in the late 1970s. Klecko stated, "I would guess between 65% and 75% were using AS in 1987" (Klecko & Fields, 1989). Klecko added, "I used AS when I wanted to be bear strong for the three NFL ('Strongest Man in Football') contests I entered in the off-season 1979–1981."

In a 1986 article in *Sports Illustrated* (Zimmerman, 1986), Los Angeles Raider defensive end Howie Long estimated the level of steroid use in the NFL: "At least 50% of the big guys. The offensive lines 75%, defensive line 40%, plus 35% of the linebackers. I don't know about the speed positions, but I've heard that they're used there too" (p. 18). From the same article, "Anabolic steroids are the worst problem in the NFL," said Indianapolis linebacker Johnny Cookes (p. 18).

Steve Courson (1988), who played for the Pittsburgh Steelers and Tampa Bay Buccaneers from 1977 to 1985, stated, "My educated guess is that 50% of the linemen use steroids." While testifying before the U.S. Senate Judiciary Committee in 1989, the Atlanta Falcon's All-Pro lineman Bill Fralic described steroid use in the NFL as rampant: "I would say that the guys I play against—that is, excluding the quarterbacks, and defensive backs and wide receivers, it is probably about 75%" (Fralic, 1989).

In 1991, prior to his death, NFL All-Pro lineman Lyle Alzado (1991) charged that NFL officials have known about extensive use of anabolic steroids by the players but have chosen to ignore it. He said that he used drugs during his entire career in the NFL, which spanned nearly two decades. Alzado also said he believed the teams' coaches knew that he and others were taking drugs, but they "just coached and looked the other way" (Alzado, 1991, p. 27). One of Alzado's coaches admitted that he knew about Alzado's drug use. "When I was coaching him, I was aware that he was using steroids," former Oakland Raiders coach Tom Flores told Steve Kelley of the *Seattle Times* (Kelley, 1991).

The current drug advisor to the NFL, Dr. John Lombardo, has stated that, "In the late '70s and the '80s, use of steroids was unbridled, uncontrolled. . . . People felt they had to take them to compete" (Miller, 1996). The precise level of steroid use in the NFL during the 1970s and 1980s probably will never be known, but it appears that steroid use was quite substantial. Unfortunately, the question of performance-enhancing drug use in the NFL persists in the 1990s. Continued speculation of epidemic levels of drug use has been fueled further by the dramatic increase in the size of NFL players, from quarterbacks to offensive linemen (Keteyian, 1998). In 1987 only 27 NFL players weighed more than 300 pounds, while in 1997 there were approximately 240 players over 300 pounds (Noonan, 1997). Some argue that the size increase is a consequence of high-calorie diets and food supplements such as creatine (Noonan, 1997), while others point their finger at anabolic steroids and human growth hormone (hGH) as the cause (Bamberger & Yaeger, 1997; Keteyian, 1998).

NFL officials counter that its year-round, random drug testing program has limited steroid use to a few marginal players (Noonan, 1997). However, the very integrity of the NFL drug testing program has been brought into question. Accusations have been made of covering up positive tests of star players, allowing players to "come back tomorrow" to give their urine sample, or allowing someone else to give "your" sample (Almond, 1993, 1995; "Dangers of Steroids," 1991): if true, all of these are flagrant violations of accepted testing policies. Even more disturbing is the revelation of Eric Moore, an offensive lineman for the New York Giants who was arrested in 1993 for possession of anabolic steroids with intent to deliver. During his interrogation by a Drug Enforcement Administration (DEA) agent,

> *Moore told the agent that he was usually given advance warning of any test, the centerpiece of the NFL's drug program. Moore said he was allowed to enter the testing room alone and that he kept a clean vial of urine in his jock strap to substitute for his own specimen (Almond, 1995).*

All this is consistent with the comments of Dr. Forrest Tennant, the former NFL drug advisor:

> *When I was dealing with cocaine, marijuana, and alcohol, no problem. Everybody supported cleaning that problem up. But when we decided to move into dealing with steroids, that is when you found out how many people around the league knew they worked, knew they wanted to see certain players keep taking them, and you would run into those pockets of resistance ("Now It Can Be Told," 1992).*

The potential problems with the integrity of the testing program, combined with the fact that there is no effective test for hGH and that the tests for testosterone can be circumvented (see chapter 13), argue that performance-enhancing drug use remains a significant and widespread problem in the NFL.

College

Although the National Collegiate Athletic Association (NCAA) outlawed in principle the use of anabolic steroids in 1973, it was not until 1986 that a testing program was initiated—10 years after the International Olympic Committee (IOC) began testing for these drugs (see chapter 12).

The diffusion of steroid use in college football was undoubtedly delayed by the perceptions that many coaches held during the 1950s and 1960s that increased muscle mass and basic strength conditioning did not afford an advantage; some coaches persisted in this thinking even in the early 1970s. Soon after, however, coaches appeared to dismiss the "muscle bound" theory, and elaborate weight-training facilities and professional strength coaches became an integral part of college football.

Jim Calkins, the co-captain of the 1969 University of California football team, claimed that he was given anabolic steroids by the team physician in order to gain weight to play tight end (Scott, 1971). Steve Courson (1988), during his playing days at the University of South Carolina, was prescribed Dianabol by the team physician in 1974. During the 1980s, football players at Stanford, the University of Oklahoma, North Dakota State University, Salisbury State, the University of Nevada-Reno, Georgia Southern College, the University of Southern California, the University of Tennessee, Louisiana State University, the University of Pittsburgh, Northwestern University, the University of Texas, the University of Minnesota, and Vanderbilt were all involved in steroid use (Huffman, 1990; "Player Claims," 1985; Wadler & Hainline, 1989; Yaeger & Looney, 1993). Furthermore, two of the most famous schools in college football, the University of Nebraska and Notre Dame, have been implicated in widespread steroid use (Keteyian, 1987; Yaeger & Looney, 1993).

The University of Nebraska has been at the cutting edge in strength training at the collegiate or professional levels for over three decades. Unfortunately, "no school has a bigger reputation for clandestine steroid involvement than the University of Nebraska" (Yaeger & Looney, 1993). The program placed a great deal of emphasis on strength, speed, and power. "Nebraska at times resembled less of a football team and more of a powerlifting club . . . the powerlifting mind-set that eventually permeated the squad—that led Nebraska players closer and closer to the S-word. Not strength . . . but steroids" (Keteyian, 1987).

One of the largest criminal investigations into steroid trafficking in the United States touched Lincoln, Nebraska. According to the U.S. Attorney's Office in San Diego, where the case was prosecuted, the investigation led to the conviction of Tony Fitton, whom the Feds considered the "kingpin" of steroids in the 1980s. Fitton admitted supplying Nebraska players with steroids (Yaeger & Looney, 1993).

In another report, a former drug dealer described steroid use at Nebraska as "massive," and estimated use on the 1983 and 1984 teams as high as 85% (Keteyian, 1987). Additional evidence of rampant steroid use derives from a number of journalistic investigations implicating such Cornhusker greats as Dean Steinkuhler, Dave Remington, Danny Noonan, Neil Smith, and Lawrence Pete, who have admitted using steroids while at Nebraska (Keteyian, 1987; Yaeger & Looney, 1993).

Regarding steroid use at Notre Dame, Yaeger and Looney (1993) concluded the following:

First Lou Holtz arrived at Notre Dame. Then a lot of steroids did. The connection is inescapable. It also has been devastating. The football team quickly became awash in anabolic steroids, starting in 1986.

The authors also showed a Nebraska "connection," in that Holtz, on his arrival, hired as his strength coach Scott Raridon, who was a starting offensive guard for Nebraska in 1983.

Based on the results of an anonymous survey of Division I–III athletes, sponsored by the NCAA in 1989, one could expect that on a team with 100 football players, on average 10 (i.e., 10%) would have used steroids in the prior 12 months (Anderson et al., 1991). A more recent survey of NCAA intercollegiate athletes shows that steroid use is on the decline in football (i.e., down to 2%) as well as in other sports ("Survey Shows," 1997). As in the case of professional football, the purported decrease in steroid use among college football players is not consistent with the significant increases in the size of players and a drug-testing program full of loopholes. Moreover, the validity of anonymous surveys of any group of elite athletes has to be carefully scrutinized, because admitting to steroid use poses a potential threat to the athlete's scholarship and future livelihood. In addition, the fear of guilt by association and its potential to adversely affect the athlete's place in sport history may result in a hesitancy to volunteer or be truthful. (For more information on the validity of surveys of drug use, see chapter 3.)

In addition to football, other collegiate men's sports have been linked with anabolic steroid use: these include track and field, baseball, basketball, gymnastics, lacrosse, swimming, volleyball, wrestling, soccer, and tennis (Anderson et al., 1991; "Survey Shows," 1997; Yesalis et al., 1990; see chapter 3).

High School

Use of anabolic steroids by high school athletes is rumored to have begun as early as 1959 when a physician in Texas allegedly administered Dianabol to a high school football team for an entire season (Morris, personal communication, 1989). As part of a clandestine "research" program in the early 1960s, a high school football team was reportedly given steroids by a team physician working in cooperation with a pharmaceutical company (Gilbert, 1969b). In 1965, a physician in Bloomington, California, oversaw a study in which three different commercial brands of anabolic steroids were administered to 10th- and 11th-grade football players (Gilbert, 1969b). Prior to 1972, some high school coaches in Alabama were rumored to have advised football players to take Dianabol to help them gain weight (Wade, 1972). By the late 1980s anabolic steroid use had been reported in high school baseball, basketball, track and field, and wrestling (Buckley, Yesalis, Friedl, Anderson, Streit, & Wright, 1988). The spread of steroid use to adolescents likely has involved a variety of paths over the past four decades, including interactions with older athletes, coaches, physicians, and even parents. For further information on the use of anabolic steroids by adolescents, refer to chapters 3 and 4.

Other Sports

Due to the competitive nature of our culture and, in some instances, lucrative financial rewards, anabolic steroid use has diffused to a variety of other sports and activities. For example, there appears to be an eerie parallel between the spread of anabolic steroids in various types of horse racing and their use in human athletics (Cotolo, 1992). As in human athletics, rumors and accusations abound that performance-enhancing drug use is epidemic in horse racing, while others say the problem is overstated; some say drug testing is behind the times and refer to "designer" drugs, while others argue that testing is working; some critics say a get-tough-on-cheaters policy is long overdue, while others propose that drug use should be allowed, but in a controlled fashion; and some veterinarians even argue that anabolic steroids really do not confer a competitive advantage (Cotolo, 1992).

As with football players, the size and strength of professional baseball players appears to have increased markedly over the past decade. As a consequence, suspicions of anabolic steroid use have arisen. In 1995, Randy Smith, general manager of the San Diego Padres stated, "We all know there's steroid use, and it's definitely become more prevalent." Smith estimated the prevalence of use at 10–20% of players, while an anonymous American League general manager said, "I wouldn't be surprised if it's closer to 30%" (Nightengale, 1995). In 1998, an anonymous American League front-office executive stated:

> *It (anabolic steroid use) is absolutely rampant right now.... Steroids have completely changed the game. Guys try to cover it up by saying they're using creatine (a muscle enhancer). Or they're just lifting weights now. Come on. It's a completely different look. I can pick out a kid using creatine from a kid on 'roids (Rosenthal).*

Other sports and activities now under the shadow of anabolic steroid use include rugby, professional wrestling, Paralympics, and even pigeon racing ("Hulkster Admits," 1994; O'Brien, 1993; Reuter, 1995; Struman, 1992; "Briefly," 1992).

Conclusions

Although it has taken five decades, there now appears to be a consensus among various interest groups—including athletes, physicians, coaches, administrators, and spectators—that performance-enhancing drug use in most sports, in particular anabolic steroid use, is a serious and growing problem. Several national meetings and a variety of books and reports have been devoted exclusively to this issue (Dubin, 1990; Haislip, 1994; Lin & Erinoff, 1990; National Steroid Consensus Meeting, 1989; Voy, 1990; Yesalis & Cowart, 1998).

As with many problems that are long-standing and vexing, society seeks not only solutions but also someone or something to blame. Most if not all the blame to date has been laid at the feet of the athlete by politicians, the press, sport federations, and the medical community.

In this regard, when we review the history of anabolic steroid use in sport and exercise, a number of ironies present themselves. Not only did the medical community develop these drugs, but it played a role early on in "selling" this potential fountain of youth. It was a physician and some officials and supporters of the U.S. weightlifting team who initiated use of the drugs in this country. It was government scientists and sport federation officials who institutionalized use in Eastern European Communist bloc countries. In a number of instances it was physicians and/or coaching staffs at the professional, collegiate, or high school levels who provided, facilitated, or encouraged the use of steroids. It was physicians who, until at least the late 1980s, served as the primary source of these drugs for over one-third of the steroid users in this country (Scott, 1971; Yesalis et al., 1990). It was, and is, a number of sport federations that for decades have covered up this problem, conveniently looked the other way, or instituted drug-testing programs that were designed to fail (Dubin, 1990; Franke & Berendonk, 1997; Voy, 1990; Yesalis & Cowart, 1998). It was, and is, our society that emphasizes and rewards speed, strength, size, aggression, and, above all, winning.

References

Allen, K. (1998, June 4). China's road to success hits its share of hurdles. *USA Today,* p. 5E.

Almond, E. (1993, January 29). TV report in 1990 zeroed in on drugs. *Los Angeles Times,* p. 8c.

Almond, E. (1995, January 23). Drug testing in NFL under a microscope; pro football: Health officials, former players question efforts to detect steroids as athletes continue to get bigger, stronger. *Los Angeles Times,* p. 1c.

Alzado, L. (1991, July 8). I'm sick and I'm scared. *Sports Illustrated,* 20–27.

Anderson, W.A., Albrecht, M.A., McKeag, D.B., Hough, D.O., & McGrew, C.A. (1991). A national survey of alcohol and drug use by college athletes. *The Physician and Sportsmedicine, 19*(2), 91–104.

Athletes live with steroids' toll. (1997, October 5). *Des Moines Sunday Register,* p. 12a.

Bamberger, M., & Yaeger, D. (1997, April 14). Over the edge. *Sports Illustrated, 86*(15), 60–70.

Ban for steroid user. (1995, June 25). *New York Times,* pp. 14, 10s.

Bøje, O. (1939). Doping. *Bulletin of the Health Organization of the League of Nations, 8,* 439–469.

Briefly. (1992, September 9). *USA Today,* p. 2c.

Brown, J., & Tait, G. (1973). Anabolic steroids—the views of users. *Track Techniques, 54,* 1713–1716.

Buckley, W., Yesalis, C., Friedl, K., Anderson, W., Streit, A., & Wright, J. (1988). Estimated prevalence of anabolic steroid use among male high school seniors. *Journal of the American Medical Association, 260,* 3441–3445.

Butenandt, A., & Hanisch, G. (1935). Über Testosteron Umwandlung des Dehydroandrosterons in Androstenediol und Testosteron; ein Weg zur Darstellung des Testosteron aus Cholesterin [Concerning testosterone conversion of dehydroandrosterone in androstenediol and testosterone: A way to the production of testosterone out of cholesterin]. *Zeitschrift Physiologische Chemie, 237,* 89–97.

Chinese swimmers, lifters dominate. (1994, October 5). *USA Today,* p. 9c.

Cotolo, F. (1992). Better racing through chemistry. *Times: In harness*. (Eight-part series) February 8, 22, March 7, 21, April 4, 18, May 2, 16.

Courson, S. (1988, November 14). Steroids: A different perspective. *Sports Illustrated,* 106.

Courson, S. (1991). *False glory.* Stamford, CT: Longmeadow Press.

The dangers of steroids are becoming more apparent. (1991, July 22). *Sports Illustrated,* 10.

David, K., Dingemanse, E., Freud, J., & Laqueur, E. (1935). Über krystallinisches männliches Hormon aus Hoden (Testosteron) wirksamer als aus Harn oder aus Cholesterin bereitetes Androsteron [Crystalline male hormone from testes (testosterone) more active than androsterone preparations from urine or cholesterol]. *Zeitschrift Physiologische Chemie, 233,* 281–293.

de Kruif, P. (1945). *The male hormone.* Orlando, FL: Harcourt, Brace, & Co.

Drugs detected. (1995, March 21). *USA Today,* p. 2c.

Dubin, C. (1990). Commission of inquiry into the use of drugs and banned practices intended to increase athletic performance (Catalogue No. CP32-56/1990E, ISBN 0-660-13610-4). Ottawa, ON: Canadian Government Publishing Center.

Duchaine, D. (1982). *Underground steroid handbook.* Santa Monica, CA: OEM.

Duchaine, D. (1989). *Underground steroid handbook II.* Venice, CA: HLR Technical Books.

East German says he gave out steroids. (1998, July 7). *USA Today,* p. 3c.

Edelman, R. (1993). *Serious fun: A history of spectator sports in the USSR.* New York: Oxford University Press.

Fair, J. (1988). Olympic weightlifting and the introduction of steroids: A statistical analysis of world championship results, 1948–72. *International Journal of the History of Sport, 5,* 96–114.

Fair, J. (1993). Isometrics or steroids? Exploring new frontiers of strength in the early 1960s. *Journal of Sport History, 20,* 1–24.

Fish, M. (1993, September 29). Experts suspect "a whole country" may be cheating. *The Atlanta Journal/The Atlanta Constitution,* p. E3.

Fish, M. (1994, April 17). China's Olympic obsession. *The Atlanta Journal/The Atlanta Constitution,* pp. A1, A8–9.

Fralic, W. (1989, April 3, May 9). Testimony before U.S. Senate, Committee on the Judiciary. *Hearings on steroids in amateur and professional sports—the medical and social costs of steroid abuse.* 101st Congress, 1st sess.

Francis, C. (1990). *Speed trap.* New York: St. Martin's Press.

Franke, W., & Berendonk, B. (1997). Hormonal doping and androgenization of athletes: A secret program of the German Democratic Republic government. *Clinical Chemistry, 43,* 1262–1279.

Fussell, S.W. (1990). *Muscle: Confessions of an unlikely bodybuilder.* New York: Poseidon Press.

Gilbert, B. (1969a, June 23). Drugs in sport: Part 1. Problems in a turned-on world. *Sports Illustrated,* 64–72.

Gilbert, B. (1969b, June 30). Drugs in sport: Part 2. Something extra on the ball. *Sports Illustrated,* 30–42.

Gilbert, B. (1969c, July 7). Drugs in sport: Part 3. High time to make some rules. *Sports Illustrated,* 30–35.

Gilmour, J. (1998, April 24–25). *Response to "A comparative analysis of doping scandals: Canada, Russia, and China" by Kidd, Brownell, and Edelman.* Paper presented at Doping in Elite Sport Conference, Amateur Athletic Foundation of Los Angeles.

Haislip, G.R. (1994). *Conference Report: International Conference on the Abuse and Trafficking of Anabolic Steroids.* Washington, DC: U.S. Drug Enforcement Administration, Office of Diversion Control.

Hearings before the Subcommittee to Investigate Juvenile Delinquency of the Committee on the Judiciary, U.S. Senate, 93rd Cong., 1st Sess.. (1973, June 18, July 12, 13) (testimony of H. Connolly).

Hearings on steroids in amateur and professional sports—the medical and social costs of steroid abuse before the Committee on the Judiciary, U.S. Senate, 101st Cong., 1st Sess. (1989, April 3 and May 9) (testimony of P. Connolly).

Hendershott, J. (1969). Steroids: Breakfast of champions. *Track and Field News, 22*(3).

Hersh, P. (1993a, November 16). China's swimming success raises specter of East Germany. *Chicago Tribune,* sec. 4, p. 4.

Hersh, P. (1993b, August 26). Too far, too fast. *Chicago Tribune,* pp. 1, 6.

Hoberman, J. (1992a). *Mortal engines*. New York: Free Press.

Hoberman, J. (1992b). The early development of sports medicine in Germany. In J.W. Berryman & R.J. Park (Eds.), *Sport and exercise science: Essays in the history of sports medicine.* Champaign: University of Illinois Press.

Hoberman, J., & Todd, T. (1992, June 7). Chinese regime is hiding atrocities behind a facade of athletic utopia. *Austin American-Statesman,* p. E16.

Huffman, S. (1990, August 27). I deserve my turn. *Sports Illustrated,* 26–31.

Hulkster admits to steroid use. (1994, July 15). *Chicago Sun-Times,* p. 109.

Johnson, W. (1985, May 13). Steroids: A problem of huge dimensions. *Sports Illustrated,* 38–61.

Johnston, R. (1974, October 14). The men and the myth. *Sports Illustrated,* 106–120.

Kearns, B., Harkness, R., Hobson, V., & Smith, A. (1942). Testosterone pellet implantation in the gelding. *Journal of the American Veterinary Medicine Association, C/780,* 197–201.

Kelley, S. (1991, July 10). This chapter of Alzado's story is sad. *Seattle Times.*

Kenyon, A., Knowlton, K., Sandiford, I., Koch, F., & Lotwin, G. (1940). A comparative study of the metabolic effects of testosterone propionate in normal men and women and in eunuchoidism. *Endocrinology, 26,* 26–45.

Kenyon, A., Sandiford, I., Bryan, A., Knowlton, K., & Koch, F. (1938). The effect of testosterone propionate on nitrogen, electrolyte, water and energy metabolism in eunuchoidism. *Endocrinology, 23,* 135–153.

Keteyian, A. (1987, January 5). A former husker fesses up. *Sports Illustrated,* 24.

Keteyian, A. (1998, August) Mass deception: Today's athlete is getting bigger, stronger, faster . . . unnaturally. *Sport,* 38–39.

Kidd, B., Edelman, R., & Brownell, S. (1998, April 24–25). *A comparative analysis of doping scandals: Russia, Canada, China.* Paper presented at Doping in Elite Sport Conference, Amateur Athletic Foundation of Los Angeles.

Klecko, J., & Fields, J. (1989). *Nose to nose: Survival in the trenches in the NFL.* New York: Morrow.

Klein, A. (1986). Pumping irony: Crisis and contradiction in bodybuilding. *Sociology of Sport Journal, 3,* 112–133.

Klein, A. (1993). Of muscles and men. *The Sciences, 33,* 32–37.

Kochakian, C. (Ed.). (1976). *Anabolic-androgenic steroids.* New York: Springer-Verlag.

Kochakian, C., & Murlin, J. (1935). The effect of male hormone on the protein and energy metabolism of castrate dogs. *Journal of Nutrition, 10,* 437–459.

Kruskemper, H. (1968). *Anabolic steroids.* New York: Academic Press.

Leigh, W. (1990). *Arnold: The unauthorized biography.* New York: Congdon-Weed.

Lifetime drug ban. (1998, April 8). *USA Today,* p. 3c.

Lin, G., & Erinoff, L. (Eds.). (1990). *Anabolic steroid abuse* (National Institute on Drug Abuse Research, Monograph 102, DHHS publication number ADM 90-1720). Rockville, MD: U.S. Department of Health and Human Services, Public Health Service.

Miller, A. (1996, May 3). Reports of steroid use down, but abuse not over, some say. *The Atlanta Journal/The Atlanta Constitution,* p. G4.

Mix, R. (1987, October 19). So little gain for the pain. *Sports Illustrated.*

Montville, L. (1994, September 19). Flora and furor. *Sports Illustrated,* 40–42.

Moore, K. (1993, September 27). Great wall of doubt. *Sports Illustrated,* 20–21.

Nack, W. (1998, May 18). The muscle murders. *Sports Illustrated,* 86–106.

National Steroid Consensus Meeting. (1989, July 30–31). Sponsored by the United States Olympic Committee, the National Collegiate Athletic Association, the National Federation of State High School Associations and the Amateur Athletic Foundation, Los Angeles.

Nightengale, B. (1995, July 15). Many fear performance-enhancing drug is becoming prevalent and believe something must be done. *Los Angeles Times,* p. 1c.

Nightline, ABC News. (1998, July 6). Cheating at the Olympics: Should history be rewritten?

Noden, M. (1993, March 15). Shot down. *Sports Illustrated.*

Noonan, D. (1997, December 14). Really big football players. *New York Times Magazine,* pp. 64–69.

Now it can be told. (1992, January 22). Burrelle's Info Services.

O'Brien, R. (1993, December 13). Grappling with decline. *Sports Illustrated.*

Out of action. (1997, April 29). *USA Today,* p. 1c.

Patrick, D. (1993, September 16). Sudden burst encourages drug rumors. *USA Today,* pp. 1–2c.

Patrick, D. (1997, October 24). Breaking the standards. *USA Today,* p. 3c.

Payne, A.H. (1975). Anabolic steroids in athletics. *British Journal of Sports Medicine, 9,* 83–88.

Phillips, W. (1990). *Anabolic reference guide* (5th ed.). Golden, CO: Mile High.

Player claims druggist used Vandy weight room. (1985, January 13 and 23). *Tampa Bay Tribune.*

Rosellini, L. (1992, February 17). The sports factories. *U.S. News & World Report,* 48–59.

Rosenthal, K. (1998). Steroids: Baseball's darkest secret. *MSNBC on the Internet.*

Rugby: Three players fail World Cup drug test. (1995, October 12). London: Reuter.

Scott, J. (1971, October 17). It's not how you play the game, but what pill you take. *New York Times Magazine.*

Simonson, E., Kearns, W., & Enzer, N. (1941). Effect of oral administration of methyltestosterone on fatigue in eunuchoids and castrates. *Endocrinology, 28,* 506–512.

Simonson, E., Kearns, W., & Enzer, N. (1944). Effect of methyltestosterone treatment on muscular performance and the central nervous system of older men. *Journal of Clinical Endocrinology and Metabolism, 4,* 528–534.

Starr, B. (1981). *Defying gravity: How to win at weightlifting.* Wichita Falls, TX: Five Starr Productions.

Steroid information given to athletes. (1984, July 2). *Tampa Bay Tribune.*

Struman, M. (1992, December 17). Bulky pigeons face drug-testing. *USA Today,* p. 2c.

Survey shows steroid use on the decline. (1997, September 15). *NCAA News,* 1.

Todd, T. (1987). Anabolic steroids: The gremlins of sport. *Journal of Sport History, 14,* 87–107.

Voy, R. (1991). *Drugs, sport, and politics.* Champaign, IL: Leisure Press.

Wade, N. (1972). Anabolic steroids: Doctors denounce them, but athletes aren't listening. *Science, 176,* 1399–1403.

Wadler, G., & Hainline, B. (1989). *Drugs and the athlete.* Philadelphia: Davis.

We'll take it. (1997, October 1). *USA Today,* p. 3c.

Whitten, P. (1994). China's short march to swimming dominance: Hard work or drugs? *Swimming World and Junior Swimmer,* 34–39.

Williams, D. (1989, April 3, May 9). Testimony before U.S. Senate, Committee on the Judiciary. *Hearings on steroids in amateur and professional sports—the medical and social costs of steroid abuse.* 101st Congress, 1st sess.

Wright, J. (1978). *Anabolic steroids and sports.* Natick, MA: Sports Science Consultants.

Yaeger, D., & Looney, D. (1993). *Under the tarnished dome: How Notre Dame betrayed its ideals for football glory.* New York: Simon & Schuster.

Yesalis, C., Anderson, W., Buckley, W., & Wright, J. (1990). Incidence of the nonmedical use of anabolic-androgenic steroids. In G. Lin & L. Erinoff (Eds.), *Anabolic steroid abuse* (National Institute on Drug Abuse Research, Monograph 102, DHHS Publication No. ADM 90-1720). Rockville, MD: U.S. Department of Health and Human Services, Public Health Service.

Yesalis, C., & Cowart, V. (1998). *The steroids game.* Champaign, IL: Human Kinetics.

Zimmerman, P. (1986, November 10). The agony must end. *Sports Illustrated,* 17–21.

CHAPTER

3

Incidence of Anabolic Steroid Use: A Discussion of Methodological Issues

Charles E. Yesalis, ScD; Michael S. Bahrke, PhD;
Andrea N. Kopstein, PhD;
and Camille K. Barsukiewicz, PhD

A lot of guys won't talk about their steroid use. They won't even tell their wives. I'm talking about it because I don't want to be hypocritical, because I believe in telling the truth.

Steve Courson
Pittsburgh Steelers, 1977–1983
Tampa Bay Buccaneers, 1984–1985
Sports Illustrated, May 13, 1985

Portions of this chapter are reprinted from *Clinical Sports Medicine* 1990; see credits page for more information.

Our concern over drug use in sport and exercise is generally founded in one or more of the following moral and ethical issues: (1) The athlete may suffer physical or psychological harm as a result of drug use; (2) the use of drugs by one athlete may coerce other athletes to use drugs to maintain parity; (3) the use of drugs in sport is unnatural in that any resulting success is due to external factors; and (4) the athlete who uses drugs has an unfair advantage over athletes who do not use them (see introduction). Given these concerns, it is important to be able to accurately assess the magnitude of drug use in sport. If we underestimate drug use (i.e., false negatives), the above-stated concerns will likely, at least in part, be realized. If we overestimate drug use (i.e., false positives), we could wrongly affect the reputations of individuals, teams, or even nations.

Until the mid-1970s, all that was known regarding the incidence of performance-enhancing drug use in sport was based on anecdotes, testimonials, and rumors reported by journalists and others (Gilbert, 1969a–c; Scott, 1971; Wade, 1972; Wright, 1978). High levels of steroid use were reported in weightlifting, powerlifting, bodybuilding, professional football, and the throwing events in track and field; even use by high school athletes was reported as early as 1959 (Frazier, 1973; Gilbert, 1969a–c). Although investigative journalism is still a valuable source of information about the level of drug use in sport, other sources are available. These include government records and investigations, as well as the results of systematic surveys and of drug testing associated with athletic competition.

The purpose of this chapter is to discuss the difficulties faced in accurately estimating the prevalence of drug use among athletes by examining the four major methods generally employed in estimating usage: investigative journalism, government investigation, drug testing, and surveys. In addition, the results of surveys of anabolic steroid use among adolescents, collegiate, professional, and Olympic athletes will be presented, with particular attention given to the veracity of responses to survey questions.

Investigative Journalism

Journalists, using primarily the personal observations, accounts, or opinions of self-selected informants, both anonymous and attributed, have detailed during the past four decades a sustained epidemic of drug use in sport at the professional, Olympic, collegiate, and even high school levels (Bamberger &Yaeger, 1997; Fish, 1993a; Gilbert, 1969a–c; Janofsky, 1988; Johnson, 1985; Kelley, 1991; Keteyian, 1989; Litsky, 1993; Rosellini, 1992; Scott, 1971; Todd, 1983; Wade, 1972; Zimmerman, 1986). The writings and testimonials of former athletes and others in, or around, sport generally have confirmed that doping in sport is a serious and continuous problem (Alzado, 1991; Courson, 1991; Francis, 1990; Hoberman, 1992; Huizenga, 1994; Klecko & Fields, 1989; Mix, 1987; Voy, 1991).

While using investigative methods to assess the incidence of performance-enhancing drug use in sport is often less expensive and time consuming than the other methods, it is fraught with methodological limitations. Individuals who use or have used drugs and who serve as informants may project their behavior onto others in an attempt to rationalize their drug use—"Everybody does it" (see below). This may result in an overestimate of the level of drug use. Conversely, athletes, coaches, team physicians, and others may either refuse to cooperate with journalists or deny drug use not only to protect themselves but to protect their teammates, school, conference, or even the reputation of their sport. In fact, the Dubin Commission (1990, see below) refers to a "conspiracy of silence" and a "pact of ignorance" among those in sport when it comes to discussing drug use. Testimonials on drug use in sport are generally limited to former athletes, because current athletes fear possible retribution from coaches, teammates, or sport federation officials. Even former athletes could be reticent to discuss drug use because they could be ostracized by the news media, as well as by their fans and former teammates. In turn, this could affect their livelihood by, for example, adversely impacting paid speaking engagements, autograph signings, and induction into halls of fame. Each of these disincentives could result in an underestimate of drug use in sport.

Similarly, sport federation officials, when interviewed, most often have tended to deny that a major doping problem exists within sport, or have at least downplayed its magnitude ("ITF Disputes," 1994; "NFL," 1993; "Drug Testing," 1996). When pushed, sport officials frequently have stated, "we've had problems in the past, but now things are different" ("USOC Officials," 1995; "Drugs," 1992; "IOC Mum," 1998; Yesalis, 1996).

Another potential problem of investigative journalism is the scope of the investigation and its effect on the generalizability of the findings. Often, reports will focus on a few athletes, teams, or sports. Even if the findings are valid, they most likely cannot be legitimately generalized beyond the scope of the investigation.

Government Investigations

During the past three decades, the U.S. Congress has held several hearings on performance-enhancing drug use in sport (*Legislation to Amend,* 1988; *Anabolic Restriction Act,* 1989; *Abuse of Steroids,* 1990; *Hearings Before the Subcommittee,* 1973; *Hearings on Steroid Abuse,* 1989). During these hearings, current and former athletes, as well as some coaches and sport federation officials, with few exceptions, have supported the notion that there is a significant doping problem. However, from a methodological perspective, once again, the volunteered opinions and observations of a relatively small sample of individuals, selected in a nonrandom manner, have been used to estimate the extent of doping in a relatively small number of sports at various levels of competition.

Spawned by the Ben Johnson doping incident in the 1988 Seoul Olympic Games, the Dubin Commission (1990) in Canada investigated the extent of drug use in Olympic sport. While the proceedings employed a more aggressive legal format, including cross-examination of witnesses under oath, it fell well short of the adversarial format of a trial, and relied heavily on the veracity and recall of selected witnesses. Nevertheless, after 91 days of testimony from a parade of witnesses, the Commission concluded the following:

> *Unfortunately, the noble sentiments and lofty ideals proclaimed in the Olympic Charter are a far cry from the reality of international competition. This reality has not until recently been widely known, but the conspiracy of silence has now been broken and the truth revealed. Truth is not always pleasant.*

Franke and Berendonk's (1997) analysis of a large cache of captured Stasi files from the former German Democratic Republic (GDR) paints a chilling picture of sustained collusion among high level government, sports medicine, drug testing, sport federations, and GDR Olympic officials to systematically dope GDR athletes. Even though the face validity of these data is seemingly great, at least 15 of those "accused" by the authors of collaborating in this doping conspiracy have sought relief in the German courts (Franke, 1998). However, to date, all have lost. In fact, these Stasi files have served as primary evidence for a wide-scale criminal prosecution of the above-mentioned individuals ("Athletes Live," 1997; Franke, 1998; "Coaches Charged," 1997).

While the internal validity of Franke and Berendonk's conclusions appears quite strong, the external validity (generalizability) is brought into question in that all the data involve one, now defunct, country. Notwithstanding, the temptation to draw parallels with the sport systems of the former Soviet Union and current Communist China is great.

Drug Testing

During the past ten years, less than 3% of NCAA, Olympic, and NFL athletes who were tested were shown to be positive for banned substances

(Catlin & Murray, 1996; "Drug-Testing," 1998). The level of drug use implied by these test results is at great odds with most of the conclusions of investigations conducted by journalists and the government organizations discussed above. This is likely due to the fact that drug testing as a method of estimating the level of performance-enhancing drug use is seriously flawed, in that testing can often be circumvented by the user, increasing the probability of a false negative. In the case of drug testing only at competitive events, athletes usually can determine when to discontinue use of training drugs (such as anabolic steroids) prior to testing so as to allow the metabolites of the drugs to clear the body and, thus, avoid a positive test (Yesalis & Cowart, 1998; see chapter 13). When faced with unannounced, out-of-competition testing, the drug-using athlete has available a number of strategies to successfully circumvent the testing process (Longman, 1995; Yesalis, 1996; Yesalis & Cowart, 1998; see chapter 13). For example, the athlete can titrate his or her dose by using transdermal patches or skin creams containing testosterone, and, combined with the results of self-testing from private laboratories, remain below the maximum allowable testosterone/epitestosterone (T/E) ratio of 6:1 (Longman, 1995; Yesalis & Cowart, 1998; see chapter 13).

Another factor allowing drug-using athletes to escape detection is the lack of effective tests for certain performance-enhancing drugs. At present, there is no effective (i.e., confirmatory) test to detect the presence of exogenous human growth hormone (hGH), which is used by power, strength, and sprint athletes for its anabolic (muscle-building) effects. According to a *Sports Illustrated* investigative report on doping in sport (Bamberger & Yaeger, 1997), some athletes jokingly referred to the Atlanta Olympics as the "Growth Hormone Games." A related anabolic hormone, insulinlike growth factor (IGF-1), is also available to athletes, and as with hGH, there is no effective test for detecting its use. There is also no viable test as yet for erythropoietin (EPO), which is used by some athletes to increase their number of red blood cells, thus improving the oxygen-carrying capacity of their blood and ultimately their endurance performance (see chapter 13). Significant numbers of high school, collegiate, and Olympic athletes have probably used creatine, a substance found naturally in the body that has been demonstrated to enhance performance (Volek & Kraemer, 1996). Because it is a food supplement, it does not appear on the list of banned drugs. However, a person would need to eat more than 10 to 20 pounds of meat daily to equal the standard loading dose now being taken by athletes: easy for a tiger, tough for a human! Is creatine a performance-enhancing substance? The data would appear to indicate that it is.

Although the results of drug testing appear to significantly underestimate the level of use of steroids and other performance-enhancing drugs among athletes, these tests have documented steroid use by both men and women in a large variety of sports, from swimming to weightlifting (Dubin, 1990). For more information on drug testing, see chapters 12 and 13.

Surveys

The vast majority of survey research on the use of performance-enhancing drugs has focused on anabolic steroid use among adolescents. While there has been an ongoing series of cross-sectional surveys of drug use among NCAA athletes and a modest number of studies of bodybuilders, only a handful of surveys have explored this issue among professional and Olympic athletes.

Junior High and High School

Corder, Dezelsky, Toohey, and DiVito (1975) surveyed students in 10 Arizona high schools in 1971 and 1975 and found among the general student body a prior, or lifetime, anabolic steroid use rate of less than 1%; 4% of athletes in the 1975 survey reported previous use of anabolic steroids. The authors did not report their findings according to the subjects' gender. In a 1986 study of 8th, 10th, and 12th graders in 11 public school districts in Michigan, 3%, 2%, and 2% of students, respectively, reported previous steroid use, whereas 1% of respondents in each of the grades acknowledged use in the prior month (Newman, 1986). The lifetime anabolic steroid use rate among seniors was 5% for boys and 1% for girls.

Polen, Schnider, Sirotowitz, and West (1986) surveyed 200 randomly selected students at a Florida high school with an enrollment of 2,000; 18% of males (but no females) reported prior steroid use. Of 190 varsity football players in six high schools in Oregon, only 1.1% admitted steroid use (Bosworth, Bents, Trevisan, & Goldberg, 1987).

In 1987, the first nationwide study of anabolic steroid use at the high school level was conducted by Buckley, Yesalis, Friedl, Anderson, Streit, and Wright (1988), who found that 6.6% of male high school seniors reported having used these drugs. There was no difference in the levels of reported anabolic steroid use between urban and rural areas, but there was a small but significant difference by size of enrollment: Students at larger high schools had a higher rate of reported anabolic steroid use. Almost 40% of the anabolic steroid users reported five or more cycles of use. In addition, of the self-reported anabolic steroid users, 38% had initiated use before age 16, 44% used more than one steroid at a time (stacking), and 38% used injectable anabolic steroids. More than one-third of the anabolic steroid users did not intend to participate in interscholastic sports. Only 15% of the public and private high schools that participated in this study had no reported anabolic steroid use. However, in a survey of 472 head football coaches in Michigan high schools, only 12% admitted that they knew of at least one player who used anabolic steroids before 1988—or suspected as much (Duda, 1988).

State and Local Surveys

Table 3.1 summarizes basic methodological information for state and local surveys, most of which were conducted since 1990. Although specific methods used in each study differ, all studies employed cross-sectional designs and used self-administered questionnaires. Some surveys focused on steroid use, while other surveys included alcohol, cigarettes, and other drugs as well as steroids. Most questionnaires specified steroid use without a physician's prescription in order to differentiate steroids used for performance enhancement from those employed in prescribed medical treatment (e.g., for asthma). All surveys emphasized the confidential nature of responses to participating students. For some surveys, anonymity was enhanced by research team members administering the survey (as opposed to school personnel).

Current Trends

A number of local and statewide surveys have confirmed the findings of the study by Buckley and colleagues (1988), indicating that 3% to 12% of high school males admit to using steroids some time during their lives (Hubbell, 1990; Johnson, Jay, Shoup, & Rickert, 1989; Komoroski & Rickert, 1992; Krowchuk et al., 1989; Ringwalt 1989; Ross, Winters, Hartmann, Robb, & Dillemuth, 1989; Terney & McLain, 1990; Vaughan, Walter, & Gladis, 1991; Whitehead, Chillag, & Elliott, 1992; Windsor & Dumitru, 1989). Although these studies primarily involved males, some have examined the use of anabolic steroids among adolescent females, usually finding that 0.5% to 2% report having used steroids (Yesalis & Bahrke, 1995). More recent individual studies (table 3.2) provide evidence of continued steroid use despite legal regulation/restriction and educational interventions. However, between-study conclusions regarding changes in levels of steroid use are complicated by methodological issues such as differences in study populations and sampling techniques and survey designs. In addition, identifying specific reasons for any change in steroid use is confounded by the introduction at different times of state and federal regulations and varied educational interventions across localities. While still problematic, individual state- and national-level studies that measure anabolic steroid use at multiple points in time are more useful regarding trend analysis.

Single-Year State Studies

The data discussed in this section are presented in table 3.2. A 1991 study of 7th graders in Modesto, California, showed that 4.7% of males and 3.2% of females admitted using steroids (Radakovich, Broderick, & Pickell, 1993). A 1992–1993 survey at ten Denver high schools found the overall prevalence of anabolic steroids was 2.7%, with a rate of 4% for males and 1.3%

Table 3.1 Research Methods of State and Local Studies

References	Setting	Survey year	Participants/ response rate	Instrument features
Radakovich et al., 1993	Modesto, CA	1991	7th grade students. 810 respondents, 48% of those surveyed.	Questionnaire (based on others' research), steroids as main focus
Tanner et al., 1995	Denver, CO	1992–93	General student body. 6,930 respondents, 96.6% of those surveyed.	Questionnaire (based on Terney & McLain, 1990), steroids as main focus
Luetkemeier et al., 1995	Salt Lake City, UT	1995	General student body. 1,907 respondents, 87% of those surveyed.	Questionnaire (based on others' research), steroids as main focus
Stilger & Yesalis, 1999	Indiana, statewide	1993	Football players. 873 randomly selected respondents, no response rate reported.	Questionnaire (based on others' research), steroids as main focus
Ringwalt, 1989	North Carolina, statewide	1989	7th–12th graders, general student body. 11,531 respondents, no response rate reported.	Questionnaire (based on previous research), steroid use as part of alcohol and drug use study
North Carolina, 1991	North Carolina, statewide	1991	7th–12th graders, general student body. 10,848 respondents, 99.7% of those surveyed.	Questionnaire (same as 1989)
South Carolina, 1989–90	South Carolina, statewide	1989	7th–12th graders, general student body. 223,663 respondents, no response rate reported.	Questionnaire (modeled on similar national and state questionnaires), steroid use as part of alcohol and drug use study
South Carolina, 1992–93	South Carolina, statewide	1992	7th–12th graders, general student body. 232,304 respondents, no response rate reported.	Questionnaire (same as 1989)
Windsor & Dumitru, 1989	Texas, unnamed metropolitan area	1988	General student body. 901 respondents, 89% of those surveyed.	Questionnaire specific to steroid use

Texas, 1995	Texas, statewide	1990	7th–12th graders, general student body. Numbers of participants and response rate not reported.	Texas School Survey (extensively modified from a New York instrument), steroid use as part of alcohol and drug use study
Texas, 1995	Texas, statewide	1992	7th–12th graders, general student body. 73,073 respondents, no response rate reported.	Some questions added to 1990 survey
Texas, 1995	Texas, statewide	1994	7th–12th graders, general student body. 107,093 respondents, 85% of those surveyed.	Some questions and modifications to the 1992 survey
DuRant et al., 1993	Richmond County, Georgia	1990	9th graders. 1,881 respondents, 100% of those surveyed.	Questionnaire (modified version of CDC Secondary School Health Risk Survey and YRBSS), steroid use as part of general drug and alcohol use survey
DuRant, 1994	Richmond County, Georgia	1991	9th graders. 1,422 repondents, 100% of those surveyed.	Questionnaire (same as 1990)
Terney & McLain, 1990	Chicago, Illinois	1988	9th–12th graders, general student body. 2,113 respondents, 66% of those surveyed.	Questionnaire developed by authors, steroids as main focus
Gaa et al., 1994	Illinois, statewide	1991	9th and 12th graders, general student body. 3,047 respondents, 81% of those surveyed.	Questionnaire developed and tested by authors, steroids as main focus
Maryland, 1989	Maryland, statewide	1989	12th graders, general student body. 13,461 respondents, no response rate given.	Questionnaire (based on previous research), steroid use as part of alcohol and drug use study
Maryland, 1992	Maryland, statewide	1992	12th graders, general student body. 18,218 respondents, no response rate given.	Questionnaire (same as 1989)

Table 3.2 State and Local Studies of Anabolic Steroid Use by Adolescents

References	State study (study year)	Prevalence % males	Prevalence % females	Prevalence % overall
Radakovich et al., 1993	California (1991)	4.7	3.2	
Tanner et al., 1995	Colorado (1992–93)	4.0	1.3	2.7
Luetkemeier et al., 1995	Utah (1995)	4.0	1.4	3.3
Stilger & Yesalis, 1999	Indiana (1993)	6.3		
Ringwalt, 1989	North Carolina (1989)	3.2	0.5	1.9
North Carolina, 1991	North Carolina (1991)			1.6
South Carolina, 1994	South Carolina (1989–90)			2.8
South Carolina, 1994	South Carolina (1992–93)			1.6
Windsor & Dumitru, 1989	Texas (1988)	5.0	1.4	3.0
Texas, 1995	Texas (1992)	2.6	0.7	1.7
DuRant et al., 1993	Georgia (1990)	6.5	1.9	4.2
DuRant et al., 1994	Georgia (1991)	4.8	2.9	3.8
Terney & McLain, 1990	Illinois (1988)	6.5	2.5	4.4
Gaa et al., 1994	Illinois (1991)	3.0	1.0	1.9
Maryland, 1989	Maryland (1989)			3.1
Maryland, 1992	Maryland (1992)			1.9

for females (Tanner, Miller, & Alongi, 1995). A disturbing finding of this study was that 56% of those who acknowledged being steroid users cited their coaches, physicians, or parents as primary sources of these drugs.

A 1995 survey of 2,200 junior and senior high school students in Salt Lake City, Utah, showed an overall prevalence of anabolic steroid use of 3.3%, with a rate of 4% for males and 1.4% for females (Luetkemeier, Bainbridge, Walker, Brown, & Eisenman, 1995). The researchers found these results surprising because of the traditional conservatism generally exhibited by Utah citizens. Citizens of Utah usually rank high on issues of health awareness, and Utah high school seniors rank well below the national average in the use of other substances such as alcohol, tobacco, marijuana, and cocaine. Indiana high school football players were surveyed in 1993, and 6.3% were found to be current or former anabolic steroid users (Stilger & Yesalis, 1999).

Multi-Year State Studies

A 1989 survey of 7th through 12th grade students in North Carolina public schools revealed a lifetime steroid use rate of 1.9% (Ringwalt, 1989; table 3.2). Anabolic steroid use was reported by 3.2% of male students and 0.5% of females. A similar study was conducted in 1991 (North Carolina Department of Public Instruction, 1991) and revealed a lifetime prevalence rate of 1.6%, a drop of 16% since the time of the 1989 survey. A male/female breakdown of steroid use was not available for the 1991 study.

A study conducted in 1989 in South Carolina revealed that 2.8% of 7th through 12th grade students had used anabolic steroids at least once in their lives (South Carolina Department of Education and Commission on Alcohol and Drug Abuse, 1994). A similar study conducted in 1992 found a steroid use rate of 1.6% among 7th–12th grade students, a 43% decrease from the 1989 study.

A 1988 survey of high school students in one metropolitan area in Texas demonstrated an overall lifetime steroid use of 3% (5% in males and 1.4% in females) (Windsor & Dumitru, 1989). A 1995 report by the Texas Commission on Alcohol and Drug Abuse found a lifetime use rate of 1.7% (2.6–2.8% among males and 0.7–0.9% among females) in surveys administered consecutively in 1990 and 1992, and a 1.9% use rate (2.8% among males and 0.9% among females) in 1994 (Texas Commission on Alcohol and Drug Abuse, 1995).

DuRant, Rickert, Ashworth, Newman, and Slavens (1993) studied anabolic steroid use among participants in 9th grade health science classes in Richmond County, Georgia. The November 1990 survey indicated a lifetime use of 4.2% (6.5% among males and 1.9% among females). Readministered in February 1991, the survey indicated a lifetime use rate of 3.8% (4.8% among males and 2.9% among females) (DuRant, Ashworth, Newman, & Rickert, 1994), representing a decrease in total use of 10% (a 26% drop among males but a 53% increase in use among females).

Unfortunately, the responses were anonymous and subjects could not be matched for reliability of response across surveys.

A 1988 survey of 9th through 12th grade physical education, driver education, and health classes in 47 Chicago area schools revealed a lifetime anabolic steroid use rate of 4.4% (6.5% among males and 2.5% among females) (Terney & McLain, 1990). In 1991 an additional study of adolescent steroid use was conducted using a different sampling method than the 1988 study. The stratified random sample of 38 high schools across the state revealed an overall 1.9% steroid use rate among 9th and 12th graders (3.0% of males and 1.0% of females) (Gaa, Griffith, Cahill, & Tuttle, 1994).

The Maryland Department of Education has conducted biennial surveys since 1973 on adolescent drug use (Ross et al., 1989; Maryland, 1992). Students admitting to having ever used steroids decreased among 12th-grade students from 3.1% in 1989 to 1.9% in 1992, a decrease of 39%.

In summary, the results of state-level studies show a downward trend in adolescent steroid use rates between 1988 and 1994. However, the reader is cautioned that relatively small increases or decreases in initially low rates can result in a substantial percent change in steroid use and that no tests of the statistical significance of these percent changes in the rate of use were computed.

National Surveys

Tables 3.3 and 3.4 present data from three national surveys (the Monitoring the Future study, the Youth Risk and Behavior Surveillance System, and the National Household Survey on Drug Abuse) that provide multiyear information on anabolic steroid use among adolescents. The following paragraphs describe these surveys.

The Monitoring the Future Study (MTF)

The MTF study is a national-level epidemiological survey that has been conducted annually since 1975 through the National Institute on Drug Abuse research grants awarded to the Institute for Social Research (ISR) at the University of Michigan (Johnston, O'Malley, & Bachman, 1996). Its purpose is to determine the prevalence of students' use of drugs and their related attitudes and beliefs. The study comprises three substudies: (1) an annual survey of high school seniors, initiated in 1975; (2) ongoing panel studies of representative samples of each graduating class (conducted by mail since 1976); and (3) annual surveys of 8th and 10th graders initiated in 1991. The MTF study uses a multistage probability sample: stage one, the selection of specific geographic areas; stage two, the selection of one or more schools in the area; and stage three, student selection. To increase privacy, data are collected using self-administered questionnaires distributed in the classroom by representatives of the ISR when the teacher is not present. Approximately 50,000 8th, 10th, and 12th graders are surveyed each year. Dropouts and students absent on the day of survey administration are excluded. Recognizing the dropout population may be at greater risk for drug use, this survey was expanded to include nationally representative samples of 8th and 10th graders in 1991. National statistics indicate the majority of dropouts leave school after the 10th grade.

The Youth Risk and Behavior Surveillance System (YRBSS)

The YRBSS monitors health risk behaviors among youth, including the use of alcohol, tobacco, and other drugs (Kann et al., 1995, 1996). This system includes a national school-based survey and surveys conducted in 35 states and territories. The data presented here are from the national survey. The YRBSS, which is sponsored by the Centers for Disease Control and Prevention (CDC), was initiated in 1990 and began collecting information on anabolic steroid use in 1991. Since 1991, the survey has been conducted on a biennial basis. Participants in this survey are selected using a three-stage, cluster sampling design. The number of students included in each survey has ranged from 16,000 in the 1993 YRBSS to 11,000 for the 1995 survey. The students are representative of grades 9 through 12, attending public and private schools in all 50 states and the District of Columbia. The YRBSS is conducted in classrooms (the 1992 survey being the exception) and uses anonymous, self-administered questionnaires and answer sheets.

The National Household Survey on Drug Abuse (NHSDA)

The NHSDA began in 1971 under the auspices of the National Commission on Marijuana and Drug Abuse (U.S. Department of Health and Human Services [USDHHS], 1992). From 1974 to 1992, this survey was sponsored by the National Institute on Drug Abuse. Since October 1992, the Substance Abuse and Mental Health Services Administration (SAMHSA) has sponsored the NHSDA. The target population for this ongoing survey is all civilian residents of households and noninstitutional group quarters (e.g., college dormitories, homeless shelters, and rooming houses) in the contiguous United States. Hawaii and Alaska have been included since 1991. The survey design is a stratified, multistage probability sample. Blacks, Hispanics, youths, and six metropolitan areas are oversampled. Persons participating in the survey are interviewed in their homes and, for respondents under age 18, parents may remain in the room during the interview. To enhance anonymity, drug use questions are answered on a self-administered answer sheet. Substantially higher prevalence rates for some drugs (including the use of anabolic steroids) in both the MTF and the YRBSS have been attributed to youths being more willing to admit to use in the relative privacy of the school setting than at home, where parents may be present (SAMHSA, 1993, 1994, 1995). Note that although only one survey (i.e., the NHSDA) specifically identifies the substance of interest as "anabolic steroids" (the MTF and YRBSS use the term "steroids"), all three surveys specify the nonmedical use of steroids, which differentiates performance-enhancement steroids from those used in medicinal therapy.

The data presented from all three surveys (MTF, YRBSS, and NHSDA) refer to participants reporting having used steroids at least once in their lifetime (table 3.3). The MTF study also provides information on steroid use in the past year and in the 30 days prior to the survey (table 3.4).

Table 3.3 National Studies of Lifetime Anabolic Steroid Use by Adolescents

Study	Year	Sample size	Grade level/ age	Total use %	Males %	Females %
YRBSS	1991	12,267	9–12	2.7	4.1	1.2
YRBSS	1993	16,267	9–12	2.2	3.1	1.2
YRBSS	1995	10,904	9–12	3.7	4.9	2.4
MTF	1989	2,283	12	3.0	4.7	1.3
MTF	1990	2,533	12	2.9	5.0	0.5
MTF	1991	2,500	12	2.1	3.6	0.4[2]
MTF	1992	2,633	12	2.1	3.5[3]	0.7
MTF	1993	2,716	12	2.0	3.5	0.6
MTF	1994	2,567	12	2.4	3.8	0.9
MTF	1995	2,567	12	2.3	3.8	0.8
MTF	1996	2,275	12	1.9	3.2[5]	0.6
MTF	1997	2,566	12	2.4	4.1[1,4]	0.9[5]
NHSDA	1991	8,005	12–17 y	0.6	1.0	0.2
NHSDA	1992	7,254	12–17 y	0.3	0.4	0.1
NHSDA	1993	6,978	12–17 y	0.2	0.3[6]	0.1
NHSDA	1994	4,678	12–17 y	0.7	0.7	0.6[7]

[1] 1989–97 significant ($p < .05$)

[2] 1989–91 significant ($p < .001$)

[3] 1990–92 significant ($p < .001$)

[4] 1993–97 significant ($p < .01$)

[5] 1991–97 significant ($p < .05$)

[6] 1991–93 significant ($p < .05$)

[7] 1991–94 significant ($p < .05$)

Table 3.4 Trends in the Prevalence of Steroid Use Among 8th, 10th, and 12th Graders by Sex (%)

	Lifetime						
	91	**92**	**93**	**94**	**95**	**96**	**97**
8th Grade	1.9	1.7	1.6	2.0	2.0	1.8	1.8
Male	3.0	2.6	2.5	2.8	2.6	2.1	2.4[1]
Female	0.8	0.9	0.8	1.1	1.3	1.4	1.2[1]
10th Grade	1.8	1.7	1.7	1.8	2.0	1.8	2.0
Male	3.1	2.9	2.8	3.0	3.3	2.6	2.9
Female	0.5	0.5	0.6	0.7	0.8	1.1	1.1[1]
12th Grade	2.1	2.1	2.0	2.4	2.3	1.9	2.4
Male	3.6	3.5	3.5	3.8	3.8	3.2	4.1[1]
Female	0.4	0.7	0.6	0.9	0.8	0.6	0.9[2]
	Past year						
	91	**92**	**93**	**94**	**95**	**96**	**97**
8th Grade	1.0	1.1	0.9	1.2	1.0	1.0	1.0
Male	1.8	1.7	1.4	1.8	1.3	1.1	1.3[1]
Female	0.3	0.5	0.3	0.6	0.8	0.7	0.7[1]
10th Grade	1.1	1.1	1.0	1.1	1.2	1.2	1.2
Male	1.9	1.9	1.7	1.9	2.0	1.7	1.8
Female	0.3	0.3	0.3	0.4	0.5	0.6	0.6[1]
12th Grade	1.4	1.1	1.2	1.3	1.5	1.4	1.4
Male	2.4	2.1	2.5	2.1	2.4	2.2	2.5
Female	0.2	0.1	0.1	0.5	0.6	0.4	0.5[1]
	Past month						
	91	**92**	**93**	**94**	**95**	**96**	**97**
8th Grade	0.4	0.5	0.5	0.5	0.6	0.4	0.5
Male	+	0.9	0.8	0.9	0.7	0.6	0.7
Female	+	0.2	0.2	0.2	0.3	0.2	0.2

(continued)

Table 3.4 *(continued)*

	Past month						
	91	**92**	**93**	**94**	**95**	**96**	**97**
10th Grade	0.6	0.6	0.5	0.6	0.6	0.5	0.7
Male	+	1.0	0.9	1.0	1.0	0.8	1.0
Female	+	0.1	0.1	0.2	0.2	0.2	0.3
12th Grade	0.8	0.6	0.7	0.9	0.7	0.7	1.0
Male	+	1.1	1.4	1.2	0.8	1.1	1.8[2]
Female	+	0.1	—	0.3	0.5	0.3	0.2

[1] 1991 versus 1997 — significant ($p < .05$)
[2] 1991 versus 1997 — significant ($p < .01$)
+ not available
— less than 0.05%

Data from Johnston, O'Malley, & Bachman 1998.

Data are shown in table 3.3 for the 1991, 1993, and 1995 YRBSS national surveys. Over this period, the proportion of adolescent males reporting ever using steroids in their lifetime has increased slightly: reported use rose from 4.1% in 1991 to 4.9% in 1995 (not statistically significant). Likewise, the proportion of females reporting the use of steroids doubled during this same time period, from 1.2% in 1991 to 2.4% in 1995, but this increase is not statistically significant.

Data on the lifetime use of anabolic steroids among participants in the MTF study are shown in tables 3.3 and 3.4. Long-term trends, from 1989 to 1997, show statistically significant declines ($p < .05$) in lifetime use of anabolic steroids for 12th-grade males. The change between 1989 and 1997 is not statistically significant for females. Lifetime use of steroids among 12th-grade males peaked in 1990 at 5% and then significantly decreased to a low point of 3.5% ($p < .001$) in 1992 and in 1993. Subsequently, lifetime use of steroids among 12th-grade males increased significantly (from 3.5% in 1993 to 4.1% in 1997 ($p < .01$). Lifetime use among 12th-grade females was highest in 1989 (1.3%) and then decreased significantly to a low point of 0.4% ($p < .001$) in the 1991 survey. Subsequent to 1991, lifetime use among female seniors increased from 0.4% to 0.9% in 1997 ($p < .05$). Lifetime use for 8th-grade males decreased significantly ($p < .05$) between 1991 and 1997, while the prevalence of steroid use for 10th-grade males remained fairly stable. During the same period, steroid use among females in the 8th and 10th grades increased significantly ($p < .05$) (table 3.4).

Past-year use (using at least once in the 12 months prior to survey) for anabolic steroids among 8th, 10th, and 12th graders is shown annually for 1991 to 1997 in table 3.4. For 8th-grade males, past-year use decreased significantly, with 1.8% reporting use in 1991 dropping to 1.3% in 1997 ($p < .05$). Among female 8th graders, the increase from 0.3% in 1991 to 0.7% in 1997 is significant ($p < .05$). Tenth-grade males have reported stable rates of past-year steroid use from 1991 to 1997. The proportion of 10th-grade females reporting past-year steroid use increased significantly over this 6-year period, 0.3% in 1991 and 0.6% in 1997 ($p < .05$). For seniors, past-year use has been stable between 1991 and 1997 for males and increased among females ($p < .05$).

Past-month use (any use in the 30 days prior to survey) for anabolic steroids among 8th, 10th, and 12th graders is shown for 1992 to 1997 in table 3.4. Past-month use is commonly referred to as current use of a particular substance. Past-month use has been relatively stable for all three grades and both sexes. The only exception was a significant increase, from 1.1 % in 1992 to 1.8% in 1997 ($p < .01$) for 12th-grade males.

The NHSDA is a primary source of statistical information on the use of illegal drugs in the United States for persons 12 years of age and older (USDHHS, 1992; SAMHSA, 1993, 1994, 1995). Examining the data on lifetime use of steroids in table 3.3, 0.6% of 12 to 17 year olds in the NHSDA reported steroid use overall in 1991, the first year these drugs were included in the survey. The 1994 survey found that 0.7% of this same age group reported using steroids at least once. This is a stable trend, but the intervening years have lower estimates of use. Male steroid use declined, although not significantly, from 1991 to 1994, whereas steroid use by females increased significantly ($p < .05$) during this same period. The 1994 survey was the last year the NHSDA included questions related to steroid use, due to reliability concerns caused by the very low numbers of steroid-using respondents.

In summary, the only comparable years for the national data sets are 1991 through 1995 (1991–1994 for the NHSDA). Among male adolescents, the 5-year trend for use of anabolic steroids at least once in one's lifetime (lifetime use) is generally statistically stable. For the YRBSS, lifetime use among males was 4.1% in 1991, increasing to 4.9% in the 1995 survey (not significant). Use among females did increase, although not significantly during this same period. The MTF data indicate that 3.6% of male seniors used anabolic steroids in 1991. In this data set, the proportion of male seniors reporting anabolic steroid use has also remained stable from 1991 through 1995, ranging from 3.5% to 3.8%. None of these fluctuations is statistically significant. Likewise, lifetime steroid use rates for 8th- and 10th-grade males were stable from 1991 to 1995. Past-year use among males was reasonably stable for two of these same three groups during this same period (use among 8th-grade males decreased significantly, $p < .05$). Lifetime anabolic steroid use increased ($p < .05$) for 8th-, 10th-, and 12th-grade females, as was the case for past-year steroid use, with the exception of 10th graders (n.s.) (table 3.4). For the NHSDA, male lifetime steroid use was 1.0% in 1991 and 0.7% in 1994, a nonsignificant difference. In the intervening survey years of 1992 and 1993, male steroid use had significantly declined ($p < .05$) and then increased. Finally, during the comparable periods for the three surveys, use among adolescent males appears generally stable. However, among females in the three surveys, the trend for anabolic steroid use between 1991 and 1995 reveals consistent increases in use, with some of the increases being statistically significant.

International Surveys of Adolescent Steroid Use

It should be noted that the use of anabolic steroids by adolescents is not limited to the United States (table 3.5). Three Canadian studies (Adalf & Smart, 1992; Canadian Centre for Drug-Free Sport, 1993; Killop & Stennett, 1990), two South African surveys (Lambert, Titlestad, and Schwellnus, 1998; Schwellnus et al., 1992), one British study (Williamson, 1993), two Swedish surveys (Kindlundh, Isacson, Berglund, & Nyberg, 1998; Nilsson, 1995), and one Australian study (Handelsman & Gupta, 1997) have reported overall prevalence rates for high school students to range between 1% and 3% (table 3.5), which approximate those reported in the United States and reflect the cross-cultural impact of steroids on performance and appearance.

College Students

Of 67 intercollegiate swimmers (male and female) from six universities surveyed in 1981, only one athlete (a male) reported prior use of anabolic steroids (Toohey & Corder, 1981). Dezelsky, Toohey, and Shaw (1985), in a study of nonmedical drug use among students at five public universities in 1970 and 1984, found that only 1% of nonathlete students reported using anabolic steroids in 1984. However, the percentage of intercollegiate athletes who reported anabolic steroid use rose from 15% in 1970 to 20% in 1984 (table 3.6). Anabolic steroid use rates were not reported separately for males and females, nor were they reported by sport.

Of the 1,010 respondents in a survey of college men at three eastern U.S. universities, 2% acknowledged anabolic steroid use, whereas 9.4% of the 147 varsity athletes in the sample reported using these drugs (Pope, Katz, & Champoux, 1988; table 3.6).

Anderson and McKeag (1985) surveyed 2,039 NCAA male and female athletes at 11 NCAA-member colleges and universities nationwide regarding alcohol and drug use (table 3.6). The heaviest anabolic steroid use (defined as use in the past 12 months) was among football players (9%), whereas 4% of the male track-and-field athletes reported prior use. Men's

Table 3.5 Anabolic Steroid Use Among International High School–Age Students

Reference	Site	Sample size	Age/Grade (%)	Male (%)	Female (%)	Total	Time span
Killop & Stennett, 1990	London, Ontario, Canada, secondary schools	2,972	Overall	5.3	0.6	3.0	Past 12 months
			Grade 9	5.5	1.3	3.7	
			Grade 10	5.7	0.0	3.1	
			Grade 11	4.5	0.4	2.4	
			Grade 12	4.6	1.4	2.9	
			Grade 13	5.9	0.0	2.6	
Candian Ctr for Drug-Free Sport, 1993	Canada, 5 regions, 107 schools	16,169	Overall	4.1	1.5	2.8	Past 12 months
			11–13 y	2.8	1.1	2.0	
			14–15 y	3.9	2.1	3.1	
			16+ y	5.5	1.5	3.5	
Adalf & Smart, 1992	Ontario, Canada	3,915	Grades 7, 9, 11, 13	2.1	0.2	1.1	Past 12 months
Schwellnus et al., 1992	Cape Peninsula, South Africa	1,361	High school	1.2	0.0	0.6	Not specified
Lambert et al., 1998	South Africa, 2 regions	2,772	16–18 y	2.8	0.7	1.4	Not specified
Williamson, 1993	England, College of Technology	633	61% < 19 y	4.4	1.0	2.8	Lifetime
						1.4	Current
Nilsson, 1995	Falkenburg, Sweden	1,383	14–19 y	5.8	1.0	—	Lifetime
Kindlundh et al., 1998	Uppsala, Sweden	2,742	16–19 y	2.7	0.4	1.6	Lifetime
Handelsman & Gupta, 1997	NSW & Victoria, Australia, 203 schools	13,355	12–19 y	3.2	1.2	—	Lifetime

Table 3.6 Anabolic Steroid Use Among U.S. College Athletes

Reference	Site	Sample size	Group	Incidence of Use (%)
Dezelsky et al., 1985	5 universities	4,171	Athletes, 1970	15.0
			Athletes, 1984	20.0
			Nonathletes, 1984	1.0
Anderson & McKeag, 1985	11 universities, intercollegiate athletes	2,039	Football	8.4
			Division I	4.9
			Division II	4.2
			Division III	2.2
			Men's baseball	3.5
			Men's basketball	3.6
			Men's tennis	3.6
			Men's track and field	4.7
			Women's basketball	0.0
			Women's softball	0.0
			Women's swimming	0.7
			Women's tennis	0.0
			Women's track and field	0.0
Anderson et al., 1991	11 universities, intercollegiate athletes	2,282	Football	9.7
			Division I	4.8
			Division II	5.3
			Division III	4.3
			Men's baseball	2.2
			Men's basketball	1.6
			Men's tennis	2.2
			Men's track and field	4.1
			Women's basketball	0.8
			Women's softball	0.0
			Women's swimming	1.0
			Women's tennis	0.0
			Women's track and field	1.2
Anderson et al., 1993	11 universities, intercollegiate athletes	2,505	Football	5.0
			Division I	1.9
			Division II	4.3
			Division III	1.9
			Men's baseball	0.7
			Men's basketball	2.6
			Men's tennis	0.0
			Men's track and field	0.0
			Women's basketball	1.5
			Women's softball	1.7
			Women's swimming	0.6
			Women's tennis	2.7
			Women's track and field	2.7

Reference	Site	Sample size	Group	Incidence of Use (%)
NCAA, 1997	637 NCAA institutions, intercollegiate athletes	13,914	Football	2.2
			Division I	1.2
			Division II	1.1
			Division III	1.3
			Men's baseball	1.9
			Men's basketball	0.6
			Men's tennis	0.5
			Men's track and field	1.3
			Women's basketball	0.4
			Women's softball	0.9
			Women's swimming	0.8
			Women's tennis	0.3
			Women's track and field	0.6
Pope et al., 1988	3 universities	1,010	Men	2.0
			Varsity athletes ($N = 147$)	9.4

sports not typically associated with anabolic steroid use but found to have some anabolic steroid users were baseball (3%), basketball (4%), and tennis (4%). For women, only one sport was associated with anabolic steroid use—swimming (1%). Overall, 5% of Division I athletes, 4% of Division II athletes, and 2% of Division III athletes reported anabolic steroid use in the year prior to the survey.

Anderson, Albrecht, McKeag, Hough, & McGrew (1991) replicated the Anderson and McKeag (1985) study of athletes during the 1988–1989 academic year (table 3.6). Data were collected from 2,282 male and female athletes at 11 colleges and universities. Seven of the original 11 universities participated in the second study. Overall, anabolic steroid use had increased only slightly over the preceding four years. For Division I athletes, reported anabolic steroid use remained at 5%. However, for Division II and Division III athletes, anabolic steroid use rose to 5% and 4%, respectively.

Across Divisions I–III, the highest incidence of reported anabolic steroid use was again among football players (10%). Anabolic steroid use remained the same for men's track and field (4%), but declined in baseball (2%), basketball (2%), and tennis (2%). Unlike the Anderson and McKeag (1985) study, which found anabolic steroid use in only one sport for women, the 1991 survey by Anderson and colleagues revealed three women's sports associated with anabolic steroid use: track and field (1%), basketball (1%), and swimming (1%). Refer to table 3.6 for Division I use rates for selected sports. For those athletes using steroids, 25% began use before college, 25% initiated use during the first year of college, and 50% began after the first year of college (Anderson et al., 1991).

In 1993, Anderson and his colleagues again repeated their study, observing a significant decline in anabolic steroid use among male athletes, although football players continued to have the highest level of self-reported use (table 3.6). However, female athletes surveyed showed considerable increases in steroid use relative to the 1985 and 1989 surveys. Yet another survey was conducted in 1997 (NCAA Research Staff), using a substantially different sampling method, and showed a further decline in steroid use in most sports. Football players, again, reported the highest level of use, at 2.2%, although this is a substantial decline from the previous surveys.

With a significantly different methodology than the self-report format discussed above, Yesalis, Buckley, Anderson, Wang, Norwood, Ott, and colleagues (1990) employed projected-response survey techniques with collegiate athletes and used indirect questions. Thus respondents were asked to estimate the level of their competitors' steroid use. Over 1,600 male and female athletes at five NCAA Division I institutions participated in this study during the 1989–1990 academic year. The mean overall projected rate of any prior use of anabolic steroids across all sports surveyed was 14.7% for male athletes and 5.9% for females. Among men's sports, football reported the highest projected lifetime anabolic steroid use rates with 29.3%, followed by track and field with 20.6%. The greatest projected steroid use rate for women's sports was for track and field (16.3%). The overall projected rate of steroid use during the past 12 months reported was approximately three times greater than the rate obtained from self-reports by Anderson and colleagues (1991) (table 3.7).

Other Athletes

Silvester (1973) surveyed track-and-field athletes who participated in the 1972 Olympics and found that 68% of the participants reported prior anabolic steroid use, with 61% having used steroids within 6 months of the games (table 3.8). In 1975, Ljungqvist surveyed elite Swedish male track-and-field athletes and found that 31% admitted prior anabolic steroid use (Ljungqvist, 1975). None of the middle- or long-distance runners admitted anabolic steroid use, but 75% of the throwers did (table 3.8). In a survey of 155 U.S. Olympians who participated in the 1992 Winter Games, 80% of the athletes classified steroid use among Olympic competitors as a very serious or somewhat serious problem; just 5% thought that it was not a problem (Pearson & Hansen, 1992). When asked to estimate the level of steroid use in their own sport, 43% of the respondents estimated 10% or more, while 34% estimated 1% to 9%. Only 23% of the athletes surveyed believed that there was no steroid use in their sport. In a survey of former Olympians (Pearson, 1994), 75% of the medalists and 63% of the nonmedalists stated that more athletes use performance-enhancing drugs than when they competed.

Table 3.7 Estimates of Anabolic Steroid Use During Past 12 Months Among Division I NCAA Athletes (%) (Self-Reported vs. Projected Use)

	Male					
Reference	**Baseball**	**Basketball**	**Football**	**Tennis**	**Track and field**	**Weighted mean**
Anderson et al., 1991	2.6	1.6	9.6	0	2.3	6.2
Yesalis, Buckley et al., 1990	6.7	6.9	22.4	2.8	16.0	16.4
	Female					
	Softball	**Basketball**	**Swimming**	**Tennis**	**Track and field**	**Weighted mean**
Anderson et al., 1991	0	0	0	0	1.5	0.6
Yesalis, Buckley, et al., 1990	2.9	6.3	5.3	5.6	9.5	6.4
	All sports, male and female combined					
Anderson et al., 1991		Self-reported use				4.8
Yesalis, Buckley, et al., 1990		Projected use				14.1

Table 3.8 Anabolic Steroid Use Among Other Athletes

Reference	Site	Sample size	Group	Incidence of Use (%)
Silvester, 1973	Olympians in track and field from 7 countries	—	Lifetime Past 6 months	68 61
Ljungqvist, 1975	Elite Swedish male track-and-field athletes	99	Lifetime, all Throwers only	31 75
Frankle et al., 1984	Weightlifters in 3 Chicago gyms	250	Lifetime	44
Newman, 1987	Elite female athletes in over 15 sports, U.S.	271	Lifetime Past 12 months	3 1
McKillop, 1987	Male amateur bodybuilders in 1 gym in Scotland	41	Lifetime	19
Yesalis et al., 1988	Elite powerlifters, U.S.	45	Questionnaire ($N = 45$) Telephone ($N = 20$) Lifetime	33 55
Tricker et al., 1989	Amateur, competitive bodybuilders in Missouri and Kansas	176	Males ($N = 108$) Females ($N = 68$) Current	55 10
Kisling et al., 1989	Bodybuilders in 1 gym, Denmark	138	Males Time span not specified	62
Lindstrom et al., 1990	Swedish bodybuilders in 1 gym	171	Males ($N = 138$) Females ($N = 33$) Current	38 9
Yesalis & Courson, 1990	Professional American football players	120	Lifetime Past 12 months	28 3
Perry et al., 1992	Weightlifters in private gyms in Great Britain	160	Total Time span not specified	39
Korkia & Stimson, 1993	21 gyms in Great Britain	1,669	Males ($N = 1,310$) Females ($N = 349$) 10 not identified	9 lifetime 6 current 2 lifetime 1 current
Kersey, 1993	Weight trainers at 5 health clubs/gyms, U.S.	178	Males (N = 139) Females (N = 39) Lifetime	18 3
Ohaeri et al., 1993	Professional Nigerian athletes	250	Total, lifetime	1

Reference	Site	Sample size	Group	Incidence of Use (%)
Delbeke et al., 1995	Competitive body-builders in Flanders	379	Males & females (urinalysis) Current	42
Wagman et al., 1995	Elite powerlifters, U.S.	15	Males, lifetime	67

Newman (1987) surveyed elite female athletes in more than 15 sports and found that lifetime incidence of anabolic steroid use was 3%, but only 1% of the athletes acknowledged using these drugs in the preceding year (table 3.8). The lifetime use rate was slightly higher for those over the age of 26 (4%) and members of professional teams (5%). The prevalence of lifetime use of anabolic steroids among 250 Nigerian professional sports men and women has been reported as 1.2% (Ohaeri et al., 1993).

In 1988, Yesalis, Herrick, Buckley, Friedl, Brannon, and Wright surveyed elite powerlifters at a major contest, using both questionnaires and follow-up telephone interviews. One-third of the questionnaire respondents admitted prior anabolic steroid use, but 55% of those interviewed later by telephone conceded steroid use (table 3.8). Among elite powerlifters in the United States surveyed by Wagman, Curry, and Cook (1995), 67% were identified as current and/or previous anabolic steroid users.

Frankle, Cicero, and Payne (1984) questioned weight trainers in three gymnasiums in the Chicago area and found that 44% reported prior anabolic steroid use (table 3.8). Of a subsample of 50 anabolic steroid users interviewed in-depth, only 44% were competing in athletics. Anabolic steroid use rates by sex were not reported. In a study of amateur competitive bodybuilders, over half of the men and 10% of the women reported using anabolic steroids at some time in their lives (Tricker, O'Neill, & Cook, 1989; table 3.8). Of 185 weight trainers in gyms and health clubs in a southwestern U.S. city, 18% of men and 3% of women acknowledged they had used or were currently using anabolic steroids (Kersey, 1993).

In 1985 McKillop surveyed bodybuilders in a gymnasium in Scotland, of whom 19.5% acknowledged prior steroid use (McKillop, 1987; table 3.8). Similarly, two single-gym studies of bodybuilders revealed high lifetime use rates among men (62% and 38.4%) (Kisling, Fauner, Larsen, & Nielsen, 1989; Lindstrom, Nilsson, Katzman, Janzon, & Dymling, 1990; table 3.8). A relatively high rate of anabolic steroid use (9.1%) was reported by female bodybuilders in one of these studies (Lindstrom et al., 1990).

Participants in a study of 21 gymnasiums in Great Britain reported only a 9.1% use rate for males and 2.3% for females over their lifetime (Korkia & Stimson, 1993). Use did vary among the gyms, however, ranging from no use at one gym to a high of 46% in another. Likewise, results from another British survey of private gymnasium members indicated a 38.8% steroid use rate for survey participants (Perry, Wright, & Littlepage, 1992; table 3.8). Competitive bodybuilders in Flanders were subject to unannounced testing for steroids during national and international competitions from 1988 to 1993. The results of this testing revealed a steroid use rate of about 42% (Delbeke, Desmet, & Debackere, 1995; table 3.8).

In 1990, an attempt was made to survey 1,600 NFL players via mail by the NFL Players Association and the Olympia Steele Management Group (Yesalis & Courson, 1990; table 3.8). Only 120 players (~7.5%) elected to participate, however. Twenty-eight percent of all respondents and 67% of offensive linemen reported prior use of anabolic steroids. Only 3% of the participants reported steroid use in the past 12 months. When the participants were asked what percent of their fellow NFL players did they believe had ever used anabolic steroids, the mean response was 32%; the estimate of use among fellow players for the past 12 months was 19%.

Methodological Issues

Survey research is dependent on self-reported data about the attitudes, motivations, beliefs, and behaviors known only to the respondent. A frequent concern about survey research, especially surveys dealing with illegal, controversial, or socially stigmatized behaviors, is the veracity of responses given by the participants. Illicit drug use, including the use of anabolic steroids and many other performance-enhancing drugs that are also illegal and socially stigmatized, is no different. Thus, the extent to which athlete-respondents honestly report their drug use is unknown.

The focus on the validity of self-report is not new. In a 1944 article titled "Do They Tell the Truth?" Hyman evaluated how willing people were to admit they cashed war bonds, a socially unacceptable behavior at the time. Hyman found many people who were documented as having redeemed war bonds subsequently denied their behavior (Harrell, 1985).

Social Desirability

According to social desirability theory (Crowne & Marlowe, 1960; Edwards, 1957), distortion of self-reports occurs as a function of the perceived social acceptability of the behavior in question. Survey respondents may underreport their drug use to conceal their behaviors from the interviewer, the general public, sponsors of the survey, and other members of their households in order to present themselves, or perhaps their sport, in a way they feel is more socially acceptable. Conversely, respondents who view substance use positively may exaggerate reported use in order to impress others or to live up to a positive self-image (Schuman & Presser, 1981).

The mode of administering survey questions affects the reporting of sensitive topics. So it is important to have a good understanding of how privacy or lack of privacy during an interview affects the veracity of reporting. Literature on substance-use survey questions indicates self-administration increases levels of reporting compared to administration of the same question by an interviewer. Respondents of all ages are generally reluctant to admit that they have engaged in illegal and/or embarrassing activities to an interviewer (Tourangeau & Smith, 1996; Tourangeau, Smith, & Rasinski, 1997). In addition to self-administration, privacy is one explanation for the much higher rates of drug use reported in school-based surveys like the MTF and the YRBSS as compared to the NHSDA (Gfroerer, Wright, & Kopstein, 1997). The NHSDA does provide a self-administered answer sheet for substance use, but adults are allowed to stay in the room when the respondent is 12 to 17 years of age.

Factors related to social desirability also threaten the validity of self-reporting. Respondents may be reluctant to disclose behaviors that have specific legal and social consequences. Most drugs that have been shown to enhance physical performance are used in violation of the rules of sport federations (Wadler & Hainline, 1989) and state and federal laws (Yesalis, Barsukiewicz, Kopstein, & Bahrke, 1997).

Individual Variation

Studies that have examined the validity of self-report have consistently found that not everyone is equally likely to provide inaccurate information. In 1944, Hyman found certain subgroups of the population were more likely to deny war bond redemption. Persons with higher incomes were more likely than those with low incomes to distort their responses. Following analysis of data from the Denver Validity Study, Cahalan (1968) reported distorted responses differed by gender, age, and socioeconomic status. Women were less likely than men to exaggerate their contributions to the Community Chest. Cahalan found that younger people were more likely than older ones to exaggerate socially desirable behaviors like charitable contributions and voting. When Weiss looked at self-reported voter registration and voting among African-American welfare mothers in 1968, she found differences by age, education, and social status. Older women with more education were more likely to exaggerate information related to voting. Weiss felt this was because they valued voting and wanted to present a more positive picture of themselves (Weiss, 1968).

Drug use may vary substantially among different populations, such as high school, college, Olympic, and professional athletes, and the accuracy of their self-reports may also vary. Arguably, adolescents may be more forthcoming regarding their illicit performance-enhancing drug use because they have less to lose than college, elite, or professional athletes whose scholarships or livelihoods depend on their participation and success in sport. The fear of guilt by association and its potential to adversely affect one's place in sport history may cause the athlete to hesitate to volunteer or be truthful.

Validity of self-report appears in many instances to be a function of personal norms and self-expectations. For example, because of the virilizing qualities of anabolic steroids (Kochakian, 1976), women might be more secretive about their anabolic steroid use than men or even adolescents.

Drug use may be reported inaccurately because of variation in memory among respondents. For example, rare behaviors are often recalled but routine behaviors cannot always be recalled to immediate memory (Bradburn, Rips, & Shevell, 1987). Respondents may have difficulty accurately recalling the number of times they use cigarettes or alcohol in an interval as long as a year. In the experience of the authors, athletes have a strong recollection as to whether or not they have ever used a particular type of performance-enhancing drug. However, their memory is limited when they are asked to recall the specific name of a drug (generic/brand name), dosage, number of episodes of use (cycles), time frames for drug use, and so on.

Respondents may vary in understanding the question being asked in a particular survey, and some respondents may have reading difficulties that preclude an accurate response. The complexity of the scales for reporting frequencies and amounts of drug use can also be a source of confusion and variation.

Type of Drug

Findings from a series of methodological studies conducted in conjunction with the NHSDA indicate that the more stigmatized the drug, the more likely the respondent will deny use. This finding has been replicated in a number of other studies. Marijuana use is reported more validly than cocaine (Harrison, 1992, 1997; Fendrich & Xu, 1994; Mieczkowski, 1990). Among an arrestee population, Harrison found that respondents were most willing to report marijuana, followed by opiates, amphetamines, and then cocaine (Harrison, 1992).

While the use of traditional "street" drugs may constitute misdemeanor violations of state and federal laws, it is the violation of sport rules that could have, at least from the perspective of the athlete, a greater impact on their life, including the loss of a scholarship, income, and so on. Thus, in sport some drugs may be more stigmatized than others. For example, it can be argued that athletes will acknowledge marijuana use before anabolic steroid use, because marijuana use, while stigmatized, is, unfortunately, not a rare behavior, and society does not view this drug as enhancing athletic performance. Perhaps this explains, in part, the International Court of Arbitration for Sport overturning Canadian snowboarder Ross Rebagliati's positive drug test for marijuana at the Nagano Olympic Games and the reinstatement of his gold medal ("Drug Wars," 1998).

Accuracy

There is a wide array of inferential evidence for the validity of self-reported drug use. As contained in a report of the U.S. General Accounting Office (U.S. GAO, 1993), examples of such evidence include the considerable proportion of respondents that *do admit* to illegal drug use, the general completion of survey items concerning sensitive behaviors, the statistical demonstrations of predictable relationships between drug use and items concerning drug use, attitudes, and delinquent activities, similar prevalence rates obtained through an assortment of surveys, and the failure of people to report the use of a fictitious drug (which is included on most substance use surveys).

The large numbers of people who admit to drug use is readily demonstrated by looking at the data available from the national surveys on this topic. In 1997, the MTF study revealed that more than half (54.3%) of seniors in high school had used some sort of illicit drug at least once in their lives (Johnston, O'Malley, & Bachman, 1998). In the 1996 NHSDA, 6.1% of the respondents reported current use (current use refers to using at least once in the 30 days prior to the survey) of an illicit drug, which corresponds to an estimated 13 million Americans age 12 and older.

However, accuracy of reporting among adolescents, at least as it applies to anabolic steroid use, is somewhat suspect given the results of a 1988 study of high school athletes. Among the participants, 39% of male athletes and 56% of female athletes denied that they had even *heard of* using anabolic steroids to aid performance. This unawareness is noteworthy given that the study took place during a decade marked by significant media attention to drug use among athletes.

The reliability of surveys used in determining the prevalence of drug use among adolescents has been tested by DuRant and colleagues (1993, 1994). Although DuRant and colleagues (1994) have reported that self-report measurements on substance use by ninth-grade students provide a reliable method of determining drug use, they found self-reported lifetime anabolic steroid use had significantly decreased (5.4% to 4.8%) for males, and significantly increased for females (1.5% to 2.9%) when they readministered their questionnaire four months later. Unfortunately, since the two questionnaires were administered anonymously, the two surveys could not be paired.

In an anonymous, self-administered survey of elite (adult) powerlifters, only 33% reported having ever used anabolic steroids (Yesalis et al., 1988)—this in a sport in which many believe the use of these drugs is virtually universal (Starr, 1981; Todd, 1987; Wright, 1982). When a co-investigator, whom the study participants knew, again questioned (via telephone) some of the athletes about their steroid use, 55% admitted prior use. Thus it is possible that the level of trust the subjects felt with the interviewer was a more important factor to them than anonymity.

In 1990, an attempt was made to survey 1,600 NFL players via mail from the NFL Players Association (Courson, 1991). However, only 120 players (7.5%) were willing to participate. This extremely low response rate is notable since the survey was endorsed strongly by the players' own professional association and the anonymity of respondents was guaranteed. Nevertheless, of those who did participate, 28% of all respondents and 67% of offensive linemen reported prior use of anabolic steroids. Only 3% of the participants reported steroid use in the past 12 months. When the participants were asked what percent of their fellow NFL players did they believe had ever used anabolic steroids, the mean response was 32%; the estimate of use among fellow players for the past 12 months was 19%. This indirect survey technique (i.e., in which respondents estimate their competitors' anabolic steroid use level) relies to some extent on hearsay as well as the opportunity to project one's own behavior onto others, and the resulting estimates of use probably represent an upper bound or overestimation of use (Tricker, O'Neill, & Cook, 1989; Yesalis, Buckley, et al., 1990). This indirect survey method is probably less threatening to the athlete in that it does not require the respondent to divulge information about himself or herself or about specific teammates; this method likely results in a higher level of participation in the study. Undoubtedly a certain amount of projection also takes place (Semeonoff, 1976). That is, the respondent protects himself or herself from anxiety by projecting or externalizing inappropriate behaviors to others, as if by projecting these behaviors (in this case, anabolic steroid use) to someone else, one denies or rationalizes their existence within oneself. Also, anxiety related to one's own inappropriate behavior may be diluted if the behavior can be projected toward others in an effort to characterize the activity as less atypical or more mainstream. Thus, the true level of anabolic steroid use among athletes probably lies somewhere between the lower-bound estimates from self-reports and the upper-bound estimates obtained from the projective response techniques.

Apparently, only one study has examined the validity of self-report in identifying anabolic steroid use among athletes. To determine the validity of self-report in the detection of steroid use among weightlifters, Ferenchick (1996) compared self-report with assay results of simultaneous urine samples from 48 male weightlifters. The sensitivity of self-report in the detection of steroid use was 74% (a value that increased to 90% when lifetime use was considered) and specificity was 82%. Also, 22 of 23 participants in the study who declared current steroid use had at least one undeclared steroid identified in their urine. (However, this may not be unusual, since several studies [Debruyckere, de Sagher, & Van Peteghem, 1992; Kicman et al., 1994] have found steroid-positive urine following the dietary consumption of meat contaminated with anabolic steroids.) In addition, 15 participants reported at least one drug that was not detected in the urine. (Again, this may not be unusual given the lack of purity and questionable content of black-market drugs [Colman, A'Hearn, Taylor, & Le, 1991; Fish, 1993a; Musshoff, Daldrup, & Ritsch, 1997; Walters, Ayers, & Brown, 1990] that may constitute as much as 50 to 80% of the anabolic steroids used by athletes [Haislip, 1994]). Furthermore, 3 of 17 declared nonusers had objective evidence of steroids in their urine. All of this led Ferenchick to conclude that the validity of self-report may be inadequate to differentiate reliably between steroid users and nonusers. Whether these conclusions are applicable to elite athletes is questionable in that it can be argued that elite athletes have greater access to pharmaceutical grade steroids prescribed by physicians.

Time Frame

Another issue deserving comment is that some studies have focused their attention on anabolic steroid use during the past month or 12 months (Anderson et. al., 1991; Anderson, Albrecht, & McKeag, 1993; Anderson & McKeag, 1985; "Survey," 1997) rather than focusing on any past use of these drugs. Anabolic steroids are not necessarily temporary performance enhancers; they are capable of providing the athlete with increased muscle mass and strength, much of which can be maintained for a number of years through training alone. One might then argue that once a strength athlete uses anabolic steroids, he is never really the same person. Consequently, is there a difference between a college football player who does not currently use steroids but used them in high school to gain enough weight to win a scholarship, and a college player who used the drugs during the summer season to retain his starting position in the fall?

Nonresponders

A review of studies of the use of anabolic steroids across various levels of competition showed response rates that ranged from 7.5 to 99.5% or were not reported (Yesalis & Bahrke, 1995; Courson, 1991). There is no information on individuals who chose not to volunteer information, but it is reasonable to hypothesize, based on the above discussion, that a disproportionate number of those who did not participate were anabolic steroid users, which would result in an underreporting bias.

Credibility

For some time there has been a lack of trust and communication between members of the athletic community and the scientific and medical communities regarding anabolic steroids and other performance-enhancing drugs. In part, this is a function of a poor understanding by clinicians and researchers of the motivations of athletes, and vice versa.

The medical community has lost much credibility as a result of repeated denials that anabolic steroids significantly enhance performance (American College of Sports Medicine [ACSM], 1977; Elashoff, Jacknow, Shain, & Braunstein, 1991). For the past three decades, some physicians and scientists have dogmatically reported that any weight an athlete gains while taking steroids is mainly the result of fluid retention and that any strength gain is largely psychological (a placebo effect). Along the same line, some members of the sports medicine community have, with the best of intentions, adopted an overly aggressive educational strategy and have made strong, but often unfounded, pronouncements regarding the adverse health effects of anabolic steroids. Athletes, on the other hand, simply have not witnessed longtime steroid users "dropping like flies." This credibility gap has been exacerbated by the apparent contradiction between warnings of dire health consequences and clinical applications of these drugs, such as the 10-center worldwide trial sponsored by the World Health Organization to test the efficacy of anabolic steroids as a male contraceptive (World Health Organization Task Force, 1996) and multicenter trials to assess the effects of testosterone supplementation in older men ("Testosterone," 1996). The doses used in these studies equal or exceed those used by endurance and sprint athletes, among others (see introduction).

Validation

An approach for determining the validity of self-reported drug use is to evaluate responses that should be consistent over time. Lifetime use of a substance should logically never decline. Therefore, one can look at the rates of recanting of earlier lifetime use. For anabolic steroids use, one can look at the lifetime use reported in the MTF study by cohorts of students (table 3.9). An example is the 8th graders who were surveyed in 1991. These same students were 10th graders in the 1993 survey and seniors in the 1995 survey.

Validation of self-report requires comparing study results to some method that is more accurate. Research on the use of self-report methods has shown them to be valid for documenting recreational drug use,

Table 3.9 Lifetime Use of Anabolic Steroids by Cohort

Cohort	8th grade	10th grade	12th grade
1991 8th graders	1.9	1.7	2.3
1992 8th graders	1.7	1.8	1.9
1993 8th graders	1.6	2.0	2.4
1994 8th graders	2.0	2.0	(not available)

especially for adolescents (McClary & Lubin, 1985; Smart & Blair, 1978). When the recreational drug use rates from self-report studies have been compared with external methods of documenting drug use (e.g., reports by others, or blood and urine samples), the self-report use rates have been similar to or only slightly lower than the rates derived by the other methods (Ausel et al., 1976; Bonito, Nucro, & Schaffer, 1976; Deaux & Callaghen, 1984; Petzel, Johnson, & McKillip, 1973; Stacy, Widaman, & Hays, 1985). Unfortunately, due to the shortcomings of testing for drugs in sport, discussed above, the applicability of this validation strategy is somewhat limited.

Recommendations

Researchers need to concentrate on making self-reported data better. To help maximize accurate reporting, the Committee on Privacy and Confidentiality of the American Statistical Association (1429 Duke Street, Alexandria, Virginia, 22314-3402) recommends that sponsors of surveys should do the following:

1. Assure participants that the information provided will be kept confidential.
2. Ensure participants' responses will be used only for statistical purposes.
3. Provide participants with information so they can make an informed decision about whether or not to participate (informed consent).

Additional strategies for reducing concealment or underreporting include the following:

1. Establishing rapport with the respondent by choosing skillful interviewers and enlisting respondent support by giving them the objectives of the study
2. Concentrating more on recent events, because there are definite limits to the type and amount of detailed information that respondents can recall
3. Carefully constructing questionnaire and fieldwork procedures to evaluate potential response bias associated with method of inquiry—this usually requires pretesting the questionnaire

Summary

The level of anabolic steroid use has increased significantly over the past three decades, and it is no longer limited to elite athletes or men. Although higher rates of anabolic steroid use are reported by competitive athletes, a significant number of recreational athletes appear to be using these drugs, probably to improve their appearance. The use of anabolic steroids has trickled down from the Olympic, professional, and college levels to the high schools and the junior high schools. Steroid use has been reported by adolescents in both urban and rural areas and in schools of all sizes, and it is believed that among high school seniors 3 to 12% of males and 0.5 to 2% of females have used anabolic steroids at some time.

It is important for us to be able to accurately assess the prevalence of drug use in sport, primarily to protect the health of athletes and maintain a "level playing field." Unfortunately, the four major methods (investigative journalism, government investigation, drug testing, and surveys of athletes) used in determining the prevalence of drug use among athletes suffer from significant methodological weaknesses, often precluding accurate assessment. In particular, the responses of athletes to the questions of journalists, drug use surveys, or even government investigations may be influenced by any or all of the following: the athlete's desire to respond to the questions in a socially desirable manner, memory lapse; the illegal nature of the substances being surveyed, and a general distrust of those doing the questioning. Drug testing, at the very least, is hamstrung by significant limitations in technology. All these limitations would likely result in a significant underreporting bias. Future investigations and research will need to address these shortcomings if a more accurate estimate of drug use among athletes is to be obtained.

References

The abuse of steroids in amateur and professional athletics: Hearings before the Subcommittee on Crime of the Committee on the Judiciary, House of Representatives, 101st Cong., 2nd Sess. (1990, March 22).

Adalf, E., & Smart, R. (1992). Characteristics of steroid users in an adolescent school population. *Journal of Alcohol and Drug Education, 38,* 43–49.

Alzado, L. (1991, July 8). I'm sick and I'm scared. *Sports Illustrated,* 20–27.

American College of Sports Medicine (ACSM). (1977). Position statement on the use and abuse of anabolic-androgenic steroids in sports. *Medicine and Science in Sports and Exercise, 9,* 11–13.

The Anabolic Steroid Restriction Act of 1989: Hearing on H.R. 995 before the Subcommittee on Crime of the Committee on the Judiciary, House of Representatives, 101st Cong., 1st Sess. (1989, March 23).

Anderson, W., Albrecht, M., & McKeag, D. (1993). Second replication of a national study of the substance use/abuse habits of college student-athletes. Final report. *NCAA News.*

Anderson, W.A., Albrecht, M.A., McKeag, D.B., Hough, D.O., & McGrew, C.A. (1991). A national survey of alcohol and drug use by college athletes. *The Physician and Sportsmedicine, 19,* 91–104.

Anderson, W., & McKeag, D. (1985). *The substance use and abuse habits of college student-athletes* (Research Paper No. 2). Mission, KS: National Collegiate Athletic Association.

Athletes live with steroids' toll. (1997, October 5). *Des Moines Sunday Register,* p. 12a.

Ausel, S., Mandell, W., Mathias, L., et al. (1976). Reliability and validity of self-reported illegal activities and drug use collected from narcotic addicts. *International Journal of the Addictions, 11,* 325–336.

Bamberger, M., & Yaeger, D. (1997, April 14). Over the edge. *Sports Illustrated, 86,* 60–70.

Bonito, A., Nucro, D., & Schaffer, J. (1976). The veridicality of addicts' self-reports in social research. *International Journal of the Addictions, 11,* 719–724.

Bosworth, E., Bents, R., Trevisan, L., & Goldberg, L. (1987). Anabolic steroids and high school athletes. *Medicine and Science in Sports and Exercise, 20*(2)(Suppl.), S3, 17.

Bradburn, N., Rips, L., & Shevell, S. (1987). Answering autobiographical questions: The impact of memory and inference on surveys. *Science, 236,* 157–161.

Buckley, W., Yesalis, C., Friedl, K., Anderson, W., Streit, A., & Wright, J. (1988). Estimated prevalence of anabolic steroid use among male high school seniors. *Journal of the American Medical Association, 260,* 3441–3445.

Cahalan, D. (1968). Correlates of respondent accuracy in the Denver validity survey. *Public Opinion Quarterly, 32,* 607–621.

Canadian Centre for Drug-free Sport. (1993). *National School Survey on Drugs and Sport: Final report.* Gloucester.

Catlin, D., & Murray, T. (1996). Performance-enhancing drugs, fair competition, and Olympic Sport. *Journal of the American Medical Association, 276,* 231–237.

Coaches charged. (1997, October 15). *USA Today,* p. 3C.

Colman, P., A'Hearn, E., Taylor, R., & Le, S. (1991). Anabolic steroids—analysis of dosage forms from selected case studies from the Los Angeles County Sheriff's Scientific Services Bureau. *Journal of Forensic Sciences, 36,* 1079–1088.

Corder, B.W., Dezelsky, T.L., Toohey, J.V., & DiVito, C.L. (1975). Trends in drug use behavior at ten Central Arizona high schools. *Arizona Journal of Health, Physical Education, Recreation and Dance, 18,* 10–11.

Courson, S. (1991). *False glory.* Stamford, CT: Longmeadow Press.

Crowne, D., & Marlowe, D. (1960). A new scale of social desirability independent of psychopathology. *Journal of Counseling Psychology, 24,* 349–354.

Deaux, E., & Callaghen, J. (1984). Estimating statewide health risk behavior: A comparison of telephone and key information survey approaches. *Evaluation Review, 8,* 467–492.

Debruyckere, G., de Sagher, R., & Van Peteghem, C. (1992). Clostebol-positive urine after consumption of contaminated meat. *Clinical Chemistry, 38,* 1869–1873.

Delbeke, F., Desmet, N., & Debackere, M. (1995). The abuse of doping agents in competing body builders in Flanders (1988–1993). *International Journal of Sports Medicine, 16,* 66–70.

Dezelsky, T., Toohey, J., & Shaw, R. (1985). Non-medical drug use behavior at five United States universities: A 15-year study. *Bulletin on Narcotics, 27,* 45–53.

Drugs still mystery Olympic ingredient. (1992, July 22). *Chicago Tribune,* pp. 1, 7.

Drug-testing results for 1997 improve from previous year. (1998, August 31). *NCAA News,* 12.

Drug testing results in Atlanta confound expectations. (1996, September). *Sports Medicine Digest,* 103.

Drug wars. (1998, February 4). *USA Today,* p. 10C.

Dubin, C. (1990). *Commission of inquiry into the use of drugs and banned practices intended to increase athletic performance* (Catalogue No. CP32-56/1990E, ISBN 0-660-13610-4). Ottawa, ON: Canadian Government Publishing Center.

Duda, M. (1988). Gauging steroid use in high school kids. *The Physician and Sportsmedicine, 16,* 16–17.

DuRant, R., Rickert, V., Ashworth, C., Newman, C., & Slavens, G. (1993). Use of multiple drugs among adolescents who use anabolic steroids. *New England Journal of Medicine, 328,* 922–926.

DuRant, R., Ashworth, C., Newman, C., & Rickert, V. (1994). Stability of the relationships between anabolic steroid use and multiple substance use among adolescents. *Journal of Adolescent Health, 15,* 111–116.

Edwards, A. (1957). *The social desirability variable in personality assessment and research.* New York: Dryden.

Elashoff, J., Jacknow, A., Shain, S., & Braunstein, G. (1991). Effects of anabolic-androgenic steroids on muscular strength. *Annals of Internal Medicine, 115,* 387–393.

Fendrich, M., & Xu, Y.C. (1994). The validity of drug-use reports from juvenile arrestees. *International Journal of the Addictions, 29,* 971–985.

Ferenchick, G. (1996). Validity of self-report in identifying anabolic steroid use among weightlifters. *Journal of General Internal Medicine, 11,* 554–556.

Fish, M. (1993a, September 28). Steroids: Riskier than ever. *Atlantic Journal/Constitution,* p. D1.

Fish, M. (1993b, September 29). Experts suspect "a whole country" may be cheating. *The Atlanta Journal/Constitution,* p. E3.

Francis, C. (1990). *Speed trap.* New York: St. Martin's Press.

Franke, W. (1998, February 9–14). *Hormonal doping of athletes: The German Democratic Republic's secret program.* Paper presented at Drugs and Athletes: A Multidisciplinary Symposium. American Academy of Forensic Sciences, San Francisco.

Franke, W., & Berendonk, B. (1997). Hormonal doping and androgenization of athletes: A secret program of the German Democratic Republic government. *Clinical Chemistry, 43,* 1262–1279.

Frankle, M., Cicero, G., & Payne, J. (1984). Use of androgenic anabolic steroids by athletes [Letter to the editor]. *Journal of the American Medical Association, 252,* 482.

Frazier, S. (1973). Androgens and athletes. *American Journal of Diseases of Children, 125,* 479–480.

Gaa, G., Griffith, E., Cahill, B., & Tuttle, L. (1994). Prevalence of anabolic steroid use among Illinois high school students. *Journal of Athletic Training, 29,* 216–222.

Gfroerer, J., Wright, D., & Kopstein, A. (1997). Prevalence of youth substance use: The impact of methodological differences between two national surveys. *Drug and Alcohol Dependence, 47,* 19–30.

Gilbert, B. (1969a, June 23). Drugs in sport: Part 1. Problems in a turned-on world. *Sports Illustrated,* 64–72.

Gilbert, B. (1969b, June 30). Drugs in sport: Part 2. Something extra on the ball. *Sports Illustrated,* 30–42.

Gilbert, B. (1969c, July 7). Drugs in sport: Part 3. High time to make some rules. *Sports Illustrated,* 30–35.

Haislip, G.R. (1994). *Conference report: International Conference on the Abuse and Trafficking of Anabolic Steroids.* Washington, DC: U.S. Drug Enforcement Administration, Office of Diversion Control.

Handelsman, D., & Gupta, L. (1997). Prevalence and risk factors for anabolic-androgenic steroid abuse in Australian high school students. *International Journal of Andrology, 20,* 159–164.

Harrell, A. (1985). Validation of self-report: The research record. In B.A. Rouse, N.J. Kozel, & L.G. Richards (Eds.), *Self-report methods of estimating drug use: Meeting current challenges to validity* (NIDA Research Monograph 57, pp. 12–21). Washington, DC: Department of Health and Human Services.

Harrison, L. (1992). Trends in illicit drug use in the USA: Conflicting results from national surveys. *International Journal of Addiction, 27,* 817–847.

Harrison, L. (1997). The validity of self-reported drug use in survey research: An overview and critique of research methods. In L. Harrison & A. Hughes (Eds.), *The validity of self-reported drug use: Improving the accuracy of survey estimates* (NIDA Research Monograph 167, pp. 17–36; NIH Pub. No. 97-4147). Washington, DC: Department of Health and Human Services.

Hearing on steroid abuse in America before the Committee on the Judiciary, U.S. Senate, 101st Cong., 1st Sess. (1989, April 3).

Hearings before the Subcommittee to Investigate Juvenile Delinquency of the Committee on the Judiciary, U.S. Senate, 93rd Cong., 1st Sess. (1973, June 18, July 12, 13).

Hoberman, J. (1992). The early development of sports medicine in Germany. In J. Berryman & R. Park (Eds.), *Sport and exercise science: Essays in the history of sports medicine.* Champaign: University of Illinois Press.

Hubbell, N. (1990). *The use of steroids by Michigan high school students and athletes: An opinion research study of 10th and 12th grade high school students and varsity athletes,* November 1989 through January 1990. Lansing: Michigan Department of Public Health, Chronic Disease Advisory Committee.

Huizenga, R. (1994). *You're OK it's just a bruise.* New York: St. Martin's Press.

Hyman, H. (1944). Do they tell the truth? *Public Opinion Quarterly, 8,* 557–559.

IOC mum on latest positive drug test. (1998, February 20). *USA Today,* p. 13E.

ITF disputes Becker charges. (1994, January 27). *Chicago Sun-Times,* p. 6.

Janofsky, M. (1988, November 17). System accused of failing test posed by drugs. *New York Times,* pp. 1, D31.

Johnson, M., Jay, M., Shoup, B., & Rickert, V. (1989). Anabolic steroid use in adolescent males. *Pediatrics, 83,* 921–924.

Johnson, W. (1985, May 13). Steroids: A problem of huge dimensions. *Sports Illustrated,* 41–61.

Johnston, L., O'Malley, P., & Bachman, J. (1996). *National survey results on drug use from the Monitoring the Future study, 1989–1995: Vol. I. Secondary school students*. Washington, DC: U.S. Department of Health and Human Services, National Institute on Drug Abuse.

Johnston, L., O'Malley, P., & Bachman, J. (1998). *National survey results on drug use from the Monitoring the Future study, 1975–1997: Vol. I. Secondary school students*. Rockville, MD: U.S. Department of Health and Human Services, National Institutes of Health, National Institute on Drug Abuse.

Kann, L., Warren, C., Harris, W., et al. (1995, March 24). Youth risk behavior surveillance—United States, 1993. *Morbidity and Mortality Weekly Report (MMWR), 44,* SS-1.

Kann, L., Warren, C., Harris, W., et al. (1996, September 27). Youth risk behavior surveillance—United States, 1995. *Morbidity and Mortality Weekly Report (MMWR), 45,* SS-4.

Kelley, S. (1991, July 10). This chapter of Alzado's story is sad. *Seattle Times.*

Kersey, R. (1993). Anabolic-androgenic steroid use by private health club/gym athletes. *Journal of Strength and Conditioning Research, 7,* 118–126.

Keteyian, A. (1989). *Big red confidential: Inside Nebraska football.* New York: Contemporary Books.

Kicman, A., Cowan, D., Myhre, L., Nilsson, S., Tomten, S., & Oftebro, H. (1994). Effect on sports drug tests of ingesting meat from steroid (methenolone)-treated livestock. *Clinical Chemistry, 40,* 2084–2087.

Killop, S., & Stennett, R. (1990). *Use of performance-enhancing substances by London secondary school students* (Report no. 90-03). London, ON: Board of Education for the City of London.

Kindlundh, A., Isacson, D., Berglund, L., & Nyberg, F. (1998). Doping among high school students in Uppsala, Sweden: A presentation of the attitudes, distribution, side effects, and extent of use. *Scandinavian Journal of Social Medicine, 26,* 71–74.

Kisling, A., Fauner, M., Larsen, O.G., & Nielsen, S. (1989). Medicinmisbrug blandt bodybuildere [Drug abuse in body builders: A questionnaire study]. *Journal of Danish Medicine, 151,* 2582–2584.

Klecko, J., & Fields, J. (1989). *Nose to nose: Survival in the trenches in the NFL*. New York: Morrow.

Kochakian, C. (Ed.). (1976). *Anabolic-androgenic steroids.* New York: Springer-Verlag.

Komoroski, E., & Rickert, V. (1992). Adolescent body image and attitudes to anabolic steroid use. *Sports Medicine, 146,* 823–828.

Korkia, P., & Stimson, G. (1993). *Anabolic steroid use in Great Britain: An exploratory investigation.* London: Centre for Research on Drugs and Health Behavior.

Krowchuk, D., Anglin, T., Goodfellow, D., Stancin, T., Williams, P., & Zimet, G. (1989). High school athletes and the use of ergogenic aids. *American Journal of Diseases of Children, 143,* 486–489.

Lambert, M., Titlestad, S., & Schwellnus, M. (1998). Prevalence of androgenic-anabolic steroid use in adolescents in two regions of South Africa. *South African Medical Journal, 88,* 876–880.

Legislation to amend the controlled substance act to make the anabolic steroid methandrostenolone a Schedule I Controlled Substance:Hearing on H.R. 3216 before the Subcommittee on Crime of the Committee on the Judiciary, House of Representatives, 100th Cong., 2nd Sess. (1988, July 27).

Lindstrom, M., Nilsson, A., Katzman, P., Janzon, L., & Dymling, J. (1990). Use of anabolic-androgenic steroids among body builders—frequency and attitudes. *Journal of Internal Medicine, 227,* 407–411.

Litsky, F. (1993, January 15). D.E.A. says more players at risk. *New York Times,* p. B9.

Ljungqvist, A. (1975). The use of anabolic steroids in top Swedish athletes. *British Journal of Sports Medicine, 9,* 82.

Longman, J. (1995, April 9). U.S.O.C. experts call drug testing a failure. *New York Times,* p. 11.

Luetkemeier, M., Bainbridge, C., Walker, J., Brown, D., & Eisenman, P. (1995). Androgenic steroids: Prevalence, knowledge, and attitudes in junior and senior high school students. *Journal of Health Education, 26,* 4–9.

Maryland Department of Health and Mental Hygiene, Alcohol and Drug Abuse Administration, and the Juvenile Justice Advisory Council of Maryland (1989). *1988–1989 survey of substance abuse among Maryland adolescents.*

Maryland State Department of Education. (1992). *1992 Maryland adolescent drug survey*. Baltimore: Author.

McClary, S., & Lubin, B. (1985). Effects of type of examiner, sex, and year in school on self-report of drug use by high school students. *Journal of Drug Education, 15,* 49–55.

McKillop, G. (1987). Drug abuse in bodybuilders in the west of Scotland. *Scottish Medical Journal, 32,* 39–41.

Mieczkowski, T. (1990). The accuracy of self-reported drug use: An evaluation and analysis of new data. In R. Weisheit (Ed.), *Drugs and crime and the criminal justice system*. Cincinnati, OH: Anderson.

Mix, R. (1987, October 19). So little gain for the pain. *Sports Illustrated,* 54–59.

Musshoff, F., Daldrup, T., & Ritsch, M. (1997). Anabole steroide auf dem deutschen Schwarzmarkt [Anabolic steroids on the German black market]. *Archiv fur Kriminologie, 1916,* 152–158.

NCAA Research Staff. (1997). *NCAA study of substance use and abuse habits of college student-athletes.* Overland, KS: NCAA.

Newman, M. (1986). *Michigan Consortium of Schools student survey.* Minneapolis, MN: Hazelden Research Services.

Newman, M. (1987). *Elite women athletes survey results.* Center City, MN: Hazelden Research Services.

NFL drug users find invisible assistance. (1993, July 12). *Milwaukee Sentinel,* p. 7B.

Nilsson, S. (1995). Androgenic anabolic steroid use among male adolescents in Falkenburg. *European Journal of Clinical Pharmacology, 48,* 9–11.

North Carolina Department of Public Instruction, Alcohol and Drug Defense Program. (1991). *Alcohol and other drug use patterns among students in North Carolina public schools, grade 7–12.* Raleigh, NC: Author.

Ohaeri, J., Ikpeme, E., Ikwuagwu, P., et al. (1993). Use and awareness of effects of anabolic steroids and psychoactive substances among a cohort of Nigerian professional sports men and women. *Human Psychopharmacology, 8,* 429–432.

Pearson, B. (1994, February 7). Olympic survey: Olympians of winters past. *USA Today,* p. C5.

Pearson, B., & Hansen, B. (1992, February 5). Survey of U.S. Olympians. *USA Today,* p. 10C.

Perry, H., Wright, D., & Littlepage, B. (1992). Dying to be big: A review of anabolic steroid use. *British Journal of Sports Medicine, 26,* 259–261.

Petzel, T., Johnson, J., & McKillip, J. (1973). Response bias in drug surveys. *Journal of Consulting and Clinical Psychology, 40,* 437–439.

Polen, L., Schnider, L., Sirotowitz, A., & West, J. (1986, October). Teenage drug epidemics: Build up on steroids. *Sword and Shield.* (Available from South Plantation High School, Broward County, FL.)

Pope, H., Katz, D., & Champoux, R. (1988). Anabolic-androgenic steroid use among 1,010 college men. *The Physician and Sportsmedicine, 16,* 75–81.

Radakovich, J., Broderick, P., & Pickell, G. (1993). Rate of anabolic androgenic steroid use among students in junior high school. *Journal of the American Board of Family Practice, 6,* 341–345.

Ringwalt, C. (1989). *Alcohol and other drug use patterns among students in North Carolina public schools, grades 7–12: Results of a 1989 student survey.* Raleigh, NC: North Carolina Department of Public Instruction, Alcohol and Drug Defense Section, Division of Student Services.

Rosellini, L. (1992, February 17). The sports factories. *U.S. News & World Report,* 48–59 .

Ross, J., Winters, F., Hartmann, K., Robb, W., & Dillemuth, K. (1989). *1988–89 survey of substance abuse among Maryland adolescents.* Baltimore: Maryland

Department of Health and Mental Hygiene, Alcohol and Drug Abuse Administration.

Schuman, H., & Presser, S. (1981). *Questions and answers in attitude surveys. Experiments on question form, wording and context.* New York: Academic Press.

Schwellnus, M., Lambert, M., Todd, M., et al. (1992). Androgenic anabolic steroid use in matric pupils. *South African Medical Journal, 82,* 154–158.

Scott, J. (1971, October 17). It's not how you play the game, but what pill you take. *New York Times Magazine,* 40–41, 106–114.

Semeonoff, B. (1976). *Projective techniques.* London: Wiley.

Silvester, L. (1973). Anabolic steroids at the 1972 Olympics. *Scholastic Coach, 43,* 90–92.

Smart, R., & Blair, N. (1978). Test-retest reliability and validity information for a high school drug use questionnaire. *Drug and Alcohol Dependence, 3,* 265–271.

South Carolina Department of Education and South Carolina Commission on Alcohol and Drug Abuse. (1994). *The youth survey results regarding alcohol and other drug use in South Carolina: 1989–90 and 1992–93 school years.* N.p.: Author.

Stacy, A., Widaman, K., & Hays, R. (1985). Validity of self-reports of alcohol and other drug use. A multitrait-multimethod assessment. *Journal of Personality and Social Psychology, 49,* 219–232.

Starr, B. (1981). *Defying gravity: How to win at weightlifting.* Wichita Falls, TX: Five Starr Productions.

Stilger, V., & Yesalis, C. (1999). Anabolic-androgenic steroid use among high school football players. *Journal of Community Health, 24*(2) 131–145.

Substance Abuse and Mental Health Services Administration (SAMHSA). (1993, 1994, 1995). *National Household Survey on Drug Abuse: Population estimates, 1992, 1993, and 1994* (DHHS Publication Nos. [SMA]93-2053, [SMA]94-3017, and [SMA]95-3063). Rockville, MD: Author.

Survey shows steroid use on decline. (1997, September 15). *NCAA News,* 1.

Tanner, S., Miller, D., & Alongi, C. (1995). Anabolic steroid use by adolescents: Prevalence, motives and knowledge of risks. *Clinical Journal of Sports Medicine, 5,* 108–115.

Terney, R., & McLain, L. (1990). The use of anabolic steroids in high school students. *American Journal of Diseases of Children, 144,* 99–103.

Testosterone replacement therapy: May improve life for aging males. (1996, February). *Endocrine News, 21,* 1–7.

Texas Commission on Alcohol and Drug Abuse. (1995). *1994 Texas School Survey of Substance Abuse Among Students: Grades 7–12.* Austin, TX: Author.

Todd, T. (1983, August). The steroid predicament. *Sports Illustrated,* 66–77.

Todd, T. (1987). Anabolic steroids: The gremlins of sport. *Journal of Sport History, 14,* 87–107.

Toohey, J., & Corder, B. (1981). Intercollegiate sports participation and nonmedical drug use. *Bulletin on Narcotics, 23*(3), 23–26.

Tourangeau, R., & Smith, T. (1996). Asking sensitive questions. *Public Opinion Quarterly, 60,* 275–304.

Tourangeau, R., Smith, T., & Rasinski, K. (1997). Motivation to report sensitive behaviors on surveys: Evidence from a bogus pipeline experiment. *Journal of Applied Social Psychology, 27,* 209–222.

Tricker, R., O'Neill, M., & Cook, D. (1989). The incidence of anabolic steroid use among competitive bodybuilders. *Journal of Drug Education, 19,* 313–325.

U.S. Department of Health and Human Services, National Institute on Drug Abuse. (1992). *National Household Survey on Drug Abuse: Population estimates, 1991* (DHHS Publication No. ADM-92-1887). Rockville, MD: Author.

U.S. General Accounting Office (GAO). (1993). *Drug use measurement strengths, limitations, and recommendations for improvement* (Report GAO-PEMD 93-18). Washington, DC: Superintendent of Documents, U.S. Government Printing Office.

USOC officials cite test failures. (1995, April 9). *News-Gazette,* (Champaign, IL) p. D7.

Vaughan, R., Walter, H., & Gladis, M. (1991). Steroid use among adolescents: Another look. *AIDS, 5,* 112–113.

Volek, J., & Kraemer, W. (1996). Creatine supplementation: Its effect on human muscular performance and body composition. *Journal of Strength and Conditioning Research, 10,* 200–210.

Voy, R. (1991). *Drugs, sport, and politics.* Champaign, IL: Leisure Press.

Wade, N. (1972). Anabolic steroids: Doctors denounce them, but athletes aren't listening. *Science, 176,* 1399–1403.

Wadler, G., & Hainline, B. (1989). *Drugs and the athlete.* Philadelphia: Davis.

Wagman, D., Curry, L., & Cook, D. (1995). An investigation into anabolic androgenic steroid use by elite U.S. powerlifters. *Journal of Strength and Conditioning Research, 9,* 149–154.

Walters, M., Ayers, R., & Brown, D. (1990). Analysis of illegally distributed steroid products by liquid chromatography with identity confirmation by mass spectrometry or infrared spectrophotometry. *Journal of the Association of Official Analytical Chemists, 73,* 904–926.

Weiss, C. (1968). Validity of welfare mothers: Interview responses. *Public Opinion Quarterly, 32,* 622–633.

Whitehead, R., Chillag, S., & Elliott, D. (1992). Anabolic steroid use among adolescents in a rural state. *Journal of Family Practice, 35,* 401–405.

Williamson, D. (1993). Anabolic steroid use among students at a British college of technology. *British Journal of Sports Medicine, 27,* 200–201.

Windsor, R., & Dumitru, D. (1989). Anabolic steroid use by adolescents: Survey. *Medicine and Science in Sports and Exercise, 21,* 494–497.

World Health Organization Task Force on Methods for the Regulation of Male Fertility. (1996). Contraceptive efficacy of testosterone-induced azoospermia and oligozoospermia in normal men. *Fertility and Sterility, 65,* 821–829.

Wright, J. (1978). *Anabolic steroids and sports.* Natick, MA: Sports Science Consultants.

Wright, J. (1982). *Anabolic steroids and sports II.* Natick, MA: Sports Science Consultants.

Yesalis, C. (1996, August 1). No medals for drug testing. *New York Times,* p. A27.

Yesalis, C.E., Anderson, W.A., Buckley, W.E., & Wright, J.E. (1990). Incidence of the nonmedical use of anabolic-androgenic steroids. In G. Lin & L. Erinoff (Eds.), *Anabolic steroid abuse* (National Institute on Drug Abuse Research, Monograph 102, DHHS Publication No. ADM 90-1720). Rockville, MD: U.S. Department of Health and Human Services, Public Health Service.

Yesalis, C., & Bahrke, M. (1995). Anabolic-androgenic steroids: Current issues. *Sports Medicine, 19,* 326–340.

Yesalis, C., Barsukiewicz, C., Kopstein, A., & Bahrke, M. (1997). Trends in anabolic-androgenic steroid use among adolescents. *Archives of Pediatric and Adolescent Medicine, 151,* 1197–1206.

Yesalis, C.E., Buckley, W.A., Anderson, W.A., Wang, M.O., Norwig, J.A., Ott, G., Puffer, J.C., & Strauss, R.H. (1990). Athletes' projections of anabolic steroid use. *Clinical Sports Medicine, 2,* 155–171.

Yesalis, C., & Cowart, V. (1998). *The steroids game.* Champaign, IL: Human Kinetics.

Yesalis, C.E., & Courson, S.P. (1990). [Anabolic steroid use among a self-selected sample of NFL players]. Unpublished data.

Yesalis, C., Herrick, R., Buckley, W., Friedl, K., Brannon, D., & Wright, J. (1988). Self-reported use of anabolic-androgenic steroids by elite power lifters. *The Physician and Sportsmedicine, 16,* 91–100.

Zimmerman, P. (1986, November 10). The agony must end. *Sports Illustrated,* 17–21.

CHAPTER

4

Prevention of Anabolic Steroid Use

Linn Goldberg, MD, and Diane L. Elliot, MD

People like to think that things are better since Ben Johnson. I argue the opposite. If anything, Ben Johnson's getting caught promoted drug use. He won.

Dutch track coach Henk Kraayenhof
Sports Illustrated
April 14, 1997

This manuscript was supported in part by a grant DA-07356 from the National Institute on Drug Abuse.

Anabolic steroids (AS) are used by athletes to enhance muscle growth and strength and to improve physical performance (American Medical Association [AMA], 1990; Wade, 1972; Beckett & Cowan, 1979; Wilson & Griffin, 1980; AMA, 1988). Unlike the use of other controlled and illicit drugs, AS use typically does not have an antisocial goal and is not intended as a means to lose contact with reality (e.g., "get high"). In fact, most AS use is aimed at prosocial achievements, such as playing on a team, excelling in sports, gaining a college scholarship or professional contract, and/or developing a more "attractive" or perceived ideal appearance (AMA, 1990; Wilson & Griffin, 1980; Buckley et al., 1988). Because of the unique aspects of AS use and differences from other drugs of abuse (alcohol, marijuana, cocaine, etc.), preventing AS use requires targeted intervention methods that differ from traditional drug education techniques.

Scope of the Problem

Athletics have been thought to provide a safe haven for students, resulting in a nurturing atmosphere with an emphasis on teamwork, fair play, and ethical behavior (Coakley, 1993). Physical activity and competition in school sports is believed to help insulate adolescents from many deviant and harmful health behaviors (Levin et al., 1995; Aaron, Dearwater, & Anderson, 1995; Cowart, 1990; Du Rant, Escobedo, & Heath, 1995; Kokotailo et al., 1996). Unfortunately, there is little evidence to support this contention. In fact, for males, sports that feature aggressive contact may increase the risk of engaging in a number of health risk behaviors (Coakley, 1993). This includes use of chewing tobacco, physical violence, less frequent condom use, and not using a seat belt (Levin et al., 1995; Aaron, Dearwater, & Anderson, 1995; Kokotailo et al., 1996). In addition, adolescent athletes (male and female) are more likely to use anabolic steroids than their nonathletic counterparts (AMA, 1990; AMA, 1988; Buckley et al., 1988; Cowart, 1990).

In the early 1990s, approximately 1 million individuals in the United States used anabolic steroids for athletic achievement or to assist in gaining a more muscular physical appearance (Melchert & Welder, 1995). During the same period, use of anabolic steroids by U.S. high school students was estimated to be between one-quarter and one-half million (Cowart, 1990); the group with the highest number of users was engaged in high school football (AMA, 1988; Cowart, 1990; Committee on Sports Medicine, 1989). More recent assessments of AS use by the Youth Risk Behavior Survey (Centers for Disease Control, 1996) shows that nearly 5% of all adolescent males and 2.5% of all adolescent females (grades 9–12) report having used anabolic steroids, while the Monitoring the Future study (Johnston, O'Malley, & Bachman, 1990–1996) found 3.2% of males and 0.6% of females in high school use anabolic steroids. Overall, use by adolescents has recently increased (Greenberg, 1999), while most other illicit drug use has remained constant.

Despite its potential benefits in enhancing athletic performance, AS use can have many adverse physical and emotional consequences, and some of these are severe and irreversible (Goldberg, 1996). Problems associated with AS use include various malignancies, myocardial infarction, coagulation disorders, male pattern baldness, acne, liver disease, height stunting, lipid abnormalities, stroke, and pathological mood disorders (Melchert & Welder, 1995; Goldberg, 1996; Haupt & Rovere, 1984; Bierly, 1987; Pope & Katz, 1988). National and international athletic associations, including the U.S. Olympic Committee (USOC), International Olympic Committee (IOC), and National Collegiate Athletic Association (NCAA), and health organizations, such as the American Medical Association (AMA), American College of Sports Medicine (ACSM), and American Academy of Pediatrics, have denounced AS use because of the potential of creating an unfair advantage and/or the possible harm to the user (AMA, 1988; Committee on Sports Medicine, 1989; ACSM, 1987; Fuentes, Rosenberg, & Davis, 1995).

Currently, there are no studies to assess the effect of drug treatment programs to intervene with those who currently use anabolic steroids. Since there are gender-specific mediators to anabolic steroids and other drugs of abuse, we believe it is important to establish education curricula that directly impact these unique factors for drug prevention (Elliot et al., 1997; Center on Addiction and Substance Abuse, 1996; Aaron, Dearwater, & Anderson, 1995). This chapter will deal with prevention efforts among male adolescent athletes, a vulnerable group with the highest AS use.

Drug-Testing Policy

The usual response to athletes' drug abuse behaviors is drug surveillance (Fuentes, Rosenberg, & Davis, 1995; Husch, 1933; USOC, 1996). Drug testing in international Olympic competition began during the Mexico City Olympics in 1968. Testing for anabolic steroids started in 1976. Although drug testing of elite, professional, and college athletes is now routine, mandatory random drug testing of adolescents engaged in middle school and high school sport is controversial. However, a recent Supreme Court decision supported drug testing as an appropriate deterrent for adolescent athletes (*Vernonia School District 47 v. Acton,* 1995). This legal policy is being considered and adopted by a number of school districts throughout the United States (Elsner, 1990; American Academy of Pediatrics, 1996; Fuller, 1996; "High School Athletes," 1997; Taylor, 1997). The majority decision, written by Justice Antonin Scalia, states,

It seems self-evident that a drug problem, largely fueled by the "role model" effect of athletes' drug use, and of particular danger to athletes, is effectively addressed by making sure that athletes do not use drugs.

The Court believes that a drug-testing policy is reasonable when comparing "negligible" individual interest against this "compelling" public interest.

The policy of drug testing is found in many other societal sectors besides sport, including the military, private business, and federal agencies (Fuentes, Rosenberg, & Davis, 1995; Husch, 1933; USOC, 1996; Peat, 1995; Normand, Lempert, & O'Brien, 1994). These policies provide a model for drug testing in school athletic programs. Some school districts have initiated a policy of random drug testing to deter substance abuse among adolescents (*Vernonia School District 47 v. Acton,* 1995; Elsner, 1990; "Drug, Alcohol Use," 1996), in part due to the ineffectiveness of many drug prevention programs and because of the widespread use of drugs by young athletes (ACSM, 1987; Faulkner & Slattery, 1990). By upholding random drug testing of middle school and high school athletes (*Vernonia School District 47 v. Acton,* 1995), the Court invoked the Fourth Amendment balancing test, suggesting that "students have a diminished expectation of privacy, and this is especially true in the context of athletic competition." The majority opinion characterized the surveillance system of urine testing as only a "minor intrusion."

Although testing for AS use was not a consideration in the Supreme Court case, it is logical to assume that adding anabolic steroid to the drug-testing list would be justifiable. Unfortunately, it is not clear whether a policy of school-based drug testing has any merit for adolescents. There has never been a prospective controlled study to determine the efficacy of a drug surveillance policy to retard initiation and use of drugs among adolescents (Jacobs & Morag, 1992). In fact, despite spending over $1.2 billion for drug tests in the workplace, no scientific assessments of preventive measures have ever been performed on this large population (Normand, Lempert, & O'Brien, 1994). Even if effective, a drug-testing policy may be of use only during the athlete's sport season or school year, and its ability to alter behavior during the rest of the year or the future is unknown. There may be no sustaining benefit when the student is placed in another environment without the necessary knowledge and skills to resist future drug use.

Another argument against drug-testing approaches is that surveillance programs fail to provide training in healthy and socially acceptable alternative behaviors and lead targeted subjects to become more adept at concealing undesirable behavior, rather than reducing drug use (Fuentes, Rosenberg, & Davis, 1995; "Drug, Alcohol Use," 1996). The American Academy of Pediatrics Committee on Substance Abuse suggests that involuntary testing is not appropriate for children and adolescents (American Academy of Pediatrics, 1996). In any event, those schools who initiate a drug-testing program have no evidence that it works, and some may be responding to pressures to "just do something."

Alternatively, there may be environmental factors at work when schools adopt a drug-testing program. Although these factors are theoretical at present, the influence of the school environment is paramount in predicting drug use among teens. High school students indicate that the degree of concern by school personnel (principals, teachers) influences drug-use behaviors (National Center on Addiction and Substance Abuse, 1997). When a school environment suggests to students that a "drug-free" policy exists, significantly less drug use occurs. By adopting a policy of drug surveillance among "role model" athletes, school officials and coaches may be sending a clear message that AS use and/or other drug use is not tolerated. We, along with others, have found that drug testing athletes in high school and at the collegiate level is highly acceptable, both to the athletes and their school administrators (National Center on Addiction and Substance Abuse, 1997; Anderson, Albrech, & McKeag, 1991).

Educational Strategies

Most large-scale drug-abuse interventions have been limited to tobacco, alcohol, and other psychoactive substances (Hansen et al., 1988; Labouvie, Pandina, & Johnson, 1991; U.S. Department of Health and Human Services [USDHHS], 1997; Bangert-Drowns, 1988; Botvin, 1986). There have been three major types of educational strategies used to prevent drug abuse behaviors: (1) knowledge-only approach, (2) cognitive-affective programs, and more recently, (3) social-psychological interventions (USDHHS, 1997; Bangert-Drowns, 1988; Botvin, 1986). The results of implementing some of these programs have been contradictory, especially for the cognitive (fact-only) and affective approaches. The knowledge-only approach is not effective in reducing either drug-use intentions or abuse of drugs (Bangert-Drowns, 1988). Likewise, programs that attempt to discourage use by emphasizing only the adverse effects of drugs also are ineffective (Botvin et al., 1990). Fortunately, newer social-psychological programs have been increasingly successful. (USDHHS, 1997; Bangert-Drowns, 1988; Botvin, 1986).

Recent drug-prevention strategies have capitalized on a number of features that guide effective programs. The principles for school-based programs have been delineated by the National Institutes of Health publication entitled *Preventing Drug Use Among Children and Adolescents: A Research Based Guide* (USDHHS, 1997). In general, the program should be age appropriate, contain multiple years of intervention (an initial year and subsequent booster sessions for each successive year), have detailed lesson plans and student materials, provide training in drug-resistance skills and self-efficacy, teach actual norms of drug use, and use interactive teaching methods. The activities are intended to promote positive peer influences, empower students, and allow enough instructional dose effect (10–15 class sessions) to achieve these effects.

AS Education: The ATLAS Study

To date, our research is the only empirically tested AS prevention program (Goldberg et al., 1996a; Goldberg et al., 1996b). As we completed stepwise prevention research to observe what works and which interventions are not successful, we were able to develop a comprehensive curriculum, entitled ATLAS (Adolescents Training and Learning to Avoid Steroids) (Goldberg et al., 1996b). Initially, we used a fact-only prevention strategy for anabolic steroid use among adolescent athletes (Goldberg et al., 1990). This was done to assess whether a balanced risk-and-benefit knowledge approach would change attitudes or intentions to use anabolic steroids, even in the short term (e.g., immediately after program delivery). We found that despite knowledge improvements, no alteration in attitudes or intentions to use steroids occurred, similar to the lack of efficacy of other cognitive-based drug-prevention programs (Bangert-Drowns, 1988; Berberian, Lovejoy, & Paparella, 1976).

In our next attempt to reduce young athletes' intentions to use anabolic steroids, we performed a randomized, controlled study to assess an approach that stressed only the negative side effects of anabolic steroids (a method referred to as "scare tactics") (Goldberg et al., 1991). This was consistent with the recommendations by the Council of Scientific Affairs of the American Medical Association (AMA, 1990). This curriculum did not acknowledge any potential benefits of the use of anabolic steroids. After the intervention, no change in knowledge, attitudes, or intentions were observed. In fact, there was a trend toward increased desire to use anabolic steroids among those who received the "risk-only" approach. Despite these apparent failures, we began to develop a theoretical model of AS use prevention, with the help of correlational data and the findings of other investigations (USDHHS, 1991; Thompson et al., 1991; Bents et al., 1990; Carlson et al., 1991; Folker et al., 1992; Jarrett et al., 1992; Bandura, 1977; Fishbein & Ajzen, 1975; Jessor & Jessor, 1977). This allowed us to design a program that focused on risk and protective factors of AS use, which could potentially change intentions to use anabolic steroids and/or the onset of AS use.

Risk Factors

Drug-prevention research studies (Hansen et al., 1988; Labouvie, Pandina, & Johnson, 1991; USDHHS, 1997; Botvin et al., 1990; Goldberg et al., 1996a) have shown that certain risk factors promote substance abuse, such as dysfunctional families, poor social skills, inability to turn down a drug offer, perception of peer approval, and misperception of normative behaviors.

Other factors protect or buffer the potential user from substance abuse, including the ability to turn down a drug offer, parental disapproval of drug use, understanding actual drug use prevalence, and belief in peer intolerance to drug use. We postulated that these risk and protective factors appear to be present for AS use as well. Our data suggested that anabolic steroid use is a goal-directed activity that is reinforced by (1) peers and nonpeers (family, coaches, sport figures, media), (2) the belief in potential beneficial effects of AS use, and (3) the lack of belief in personal adverse effects of use (Goldberg et al., 1996a). Factors other than peer and nonpeer influences and positive reinforcement due to steroids' muscle building effects (USDHHS, 1991; Folker et al., 1992; Gaa, Griffith, & Cahill, 1992) have been suggested: perceived normative use behavior, "win-at-all-costs" attitudes, specific knowledge deficits about side effects of AS use (testicular atrophy, stunted growth) (Thompson et al., 1991), lack of personal vulnerability to unwanted effects (Smith, 1980), impulsive and hostile behaviors, reduced ability to "resist" an offer of anabolic steroids, poor body image, and lack of antisteroid attitudes (Goldberg et al., 1996a).

The intervention we designed was a primary prevention program aimed at modifying those factors that increased the desire of young athletes to use anabolic steroids. In addition, sport nutrition and strength training alternatives to anabolic steroids were stressed, based on our preliminary findings that these are essential ingredients to altering adolescent intentions toward AS use (Bents et al., 1990). Because of the success of peer educators (Botvin et al., 1990; Klepp, Halper, & Perry, 1986) and the potentially powerful effect of the coach and social influences in the team setting, we capitalized on a team-centered approach to exert positive peer pressure and role modeling. We hypothesized that after the intervention, adolescents enrolled in an experimental program would reduce many of the risk factors that promote AS use, and over time this would lead to a reduction in AS use.

We studied 31 high school teams, randomized to 15 experimental and 16 control schools, in a study funded by the National Institutes on Drug Abuse (Goldberg et al., 1996b). With a data set of over 1,500 adolescent athletes, we were able to correlate potential risk factors with students' intentions to use anabolic steroids in the future (e.g., the high-risk group).

We observed that 10 factors were significantly different in this group. These athletes were more likely to believe

- that there are more good reasons to use anabolic steroids than reasons not to use them,
- that anabolic steroids do not have many adverse effects,
- that they will personally not likely suffer from the negative effects of AS use,
- that more of their friends use drugs,
- that more people are using anabolic steroids than actually do,
- in winning at all costs,
- that their coach is more tolerant of AS use,
- in their athletic potential and ability,
- in a positive image of AS users, and
- that they have less ability to control their emotions and exhibit more impulsive behavior.

Pilot Research

Prior to implementation of our large randomized, controlled study, a feasibility trial was performed with two urban high schools, consisting of 70 students (Goldberg et al., 1996a). The intervention scheme initially consisted of 16 forty-five minute sessions, 8 in the classroom and 8 in the weight room. The coach and peer leaders led the class in the intervention after being trained by research staff. The topics included in the intervention are found in figure 4.1. The project's strength trainers directed the weight-training sessions.

The results showed that those who completed the ATLAS program had less desire to use anabolic steroids, even if their friends used them, were less likely to believe that AS use was a good idea, believed steroids were more dangerous, improved their body image, had a greater understanding of alternatives to steroid use, and had less belief that dietary supplements were beneficial. After reviewing the program components, we were able to refine and condense the intervention to a 7-week curriculum. This provided a better fit to the school athletic season and the necessary research requirements: informed consent, preprogram questionnaires, postprogram questionnaires, and coach and peer training periods.

The ATLAS Study Design

Our long-term study consisted of 31 Portland, Oregon, metropolitan high schools (Goldberg et al., 1996b). Fifteen schools received a 7-week prevention intervention during the sport season. The control schools re-

Classroom Session Topics

1. Adolescent testosterone production and side effects of AS use
2. Weight training for muscular endurance, strength, and power
3. Review and critique of bodybuilding magazines: finding side effects and ads to treat side effects (acne medication, surgery for gynecomastia, hair replacement ads)
4. Detecting high- and low-fat foods, high-protein and high-carbohydrate foods; how to make food choices in the supermarket and at restaurants
5. Fluid needs, pre- and post-exercise snacks, and protein and calorie requirements for adolescent athletes
6. Refusal skills with role play
7. Developing public service campaigns against anabolic steroids
8. Debunking the effects of most supplements (amino acids, protein powders, and over-the-counter "ergogenic agents")
9. The effects of other drugs (alcohol, marijuana, cocaine, amphetamines, etc.) on athletic performance
10. High school and college age norms of drug use (anabolic steroids and other drugs)

Figure 4.1 ATLAS curriculum content.

ceived a standard pamphlet about anabolic steroids during the same time frame. Both experimental and control schools were similar with respect to total school enrollment, socioeconomic status, percent minority, and number of students participating in the free-lunch program. A total of 1,506 high school football players volunteered, consented to, and completed the study. Fifteen schools (N = 704 students) were in the experimental group, and 16 schools (N = 802 students) participated in the control group. All participants were assessed three times by confidential questionnaire. Just before the 9-week sport season and about a week after the season's conclusion constituted the time period for the short-term results. The long-term follow-up occurred 9 months (for graduating 12th-grade students) and 12 months (for returning high school athletes) after initial questionnaires were completed. Parents, coaches, and other school personnel were not present during the assessments and did not have access to subject questionnaires or the coding list.

Self-Report Questionnaire

The principal assessment instrument was a self-report questionnaire of 168 items, developed for this study, using items from earlier AS investigations (Goldberg et al., 1996b; Goldberg et al., 1990; Goldberg et al., 1991). The questionnaire assessed AS use, knowledge of drug effects, attitudes toward anabolic steroids, and behavioral intent to use anabolic steroids. Questions dealing with alcohol and other drugs were taken from established national high school surveys (Johnston et al., 1987). Other portions of the questionnaire concerned nutrition and exercise knowledge, normative drug-use behaviors, belief in media messages, impulsivity, hostility, attitudes toward drug refusal, body image, feelings of athletic competence (self-efficacy), and beliefs about parents' and coaches' steroid attitudes, all considered to be potential mediators for AS use.

The major portion of the questionnaire asked students to respond to each statement by marking a 7-point agreement scale that ranged from "strongly disagree" to "strongly agree." Similar agreement scales have been used in other research instruments, measuring the intensity of belief, opinion, and behavioral intent (Goldberg et al., 1996a; Goldberg et al., 1990; Goldberg et al., 1991; Likert, 1932; Anastasi, 1976; Best, 1981). Other questionnaire items used multiple-choice and forced-response queries.

The ATLAS Program

ATLAS consisted of 7 sessions delivered in a classroom setting and 7 sessions of weightlifting instruction with team members during the football season. Classroom activities were delivered by the coaching staff and coach-designated peer leaders. Peer-delivered education has been found to be successful in other drug abuse prevention efforts (Botvin et al., 1990; Klepp, Halper, & Perry, 1986). Approximately 60% of the classroom curriculum was directed by peers to enhance program delivery. The ratio of peer leaders to student-athlete participants was approximately 1:5. Classroom sessions were directly observed by research staff to assess coach and peer-leader fidelity to the curriculum. In addition, schools were assigned a physical trainer from the ATLAS staff, who would direct the 7-session weight room intervention to enhance exercise self-efficacy and reinforce salient features of the curriculum.

The curriculum content (figure 4.1) addresses the mediators of AS use and other drug use risk factors. Figure 4.2 displays the overall curriculum process (e.g., implementation scheme) of the program. Strength training and sport nutrition alternatives to exogenous anabolic steroids are used to provide students with dietary and exercise skills to improve nutrition and weightlifting self-efficacy. Nutrition goals were practiced with homework assignments (sport nutrition goals). Skills to refuse an offer of anabolic steroids and other illicit drugs were practiced in class, as this strategy has been used to reduce smoking among adolescents (Ary et al., 1990). Antisteroid media messages were developed and presented by students using video productions, brief theatrical presentations, songs, posters, and simulated radio announcements.

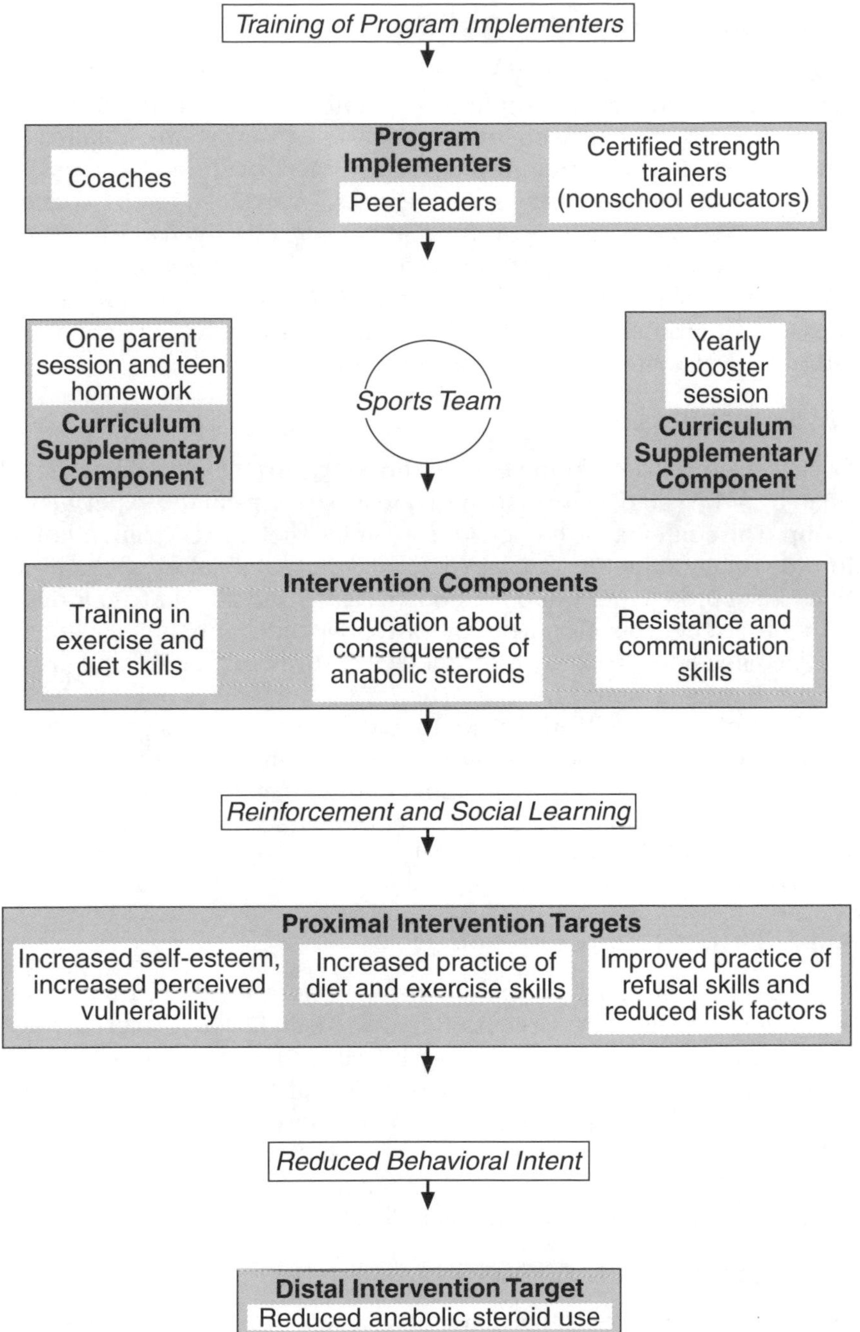

Figure 4.2 ATLAS curriculum process.

Coach and Peer Leader Training

Coaches in the experimental schools were provided with a daylong in-service and a curriculum guide to facilitate delivery of the classroom sessions. Those who missed this session were given an individualized or small group in-service that mirrored the larger coach training session. Peer leaders, referred to as "squad leaders," were selected by coaches and were trained in groups of 5 to 30 participants over a 3 to 4 hour period. These students were provided with curriculum manuals and step-by-step instruction, practicing activities that would be modeled in the classroom sessions. For their involvement, squad leaders received a letter of participation and a sweatshirt with the study logo.

Student Materials

Pocket-sized sport nutrition guides and weight-training booklets, developed by ATLAS staff, were distributed to all students in the experimental group. The contents of the booklets included dietary recommendations for adolescent athletes: low fat (below 30% of total calories), high protein (1 g of protein per pound of body weight), and adequate calories to promote strength development, the latter dependent on their weight and body composition. Healthy food choices at the supermarket and at fast-food restaurants were provided. The "ergogenic" effect of many advertised supplements with unsubstantiated claims, including protein and amino acid powders and pills, was debunked. The weight-training booklet explained techniques of strength conditioning. Safety recommendations were listed and a variety of machine and free-weight and stretching exercises were visually displayed. All students received T-shirts with the ATLAS logo to reinforce student involvement.

Parent/Guardian Involvement

Parents and guardians of student-athletes were involved by a single-evening parent meeting, organized by ATLAS staff. The discussion centered on program goals and a description of the prevention intervention. A question-and-answer session followed the presentation. Each student-athlete's parent(s) received *The Family Guide to Sports Nutrition*, a booklet developed and produced by ATLAS staff and similar to the student's nutrition guide, but with some added detail and information about meal planning and about anabolic steroids.

School Cafeteria Intervention

Most, but not all schools, participated in a school cafeteria intervention, provided by an ATLAS nutrition consultant. The cafeteria lunches emphasized ATLAS meals (less than 30% calories from fat), with high amounts of protein and carbohydrate. This allowed students to model the nutrition behaviors at the school when purchasing lunches and provided an added environmental influence.

Student members of the control school football teams received none of the enhanced intervention materials or classroom sessions, as previously described. However, these students were provided with a commercially produced pamphlet, listing the problems associated with anabolic-androgenic steroid use and the ethics of fair sportsmanship.

Results of the ATLAS Program

The intervention had significant results. Student-athletes receiving the ATLAS program reported better understanding of the effects (both positive and negative) of AS use. Importantly, these young athletes, unlike the control subjects not in the program, believed that they had greater personal vulnerability to the adverse effects of anabolic steroids, felt less impulsive, and thought that their parents and coaches had greater antisteroid attitudes. Other mediators for drug use were affected as well. ATLAS-trained students observed improved self-efficacy in strength training and sport nutrition skills, greater ability to refuse an offer of steroids, improved self-esteem, less belief in media promotional images of steroid users, and most importantly, less desire to engage in future use of anabolic steroids. Most of the short-term benefits persisted at one-year follow-up, including lowered intentions to use anabolic steroids. Although not statistically significant at just one year (prior to booster), twice as many new AS users were found in the control group. In addition, health behaviors (nutrition and exercise habits) improved among ATLAS athletes. Thus, risk for future drug use was reduced and health-promoting behaviors remained enhanced up to one year after the intervention. Use of the student food guide strongly correlated with reduced risk factors and enhanced health behaviors.

Effects During Two Successive Seasons

Since AS use is more likely to occur during the sport season when peer pressures are greatest, we combined the first and second season of the ATLAS program, adding new control and experimental students during year two of the study (Goldberg et al., 1997). The program's format was similar during both years, although we allowed ATLAS staff trainers to assist coaches in facilitating some program components.

Again, similar widespread findings were observed among the students (N = 1093) in the ATLAS program when compared to control adolescent athletes (N = 1297) who received only the standard pamphlet information. Improved knowledge of anabolic steroids, alcohol, and marijuana occurred. ATLAS-trained students believed their coach was more intolerant of anabolic steroid use, had better perception of normative AS use behaviors, acquired an enhanced ability to refuse a drug offer, developed more negative attitudes towards AS users, cited more reasons for not using anabolic steroids (as well as more reasons for using anabolic steroids), believed in greater severity of the side effects of AS use and their personal susceptibility to those effects, and had improved self-esteem. Intentions to use anabolic steroids were significantly lower for the ATLAS-trained students. After two seasons, the new use of anabolic steroids was still twice as great in the control group, with a strong trend toward being statistically significant (one-tailed, $p = 0.067$).

Conclusion

The use of anabolic steroids is reinforced by the environmental influences of peers, family, coaches, media, community, and school (Bandura, 1977; Fishbein & Ajzen, 1975; Jessor & Jessor, 1977; MacKinnon et al., 1991). Risk factors that encourage use appear to be linked to feelings of greater acceptance of AS use by parents (USDHHS, 1991; Folker et al., 1992) and coaches (USDHHS, 1991; Gaa, Griffith, & Cahill, 1992), belief of lower personal susceptibility to the drug's adverse effects (Smith, 1980), favorable opinion of AS use by others, critical knowledge deficits about anabolic steroid effects and healthy alternatives (e.g., sport nutrition and strength-training techniques) (Thompson et al., 1991), and a perception that AS use is higher than it actually is. Although anabolic steroid use among adolescents remains a national problem (Buckley et al., 1988; Cowart, 1990; Centers for Disease Control, 1996; Johnston, O'Malley, & Bachman, 1990–1996; Johnson et al., 1989), AS use is preventable among this group (Goldberg et al., 1996a; Goldberg et al., 1996b; Goldberg et al., 1997). The ATLAS sample size was large and used multiple prevention techniques. Curriculum underpinnings were guided by earlier research and refined, successful program components.

Critical differences between this intervention and typical substance abuse education may explain some of the favorable outcomes observed. Most often, adolescent drug prevention is presented in a health class setting, with loose peer relationships and a teacher who generally does not have significant contact time with students. Also, peer educators are not a common feature of many school-based substance abuse prevention programs. The ATLAS drug prevention and health promotion education intervention takes place in a team setting, with peers who share common goals and who teach a major portion of the intervention. The coaches, who facilitate program implementation, have significant contact time and investment with students and can exert considerable influence. These differences alone may account for some of the findings. Importantly, the lesson plans were scripted and easy to follow, reducing the need to "reinvent" the activities, which is a common problem in implementing school-based drug-prevention programs.

Parents were involved by receiving a family sport nutrition guide, with information about steroid use and abuse. Many attended a local evening meeting to discuss AS use, the ATLAS curriculum, and have questions answered by ATLAS staff. Parents were instructed to be explicit about their disapproval of AS, have realistic performance goals, and reinforce the healthy alternatives to performance-enhancing drugs. The findings of improved health behaviors among those in the experimental condition supports the effectiveness of the intervention model.

Prevention programs for AS use among those not engaged in team sports have never been studied. Use of the ATLAS intervention in health classes may result in similar benefits if a team-like atmosphere can be created. Although drug testing as performed in national and international competitions may be a deterrent to use of anabolic steroids and other drugs, this requires future study.

Anabolic steroid prevention can be effectively delivered in a sports-team setting, when the intervention involves peers, coaches, parents, and the school environment. The favorable findings of the ATLAS intervention suggest that the future use of anabolic steroids can be curbed and healthy behaviors may once again be fostered in sport.

References

Aaron, D.J., Dearwater, S.R., & Anderson, R. (1995). Physical activity and initiation of high-risk behaviors among adolescents. *Medicine and Science in Sports and Exercise, 27,* 1639–1645.

American Academy of Pediatrics, Committee on Substance Abuse. (1996). Testing for drugs of abuse in children and adolescents. *Pediatrics, 98,* 305–307.

American College of Sports Medicine. (1987). Position statement on the use and abuse of anabolic/androgenic steroids in sports. *Medicine and Science in Sports and Exercise, 19,* 534–539.

American Medical Association, Council on Scientific Affairs. (1988). Drug abuse in athletes: Anabolic steroids and human growth hormone. *Journal of the American Medical Association, 259,* 1703–1705.

American Medical Association, Council on Scientific Affairs. (1990). Medical and non-medical uses of anabolic-androgenic steroids. *Journal of the American Medical Association, 264,* 2923–2927.

Anastasi, A. (1976). *Psychological testing.* 4th ed. New York: Macmillan.

Anderson, W.A., Albrech, R.R., & McKeag, D.B. (1991). A national survey of alcohol and drug use by college athletes. *The Physician and Sportsmedicine, 19,* 91–104.

Ary, D., Biglan, A., Glasgow, R., Zoref, L., et al. (1990). The efficacy of social influence programs versus "standard care": Are new initiatives needed? *Journal of Behavioral Medicine, 13,* 281–296.

Bandura, A. (1977). *Social learning theory.* Englewood Cliffs, NJ: Prentice-Hall.

Bangert-Drowns, R.L. (1988). The effects of school-based substance abuse education: A meta-analysis. *Journal of Drug Education, 18,* 243–264.

Beckett, A.H., & Cowan, D.A. (1979). Misuse of drugs in sports. *British Journal of Sports Medicine, 12,* 185–194.

Bents, R., Young, J., Bosworth, E., Boyea, S., Elliot, D., & Goldberg, L. (1990). An effective educational program alters attitudes toward anabolic steroid use among adolescent athletes. *Medicine and Science in Sports and Exercise, 22,* S64.

Berberian, R.M., Lovejoy, J., & Paparella, S. (1976). The effectiveness of drug education programs: A critical review. *Health Education Monographs, 4,* 377–398.

Best, J.W. (1981). *Research in education.* 4th ed. Englewood Cliffs, NJ: Prentice-Hall.

Bierly, J.R. (1987). Use of anabolic steroids by athletes—do the risks outweigh the benefits? *Postgraduate Medicine, 82,* 67–74.

Botvin G.J. (1986). Substance abuse prevention research: Recent developments and future directions. *Journal of School Health, 56*, 369–374.

Botvin, G.J., Baker, E., Filazzola, A.D., & Botvin, E.M. (1990). A cognitive-behavioral approach to substance abuse prevention: One-year follow-up. *Addictive Behaviors, 15,* 47–63.

Buckley, W.E., Yesalis, C.E., Friedl, K.E., et al. (1988). Estimated prevalence of anabolic steroid use among high school seniors. *Journal of the American Medical Association, 260,* 3441–3445.

Carlson, H., Cleary, B., Carlson, N., et al. (1991). Ergogenic drugs among high school athletes: Trends in knowledge and abuse. *Medicine and Science in Sports and Exercise, 23,* S18.

Center on Addiction and Substance Abuse, Columbia University. (1996, June). *Substance abuse and the American woman.* New York: Author.

Centers for Disease Control. (1996, September 27). Youth risk behavior surveillance. United States, 1995. *Morbidity and Mortality Weekly Report (MMWR), 45,* SS4.

Coakley, J. (1993). Sport and socialization. In J.O. Holloszy (Ed.), *Exercise and sport sciences reviews* (Vol. 21, pp. 169–200). Baltimore: Williams & Wilkins.

Committee on Sports Medicine. (1989). Anabolic steroids and the adolescent athlete. *Pediatrics, 83,* 127–128.

Cowart, V.S. (1990). Blunting "steroid epidemic" requires alternative, innovative education. *Journal of the American Medical Association, 264,* 1641.

Drug, alcohol use cuts football season short. (1996, October 26). Hoquiam, WA: Associated Press.

Drug testing enters high schools: 4 schools in state now use program to keep kids clean. (1996, October 31). *Seattle Times.*

Du Rant, R.H., Escobedo, L.G., & Heath, G.W. (1995). Anabolic steroid use, strength training and multiple drug use among adolescents in the United States. *Pediatrics, 96,* 23–28.

Elliot, D., Goldberg, L., Moe, E., Clarke, G., Poole, L., & Witherrite, T. (1997). A validated etiologic model for adolescent girls' future disordered eating and drug use. *Medicine and Science in Sports and Exercise, 29,* S295.

Elsner, D. (1990, January 24). Drug tests for athletes off, running at Homewood Flossmoor. *Chicago Tribune,* p. C4.

Faulkner, R.A., & Slattery, C.M. (1990). The relationship of physical activity to alcohol consumption in youth. *Canadian Journal of Public Health, 81,* 168–169.

Fishbein, M., & Ajzen, I. (1975). *Belief, attitude, intention and behavior.* Reading, MA: Addison-Wesley.

Folker, R., Ganter, B., Clear, B., Carlson, H., Elliot, D., & Goldberg, L. (1992). Adolescent anabolic steroid users vs. nonusers: Differences in knowledge and attitudes. *Medicine and Science in Sports and Exercise, 24,* S44.

Fuentes, R.J., Rosenberg, J.M., & Davis, A. (Eds). (1995). *Athletic drug reference '95.* Research Triangle Park, NC: Clean Data.

Fuller, T. (1996). Drug testing enters high schools: 4 schools in state now use program to keep kids clean. *Seattle Times* [Online], October 31. Available: http://seattletimes.com [September 21, 1999].

Gaa, G.L., Griffith, E.H., Cahill, B.R., & Tuttle, L.D. (1994). Prevalence of anabolic steroid use among Illinois high school students. *Journal of Athletic Training, 29,* 216–222.

Goldberg, L. (1996). Adverse effects of anabolic steroids. *Journal of the American Medical Association, 276,* 257.

Goldberg, L., Bents, R., Bosworth, E., Trevisan, L., & Elliot, D.L. (1991). Anabolic steroid education and adolescents: Do scare tactics work? *Pediatrics, 87,* 283–286.

Goldberg, L., Bosworth, E.E., Bents, R.T., & Trevisan, L. (1990). Effect of an anabolic steroid education program on knowledge and attitudes of high school football players. *Journal of Adolescent Health Care, 11,* 1–5.

Goldberg, L., Elliot, D., MacKinnon, D., Moe, E., et al. (1997). The ATLAS (adolescents training and learning to avoid steroids) program: Effects during 2 seasons. *Medicine and Science in Sports and Exercise.*

Goldberg, L., Elliot, D.L., Clarke, G.N., MacKinnon, D.P., Zoref, L., Moe, E., Green, C., & Wolf, S.L. (1996a). The Adolescents Training and Learning to Avoid Steroids (ATLAS) Prevention Program: Background and results of a model intervention. *Archives of Pediatrics Adolescent Medicine, 150,* 713–721.

Goldberg, L., Elliot, D.L., Clarke, G.N., MacKinnon, D.P., Moe, E., Zoref, L., Wolf, S.L., Greffrath E., Miller, D.J., & Lapin, A. (1996b). Effects of a multidimensional anabolic steroid prevention intervention: The A.T. L. A. S. (Adolescents Training and Learning to Avoid Steroids) Program. *Journal of the American Medical Association, 276,* 1555–1562.

Greenberg, B. (1999, December 17). *Survey: Teen Drug Use Stable* [Press release]. Washington, DC: Associated Press. Retrieved December 19, 1999 from the

World Wide Web: http://live.av.com/scripts/editorial.dll?eeid=1256464&eetype=article&render=y.

Hansen, W.B., Graham, J.W., Wolkenstein, B.H., et al. (1988). Differential impact of three alcohol prevention curricula on hypothesized mediating variables. *Journal of Drug Education, 18,* 143–153.

Haupt, H.A., & Rovere, G.D. (1984). Anabolic steroids: A review of the literature. *American Journal of Sports Medicine, 12,* 469–484.

High school athletes could face drug testing. (1997, August 14). Sand Point, ID: Associated Press.

Husch, Jerri. (Ed.). (1933). *Programme on substance abuse: Drug use and sport; current issues and implications for public health.* Geneva: World Health Organization.

Jacobs, J.B., & Morag, B.S. (1992). The curious rejection of drug testing by America's schools. *Teachers College Record, 94,* 208–238.

Jarrett, G., Ganter, B., Carlson, H., et al. (1992). Peer delivered anabolic steroid education: Adolescent acceptability and outcomes. *Medicine and Science in Sports and Exercise, 24,* S44.

Jessor, R., & Jessor, S.L. (1977). *Problem behavior and psychosocial development.* New York: Academic Press.

Johnson, M.D., Jay, M.S., Shoup, B., & Rickert, V.I. (1989). Anabolic steroid use by male adolescents. *Pediatrics, 83,* 921–924.

Johnston, L.D., O'Malley, P.M., & Bachman, J.G. (1987). Psychotherapeutic, licit and illicit use of drugs among adolescents. *Journal of Adolescent Health Care, 8*(1), 36–51.

Johnston, L., O'Malley, P., & Bachman, J. (1990–1996). *National survey results on drug use from Monitoring the Future study, 1989–1995: Vol. 1. Secondary school students.* Rockville, MD: U.S. Department of Health and Human Services, National Institutes of Health, National Institute on Drug Abuse.

Klepp, K.L., Halper, A., & Perry, C.L. (1986). The efficacy of peer leaders in drug abuse prevention. *Journal of School Health, 56,* 407–411.

Kokotailo, P.K., Henry, B.C., Koscik, R.E., Fleming, M.F., & Landry, G.L. (1996). Substance use and other health risk behaviors in collegiate athletes. *Clinical Journal of Sports Medicine, 6,* 183–189.

Labouvie, E., Pandina, R.J., & Johnson, V. (1991). Developmental strategies of substance use in adolescence: Differences and predictors. *International Journal of Behavioral Development, 14*(3), 3–28.

Levin, D.S., Smith, E.A., Caldwell, L.L., & Kimbrough, J. (1995). Violence and high school sports participation. *Pediatric Exercise Science, 7,* 379–378.

Likert, R. (1932). A technique for the measurement of attitudes. *Archives of Psychology, 140,* 52.

MacKinnon, D.P., Johnson, C.A., Pentz, M.A., et al. (1991). Mediating mechanisms in a school based drug prevention program: First-year effects of the Midwestern Prevention Project. *Health Psychology, 10*(3), 164–172.

Melchert, R.B., & Welder, A.A. (1995). Cardiovascular effects of androgenic-anabolic steroids. *Medicine and Science in Sports and Exercise, 27,* 1252–1262.

National Center on Addiction and Substance Abuse, Columbia University. (1997, September). *Back to School 1997—CASA National Survey of American Attitudes on Substance Abuse III: Teens and Their Parents, Teachers and Principals.* New York: Author.

Normand, J., Lempert, R.O., & O'Brien, C.P. (Eds.). (1994). *Under the influence? Drugs and the American workforce.* Washington, DC: National Academy Press. ISBN 0-309-04885-0.

Peat, M.A. (1995). Financial viability of screening for drugs of abuse. *Clinical Chemistry, 41,* 805–808.

Pope, H.G., & Katz, D.L. (1988). Affective and psychotic symptoms associated with anabolic steroid use. *American Journal Psychiatry, 145,* 487–490.

Smith, G.M. (1980). *Theories on drug abuse: Selected contemporary perspectives. Perceived effects of substance use: A general theory* (National Institute on Drug Abuse Research Monograph Series No. 30, pp. 50–58). Rockville, MD: U.S. Department of Health and Human Services.

Taylor, R. (1997). Compensating behavior and the drug testing of high school athletes. *The Cato Journal, 16*(3), 1–12.

Thompson, H., Cleary, B., Folker, R., Carlson, N., Elliot, D., & Goldberg, L. (1991). Adolescent athletes and anabolic steroid abuse: Features that characterize the potential user. *Medicine and Science in Sports and Exercise, 23,* S18.

U.S. Department of Health and Human Services. (1991). *Adolescent steroid use* (Publication No. OEI-06-90-01080). Washington, DC: Department of Health and Human Services, Office of Inspector General.

U.S. Department of Health and Human Services, National Institute on Drug Abuse. (1997, March). *Preventing drug use among children and adolescents: A research-based guide* (NIH Publication No. 97-4212). Rockville, MD: Author.

United States Olympic Committee. (1996). *National Anti-Doping Program: Policies and procedures.* Colorado Springs: USOC Drug Control Administration Division.

Vernonia School District 47 v. Acton. (1995). 15 S. Ct. 2386.

Wade, N. (1972). Anabolic steroids: Doctors denounce them but athletes aren't listening. *Science, 176,* 1299–1403.

Wilson, J.D., & Griffin, J.E. (1980). The use and misuse of androgens. *Metabolism, 29,* 1278–1295.

PART II

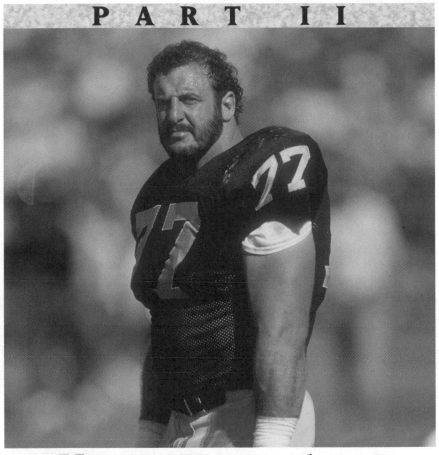

Effects, Dependence, and Treatment Issues

The background information learned in part I allows us to now turn our attention to the physical and psychological effects of anabolic steroids as well as to issues of clinical assessment and treatment.

In **chapter 5**, the author describes effects of anabolic steroid use on physical performance and body composition. He discusses the fact that androgens increase strength by enabling muscle mass gain. He also summarizes studies dealing with the effects of different doses of steroids on different types of tissue. He then explores weight gain associated with steroid use, describing changes in body composition. He also describes the converse of this, namely, body composition changes that occur with cessation of anabolic steroid use.

Adverse physical effects of anabolic steroids are discussed in **chapters 6 and 7.** Although chapter 6 concentrates on the adverse effects that are produced in normally virilized men by exogenous androgens or by pharmacological properties of the modified anabolic steroids, many of theses effects apply to women as well. Chapter 7 then focuses on the effects of anabolic steroids specific to females. Additional information on patterns of use, drugs used, and reasons for use is included as well.

In **chapter 8,** we shift our attention to psychological effects. The author discusses potential mechanisms for some androgen effects on the nervous system, the relationship between endogenous testosterone and estrogen levels and aggression, the effects of the clinical use of anabolic steroids on mood and behavior, the relationship of anabolic steroid use to mental health, and the major methodological issues involved in assessing the relationship between androgen levels and mood and behavior.

Chapter 9 reviews what we know about the potential of anabolic steroids to produce dependence, and it highlights areas for further study. The author defines *drug dependence* clinically and scientifically and discusses mechanisms, predictors, and the course of anabolic steroid dependence.

Having looked at issues of physical and psychological dependence, we now focus on clinical assessment and treatment. In **chapter 10,** the author explains the processes of identifying the steroid user in the clinical setting, assessing (or evaluating) that user, and treating the ex-user who may suffer symptoms of withdrawal.

In **chapter 11,** the authors focus on legal aspects of anabolic steroid use and abuse. They discuss the direct and indirect legal consequences of steroid use, such as drug testing, trafficking, and what constitutes criminal behavior. They also raise the issue of the legal system's role regarding steroid use.

CHAPTER

5

Effect of Anabolic Steroid Use on Body Composition and Physical Performance

Karl E. Friedl, PhD

Opinions on the efficacy of anabolic steroids tend to run parallel with respective positions on ethics.

Nicholas Wade
Science, 1972

The views, opinions, and findings in this report are those of the author and should not be construed as an official Department of the Army position, policy, or decision.

The specific competitive advantages provided to athletes by anabolic steroids have been hotly debated for several decades. A fog of confused interpretations has surrounded the same limited data (Wade, 1972). Detractors seized on the results of a large number of studies that used miniscule doses, even below replacement treatment levels, to insist that there is no effect on body composition or strength performance. On the other hand, advocates of steroid use, when faced with unpersuasive data, rationalized by arguing that benefits might not be observed if any of several complicated requirements were not met (e.g., high dietary protein intake, specific level of training, cycle of drug use, catabolic states). More recent studies on the effects of high doses of anabolic steroids provide strong experimental support for their efficacy in some types of exercise performance. Other claims based on theoretical advantages or anecdotal experience remain unsupported by the available data. This chapter reviews the current knowledge about potential advantages of anabolic steroid use by competitive male athletes.

Variations in Physiological Response to Anabolic Steroids

The principal advantages ascribed to anabolic steroids are those associated with androgenicity, or masculine traits. Upper-body strength and muscularity are two such key characteristics. In an androgen deficiency state, such as Klinefelter's syndrome, and in other states where androgens are not present in adult male levels, such as female-to-male transsexuals, anabolic steroids increase muscle mass and upper-body strength (Bhasin et al., 1997; Elbers, Asscheman, Seidell, Megens, & Gooren, 1997; Wang et al., 1996). Likewise, in adolescent males, anabolic steroid treatment is associated with increased strength and muscle mass (Gregory, Greene, Thompson, & Rennie, 1992). These are examples of the potent effects of anabolic steroids when individuals start below normal adult male levels. The effects of anabolic steroids may not simply move on a continuum from hypogonadism to hyperandrogenicity, with more of the same effect occurring in proportion to increasing steroid exposure. Hypogonadal men and castrated animals are particularly sensitive to anabolic steroids, and androgen clearance rates are lower (Bardin & Catterall, 1981; Keating & Tcholakian, 1983; Sokol et al., 1982). Thus, the important issue in this chapter, the effects of additional androgen administered to normal adult males, cannot rely on evidence from studies of clinical patients.

Anabolic steroids have effects on a wide variety of body tissues. The fundamental physiological action of anabolic steroids is thought to be exerted through hormone binding to an intracellular protein in target tissues. This hormone-receptor complex then translocates to binding sites on the chromatin, promoting gene transcription and subsequent synthesis of messenger RNA. The effects of steroid vary in different tissues according to the local environment, including enzymes present such as 5α-reductase and aromatases, and the types of receptors available. The specific biological mechanisms responsible for changes in strength and body composition are far from clear, but direct actions on the skeletal muscle are clearly a starting point. Testosterone acts directly on muscle tissue and is later eliminated as 3α-androstanediol glucuronide. There is no significant conversion to the more potent 5α-dihydrotestosterone in muscle. In other tissues, testosterone is converted to estradiol (e.g., brain) or to 5α-dihydrotestosterone (e.g., prostate), with subsequent actions through steroid receptors in those tissues, depending on the concentration of metabolite and the type and affinity of receptors in the tissue; after metabolism in these tissues, testosterone is eliminated as 5α-reduced and estrogen metabolites. Other anabolic steroids follow a similar metabolic course, to the extent that their chemical structure permits interaction with specific enzymes. Thus, plasma or urine 3α-androstanediol glucuronide is an indirect marker of peripheral androgen action in tissues such as muscle, and correlates with muscle strength changes following high-dose testosterone administration to normal men (Plymate & Friedl, 1992). An important part of the musculotrophic effect of anabolic steroids may not be directly mediated through androgen receptors but instead involves interference with catabolic effects produced by glucocorticoid hormones binding to their specific receptors. Other androgen target tissues that may be important to athletes range from neural tissue to liver and kidney, and potentially involve diverse effects, such as enhancement of IGF-1 activity, osmoregulation involving plasma volume and sodium retention, effects on immune tissues regulating cytokines, and adrenergic responses. This chapter emphasizes the empirically observed physiological effects of anabolic steroids and then considers some of the evidence for mechanisms behind these net outcomes.

Comparing Anabolic Steroid Dose and Effects

Studies must be evaluated in terms of the relative potency of the steroid. This is more difficult than it might sound because the potency of various anabolic steroids relative to testosterone may also be qualitatively different, with varying effects on different tissues according to receptor-binding properties of the compound and its metabolites. Anabolic steroids were developed expressly for the purpose of obtaining qualitative differences. They exploit the difference in actions through estrogen metabolites, 5α-reduced metabolites, and direct testosterone binding on fat and brain, reproductive tissues, and skeletal muscle, respectively (Bardin & Catterall, 1981; Michel & Baulieu, 1980). This means that any "bioequivalence" comparison of steroids needs to be carefully defined by the desired action. No dose-response study comparing various anabolic steroids in a group of resistance-training athletes has ever been conducted to assess differences in musculotrophic or strength-promoting actions.

Comparative animal studies of anabolic steroid effects on muscle size and growth are somewhat unsatisfying. For example, the Hershberger test, which has been extensively used by pharmacologists to evaluate anabolic properties of a steroid, relies on the response of the rat levator ani muscle (Hershberger, Shipley, & Meyer, 1953). The levator ani muscle was chosen to represent nonreproductive "anabolic" actions because it was more responsive to anabolic steroid than any other muscle; unfortunately, there are also important qualitative metabolic differences that make the levator ani muscle a unique responder (Knudsen & Max, 1980; Rance & Max, 1984), and it has been shown to have a 10-fold higher concentration of androgen binding sites than other muscle (Hughes & Krieg, 1988). Thus, this test may not be informative about effects on skeletal muscle.

Kochakian discovered early in his experiments that not all skeletal muscle responds to anabolic steroids equally. When he administered anabolic steroids to androgen-deficient guinea pigs, he found the predominant effect to be on upper-body muscles in the region of the shoulder girdle (see chapter 1). There are important species differences, as well. For example, the guinea pig temporal muscles are especially responsive to testosterone treatment, as are frog forearm muscles (Papanicolaou & Falk, 1938; Lyons, Kelly, & Rubinstein, 1986; Thibert, 1986). Nevertheless, what Kochakian observed is consistent with the stereotypical body shape of normally virilized men, with wider shoulders and larger necks than their normal female counterparts (Hamilton, 1948). In a study with a small number of men receiving testosterone or nandrolone injections for six weeks, we also found the main increases in body circumferences in the shoulders and chest (Friedl, Dettori, Hannan, Patience, & Plymate, 1991). If anabolic steroids have such different effects on specific muscle regions, then the muscle end point used to assess the effects of a compound must also be carefully defined. In other words, if upper-body musculature is most affected, strength tests involving these muscles would be most promising in a research investigation, as opposed to tests involving legs, for example.

With an incomplete understanding of how anabolic steroids exert their effects on skeletal muscle, nitrogen balance at least provides an approximate index of muscle protein status and provides a noninvasive method for human studies. Changes in body weight provide another measure of anabolism. When these effects were compared between orally active anabolic steroids in human studies, oxymetholone (Anadrol) and fluoxymesterone (Halotestin) were 3 times more potent, oxandrolone (Anavar) was 6 times more potent, and methandienone (Dianabol) was 10 times more potent than methyltestosterone (Liddle & Burke, 1960). As little as 1.25 mg/d methandienone produced positive nitrogen balance and weight gain in adults, and 2.5 mg/d produced higher amounts of weight gain (about 2.5 kg) in 1 month of treatment (higher doses did not produce greater weight gain). These anabolic effects occurred at doses that were lower than the 15 mg/d estimated for full androgenic replacement treatment in hypogonadal men (Liddle & Burke, 1960).

It is important to note that anabolic properties that are advantageous to an athlete are likely to extend beyond the effects defined by nitrogen retention and weight gain. Other typical "anabolic" properties range across a variety of actions, including increasing bone mineral accretion, counteracting the effects of corticosteroids to break down tissue, neurobehavioral actions related to motivation and extraversion, or simply increasing appetite. Different anabolic steroid compounds may affect each of these end points differently.

Empirical Strength Studies

In the first published strength study with normal men, Dr. Ancel Keys and his colleagues dosed 4 medical students with methyltestosterone (50 mg/d) and found no change in grip strength after 3 weeks of treatment (Samuels, Henschel, & Keys, 1942). These results must have been a great disappointment to the investigators, since much was expected from these new steroid wonder drugs. With benefit of hindsight, we know that the dependent measure was inadequate; grip strength is a convenient indicator of pubertal strength gains (Stolz & Stolz, 1951) but does not represent changes in large muscle groups and may not track change in overall muscle mass and strength in adult males (Johnson, Friedl, Frykman, & Moore, 1994). The medical students were not trained and did not engage in any grip-strength training; more recent studies demonstrate the importance of both the level of experience of the subjects and consideration of specific training during the study, appropriate to the dependent strength measures. In the 50 years since this study, methyltestosterone has not been shown to produce any great strength benefits and may be the wrong anabolic steroid on which to base conclusions about the entire class of drugs. The same study conducted with high doses of testosterone propionate (Kenyon, Knowlton, Sandiford, Kock, & Lotwin, 1940) may have radically altered the early course of this research (and athletic competition).

No other significant studies of the effects of anabolic steroids on physical performance were undertaken until 25 years after the study by Keys' group. Since then, two dozen reports, primarily from studies conducted in the 1970s, have considered the effects of anabolic steroids on strength. These studies have been repeatedly reviewed and interpreted, and at least three excellent syntheses of knowledge derived from the data have been published, reflecting the perspective of an exercise physiologist (Wright, 1980), two orthopedic surgeons (Haupt & Rovere, 1984), and an endocrinologist (Wilson, 1988). The reader is referred to these review articles for more in-depth analysis of the individual studies than will be presented here.

Strength Gains Reported With Methandienone

The best evidence for strength benefits from anabolic steroids comes from studies with methandienone (Dianabol). In contrast to methyltestosterone, methandienone has a long record of use by strength athletes with anecdotal reports of great gains. This pointed the way to the steroid with the greatest likelihood of a research payoff in investigations of steroid-induced strength effects; so, it is no coincidence that the majority of studies have been conducted with methandienone. The frequently cited review by Haupt and Rovere (1984) sorted two dozen studies into those that reported strength and body weight gains and those where there was no effect; nearly all of the studies in the group where strength gains were noted employed methandienone. Even considering only the 16 studies that had used properly blinded designs, Wilson (1988) found that the only studies reporting strength gains involved methandienone. If the same studies are considered only on the basis of muscular strength improvements measured by a single repetition maximum (1-RM) bench press, the count for strength improvement studies using methandienone is higher than reported in either of the reviews. Nearly every study concluding with significant gains in strength was also associated with an increase in body weight. Twelve studies resulting in strength improvements were performed with methandienone (Dianabol) given orally for 3 to 13 weeks in doses ranging between 5 and 100 mg/d but most using 10 mg/d (Ariel, 1973, 1974; Freed, Banks, Longson, & Burley, 1975; Hervey et al., 1981; Johnson & O'Shea, 1969; Johnson, Fisher, Silvester, & Hofheins, 1972; Loughton & Ruhling, 1977; O'Shea, 1971; Stamford & Moffatt, 1974; Tahmindjis, 1976; Ward, 1973; Win-May & Mya-Tu, 1975). These doses were above the range that is predicted to be nitrogen retaining and to produce weight gain (>5 mg/d) (Liddle & Burke, 1960). A negative study (Hervey et al., 1976) stands out as an outlier from the many studies that found improvements, particularly because of the extraordinarily high dose of methandienone employed (100 mg/d). This was one of the few methandienone studies that did not assess bench-press performance, and, although there were dramatic improvements in the leg press (with mean increases of 61 kg, along with an increase in X-ray–measured thigh muscle size), the control group also demonstrated comparable strength increases, even without the change in thigh muscles (Hervey, 1975; Hervey et al., 1976). Another methandienone study counted as negative in the review by Haupt and Rovere (1984) actually found significant improvements *only* in the 1-RM bench-press performance (Loughton & Ruhling, 1977). Only one methandienone study has been reported with no change in weight or in strength (Golding, Freydinger, & Fishel, 1974). Results of all available methandienone studies reporting data on weight gain and changes in bench-press performance are shown in table 5.1. The evidence for efficacy of this anabolic steroid for bench-press performance is compelling.

Strength Gains With Other Anabolic Steroids

At least seven studies using steroids other than methandienone have reported no significant increases in strength; only one of these seven studies noted an increase in body weight. When the relative potency of these other steroids is considered, these results also make some sense. Nearly every study in this group failed to employ a steroid dosage that would be expected to produce an effect in normal men; these other steroids did not have the history of athlete use and anecdotal dosing recommendations that is available for methandienone. The absence of weight gain in these studies is one line of evidence that the doses used were below the threshold required for important biological effects for normal men. As will be discussed in the next section, body weight is a highly consistent finding in studies employing high doses of anabolic steroids.

Two studies used injections of potentially potent nandrolone and testosterone preparations (Fahey & Brown, 1973; Crist, Stackpole, & Peake, 1983), but clearly these were conducted with inadequate doses. The doses used (100 mg/wk, or less) are at the threshold of "replacement" levels in normal men, providing a level of biological action similar to that normally provided by the endogenous androgens, the secretion of which has been suppressed by drug administration (Schulte-Beerbuhl & Nieschlag, 1980; Belkien, Schurmeyer, Hano, Gunnarsson, & Nieschlag, 1985). We used the same steroids at these low doses for control comparisons to effects at high doses (300 mg/wk). The low dose of testosterone did not raise circulating levels above normal baseline after six weekly injections, and neither one of these drugs provided the biological effects, including strength gains observed at the higher doses in the same study (Friedl et al., 1991). Rather than a dose-response relationship between these injectable esters and strength gains, all that has been demonstrated to date is a dose threshold; the studies available to Haupt and Rovere fell below this threshold of effect. More recent studies with higher doses

Table 5.1 Summary of Increases in Body Weight and 1-RM Bench Press Associated With Methandienone Administration to Healthy Young Men

Reference	Dose (mg/d)	Time (wk)	Study design	Skill level	Cont. train	Sample size	Group (#subjects)	Body weight (kg) start	Body weight (kg) Δ	Bench press (kg) start	Bench press (kg) Δ
Johnson & O'Shea, 1969	10	3	NB	UT	Y	24	Drug (12)	77.5	+2.5*	107	+16.4*
							Control (12)	80.7	+0.3	97	+6.4
O'Shea, 1971	10	4	DB	T	Y	18	Drug (9)	—	+3.9*	—	+16.9*
							Placebo (9)	—	+1.3	—	+7.4
Johnson et al., 1972	10	3	DB	UT	Y	31	Drug (12)	—	+2.4*	—	+13*
							Placebo (12)	—	+1.0*	—	+8
							Control (7)	—	+0.2	—	+5
Ward, 1973	10	4	SB	T	Y	16	Drug (8)	92.2	+1.3[1]	119	+15.6*
							Placebo (8)	87.5	+0.9	114	+4.8

Loughton & Ruhling, 1977	10 + 5	3 + 3	DB	UT/T	Y	12	T-Drug (3)	71.3	+5.6*	88.4	+23.5
							T-Con (3)	73.0	+3.0	87.7	+20.4
							UT-Drug (3)	80.4	+5.0*	66.5	+13.6
							UT-Con (3)	87.6	+1.2	81.6	+9.1
Stamford & Moffat, 1974	20	4	SB	T	Y	12[2]	Drug (6)	78.6	+2.3*	130	+7.2*
							Placebo (6)	79.4	+0.1	122	+3.8
Hervey et al., 1981	100	6	DB, X	T	Y	7	Drug (7)	87.4	+2.3*	93.9	+12.7*
							Placebo (7)	87.9	–1.3	90.0	+4.6

Time = duration of experimental group drug administration (some of the studies also included a preliminary training phase without drug); study design: NB = not blinded, SB = single-blind study, DB = double-blind study, X = crossover design; skill level: T = previous experience with resistance training, UT = exercise training–naive subjects; cont. train: Y indicates a specific physical training program was part of the drug administration phase of the study design; an asterisk indicates a statistically significant difference ($p < .05$) between control and/or placebo groups and the drug group.

[1] Body composition estimated from underwater weighing indicated +3.1 kg FFM and –1.7 kg fat mass for experimental group vs. +1.1 kg FFM and –0.1 kg fat mass for control group.

[2] Only the drug and placebo group data are shown from this study, which included other comparison groups involving a different (nonrandomized) subject population.

Others who measured body weight and maximal bench press changes with methandienone but did not specifically provide data in their reports: Ariel, 1973; Freed & Banks, 1975; and Tahmidjis, 1976. All of these also reported significant increases in body weight and strength. Golding et al., 1974 found no changes in strength or weight with 10 mg/d for 9 weeks.

of testosterone enanthate (300 mg/wk or 600 mg/wk) have demonstrated gains in weight and strength measures (Friedl et al., 1991; Bhasin et al., 1996).

The study of Bhasin and his colleagues (1996), using very high dose anabolic steroid (600 mg/wk of testosterone enanthate for 10 weeks), resulted in findings comparable to the series of methandienone studies. With methandienone (10 mg/d for 12 wk), Loughton and Ruhling found a 5.6 kg weight gain and 23.5 kg improvement in the 1-RM bench press in a small number of experienced lifters; using testosterone enanthate (600 mg/wk for 10 wks), Bhasin and colleagues found a 6.0 kg weight gain and 22 kg improvement in the 1-RM bench press in experienced lifters (the methandienone study lacked the sample size to detect differences between placebo and drug in experienced and inexperienced lifters). The results of the testosterone study also suggested additive effects of exercise and drug, with a bench-press improvement of approximately 10 kg produced by exercise or steroid, and 20 kg produced by exercise and steroid (Bhasin et al., 1996). This is an important observation that needs to be confirmed in future studies with other experimental designs. Similar results were obtained for a squat exercise, indicating that strength gains may not be limited to the upper body (figure 5.1).

Other strength studies indicate thresholds of effectiveness of various other anabolic steroids. Oxandrolone was found to be effective in increasing weight and strength in one study (O'Shea & Winkler, 1970)—the doses employed were thought to be similar in potency to those used in methandienone studies (Liddle & Burke, 1960). Three studies used oral stanozolol in doses considered appropriate for treatment of osteoporosis in elderly women without major androgenic side effects (6–8 mg/d) and apparently subthreshold for effects in normal men; a steroid-associated body weight gain was observed in two studies, but only one found a significant improvement in a strength measure (Casner, Early, & Carlson, 1971; Johnson, Roundy, Allsen, Fisher, & Silvester, 1975; O'Shea, 1974). Two studies using 1-methyl derivatives (mesterolone and methenolone acetate) produced no strength gains (Fowler, Gardner, & Egstrom, 1965; Stromme, Meen, & Aakvaag, 1974). These steroids are not demethylated in the body and may have unique properties; for example, the study with mesterolone had no effect on gonadotropins, suggesting either a relatively low biological activity at this dose or significantly different properties of this steroid (Aakvaag & Stromme, 1974; Stromme, Meen, & Aakvaag, 1974).

Methodological and Design Issues

A notable difference between studies reporting no change in strength and those finding an increase is the use of a 1-RM test. Dependent measures evaluated in these strength studies have varied from maximal grip

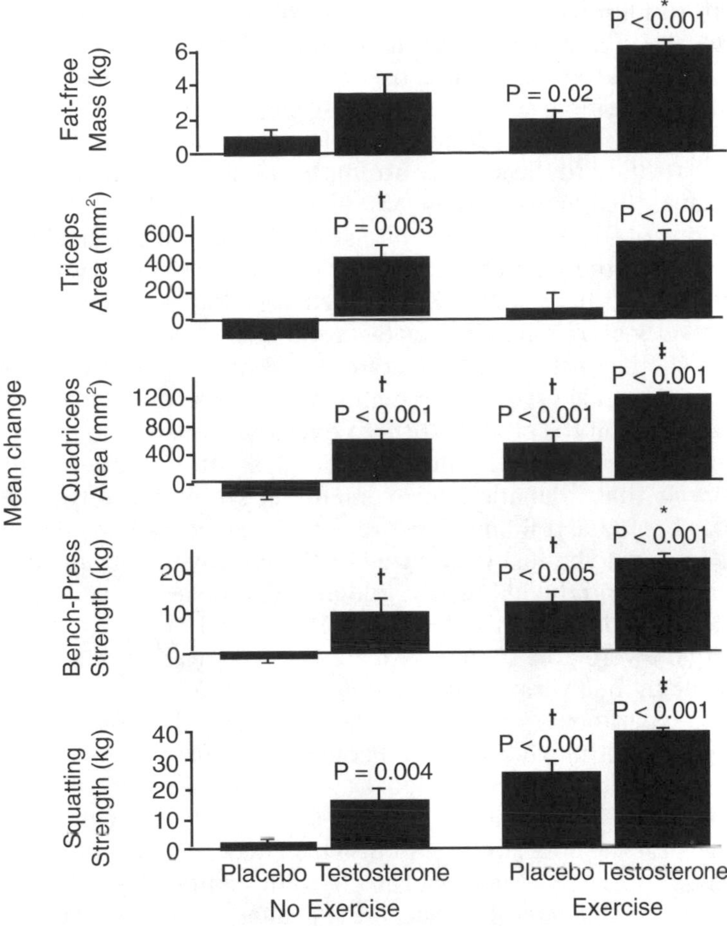

Figure 5.1 Changes from baseline measurements of fat-free mass, muscle cross-sectional areas, and strength during the experiment by Dr. Bhasin and colleagues (1996); 600 mg/wk testosterone enanthate was administered for 10 weeks. Note: The P values shown are for the comparison between the change indicated and a change of zero. The asterisks indicate $P < 0.05$ for the comparison between the change indicated and that in either no-exercise group; the daggers, $P < 0.05$ for the comparison between the change indicated and that in the group assigned to placebo with no exercise; and the double daggers, $P < 0.05$ for the comparison between the change indicated and the changes in all three other groups.

Reprinted, by permission, from S. Bhasin, T.W. Storer, N. Berman, C. Callegari, B. Clevenger, J. Phillips, T.J. Bunnell, R. Tricker, A. Shirazi, and R. Casaburi, 1996, "The Effects of Supraphysiologic Doses of Testosterone on Muscle Size and Strength in Normal Men," *The New England Journal of Medicine* 335 (6): 6.

strength to improvements in training exercises such as push-ups and pull-ups, and included cable tensiometer measurements and Cybex testing. These tend to be measures that either involve relatively small and specialized muscle groups (e.g., grip strength) or emphasize strength endurance (e.g., pull-ups). In some studies, the measured end points also had little relation to the specific strength training performed during the study; thus, the results of these studies could actually be regarded as evaluations of the effect of anabolic steroids without physical training. Irrespective of the type of training performed, nearly every study with positive findings has used a 1-RM strength test. Rather than demonstrating specificity of training, this suggests something more like a specificity of the strength effect of anabolic steroids; regardless of why this parameter is reliable, it is essential for inclusion in any future studies.

The subjects in the studies with no effect were also more likely to be inexperienced in weight training. The simplest interpretation of this observation is that dramatic improvements in strength are typically observed in the initial training of previously untrained individuals, and steroid effects could be easily obscured by the improvements in technique, coordination, and the initial physiological responses. Whatever the explanation, both Loughton and Ruhling (1977) and Hervey and colleagues (1976, 1981) were able to demonstrate larger steroid-specific effects in previously trained versus untrained men.

A good experimental design to evaluate the role of training has eluded investigators, although Bhasin and colleagues (1996) have the best yet. If only trained athletes are studied, as recommended by some researchers (Wright, 1980), the duration of any study will represent a period of detraining for the no-exercise groups. One effect of this could be to conclude inappropriately that steroid and training combined produce greater improvements than steroid alone. If the primary mechanism of strength gain is more aggressive competitive performance, training might play a relatively small role in the benefit. The alternative of recruiting sedentary subjects also confounds interpretation of changes, with large improvements expected just from learning technique and other start-up effects, including significant muscle and bone remodeling.

Future studies may demonstrate better approaches to the problems of blinding subjects to high-dose steroid treatment and teasing out the true role of exercise in the strength gains. Current studies are plagued by the problem of keeping subjects blind to their treatment to ensure that everyone has similar expectations (Ariel & Saville, 1972b; Freed et al., 1975). Discussion between subjects may unblind studies when effects involve large weight change and size differences, testicular atrophy, oily skin and acne, and subjective differences in motivation. This could be less of a problem in a dose-response study, where some of the effects such as testicular atrophy will be produced in individuals even at lower doses that produce no weight gain or strength change (Friedl et al., 1991; Young, Baker, Liu, & Seeman, 1993). In studies to understand the benefits of anabolic steroids, well-designed placebo studies help to control for the psychological effects, which appear to constitute at least one component of the performance benefit (Ariel & Saville,1972b; Johnson, Fisher, Silvester, & Hofheins, 1972).

Any future study must include measurement of anabolic steroids to assess the circulating levels of the drug and to verify that no other anabolic steroids are being used. Although assay methods were not widely available or affordable when many of the previous studies were conducted, techniques are now well established. Attached to one frequently cited strength study is an undocumented report that the drug was purchased from the test subjects by a black-market steroid distributor, and this was unknown to the investigator when the study was reported. The rumor is questionable, as the study included a placebo; however, this highlights the need to verify compliance.

Conclusions From the Empirical Strength Studies

One irrefutable conclusion from all of the available steroid strength studies is that 10 mg/d (or greater) of methandienone will produce a weight gain and an improved 1-RM bench press. In 13 separate studies employing the bench-press measure, only one did not find an improvement in the steroid-treated group (table 5.1). This occurred with or without protein supplementation and was repeatedly demonstrated in well-controlled double-blind studies. With the well-designed study by Bhasin and his colleagues (1996), it is apparent that high-dose testosterone esters can also produce improvements in bench-press strength, over and above the effect of exercise alone. It is of interest that the main drugs used by the East German sports machine in the 1970s and 1980s included an orally active compound related to methandienone, Chlorodianabol, and after drug testing was implemented in international competition, testosterone esters (Franke & Berendonk, 1997). Presumably, East German scientists were reading about the same research studies and were satisfied with the results in their drug trials with individual athletes.

Increased muscle mass is likely to be a key contributor to steroid-induced strength gains. To date, only a rough association has been demonstrated, with studies showing strength gains usually also accompanied by weight gains. More quantitative comparisons await more precise and reproducible measures of strength and of specific muscle mass changes, as discussed next.

Composition of Steroid-Induced Body Weight Gain

Anabolic steroids increase body weight. This is a universal finding and not just an effect in hypogonadal men. An early application of anabolic steroids was to induce weight gain in underweight young men and women, as well as aging veterans (Watson, Bradley, Callahan, Peters, & Kory, 1959). An application of growing interest is the use of testosterone to boost flagging testosterone levels in aging men to help maintain optimal health with better preservation of muscle mass (countering sarcopenia, or loss of muscle mass) and strength (Tenover, 1992; Urban et al., 1995; Wang et al., 1996). In male steroid contraceptive trials, the weight gain is a well-recognized effect, counted as an undesirable "side effect" to the desired contraceptive application (Swerdloff, Palacios, McClure, Campfield, & Brosman, 1978). With anabolic steroid use, normal men appear to be able to achieve a greater than normal mass. Using a height-normalized index of fat-free mass, Kouri, Pope, Katz, and Oliva (1995) demonstrated that a large sample of current steroid users presented a distinctly higher cluster of lean mass weights than did nonuser athletes or a sample of 20 Mr. America winners from the presteroid era (pre-1959). The separation of weights was distinct enough to tentatively suggest that lean mass in this upper range might even be useful in detecting steroid use.

Limits of Weight Gain

The natural limits of this weight gain are interesting to consider in light of the common response from bodybuilders after significant weight gains; invariably, they still want to be bigger. So, how much bigger can they get? Forbes has considered this question in a summary analysis of multiple studies (Forbes, 1985). He suggests that a log-dose relationship best describes the relationship between increase in lean mass and total steroid exposure. Forbes has postulated that the upper limit is around 20 kg of lean mass, equivalent to the maturational lean mass gain in adolescent males (relative to their total endogenous steroid exposure during this period of development). The highest measured increases in individuals using anabolic steroids are 9.7 kg of body weight with 140 g/d oxandrolone (Forbes, 1985) and 12.7 kg over two years in a bodybuilder using up to 100 g/d methandienone (Kilshaw, Harkness, Hobson, & Smith, 1975). However, this latter athlete also used thyroid hormone (Harkness, Kilshaw, & Hobson, 1975), which may have limited the steroid-induced gain through its catabolic effects. Although there are obvious biomechanical limits to tolerable loads on the skeleton and tendons, the mechanisms that would actually limit muscle growth are poorly defined.

The majority of short-term studies (3–10 weeks) result in 3 to 5 kg of body weight gain. The results from two of our studies are typical: a dose of 100 mg/wk of testosterone enanthate for 6 weeks was a neutral "replacement" that produced no change in weight; higher doses of testosterone enanthate, up to 300 mg/wk, and for durations up to 12 weeks, as well as lower doses of nandrolone decanoate or methyltestosterone each produced mean weight gains between 2.5 and 3 kg (Friedl, Hannon, Jones,

& Plymate, 1990; Friedl et al., 1991). Most of the methandienone studies (~10 mg/d) reported ~3 kg after 3 to 10 weeks of drug use (table 5.1).

Lean and Fat Mass Changes

The nature of this steroid-induced weight gain is still uncertain. Some of it appears to be a gain in the fat-free mass, possibly including an altered hydration; loss of fat mass is a less consistent finding and is dependent on energy balance. The primary components of the nonfat portions of body composition are water, bone mineral, protein, glycogen, and nonbone mineral, in decreasing order of their contributions by weight. Anabolic steroids are likely to affect all of these components, although no study has evaluated all of these body components at one time (table 5.2). For many athletes an increased accrual of skeletal muscle protein could be most advantageous, and this is clearly one of the effects of anabolic steroids, as demonstrated by careful studies with infusion of radiolabeled amino acid precursors of protein formation (Griggs, Kingston, Jozefowicz, Herr, Forbes, & Halliday, 1989). Increased glycogen would be useful for endurance athletes if it is available for energy utilization at the appropriate time (Jacobs, Kaiser, & Tesch, 1981). Testosterone can cause a slight weight gain through increased glycogen storage; however, rats running to exhaustion on a treadmill gained no benefit from this increased glycogen, and it appears that it may not be available for energy metabolism (Guezennec, Ferre, Serrurier, Merino, Aymonod, & Pesquies, 1984). An increase in bone mineral could be advantageous to the prevention of bone injuries in some athletes; however, the associations studied so far involve replacement therapy to hypogonadal men (Behre, Kleisch, Leifke, Link, & Nieschlag, 1997) and postmenopausal women with osteoporosis (Need, Horowitz, Bridges, Morris, & Nordin, 1989), and the effect of long-term anabolic steroid administration to healthy men may not provide the same benefit (Swartz & Young, 1988; Young et al., 1993). Increased intracellular water would not appear to be particularly advantageous to anyone, including bodybuilders, where a swelled muscle appearance is less desirable than the "cut" appearance that some competitors induce with diuretics; nevertheless, increased hydration of the lean mass remains a likely cause of weight gain, contributing to the weight gain in hypogonadal men (Bhasin et al., 1997), although this remains poorly defined for normal men.

Fat tends to increase in proportion to steroid-induced weight gains. Testosterone stimulates an increased metabolic rate but appetite also is commonly reported to increase. Welle, Jozefowicz, Forbes, and Griggs (1992) reported an increase in resting metabolic rate after 3 months of 200 mg/wk testosterone enanthate administration in three out of four normal men; however, the change could be explained by the increases in lean mass (basal metabolic rate is determined largely by the amount of

Table 5.2 Known and Suspected Effects of Anabolic Steroids on Body Composition

Component (and approx. proportions in normal man)	Effect of anabolic steroid administration
Body weight	Increase of at least several kg within several weeks of adequate anabolic steroid dosing, and possibly 20–30 kg over normal men (Forbes, 1985).
Chemical model	
Water (62%)	Appears to increase more than the increase in soft-tissue lean mass, but based only on measurements made in hypogonadal men (Bhasin et al., 1997).
Protein (17%)	Increase in protein accretion, at least acutely, in normal men; longer-term increase in total body nitrogen has also been demonstrated (Griggs et al., 1989; Hervey et al., 1981).
Fat (15%)	Changes are generally proportional to body weight change (i.e., body density remains constant) but depend on energy balance (Bhasin et al., 1996; Freidl et al., 1990).
Bone mineral (4%)	Increase, at least in hypogonadal men (Behre et al., 1997; Wang et al., 1996).
Glycogen (1%)	Increased glycogen storage in rat studies (Guezennec et al., 1984).
Nonbone mineral (1%)	Appears to increase in normal men (e.g., total body potassium concentrations are higher than seem to make sense except with greater intracellular concentration) (Hervey et al., 1976, 1981).
Morphological model	
Muscle (45%)	Increase in muscle volumes (arms and legs) and muscle fiber sizes demonstrated in normal men (Alen et al., 1984; Bhasin et al., 1996; Kuipers et al., 1993).
Bone (15%) change in	Unknown—only bone mineral has been shown to adults.
Adipose (12%)	Decrease in intra-abdominal fat stores in normal young men associated with high testosterone; subcutaneous fat tissue remains unchanged (Marin et al., 1995; Hervey et al., 1976).
Organs & other (28%)	Unknown—increases in organ weights only associated with pathology (e.g., left ventricular hypertrophy, hepatomegaly).

lean tissue). Body fat would be expected to decline as a proportion of increasing lean mass (i.e., percent body fat would decline even if fat mass were unchanged) or with increasing metabolic requirements, but only if intake remained unchanged. In castrated rats, low levels of testosterone increase appetite and stimulate weight gain; but higher doses cause weight loss (Nunez, 1982). Low doses of anabolic steroids also stimulate adipose tissue lipoprotein lipase and enhance fat storage, while higher doses, acting through estrogen metabolites, cause fat weight loss in rats (Gray, Nunez, Siegel, & Wade, 1979; Krotkiewski, Kral, & Karlsson, 1980). In normal men, testosterone is a key regulator of the distribution of fat between intra-abdominal and subcutaneous locations. A series of elegant studies by Marin has demonstrated this effect. In acute studies, after circulating levels in normal men were doubled, a greater proportion of lipid from radiolabeled milk fat was shown to be stored subcutaneously, and less went to intra-abdominal storage than in untreated men (Marin et al., 1996). A longer-term study with obese middle-aged men treated with testosterone also demonstrated a reduced triglyceride uptake in the abdominal fat (Marin, Oden, & Bjorntorp, 1995). Even if total fat mass is not reduced, testosterone has a pronounced effect on redistribution of fat away from the abdomen (Marin et al., 1992).

Total Body Potassium and Nitrogen

Several detailed studies of the composition of steroid-induced body weight gain have been conducted. Hervey and his colleagues studied 11 men in a double-blind crossover design with 100 mg/d of methandione for 6 weeks. During drug administration, the men gained 3.3 kg of weight. This increase was reflected in increases in arm, thigh, and calf circumferences, while no changes occurred during the placebo administration. Hervey concluded that the substantial increase in total body potassium indicated that the weight gain could be attributed to increased muscle mass, but it also could be intracellular water, following a steroid-induced retention of potassium (Hervey et al., 1976). Total body potassium measurements predicted that the 3.3 kg weight gain was composed of 6.3 kg lean mass gain and 2.5 kg fat loss; body density measured by underwater weighing predicted 2.4 kg lean mass gain and 0.9 kg of fat gain; skinfold thicknesses predicted no change in body fat (therefore, counting all of the weight gain against increased lean mass). A disproportionate increase in body water would have introduced an error into interpretations of body density in the direction of overestimated fat; on the other hand, a reduction of 2.5 kg of fat would certainly be expected to appear as a reduction in skinfold thickness. To help resolve the discrepancies, Hervey and his group followed this study with a second of the same design and drug dosing, but adding measurement of total body nitrogen by neutron activation analysis (unfortunately, body water measurements were lost).

In this second study, body weight gain averaged 3.6 kg and the increase in potassium was very similar to the results of the previous study. Hervey calculated that if the increased body weight reflected new muscle, body nitrogen should increase by about 100 g (Hervey et al., 1981). However, the measured increase was more than double this amount, leading the researchers to conclude that the gain was a nitrogen-rich substance that could not be described as normal muscle. Estimations about the potassium content of muscle must also remain flexible, as the conventional value of 66.6 mmol/kg of fat-free mass predict more muscle mass than was likely for either study.

Using only potassium 40 measurements to assess body composition change, Forbes and colleagues followed a group of healthy men treated with 200 mg/wk testosterone enanthate administration for 12 weeks (Forbes, Porta, Herr, & Griggs, 1992). Circulating testosterone levels were tripled by this drug regimen (Griggs et al., 1989). The average body weight gain of 4.1 kg partitioned into 7.5 kg gain of lean mass and 3.4 kg loss of fat mass, very similar to the predictions Hervey made from potassium measurements in his two studies (Hervey et al., 1976; Hervey et al., 1981). In the same study reported by Forbes, creatinine excretion was measured while the subjects were on a meat-free diet (Griggs et al., 1989). On the basis of a physiological relationship between the rate of creatinine excretion and lean mass, Forbes estimated a corresponding increase of greater than 8 kg of lean mass. This would appear to provide independent confirmation of the magnitude of lean mass increase, but this depends on the absence of a direct effect of testosterone on creatinine synthesis, an assumption that does not appear to hold true (Samuels, Henschel, & Keys, 1942). Evidence for direct effects on muscle mass was also obtained, but does not quantitatively address changes in body composition. Muscle protein synthesis rate, measured in a subset of subjects using careful tracer studies, was 25% to 30% greater than baseline measurements by the end of 12 weeks (Griggs et al., 1989).

Hydrational Changes With Anabolic Steroid Administration

After yet another series of high-dose anabolic steroid studies, we are no closer to an explanation of the steroid-specific body composition changes, but the contribution of exercise is a bit clearer. Weight changes occurred in men receiving 600 mg/wk testosterone enanthate for 10 weeks, with the largest changes (6 kg) occurring in the group also exercising during the steroid administration; men receiving steroid but not exercising gained only 3.5 kg, and placebo groups, with or without exercise, did not make appreciable gains in weight (Bhasin et al., 1996). The nature of this weight change was assessed by underwater weighing, revealing no change in body density (i.e., relative body fat may have remained constant).

Weight gain could have included an increase in hydration, but it must also have included some increase in higher density components such as protein, or body density would have decreased. MRI studies of arms and legs also confirmed an increase in muscle mass, demonstrated by an increase in muscle cross-sectional areas. These findings complemented the previously observed increase in thigh muscle width from radiographic assessments of soft tissue made by Hervey (1975).

The hydration question remains unanswered but was raised again in another study by Bhasin and his colleagues (1997) in hypogonadal men. They measured body water in a study of weight gain in hypogonadal men given replacement doses of 100 mg/wk of testosterone enanthate for 10 weeks. This is the dose that produces no change in circulating testosterone or in body weight in normal men, exactly "replacing" suppressed endogenous levels of testosterone (Friedl et al., 1991), and that brings hypogonadal men to the normal testosterone range. The men had an average weight gain of 4.5 kg; underwater weighing indicated an increase in total body density, suggesting an increase in lean mass of approximately 5 kg and a small decline in body fat; however, total body water measured by deuterium dilution increased by approximately 5.1 kg. Even with normal measurement error in the dilutional space, these results suggest an increased hydration of the soft-tissue lean mass. Interpretations of body composition from several of the standard methods of body composition, including underwater weighing (Bhasin et al., 1997) and dual-energy X-ray absorptiometry (Young et al., 1993), assume a fixed density of the lean mass; however, if lean mass properties are altered by anabolic steroid administration, these interpretations may be wrong. Future studies of healthy steroid-treated men must include careful measures of total body water and care must be taken to interpret any method in terms of the effect of hydrational changes (Friedl, 1997b).

Muscle Morphology Studies

Direct assessment of muscle tissue changes has been performed in only a few anabolic steroid studies. In the previous study, muscle biopsies were collected from the vastus lateralis of 4 subjects and no increases in muscle fiber diameter were found compared to baseline assessments; a significant increase in nonmuscular tissue was observed in the biopsies (Griggs et al., 1989). In a group of 5 Finnish athletes (powerlifters, bodybuilders, and wrestlers) self-administering a higher dose of a combination of four anabolic steroids and continued for twice as long (24 weeks), a significant increase in muscle fiber area was observed in the vastus lateralis muscle; no such change was observed in 6 control athletes (Alen, Hakkinen, & Komi, 1984). A placebo-controlled study of bodybuilders receiving nandrolone decanoate for 8 weeks also demonstrated a steroid-related increase in fiber size in the vastus lateralis muscle (Kuipers, Peeze

Binkhorst, Hartgens, Wijnen, & Keizer, 1993). These changes in muscle fiber size are important because maximal force production in a muscle is directly proportional to the cross-sectional muscle area (Ryushi & Fukanaga, 1986). However, the data from steroid studies is far from conclusive in making the connection to observed improvements in strength measurements. For example, in the Bhasin study with normal men (1996), significant increases in MRI-measured triceps and quadriceps area were observed in the two steroid-treated groups, and these men also demonstrated increases in strength performance, but the placebo-treated exercise group also demonstrated large improvements in bench-press and squat performances without changes in muscle cross-sectional areas.

Body Composition Changes After Cessation of Anabolic Steroid Use

The steroid-induced increases in body weight tend to decline over time after drug administration (Forbes et al., 1992). In the Forbes study, this decline was relatively gradual, and all but one of the subjects were sedentary subjects not specifically engaged in weight training. It may be important that steroid cessation is followed by a period of hypogonadism, while testicular function gradually returns to normal, over a period of weeks or several months (Friedl et al., 1990; Griggs et al., 1989). Although this has not been specifically studied, reduced circulating androgen during this period may help to accelerate the loss of any anabolic steroid-induced gains. How much of the gain can be sustained by physical training following drug cessation remains to be studied.

Neuromuscular and Neuropsychological Effects of Anabolic Steroid Use

Neuromuscular benefits have been suggested but remain relatively untested. On the basis of a finger-tapping test, Herrmann and Beach (1976) suggested that anabolic steroids improve psychomotor performance. These and other investigators have postulated adrenergic-like stimulant effects on the central nervous system, with close parallels to observations with amphetamines. Training alone can produce a significant shortening in patellar reflex time, and methandienone administration has also been shown to shorten patellar reflex times in weightlifters (Ariel & Saville, 1972a). However, a detailed study of a small group of elite Finnish strength athletes failed to demonstrate changes in psychomotor or motor speed tests compared to a control group not using multiple steroids in high doses (Era, Alen, & Rahkila, 1988). Both groups demonstrated improvements in isometric fast force production during 24 weeks of training, with or without anabolic steroids (Alen, Hakkinen, & Komi, 1984).

Increased aggressiveness and motivation may be very significant factors in training and competitive performance, but no detailed studies of perceived exertion or changes in training volume have been conducted. Bhasin and his colleagues detected no effects on mood or behavior after 10 weeks of high-dose testosterone treatment that increased circulating testosterone levels to 4 to 5 times greater than normal (Tricker et al., 1996). However, in another study using the same dose of testosterone ester, Pope and his colleagues found a significant increase in aggressive responses in a specially designed laboratory test (Kouri, Lukas, Pope, & Oliva, 1995). In a study with healthy young soldiers given up to 300 mg/wk for 6 weeks, we found increases on the anger subscale of the Minnesota Multiphasic Personality Inventory (MMPI) and alterations in dopamine metabolites, suggesting a biochemical basis for observed neurobehavioral changes (Hannan, Friedl, Zold, Kettler, & Plymate, 1991). Reports of uncontrolled aggression in some steroid users are too inconsistent to account for enhanced competitive performance, but investigators have frequently cited the subjective impressions of research volunteers about increased motivation levels and increased self-confidence (Hannan et al., 1991). For example, O'Shea found no changes in the objective measures of performance he applied to his swimmers, but the coaches and athletes were convinced that the swimmers had a greater recovery capacity and trained harder while using methandienone (O'Shea, 1970). These subjective observations of increased motivation and better recovery have been expressed frequently enough in other studies and in anecdotal accounts by athletes that they bear further investigation.

Individual experiments conducted by East German scientists with their athletes were also founded on this unproven belief that there is an important neuropsychological component behind the steroid advantage. In their quest to find alternative preparations that could evade drug testing at international competitions, East German scientists hit on the idea of administering anabolic steroids in a nasal spray (Franke & Berendonk, 1997). The intranasal route would require less steroid to gain maximal brain effects. Although the performance effects have not been experimentally tested, individuals reported immediate stimulatory effects (Dickman, 1991).

Sustainment of Androgenicity During Demanding Physical Training

It has been claimed that anabolic steroid use is justifiable medical treatment to sustain training-induced hypogonadism in athletes. Several leaps of faith are necessary to justify the use of anabolic steroids as "replacement" treatment in normal athletes. First, it remains to be demonstrated that episodic reductions in circulating testosterone levels produce muscle wasting or loss of strength. There is only a weak association between testosterone levels and loss of lean mass in elite male soldiers suffering very large weight losses in training (Friedl, 1997a), and the severity of hypogonadism does not correspond to the magnitude of muscle wasting in patients with myotonic dystrophy (Griggs, Kingston, Herr, Forbes, & Moxley, 1985). Furthermore, if this was important, several weeks of weakness and declining muscle mass would be observed after every cycle of steroid use, during the period when athletes are hypogonadal before their testes resume normal secretory activity. This does not seem to occur.

Secondly, a case must be made for androgen deficiency in speed and strength athletes engaged in heavy training. Studies of soldiers engaged in intensive training in scenarios with multiple stressors (Aakvaag, Sand, Opstad, & Fonnum, 1978; Opstad, 1992) have been cited as evidence that "overtraining" produces a decline in testosterone secretion. The confusion comes from the effect of a key stressor that is not typically present for athletes in training: inadequate energy intake (Opstad & Aakvaag, 1983; Guezennec, Satabin, Legrand, & Bigard, 1994). This would only be expected in some athletic specialties where food restriction to achieve or maintain low body weight or body fat is a feature of the athlete's habits—for example, wrestlers (Strauss, Lanese, & Malarkey, 1985). In strength and power sports, testosterone typically *increases* immediately after high-intensity training (Brisson et al., 1978; Kraemer et al., 1991; Kuoppasalmi, Naveri, Rehunen, Harkonen, & Adlercreutz, 1976). There are a variety of explanations for this observation, but the simplest include fluid shifts during exercise (Wilkerson, Horvath, & Gutin, 1980), which temporarily concentrates the steroid with its binding proteins in circulation, and reduced liver blood flow (Rowell, Blackmon, & Bruce, 1964), which briefly alters the balance between steroid secretion and removal rates. Catecholamines may also directly stimulate testicular secretion of testosterone (Jezova & Vigas, 1981; Frankel & Ryan, 1981; Sapolsky, 1986). Whether or not such temporary increases in circulating testosterone are of any consequence to athletic training and performance is unknown, but, clearly, anabolic steroids are not required in this group of athletes for diminished androgen levels.

Testosterone levels may be reduced in prolonged events. For example, 5 athletes participating in an 1,100 km run over 20 days demonstrated a reduction to half of normal testosterone levels by the end of the event (Schurmeyer, Jung, & Nieschlag, 1984). Reduction in plasma testosterone levels have been reported immediately following exercise for marathoners (Dessypris, Kuoppasalmi, & Adlercreutz, 1976), ultramarathoners (Morville, Pesquies, Guezennec, Serrurier, & Guignard, 1979), triathletes (Urhausen & Kindermann, 1987), and cyclists (de Lignieres, Plas, Commandre, Morville, Viani, & Plas, 1976). Although some of these reductions are relatively small, they are larger than expected from normal cyclic reductions seen through the day. Habitual distance runners, tested on a nonrunning day, were shown to have normal testosterone levels, yet these levels were lower than those of nonrunning controls (Wheeler, Wall, Belcastro, & Cumming, 1984). A similar study found even lower resting testosterone levels in runners, but also noted that 13 of the 20 subjects had lost weight since beginning their current training (Ayers, Komesu, Romani, & Ansbacher, 1985). This suggests that energy intakes that are inadequate relative to energy requirements in athletes may be one of the principal causes of decreased testosterone in sustained exercise events where it may be difficult to maintain energy balance. No mechanism has been proposed to explain an effect of physical exercise to reduce testosterone levels, while psychological stress and energy deficit have well-established effects mediated through the hypothalamus. Improved dietary intakes may be more important to these athletes than steroid supplementation.

In a setting of prolonged exercise where energy intake may be inadequate, the decline in thyroid hormones and testosterone favors a loss of fast-twitch (type II) muscle fibers and would be unfavorable to strength athletes. Muscle biopsy studies in men on ski patrol (30 km/d with backpacks) who subsisted on only one military operational meal per day for three weeks showed a significant and specific decline in fast-twitch muscle fibers in both arm and leg muscles (Schantz, Henriksson, & Jansson, 1983). This shift leads to more efficient fuel economy in semistarvation; thus, the decline in testosterone in this special setting may have a specific purpose and adaptive value. The effect of anabolic steroids in a setting of chronic energy deficiency (e.g., anorectic athlete) cannot be predicted and has not been experimentally tested, although bodybuilders have undoubtedly attempted this. One study suggests that anabolic steroid use might further reduce circulating levels of thyroid hormones that are already suppressed during energy deficit. (Deyssig & Weissel, 1993).

Countermeasures for Stress-Induced Catabolic Hormones

Androgens and glucocorticoids (such as cortisol) have opposing actions in the regulation of skeletal muscle turnover. This logically leads to the hypothesis that anabolic steroids are useful to competitive athletes because of their potential to counteract adrenal stress hormones, which promote catabolism (Gustafsson, Saartok, Dahlberg, Snochowski, Haggmark, & Eriksson, 1984; Viru & Korge, 1979). Some of the key actions of anabolic steroids, as used by athletes, may actually be mediated through effects on the cellular receptors normally designed to respond to adrenal hormones; this "crossover binding" occurs at high doses when the steroid may bind to the receptor, occupying the site without provoking the normal response (Yen et al., 1997). Some anabolic steroids bind only weakly (e.g., methanedione, stanozolol) or not at all (e.g., oxymetholone) to androgen receptors, and interference with glucocorticoid binding to glucocorticoid receptors would explain why these steroids have any effect on skeletal muscle (Hughes & Krieg, 1988). If one of the primary mechanisms for anabolic steroid effects on skeletal muscle is to shift the balance of protein turnover through interference with the glucocorticoid receptor, then a case could be made for the largest effects to occur in athletes working at a high level of training, where cortisol may be elevated. This is also a potential explanation for why experienced athletes training intensively during steroid use appear to show performance gains even at relatively low doses of steroid use (Wright, 1980); however, this effect is most likely at pharmacological doses (Salmons, 1983). It has also been suggested that increased secretion of adrenal hormones in response to stress can have a direct inhibitory effect on testicular secretion of testosterone, producing an androgen deficiency state, as previously discussed (Evain, Morera, & Saez, 1976; Sapolsky, 1985; Schaison, Durand, & Mowszowicz, 1978; Welsh & Johnson, 1981). While exercise increases cortisol levels acutely (Brandenberger & Follenius, 1975; Newmark, Himathongkam, Martin, Cooper, & Rose, 1976), hypercortisolism is usually not part of the chronic exercise response and, after an initial increase, cortisol levels usually return to normal with continued exercise (Mujika, Chatard, Padilla, Guezennec, & Geyssant, 1996; Schurmeyer, Jung, & Nieschlag, 1984). Thus, exercise itself is not likely to produce a lasting suppression of testosterone and does not explain the effect of anabolic steroids. On the other hand, the dynamic balance between anabolic and catabolic effects may be key to the actions of anabolic steroids; what happens at the receptor level is still not well understood and could be quite different from what circulating hormone levels appear to show.

Anabolic steroids may also protect injured athletes from muscle atrophy accelerated by trauma and stress hormones (Michelsen, Askanazi, Kinney, Gump, & Elwyn, 1982). Anabolic steroids have been used to benefit severely cachectic men and women suffering life-threatening losses of lean mass through diseases such as cancer and HIV infection (Berger, Pall, Hall, Simpson, Berry, & Dudley, 1996; Hengge, Baumann, Maleba, Borckmeyer, & Goos, 1996), and to prevent trauma-associated catabolism following surgery. Nitrogen loss is very high in trauma patients and in patients being treated with glucocorticoids, and these patients are helped by anabolic steroids (Michelsen et al., 1982; Mosebach, Hausmann, Caspari, & Stoeckel, 1985); however, the benefits to normal athletes are less certain. While it is likely that some muscle damage occurs in response to intensive bouts of weightlifting (Paul, DeLany, Snook, Siefert,

& Kirby, 1989; Ross, Attwood, Atkin, & Villar, 1983) and after intensive military training (Kosano et al., 1986), it is not known if anabolic steroids will prevent this damage; nor is it clear that inflammatory responses should be suppressed, as these may be beneficial to the stimulation of muscle growth (Evans & Cannon, 1991). Hakkinen and Alen (1989) considered this possible action of anabolic steroids. They found that competitive athletes using combinations of oral and injectable steroids actually had higher circulating levels of creatine kinase enzyme than nonusers who were also training intensively. In other words, based on enzyme markers of muscle cell damage, anabolic steroids did not reduce damage produced by intensive training. There are several reasons for a rise in these enzymes, separate from the muscle damage effect, which could be associated with steroid administration, such as the depot injection itself and effects on the liver from oral preparations.

Improved Aerobic Endurance Performance

In theory, aerobic and endurance capacity could be enhanced through anabolic steroid effects on oxygen transport mechanisms via effects on cardiac muscle and red cell production, and through effects on glycogen storage and metabolism. The evidence in support of any net benefit to endurance athletes is not compelling. Three empirical studies considered the effects on running or swimming performance. Johnson and O'Shea (1969) reported in *Science* that methandienone (10 mg/d for 3 wk) increased maximal oxygen uptake by 15% and significantly more than the gain in nonblinded control training partners. O'Shea did not successfully duplicate this finding with a group of swimmers, nor did the swimmers improve on swim performance over that of the control group with either methandienone (10 mg/d for 3 wk) (O'Shea, 1970) or oxandrolone (10 mg/d for 6 wk) (O'Shea & Winkler, 1970). Johnson was also unsuccessful in reproducing the improvement in aerobic capacity using methandienone (10 mg/d for 3 wk) or stanozolol (6 mg/d for 3 wk) with a running program and measurements of maximal oxygen uptake and mile run time (Johnson et al., 1975). Johnson suggested that the earlier finding with O'Shea, which relied on an estimated oxygen uptake from the Åstrand bike test, may be explained by increased leg strength rather than a real increase in aerobic capacity. The downside of anabolic steroid use in endurance athletes could well be the increased body weight; increased mass could be a great disadvantage to athletes whose primary performance involves propelling their body mass (Hoyt & Weyand, 1997).

Anabolic steroids stimulate red cell production and hemoglobin synthesis. In a study of male patients with anemia who received one of four steroids, testosterone enanthate injections provided the largest increases, raising hematocrit from a mean 20.8% to 26.4% (Neff et al., 1981).

Patients without kidneys were not responsive, indicating an effect mediated through the kidneys, whether or not direct effects on the bone to stimulate erythropoesis also occur. Two Finnish studies examining elite athletes self-administering high doses of injectable and orally active steroids showed little or no increase in hematocrit and hemoglobin concentrations (Alen, 1985; Kiraly, 1988). Researchers performing controlled experiments with high-dose anabolic steroid administration to normal men have reported the absence of increases in hematocrit and hemoglobin (Friedl, et al., 1990). This suggests that patients with low hematocrits may benefit from anabolic steroids, but increases above normal are not stimulated in normal men. Polycythemia (elevated red cell concentrations) does not appear to be a common feature even with high-dose steroid use by athletes, suggesting that this is not a likely benefit and a relatively rare risk to athletes using anabolic steroids.

Although there is no evidence of a specific action of anabolic steroids that would benefit performance of endurance athletes, other previously discussed actions that may permit a higher volume of training through enhanced psychological motivation and recovery could provide a competitive edge.

Conclusions

Anabolic steroids, as a class, produce weight gain in normal men. Typical weight gains are 3 to 5 kg after several weeks of high-dose steroid use. This appears to be a permissive action with a threshold effect, where an amount of steroid above the effective dose does not clearly produce more rapid weight gain. The nature of this weight gain is still uncertain, although an increase in muscle size and total body protein accretion is at least one component of the gain. No study to date has simultaneously studied changes in the several principal body components (e.g., water, fat, protein, bone mineral) to clearly elucidate the balance of the changes. Since different anabolic steroids may be quite different in their drug effects, care must be taken in the evaluation of the existing data with a variety of different drugs and doses. The only consistently demonstrated strength gains are based on a 1-RM bench-press test; this has been shown following several weeks of anabolic steroid administration using methandienone (10 mg/d or greater), oxandrolone (10 mg/d), and testosterone enanthate (600 mg/wk). The effects of steroids on strength performance are most clearly seen with experienced weightlifters and when strength training is performed concurrently with the steroid administration. Most studies demonstrating strength gains also demonstrate weight gains. Strength gains may occur primarily because of increased muscle mass, but other factors are also plausibly involved, such as psychological effects related to increased motivation, which permit a greater volume of high-intensity training and may enhance competitive performance. The mechanism of action for an effect on skeletal muscle is still not clear. It may involve interference with glucocorticoid binding to glucocorticoid receptors, shifting the balance of muscle protein turnover in favor of protein accrual. There is little evidence to support a beneficial role of anabolic steroids in other types of exercise performance, such as strength endurance and aerobic performance. Future studies should attempt to improve on the experimental designs, to include a proper control group as well as an effective double-blinded placebo group. The objective of these studies should be to clarify the role of training during steroid treatment, the association with changes in specific muscle mass and muscle cross-sectional areas, and the potential improvement of measures of strength other than bench-press performance.

References

Aakvaag, A., Sand, T., Opstad, P.K., & Fonnum, F. (1978). Hormonal changes in young men during prolonged physical strain. *European Journal of Applied Physiology, 39,* 283–291.

Aakvaag, A., & Stromme, S.B. (1974). The effect of mesterolone administration to normal men on the pituitary-testicular function. *Acta Endocrinologica, 77,* 380–386.

Alen, M. (1985). Androgenic steroid effects on liver and red cells. *British Journal of Sports Medicine, 19,* 15–20.

Alen, M., Hakkinen, K., & Komi, P.V. (1984). Changes in neuromuscular performance and muscle fiber characteristics of elite power athletes self-administering androgenic and anabolic steroids. *Acta Physiologica Scandanavica, 122,* 535–544.

Ariel, G. (1973). The effect of anabolic steroid upon skeletal muscle contractile force. *Journal of Sports Medicine and Physical Fitness, 13,* 187–190.

Ariel, G. (1974). Prolonged effects of anabolic steroid upon muscular contractile force. *Medicine and Science in Sports, 6,* 62–64.

Ariel, G., & Saville, W. (1972a). The effect of anabolic steroids on reflex components. *Medicine and Science in Sports, 4,* 120–123.

Ariel, G., & Saville, W. (1972b). Anabolic steroids: The physiological effects of placebos. *Medicine and Science in Sports, 4,* 124–126.

Ayers, J.W.T., Komesu, Y., Romani, T., & Ansbacher, R. (1985). Anthropomorphic, hormonal, and psychologic correlates of semen quality in endurance-trained male athletes. *Fertility and Sterility, 43,* 917–921.

Bardin, C.W., & Catterall, J.F. (1981). Testosterone: A major determinant of extragenital sexual dimorphism. *Science, 211,* 1285–1294.

Behre, H.M., Kleisch, S., Leifke, E., Link, T.M., & Nieschlag, E. (1997). Long-term effect of testosterone therapy on bone mineral density in hypogonadal men. *Journal of Clinical Endocrinology and Metabolism, 82,* 2386–2390.

Belkien, L., Schurmeyer, T., Hano, R., Gunnarsson, P.O., & Nieschlag, E. (1985). Pharmacokinetics of 19-nortestosterone esters in normal men. *Journal of Steroid Biochemistry, 22,* 623–629.

Berger, J.R., Pall, L., Hall, C.D., Simpson, D.M., Berry, P.S., & Dudley, R. (1996). Oxandrolone in AIDS-wasting myopathy. *AIDS, 10,* 1657–1662.

Bhasin, S., Storer, T.W., Berman, N., Callegari, C., Clevenger, B., Phillips, J., Bunnell, T.J., Tricker, R., Shirazi, A., & Casaburi, R. (1996). The effects of supraphysiologic doses of testosterone on muscle size and strength in normal men. *New England Journal of Medicine, 335,* 1–7.

Bhasin, S., Storer, T.W., Berman, N., Yarasheski, K.E., Clevenger, B., Phillips, J., Lee, W.P., Bunnell, T.J., & Casaburi, R. (1997). Testosterone replacement increases fat-free mass and muscle size in hypogonadal men. *Journal of Clinical Endocrinology and Metabolism, 82,* 407–413.

Brandenberger, G., & Follenius, M. (1975). Influence of timing and intensity of muscular exercise on temporal patterns of plasma cortisol levels. *Journal of Clinical Endocrinology and Metabolism, 40,* 845–849.

Brisson, G.R., DeCarufel, D., Brault, J., Valle, M.A., Audet, A., Desharnais, M., & Lefrancois, C. (1981). Circulating Δ^4-androgen levels and bicycle exercise in trained young men. 4th International Symposium on Biochemistry of Exercise, Brussels, 1979. In J. Poortmans and G. Niset (eds.) *Biochemistry of Exercise IV-B,* Baltimore, University Park Press, 1981, pp. 198–217.

Casner, S.W., Early, R.G., & Carlson, B.R. (1971). Anabolic steroid effects on body composition in normal young men. *Journal of Sports Medicine and Physical Fitness, 11,* 98–103.

Crist, D.M., Stackpole, P.J., & Peake, G.T. (1983). Effects of androgenic-anabolic steroids on neuromuscular power and body composition. *Journal of Applied Physiology, 54,* 366–370.

de Lignieres, B., Plas, J-N., Commandre, F., Morville, R., Viani, J-L., & Plas, F. (1976). Secretion testiculaire d'androgenes apres effort physique prolongé chez l'homme. *Nouvelle Presse Medicale, 5,* 2060–2064.

Dessypris, A., Kuoppasalmi, K., & Adlercreutz, H. (1976). Plasma cortisol, testosterone, androstenedione and luteinizing hormone (LH) in a non-competitive marathon run. *Journal of Steroid Biochemistry, 7,* 33–37.

Deyssig, R., & Weissel, M. (1993). Ingestion of androgenic-anabolic steroids induces mild thyroidal impairment in male body builders. *Journal of Clinical Endocrinology and Metabloism, 76,* 1069–1071.

Dickman, S. (1991). East Germany: Science in the disservice of the State. *Science, 254,* 26–27.

Elbers, J.M.H., Asscheman, H., Seidell, J.C., Megens, J.A.J., & Gooren, L.J.G. (1997). Long-term testosterone administration increases visceral fat in female to male transsexuals. *Journal of Clinical Endocrinology and Metabolism, 82,* 2044–2047.

Era, P., Alen, M., & Rahkila, P. (1988). Psychomotor and motor speed in power athletes self-administering testosterone and anabolic steroids. *Research Quarterly for Exercise and Sport, 59,* 50–56.

Evain, D., Morera, A.M., & Saez, J.M. (1976). Recepteurs de glucocorticoides dans la testicule de rat. *Annales d'Endocrinologie, 37,* 101–102.

Evans, W.J., & Cannon, J.G. (1991). The metabolic effects of exercise-induced muscle damage. *Exercise and Sports in Science Review, 19,* 99–125.

Fahey, T.D., & Brown, C.H. (1973). The effects of an anabolic steroid on the strength, body composition, and endurance of college males when accompanied by a weight training program. *Medicine and Science in Sports, 5,* 272–276.

Forbes, G.B. (1985). The effect of anabolic steroids on lean body mass: The dose response curve. *Metabolism, 34,* 571–573.

Forbes, G.B., Porta, C.R., Herr, B., & Griggs, R.C. (1992). Sequence of changes in body composition induced by testosterone and reversal of changes after the drug is stopped. *Journal of the American Medical Association, 267,* 397–399.

Fowler, W.M., Jr., Gardner, G.W., & Egstrom, G.H. (1965). Effect of an anabolic steroid on physical performance of young men. *Journal of Applied Physiology, 20,* 1038–1040.

Franke, W.W., & Berendonk, B. (1997). Hormonal doping and androgenization of athletes: A secret program of the German Democratic Republic government. *Clinical Chemistry, 43,* 1262–1279.

Frankel, A.I., & Ryan, E.L. (1981). Testicular innervation is necessary for the response of plasma testosterone levels to acute stress. *Biology of Reproduction, 24,* 491–495.

Freed, D.L.J., & Banks, A.J. (1975). A double-blind crossover trial for methandienone (Dianabol, CIBA) in moderate dosage on highly trained experienced athletes. *British Journal of Sports Medicine, 9,* 78–81.

Freed, D.L.J., Banks, A.J., Longson, D., & Burley, D.M. (1975). Anabolic steroids in athletics: Crossover double-blind trial on weightlifters. *British Medical Journal, 2,* 471–473.

Friedl, K.E. (1997a). Variability of fat and lean tissue loss during physical exertion with energy deficit. In J.M. Kinney & H.N. Tucker (Eds.), *Physiology, stress, and malnutrition: Functional correlates, nutritional intervention* (pp. 431–450). Philadelphia: Lippincott-Raven.

Friedl, K.E. (1997b). Military application of body composition assessment technologies. In S.J. Carlson-Newberry & R.B. Costello (Eds.), *Emerging technologies for nutrition research* (pp. 81–126). Washington, DC: National Academy Press.

Friedl, K.E., Dettori, J.R., Hannan, C.J., Jr., Patience, T.H., & Plymate, S.R. (1991). Comparison of the effects of high dose testosterone and 19-nortestosterone to a replacement dose of testosterone on strength and body composition in normal men. *Journal of Steroid Biochemistry and Molecular Biology, 40,* 607–612.

Friedl, K.E., Hannan, C.J., Jones, R.E., and Plymate, S.R. (1990). High-density lipoprotein cholesterol is not decreased if an aromatizable androgen is administered. *Metabolism, 39,* 69–74.

Golding, L.A., Freydinger, J.E., & Fishel, S.S. (1974). Weight, size, and strength—unchanged with steroids. *The Physician and Sportsmedicine, 2,* 39–43.

Gray, J.M., Nunez, A.A., Siegel, L.I., & Wade, G.N. (1979). Effects of testosterone on body weight and adipose tissue: Role of aromatization. *Physiological Behavior, 23,* 465–469.

Gregory, J.W., Greene, S.A., Thompson, J., & Rennie, M.J. (1992). Effects of oral testosterone undecanoate on growth, body composition, strength, and energy expenditure of adolescent boys. *Clinical Endocrinology, 37,* 207–213.

Griggs, R.C., Kingston, W., Jozefowicz, R.F., Herr, B.E., Forbes, G., & Halliday, D. (1989). Effect of testosterone on muscle mass and muscle protein synthesis. *Journal of Applied Physiology, 66,* 498–503.

Griggs, R.C., Kingston, W., Herr, B.E., Forbes, G. & Moxley, R.T. 3d. (1985). Lack of relationship of hypogonadism to muscle wasting in myotonic dystrophy. *Archives of Neurology, 42,* 881–885.

Guezennec, C.Y., Ferre, P., Serrurier, B., Merino, D., Aymonod, M., and Pesquies, P.C. (1984). Metabolic and hormonal response to short term fasting after endurance training in the rat. *Hormone and Metabolic Research, 16,* 572–575.

Guezennec, C.Y., Satabin, P., Legrand, H., & Bigard, A.X. (1994). Physical performance and metabolic changes induced by combined prolonged exercise and different energy intakes in humans. *European Journal of Applied Physiology, 68,* 525–530.

Gustafsson, J.-A, Saartok, T., Dahlberg, E., Snochowski, M., Haggmark, T., & Eriksson, E. (1984). Studies of steroid receptors in human and rabbit skeletal muscle—clues to the understanding of the mechanism of action of anabolic steroids. *Progress in Clinical and Biological Research, 142,* 261–290.

Hakkinen, K., & Alen, M. (1989). Training volume, androgen use and serum creatine kinase activity. *British Journal of Sports Medicine, 23,* 188–189.

Hamilton, J.B. (1948). The role of testicular secretions as indicated by the effects of castration in man and by studies of pathological conditions and the short lifespan associated with maleness. *Recent Progress in Hormone Research, 3,* 257–322.

Hannan, C.J., Jr., Friedl, K.E., Zold, A., Kettler, T.M., & Plymate, S.R. (1991). Psychological and serum homovanillic acid changes in men administered androgenic steroids. *Psychoneuroendocrinology, 16,* 335–343.

Harkness, R.A., Kilshaw, B.H., & Hobson, B.M. (1975). Effects of large doses of anabolic steroids. *British Journal of Sportsmedicine, 9,* 70–92.

Haupt, H.A., & Rovere, G.D. (1984). Anabolic steroids: A review of the literature. *American Journal of Sports Medicine, 12,* 469–477.

Hengge, U.R., Baumann, M., Maleba, R., Borckmeyer, N.H., & Goos, M. (1996). Oxymetholone promotes weight gain in patients with advanced human immunodeficiency virus (HIV-1) infection. *British Journal of Nutrition, 75,* 129–138.

Hermann, W.M., & Beach, R.C. (1976). Psychotropic effects of androgens: A review of clinical observations and new human experimental findings. *Pharmakopsychiatria, 9,* 205–219.

Hershberger, L.G., Shipley, E.G., & Meyer, R.K. (1953). Myotonic activity of 19-nortestosterone and other steroids determined by modified levator ani method. *Proceedings of the Society for Experimental Biology and Medicine, 83,* 175–180.

Hervey, G.R. (1975). Are athletes wrong about anabolic steroids? *British Journal of Sports Medicine, 9,* 74–77.

Hervey, G.R., Hutchinson, I., Knibbs, A.V., Burkinshaw, L., Jones, P.R., Norgan, N.G., & Levell, M.J. (1976). "Anabolic" effects of methandienone in men undergoing athletic training. *Lancet, 2,* 699–702.

Hervey, G.R., Knibbs, A.V., Burkinshaw, L., Morgan, D.B., Jones, P.R.M., Chettle, D.R., & Vartsky, D. (1981). Effects of methandienone on the performance and body composition of men undergoing athletic training. *Clinical Science, 60,* 457–461.

Hoyt, R.W., & Weyand, P.G. (1997). Advances in ambulatory monitoring: Using foot contact time to estimate the metabolic cost of locomotion. In S.J. Carlson-Newberry & R.B. Costello (Eds.), *Emerging technologies for nutrition research* (pp. 315–343). Washington, DC: National Academy Press.

Hughes, B.J., & Krieg, M. (1988). Steroid receptors and the muscular system. In P.J. Sheridan, K. Blum, & M.C. Trachtenberg (Eds.), *Steroid receptors and disease: Cancer, autoimmune, bone, and circulatory disorders* (pp. 415–433). New York: Marcel Dekker

Jacobs, I., Kaiser, P., & Tesch, P. (1981). Muscle strength and fatigue after selective glycogen depletion in human skeletal muscle fibers. *European Journal of Applied Physiology, 46,* 47–53.

Jezova, D., & Vigas, M. (1981). Testosterone response to exercise during blockade and stimulation of adrenergic receptors in man. *Hormone Research, 15,* 141–147.

Johnson, L.C., Fisher, L.J., Silvester, L.S., & Hofheins, C. (1972). Anabolic steroid: Effects on strength, body weight, oxygen uptake and spermatogenesis upon mature males. *Medicine and Science in Sports, 4,* 43–45.

Johnson, L.C., & O'Shea, J.P. (1969). Anabolic steroids: Effects on strength development. *Science, 164,* 957–959.

Johnson, L.C., Roundy, E.S., Allsen, P.E., Fisher, A.G., & Silvester, L.J. (1975). Effect of anabolic steroid treatment on endurance. *Medicine and Science in Sports, 7,* 287–289.

Johnson, M.J., Friedl, K.E., Frykman, P.N., & Moore, R.J. (1994). Loss of muscle mass is poorly reflected in grip strength performance in healthy young men. *Medicine and Science in Sports and Exercise, 26,* 235–240.

Keating, R.J., & Tcholakian, R.K. (1983). In vivo patterns of circulating testosterone following castration and intramuscular testosterone propionate injections of adult male rats. *Steroids, 42,* 63–76.

Kenyon, A.T., Knowlton, K., Sandiford, I., Kock, F.C., & Lotwin, G. (1940). A comparative study of the metabolic effects of testosterone propionate in normal men and women and in eunuchoidism. *Endocrinology, 26,* 26–45.

Kilshaw, B.H., Harkness, R.A., Hobson, B.M., and Smith, A.W.M. (1975). The effects of large doses of anabolic steroid, methandienone, on an athlete. *Clinical Endocrinology, 4,* 537–541.

Kiraly, C.L. (1988). Androgenic-anabolic steroid effects on serum and skin surface lipids, on red cells, and on liver enzymes. *International Journal of Sports Medicine, 9,* 249–252.

Knudsen, J.F., & Max, S.R. (1980). Aromatization of androgens to estrogens mediates increased activity of glucose 6-phosphate dehydrogenase in rat levator ani muscle. *Endocrinology, 106,* 440–443.

Kosano, H., Kinoshita, T., Nagata, N., et al. (1986). Change in concentrations of myogenic components of serum during 93 h of strenuous physical exercise. *Clinical Chemistry, 32,* 346–348.

Kouri, E.M., Lukas, S.E., Pope, H.G., Jr., & Oliva, P.S. (1995). Increased aggressive responding in male volunteers following the administration of gradually increasing doses of testosterone cypionate. *Drug and Alcohol Dependence, 40,* 73–79.

Kouri, E.M., Pope, H.G., Jr., Katz, D.L., & Oliva, P.S. (1995). Fat-free mass index in users and nonusers of anabolic-androgenic steroids. *Clinical Journal of Sports Medicine, 5,* 223–228.

Kraemer, W.J., Gordon, S.E., Fleck, S.J., Marchitelli, L.J., Mello, R., Dziados, J.E., Friedl, K., Harman, E., Maresh, C., and Fry, A.C. (1991). Endogenous anabolic hormonal and growth factor responses to heavy resistance exercise in males and females. *International Journal of Sports Medicine, 12,* 228–235.

Krotkiewski, M., Kral, J.G., & Karlsson, J. (1980). Effects of castration and testosterone substitution on body composition and muscle metabolism in rats. *Acta Physiologica Scandanavica, 109,* 233–237.

Kuipers, H., Peeze Binkhorst, F.M., Hartgens, F., Wijnen, J.A., & Keizer, H.A. (1993). Muscle ultrastructure after strength training with placebo or anabolic steroid. *Canadian Journal of Applied Physiology, 18,* 189–196.

Kuoppasalmi, K., Naveri, H., Rehunen, S., Harkonen, M., & Adlercreutz, H. (1976). Effect of strenuous anaerobic running exercise on plasma growth hormone, cortisol, luteinizing hormone, testosterone, androstenedione, estrone and estradiol. *Journal of Steroid Biochemistry, 7,* 823–829.

Liddle, G.W., & Burke, H.A. (1960). Anabolic steroids in clinical medicine. *Helvetica Medica Acta, 27,* 504–513.

Loughton, S.J., & Ruhling, R.O. (1977). Human strength and endurance responses to anabolic steroid and training. *Journal of Sports Medicine and Physical Fitness, 17,* 285–296.

Lyons, G.E., Kelly, A.M., & Rubinstein, N.A. (1986). Testosterone-induced changes in contractile protein isoforms in the sexually dimorphic temporalis muscle of the guinea pig. *Journal of Biological Chemistry, 261,* 13278–13284.

Marin, P., Holmang, S., Jonsson, L., Sjostrom, L., Kvist, H., Holm, G., Lindstedt, G., & Bjorntorp, P. (1992). The effects of testosterone treatment on body composition and metabolism in middle-aged obese men. *International Journal of Obesity and Related Metabolic Disorders, 16,* 991–997.

Marin, P., Lonn, L., Andersson, B., Oden, B., Olbe, L., Bengtsson, B.A., & Bjorntorp, P. (1996). Assimilation of triglycerides in subcutaneous and intraabdominal adipose tissues in vivo in men: Effects of testosterone. *Journal of Clinical Endocrinology and Metabolism, 81,* 1018–1022.

Marin, P., Oden, B., & Bjorntorp, P. (1995). Assimilation and mobilization of triglycerides in subcutaneous abdominal and femoral adipose tissue in vivo in men: Effects of androgens. *Journal of Clinical Endocrinology and Metabolism, 80,* 239–243.

Michel, G., & Baulieu, E-E. (1980). Androgen receptor in rat skeletal muscle: Characterization and physiological variations. *Endocrinology, 107,* 2088–2098.

Michelsen, C.B., Askanazi, J., Kinney, J.M., Gump, F.E., & Elwyn, D.H. (1982). Effect of an anabolic steroid on nitrogen balance and amino acid patterns after total hip replacement. *The Journal of Trauma, 22,* 410–413.

Morville, R., Pesquies, P.C., Guezennec, C.Y., Serrurier, B.D., & Guignard, M. (1979). Plasma variations in testicular and adrenal androgens during prolonged physical exercise in man. *Annales d'Endocrinologie, 40,* 501–510.

Mosebach, K.-O., Hausmann, D., Caspari, R., & Stoeckel, H. (1985). Deca-Durabolin and parenteral nutrition in post-traumatic patients. *Acta Endocrinologica, Supplementum 271,* 60–69.

Mujika, I., Chatard, J.C., Padilla, S., Guezennec, C.Y., & Geyssant, A. (1996). Hormonal responses in training and its tapering off in competitive swimmers: Relationships with performance. *European Journal of Applied Physiology and Occupational Physiology, 74,* 361–366.

Need, A.G., Horowitz, M., Bridges, A., Morris, H.A., & Nordin, B.E.C. (1989). Effects of nandrolone decanoate and antiresorptive therapy on vertebral density in osteoporotic postmenopausal women. *Archives of Internal Medicine, 149,* 57–60.

Neff, M.S., Goldberg, J., Slifkin, R.F., Eiser, A.R., Calamia, V., Kaplan, M., Baez, A., Gupta, S., and Mattoo, N. (1981). A comparison of androgens for anemia in patients on hemodialysis. *New England Journal of Medicine, 304,* 871–875.

Newmark, S. R., Himathongkam, T., Martin, R.P., Cooper, K.H., & Rose, L.I. (1976). Adrenocortical response to marathon running. *Journal of Clinical Endocrinology and Metabolism, 42,* 393–394.

Nunez, A.A. (1982). Dose-dependent effects of testosterone on feeding and body weight in male rats. *Behavioral and Neural Biology, 34,* 445.

Opstad, P.K. (1992). Androgenic hormones during prolonged physical stress, sleep, and energy deficiency. *Journal of Clinical Endocrinology and Metabolism, 74,* 1176–1183.

Opstad, P.K., & Aakvaag, A. (1983). Decreased serum levels of oestradiol, testosterone and prolactin during prolonged physical strain and sleep deprivation, and the influence of high calorie diet. *European Journal of Applied Physiology, 49,* 343–348.

O'Shea, J.P. (1970). Anabolic steroid: Effects on competitive swimmers. *Nutrition Report International, 1,* 337–342.

O'Shea, J.P. (1971). The effects of an anabolic steroid on dynamic strength levels of weightlifters. *Nutrition Reports International, 4,* 363–370.

O'Shea, J.P. (1974). A biochemical evaluation of the effects of stanozolol on adrenal, liver and muscle function in humans. *Nutrition Reports International, 10,* 381–388.

O'Shea, J.P., & Winkler, W. (1970). Biochemical and physical effects of an anabolic steroid in competitive swimmers and weightlifters. *Nutrition Reports International, 2,* 351–362.

Papanicolaou, G.N., & Falk, E.A. (1938). General muscular hypertrophy induced by androgenic hormone. *Science, 87,* 238–239.

Paul, G.L., DeLany, J.P., Snook, J.T., Siefert, J.G., & Kirby, T.E. (1989). Serum and urinary markers of skeletal muscle damage after weight lifting exercise. *European Journal of Applied Physiology, 58,* 786–790.

Plymate, S.R., & Friedl, K.E. (1992). Anabolic steroids and muscle strength. *Annals of Internal Medicine, 116,* 270.

Rance, N.E., & Max, S.R. (1984). Modulation of the cytosolic androgen receptor in striated muscle by sex steroids. *Endocrinology, 115,* 862–866.

Ross, J.H., Attwood, E.C., Atkin, G.E., & Villar, R.N. (1983). A study on the effects of severe repetitive exercise on serum myoglobin, creatine kinase, transaminases and lactate dehydrogenase. *Quarterly Journal of Medicine, 206,* 268–279.

Rowell, L.B., Blackmon, J.R., & Bruce, R.A. (1964). Indocyanine Green clearance and estimated hepatic blood flow during mild to maximal exercise in upright man. *Journal of Clinical Investigation, 43,* 1677–1690.

Ryushi, T., & Fukanaga, Y. (1986). Influence of muscle fiber composition and muscle cross-sectional area on maximal isometric strength. *Tairyoku Kagaku, 35,* 168–174.

Salmons, S. (1983). Myotrophic effects of anabolic steroids. *Veterinary Research Communications, 7,* 19–26.

Samuels, L.T., Henschel, A.F., & Keys, A. (1942). Influence of methyl testosterone on muscular work and creatine metabolism in normal young men. *Journal of Clinical Endocrinology, 2,* 649–654.

Sapolsky, R.M. (1985). Stress-induced suppression of testicular function in the wild baboon: Role of glucocorticoids. *Endocrinology, 116,* 2273–2278.

Sapolsky, R.M. (1986). Stress-induced elevation of testosterone concentrations in high ranking baboons: Role of catecholamines. *Endocrinology, 118,* 1630–1635.

Schaison, G., Durand, F., & Mowszowicz, I. (1978). Effect of glucocorticoids on plasma testosterone in men. *Acta Endocrinologica, 89,* 126–131.

Schantz, P., Henriksson, J., & Jansson, E. (1983). Adaptation of human skeletal muscle to endurance training of long duration. *Clinical Physiology, 3,* 141–151.

Schulte-Beerbuhl, M., & Nieschlag, E. (1980). Comparison of testosterone, dihydrotestosterone, luteinizing hormone, and follicle-stimulating hormone in serum after injection of testosterone enanthate or testosterone cypionate. *Fertility and Sterility, 33,* 201–203.

Schurmeyer, T., Jung, K., & Nieschlag, E. (1984). The effect of an 1100 km run on testicular, adrenal and thyroid hormones. *International Journal of Andrology, 7,* 276–282.

Sokol, R.Z., Palacios, A., Campfield, L.A., Saul, C., & Swerdloff, R.S. (1982). Comparison of the kinetics of injectable testosterone in eugonadal and hypogonadal men. *Fertility and Sterility, 37,* 425–430.

Stamford, B.A., & Moffatt, R. (1974). Anabolic steroid: Effectiveness as an ergogenic aid to experienced weight trainers. *Journal of Sports Medicine and Physical Fitness, 14,* 191–197.

Stolz, H.R., & Stolz, L.M. (1951). *Somatic development of adolescent boys* (pp. 299–315). New York: Macmillan.

Strauss, R.H., Lanese, R.R., & Malarkey, W.B. (1985). Weight loss in amateur wrestlers and its effect on serum testosterone levels. *Journal of the American Medical Association, 254,* 3337–3338.

Stromme, S.B., Meen, H.D., & Aakvaag, A. (1974). Effects of an androgenic-anabolic steroid on strength development and plasma testosterone levels in normal males. *Medicine and Science in Sports, 6,* 203–208.

Swartz, C.M., & Young, M.A. (1988). Male hypogonadism and bone fracture. *New England Journal of Medicine, 318,* 996.

Swerdloff, R.S., Palacios, A., McClure, R.D., Campfield, L.A., & Brosman, S.A. (1978). Male contraception: Clinical assessment of chronic administration of testosterone enanthate. *International Journal of Andrology, 2*(Suppl.), 731–747.

Tahmindjis, A.J. (1976). The use of anabolic steroids by athletes to increase body weight and strength. *Medical Journal of Australia, 1,* 991–993.

Tenover, J.S. (1992). Effects of androgen supplementation in the aging male. *Journal of Clinical Endocrinology and Metabolism, 75,* 1092–1098.

Thibert, P. (1986). Androgen sensitivity of skeletal muscle: Nondependence on the motor nerve in the frog forearm. *Experimental Neurology, 91,* 559–570.

Tricker, R., Casburi, R., Storer, T.W., Clevenger, B., Berman, N., Shirazi, A., & Bhasin, S. (1996). The effects of supraphysiological doses of testosterone on angry behavior in healthy eugonadal men—a clinical research center study. *Journal of Clinical Endocrinology and Metabolism, 81,* 3754–3758.

Urban, R.J., Bodenburg, Y.H., Gilkison, C., Foxworth, J., Coggan, A.R., Wolfe, R.R., & Ferrando, A. (1995). Testosterone administration to elderly men increases skeletal muscle strength and protein synthesis. *American Journal of Physiology, 269,* E820–826.

Urhausen, A., & Kindermann, W. (1987). Behaviour of testosterone, sex hormone binding globulin (SHBG), and cortisol before and after a triathalon competition. *International Journal of Sports Medicine, 8,* 305–308.

Viru, A., & Korge, P. (1979). Role of anabolic steroids in the hormonal regulation of skeletal muscle adaptation. *Journal of Steroid Biochemistry, 11,* 931–932.

Wade, N. (1972). Anabolic steroids: Doctors denounce them, but athletes aren't listening. *Science, 176,* 1399–1402.

Wang, C., Eyre, D.R., Clark, R., Kleinberg, D., Newman, C., Iranmanesh, A., Veldhuis, J., Dudley, R.E., Berman, N., Davidson, T., Barstow, T.J., Sinow, R., Alexander, G., & Swerdloff, R.S. (1996). Sublingual testosterone replacement improves muscle mass and strength, decreases bone resorption, and increases bone formation markers in hypogonadal men—a clinical research center study. *Journal of Clinical Endocrinology and Metabolism, 81,* 3654–3662.

Ward, P. (1973). The effect of an anabolic steroid on strength and lean body mass. *Medicine and Science in Sports, 5,* 277–282.

Watson, R.N., Bradley, M.H., Callahan, R., Peters, B.J., and Kory, R.C. (1959). A six-month evaluation of an anabolic drug, norethandrolone, in underweight persons. *American Journal of Medicine, 26,* 238–242.

Welle, S., Jozefowicz, R., Forbes, G., & Griggs, R.C. (1992). Effect of testosterone on metabolic rate and body composition in normal men and men with muscular dystrophy. *Journal of Clinical Endocrinology and Metabolism, 74,* 332–335.

Welsh, T.H., & Johnson, B.H. (1981). Stress-induced alterations in secretion of corticosteroids, progesterone, luteinizing hormone, and testosterone in bulls. *Endocrinology, 109,* 185–190.

Wheeler, G.D., Wall, S.R., Belcastro, A.N., & Cumming, D.C. (1984). Reduced serum testosterone and prolactin levels in male distance runners. *Journal of the American Medical Association, 252,* 514–516.

Wilkerson, J.E., Horvath, S.M., & Gutin, B. (1980). Plasma testosterone during treadmill exercise. *Journal of Applied Physiology, 49,* 249–253.

Win-May, M., & Mya-Tu, M. (1975). The effects of anabolic steroids on physical fitness. *Journal of Sports Medicine and Physical Fitness, 15,* 266–271.

Wright, J.E. (1980). Anabolic steroids and athletes. *Exercise and Sports Sciences Review, 8,* 149–202.

Yen, P.M., Liu, U., Palvimo, J.J., Trifiro, M., Whang, J., Pinsky, L., Janne, O.A., and Chin, W.W. (1997). Mutant and wild-type androgen receptors exhibit cross-talk on androgen-, glucocorticoid-, and progesterone-mediated transcription. *Molecular Endocrinology, 11,* 162–171.

Young, N.R., Baker, H.W.G., Liu, G., & Seeman, E. (1993). Body composition and muscle strength in healthy men receiving testosterone enanthate for contraception. *Journal of Clinical Endocrinology and Metabolism, 77,* 1028–1032.

CHAPTER

6

Effects of Anabolic Steroids on Physical Health

Karl E. Friedl, PhD

I know there's no written, documented proof that steroids and human growth hormone caused this cancer. But it's one of the reasons you have to look at. You have to.

Lyle Alzado
Football player, after a diagnosis of brain lymphoma,the only report of this disease in a former steroid-using athlete

The views, opinions, and findings in this report are those of the author and should not be construed as an official Department of the Army position, policy, or decision. Portions of this chapter are from Friedl 1990.

A wide variety of claims have been made about the health risks associated with the use of anabolic steroids. Many "well-established" risks are based only on anecdotal experiences and misinterpreted science. The information that is available from primary source reports of scientific studies and medical cases frequently does not support the claimed risks; but in other cases, it suggests areas of concern that have been inadequately investigated. As researchers have gained more experience with anabolic steroids, certain parallels to the health risks associated with the use of female hormonal contraception have begun to emerge; these parallels may include consequences with long latencies, perhaps adverse androgen effects involving the prostate or the heart. One key difference is that the health risks associated with the oral contraceptive pill are considered to be acceptable trade-offs to the prevention of pregnancy (which carries even greater risks to the woman); there is, as yet, no such health benefit associated with the use of anabolic steroids by healthy young males. Thus, the development of a life-threatening liver tumor in even one athlete as a consequence of anabolic steroid use should not be considered an acceptable trade-off for any advantage that the drug might bring in sport competition.

This chapter will evaluate the adverse effects associated with anabolic steroid use. It would be an oversimplification to reduce these risks to a single list, putting very diverse actions side by side, as if of equal weight, and grossly out of context. For example, the risks range from effects that are minor in terms of well-being, such as scalp hair loss, to those that are potentially lethal, such as liver tumors. Risks also include temporary effects that may be useful, such as male infertility (which may become useful in male hormonal contraception), as well as temporary effects, such as the profound suppression of serum high-density lipoprotein cholesterol (HDLC), for which it is difficult to rationalize any possible advantage. An effect that may be perceived as an inconvenient side effect in clinical use, such as weight gain, may be the main benefit sought by some athletes and by males who are self-conscious about their physique. Conversely, increasing hematocrit (another effect of steroid use) is the objective of anabolic steroid treatment of patients with severe anemia (Neff et al., 1981), whereas the same action may predispose some individuals to polycythemia (Simon, Jouet, Demory, Pollet, & Bauters, 1986; Verwilghen, Louwagie, Waes, & Vandenbroucke, 1966); the same potential complications are now being encountered by athletes using recombinant erythropoietin (Adamson & Vapnek, 1991). This chapter deals with the effects of anabolic steroid use in normal adult males, specifically the adverse effects that are produced in normally virilized men by additional androgen or by pharmacological properties of the modified anabolic steroids. This excludes some effects of virilization itself (e.g., beard growth, deepening of the voice) that are significant and undesired in a 12-year-old boy or a woman.

Distinctions Between Types and Doses of Anabolic Steroids

Not all anabolic steroids produce the same effects. The clearest distinction between groups of anabolic steroids is in the effects produced by the orally active steroids, most of which have been pharmacologically altered with an alkyl group at the 17-carbon position to slow their removal by the liver, and the anabolic steroids administered by deep intramuscular injection, which usually have a side chain ester at the 17β-carbon position to slow their release into circulation. According to various athlete surveys, the most popular of the 17-alkylated anabolic steroids are methandienone (Dianabol), oxandrolone (Anavar), stanozolol (Winstrol), and oxymetholone (Anadrol); testosterone enanthate (Delatestryl) and nandrolone decanoate (Deca-Durabolin) stand out as the most frequently injected anabolic steroid esters (Burkett & Falduto, 1984; Frankle, Cicero, & Payne, 1984; Hurley et al., 1984; Strauss, Wright, Finerman, & Catlin, 1983; Yesalis et al., 1988), and this includes their use in Olympic contestants testing positive for steroids (Catlin, Kammerer, Hatton, Sekera, & Merdink, 1987). A few exceptions to these two principal categories, such as mesterolone, testosterone undecanoate, and methenolone, so far appear to be compounds of less significance in the epidemiology of anabolic steroid abuse by athletes. We should also remember that some reported adverse effects in anabolic steroid-using athletes may coincide with other common factors. For example, bodybuilders use a wide variety of drugs, such as diuretics, thyroid hormone, and growth hormone, in addition to steroids (Weider, 1987), and they ingest many nutritional supplements, the effects of which are virtually unstudied. Other agents such as aromatase inhibitors may enhance adverse effects of steroids, such as a reduction in HDLC (Friedl, Hannan, Jones, & Plymate, 1990), or may actually block effects the athletes desire, such as the testosterone stimulation of growth factors (Hobbs, Plymate, Jones, Andress, & Patience, 1991). There is also a strong association between anabolic steroid use and use of other illicit drugs that have been shown to have adverse health consequences (Yesalis, 1993).

Some effects (e.g., thrombotic stroke) may be uniquely related to the extraordinary doses used by some athletes, for whom the dose sometimes appears to be limited only by the cost and availability of the drug. At best, most athletes set their doses based on what seems to work for their friends; unlike scientifically determined doses for desired medical treatments, there is no established dose for strength or weight gain for any anabolic steroid. Some of these athletes also equate doses between different anabolic steroids by the mass units (or even more simply, by the number of tablets!), without considering differences in potency or effects. Thus, there is no scientific basis for the doses used by athletes, which range from levels that may be lower than replacement doses to the more frequently documented doses that far exceed any experienced in clinical medicine. For example, replacement doses of testosterone enanthate for a hypogonadal man average 75 to 100 mg/wk; doses of 200 to 250 mg/wk have been used in male contraceptive trials and in the treatment of oligospermia with suppression-rebound therapy; doses reportedly used by athletes for a cycle of use lasting 6 weeks or more have exceeded 1 g/wk (Yesalis et al., 1988). Oxymetholone, an orally active 17-alkylated anabolic steroid, is used at very high doses, typically 150 mg/d, to treat life-threatening anemias; this dose is comparable to that used by some athletes in conjunction with other anabolic steroids (Friedl & Yesalis, 1989). Methandienone has produced equivocal results in many studies of muscular strength effects (Haupt & Rovere, 1984); it is usually tested at doses of less than 15 mg/d, which is estimated to give full replacement in hypogonadal men (Liddle & Burke, 1960). This drug has been self-administered in doses of 100 mg/d by athletes (Hervey et al., 1975), with doses up to 300 mg/d reportedly used by some athletes for several years (Freed, Banks, Longson, & Burley, 1975). Although anabolic steroids are generally used for short durations of several weeks at a time by bodybuilders (Friedl & Yesalis, 1989), powerlifters have been reported to use high doses of anabolic steroids continuously for up to 7 years (Cohen, Noakes, & Benade, 1988). Doses of such a high magnitude exert truly pharmacological effects and act through other nonandrogenic receptors or through a large increase in metabolites, which in normal concentrations would usually be unimportant (Janne, 1990).

Case Reports of Adverse Effects in Anabolic Steroid—Using Athletes

One way to investigate the adverse effects of anabolic steroids is to review the medical reports of cases in which anabolic steroids are known to have been used. The publication of a case report in the medical literature depends on several factors; a physician must find out that an athlete patient has used steroids and decide that the problem may be related to this steroid use, and both the physician and a journal must be interested in publishing the case as something topical or novel. Some athletes may conceal their drug use when complications arise, and the association may never be made. Other cases will be reported only because they are very unusual or because they involve serious illness or death. Clearly, this is not a suitable way to determine the health risks from steroid use by healthy athletes, but it can suggest problems worth surveillance and further research.

Suspected Disease Associations

The published case reports involving significant morbidity or mortality attributed to anabolic steroid use by athletes are summarized in table 6.1. This summary yields some important information. For one thing, a few athletes may have died as a consequence of anabolic steroid use. In some cases in which there is a questionable association with steroid use, known causative factors of the disease were also present. For example, in addition to his history of steroid use, a 22-year-old elite powerlifter with myocardial infarction weighed 330 lb and had a serum cholesterol of 596 mg/dl (McNutt, Ferenchick, Kirlin, & Hamlin, 1988). On the other hand, the case investigation of a young bodybuilder who collapsed and died in the gym revealed no predisposing factors other than a damaged heart, although this could have been explained by other factors such as a viral cardiomyopathy (Luke, Farb, Virmani, & Sample, 1990). These are interesting cases because several different mechanisms exist that support a potential risk of heart disease with high-dose anabolic steroid use (Melchert & Welder, 1995). Other cases are simply unusual—without further cases or a hint of a disease mechanism involving steroids, they remain enigmatic. For example, a case of a Wilm's tumor in a steroid user has been reported (Prat, Gray, Stolley, & Coleman, 1977). This tumor is relatively rare, especially in adults, but it has also been observed in young adult men not known to be using any anabolic steroids (Scully, Mark, & McNeely, 1981). On the other hand, two cases of hepatic adenoma (Goldman, 1985; Creagh et al., 1988), also a disorder that is rare but has been observed in young men not known to be using steroids, fit into a pattern of androgen-associated tumors observed in patients treated with anabolic steroids. As such, the hepatic adenoma was very likely a consequence of the athlete's anabolic steroid use.

Stroke: A New Association With Anabolic Steroids

Thrombotic stroke is generally unpredicted from clinical experience with anabolic steroids, but it has emerged as a possible risk of anabolic steroid abuse. Cases involving athletes (Frankle, Eichberg, & Zachariah, 1988; Laroche, 1990; Mochizuki & Richter, 1988; Lommi & Harkonen, 1991; Akhter et al., 1994) coupled with another, better documented case of a young man in a hurry to mature (Nagelberg, Laue, Loriaux, Liu, & Sherins, 1986) suggest that very high doses of anabolic steroids may produce thrombotic stroke. In the case reported by Nagelberg and colleagues, a hypogonadal man surreptitiously increased his dosing of testosterone enanthate, achieving measured plasma testosterone concentrations of

Table 6.1 Chronology of Case Reports of Serious Illness or Death in Athletes With Associated Nonmedical Androgen Use

Reference	Age/activity	Disease	Outcome	Description of androgen use
Prat et al., 1977	38 BB	Wilm's tumor	Death from cancer with metastases	Possible high-dose methandienone
Overly et al., 1984	26 BB	Hepatocellular carcinoma with metastases	Death from cancer	Many androgens for 4 y
Sklarek et al., 1984	37 BB	AIDS and hepatitis	Unknown	Shared needles in weekly steroid use
Goldman, 1985	37 BB	Hepatocellular adenoma	Surgical resection and recovery	Oxymetholone (100 mg/d for 5 y)
Edis & Levitt, 1985	27 BB	Colonic adenocarcinoma	Surgical resection and recovery	Methenolone enanthate and oxandrolone (6 m)
Roberts & Essenhigh, 1986	40 BB	Prostatic adenocarcinoma	Death from cancer with metastases	15 cycles of many androgens in 20 y
Creagh et al., 1988	27 BB	Hepatocellular adenoma	Death from hemorrhage	Anabolic steroids for at least 3 y
Frankle et al., 1988	34 BB	Cerebrovascular thrombosis	Partial recovery	Cycles of anabolic steroids for 4 y
Mochizuki & Richter, 1988	32 BB	Cerebrovascular thrombosis (?) and cardiomyopathy	Partial recovery	Many androgens since age 16; stopped 4 m before second stroke
McNutt et al., 1988	22 PL	Myocardial infarction and hypercholesterolemia	Recovery	Intramuscular and oral androgens for 6 wk
Bowman et al., 1989	23 BB	Myocardial infarction	Recovery	Anabolic steroids for 5 y

Scott & Scott, 1989	26 BB	AIDS	Unknown	Repeatedly shared a needle with infected BB injecting steroids
Luke et al., 1990 Campbell et al., 1993	21 BB	Myocardial fibrosis	Death from cardiac arrest	Injected nandrolone and testosterone esters, 2× wk [also in postmortem analysis]
Laroche, 1990	28 BB	Cerebrovascular and peripheral thromboses	Recovery	Monthly injections of many steroids for 3 y
Winwood et al., 1990	30 PL	Bleeding esophageal varices	Recovery	Stanozolol, oxandrolone, and methandienone for 18 m
Lyngberg, 1991	28 BB	Myocardial infarction and atherosclerosis	Death	[unspecified]
Ferenchick & Adelman, 1992	37 PL	Myocardial infarction	Recovery	Anabolic steroids for 7 y; injected nandrolone (200 mg/wk), testosterone, boldenone, stanozolol; ingested oxandrolone
Montine & Gaede, 1992	36 PL	Pulmonary embolism & diabetes	Death from pulmonary embolism	[unspecified]
Kennedy & Lawrence, 1993	18 SC	Sudden cardiac arrest	Death	Oxymesterone [antemortem analysis]
Kennedy & Lawrence, 1993	24 SC	Sudden cardiac arrest probably from myocarditis	Death	Oxymesterone [antemortem analysis]
Kennedy et al., 1993 Moss-Newport, 1993	27 BB	Hemorrhagic stroke and previous myocardial infarction	Death	Nandrolone and stanozolol [antemortem analysis]; used anabolic steroids for 6 y

(continued)

Table 6.1 (continued)

Reference	Age/activity	Disease	Outcome	Description of androgen use
Cabasso, 1994	27 BB	Peliosis hepatis with hemorrhage	Recovery	Oxandrolone, methandienone, nandrolone, and testosterone since age 19
Huie, 1994	25 BB	Myocardial infarction	Recovery	Nandrolone decanoate (200 mg/wk, 6 wk)
Akhter et al., 1994	21 BB	Cerebrovascular thrombosis	Recovery (?)	Ethylestrenol (6–8 mg/d, 6 wk)
Yoshida, Erb, et al., 1994	21 BB	Severe cholestasis & jaundice	Recovery	Testosterone propionate (400 mg/wk, 4 wk)
Yoshida, Karim, et al., 1994	26 BB	Severe cholestasis, jaundice, acute renal failure	Partial recovery of renal function	Stanozolol (Winstrol-V) (125 mg/wk intramuscular for at least 1 month)
Johnson et al., 1995	?	Chickenpox pneumonitis	Recovery after 34 d intensive care	Anabolic steroids for 2 y; including testosterone and nandrolone injections, norethandrolone and oxymetholone; also used ephedrine and hCG
Bryden et al., 1995	26 BB	Renal adenocarcinoma	Nephrectomy & recovery	Anabolic steroids for 6 y, including nandrolone and testosterone esters, methenolone, oxymetholone, methandienone; also used hCG
Dickerman et al., 1995	20 BB	Sudden cardiac arrest	Death	Methandione and testosterone enanthate

BB = bodybuilder; PL = powerlifter; SC = soccer player.

Adapted and updated from Friedl, 1990.

over 100 ng/ml, or 10 times normal levels. At least one of these cases was clearly identified as a cerebrovascular and peripheral thrombosis (Laroche, 1990), and several cases of thrombotic stroke have been reported in Japanese males receiving large doses of oxymetholone or fluoxymesterone for treatment of hypoplastic anemia (Shiozawa et al., 1982; Shiozawa, Tsunoda, Noda, Saito, & Yamada, 1986). Clotting abnormalities can be produced by some anabolic steroids, but the reported effects are inconsistent, with an increase in clotting factors produced by some anabolic steroids (Kruskemper, 1968); other reports suggest an increase in fibrinolytic activity (Barbosa, Seal, & Doe, 1971; Fearnley & Chakrabarti, 1962; Fearnley & Chakrabarti, 1964). A comparison between weightlifters using steroids and those confirmed (by urine assays) not to be using steroids suggests a higher prevalence of coagulation abnormalities in the steroid users, possibly increasing risk for thrombosis (Ferenchick et al., 1995). The connection may be through an estrogen effect, achieved when high doses of anabolic steroids also produce elevated estrogen levels; increased estrogenicity is supported by the occurrence of gynecomastia in some athletes using anabolic steroids, including two of the athletes with stroke (Frankle et al., 1988; Laroche, 1990). This connection is suggested by the increased risk of thrombotic stroke observed in young women taking oral contraceptives (Collaborative Group for the Study of Stroke in Young Women, 1975) and the increased risk of thromboembolism (without change in myocardial infarction rates) in male patients treated with estrogens (Coronary Drug Project Research Group, 1973).

Prostate: An Androgen Target and Potential for Disease

Some other potential risks of steroid use require special vigilance. The androgen parallel to breast cancer risk from the oral contraceptive pill may be prostate cancer, because the prostate is a target tissue for androgens and the cancer is androgen sensitive (Gittes, 1991). Prostate cancer can be induced in some special strains of rats after several months of anabolic steroid treatment (Noble, 1984), but no such connection has emerged for men more than four decades after it was first considered ("Cancer of the Prostate," 1954). However, established prostatic cancer is generally treated by reduction or complete blocking of androgens, and the disease is worsened with testosterone administration (Gittes, 1991). One study suggested that the high rate of prostate cancer in black males is linked to a purportedly higher serum testosterone level (Ross et al., 1986); but in the same theoretical terms we can argue that the risk is reduced with anabolic steroid use because sex hormone-binding globulin, which is higher in patients with prostatic carcinoma (Grasso et al.,

1990), is reduced by anabolic steroids. There is no evidence of prostate stimulation from any of the male contraceptive studies using doses of anabolic steroids up to 200 mg/wk for more than 12 months (Matsumoto, 1990; Mauss et al., 1975; Swerdloff, Palacios, McClure, Campfield, & Brosman, 1978; World Health Organization Task Force, 1990), and a key biochemical marker of prostate disease, prostate-specific antigen, is not increased by testosterone administration (Cooper et al., 1998). The one case report of prostate cancer in a bodybuilder is unusual for a relatively young white man (Roberts & Essenhigh, 1986) but this and other neoplasms involving kidney (Prat et al., 1977; Bryden et al., 1995), liver (Overly et al., 1984; Creagh et al., 1988), and colon (Edis & Levitt, 1985) may well have been promoted by the athletes' use of anabolic steroids (table 6.1). A recent study using mice exposed to continuous very high dose anabolic steroids demonstrated an increased incidence in liver and kidney tumors compared to control mice (Bronson & Matherne, 1997). Suspected, but still poorly defined, effects of some anabolic steroids on immune function (Hughes et al., 1995) and disease resistance (Johnson et al., 1995; Widder et al., 1995) could also contribute to cancer risks.

Musculoskeletal Injuries

Another group of case reports involves tendon ruptures (Bach, Warren, & Wickiewicz, 1987; David et al., 1995; Freeman & Rooker, 1995; Herrick & Herrick, 1987; Hill, Suker, Sachs, & Brigham, 1983; Kramhoft & Solgaard, 1986; Liow & Tavares, 1995; Visuri & Lindholm, 1994), which so far cannot be distinguished from the risks ordinarily faced by strength athletes with extraordinary muscle hypertrophy, even those who don't use anabolic steroids. The suggestion of an association comes primarily from animal studies. Methandienone injected into exercised mice produced collagen abnormalities (Michna, 1987); this has been interpreted as a change that might increase the risk of tendon rupture. Subsequent studies in rats also indicate steroid-induced alterations in tendon elasticity, which might explain an increased risk of tendon failure (Miles et al., 1992; Wood, Cooke, & Goodship, 1988).

Problems Indirectly Associated With Anabolic Steroids

Most of the medical case reports involve bodybuilders (table 6.1), suggesting that bodybuilders are much more likely to use steroids than all other athletes, or that bodybuilders use the drugs in ways that put them at greater risk for health consequences (e.g., higher doses, longer duration, or use with other drugs). Unfortunately, no systematic study of the medical risks of anabolic steroid use by any group of athletes has ever been conducted, and even the population of adult athletes at risk remains poorly defined. In the absence of systematic studies of steroid-using athletes, case reports and patient or subject series from special therapeutic applications form the basis of what is known of the risks possibly associated with anabolic steroids.

Case reports have also highlighted problems that are indirectly associated with steroids or with accessory drug use by bodybuilders. AIDS (Scott & Scott, 1989; Sklarek et al., 1984) and other types of infection (Rastad, Joborn, Ljunghall, & Akerstrom, 1985) are risks that come with the use of contaminated needles or contaminated black-market products when athletes inject steroids. Peripheral nerve damage (Perry, 1994) and sterile abscesses (Khankhanian, Hammers, & Kowalski, 1992) have also been associated with self-administration of parenteral steroids. The wide variety of doses, drug combinations, supplements, and other drugs used by athletes makes it difficult to pinpoint the specific agent responsible for adverse effects in anabolic steroid case reports. For example, reports in the lay press periodically suggest a relationship between steroid use and cardiac arrest, based on bodybuilders collapsing around the time of competition; the more likely proximate cause of collapse in these cases is the extreme dehydration produced with high-ceiling diuretics and associated stimulants such as amphetamines and ephedrine (Appleby, Fisher, & Martin, 1994).

Research on Health Effects

More reliable information on anabolic steroid effects is available from male contraceptive trials, in which greater than replacement doses of anabolic steroids have been tested for durations significantly greater than typical user cycles, and from therapeutic treatment of specific diseases, such as aplastic anemias with high-dose anabolic steroid treatment and male hypogonadism with replacement dose treatment. Even replacement dose treatments yield adverse effects because of pharmacological properties of the synthetic steroids (such as 17-alkylation), and some of these effects will be common to athletes abusing anabolic steroids. These known or suspected health consequences of anabolic steroid use can be divided into five main categories:

- Cosmetic effects
- Heart disease
- Liver toxicity
- Liver tumors
- Infertility

The remainder of this chapter will focus on these five areas.

Cosmetic Effects

Among the best-known side effects of anabolic steroid use in athletic circles are the cosmetic actions that include oily skin and acne, changes in hair patterns, and gynecomastia. Athletes have seen these effects with some frequency either in themselves or in others around them (Strauss et al., 1983; Yesalis et al., 1988). One of the reasons that these effects are so well acknowledged is that they are visible effects that an appearance-conscious bodybuilder may especially dread.

Hair

Body hair patterns are steroid-hormone dependent, and normal virilization includes increased facial hair growth and a gradual recession of the temporal hair line (Garn, 1951). Castration can prevent or arrest baldness in men, and treatment of castrate men with anabolic steroids again permits scalp hair loss (Hamilton, 1948). Thus, it is assumed that balding is accelerated with long-term anabolic steroid administration to normal individuals with such a genetic predisposition. Contraceptive studies lasting for up to several months have reported only slight increases in hair on the chests, backs, or lower abdomens of some subjects (Mauss et al., 1975; Swerdloff et al., 1978).

Acne

The studies of castrate men have also shown that acne is dependent on male sex steroids, because it does not occur in men castrated early in life but can be induced in some eunuchs with testosterone propionate treatment (Hamilton, 1948). The appearance of mild truncal acne or folliculitis has also been reported in male contraceptive studies involving greater than replacement doses of testosterone enanthate (Matsumoto, 1990; Mauss et al., 1975; Swerdloff et al., 1978) and with use of methyltestosterone (Bain, Rachlis, Robert, & Khait, 1980). Pharmacological doses of androgens increase sebaceous gland size and secretion rates (Strauss & Pochi, 1963), and even relatively weak androgens can markedly increase sebum production (Pochi & Strauss, 1974). These effects have also been demonstrated in athletes treating themselves with high-dose anabolic steroids, and a specific increase in skin lipid cholesterol content has been reported (Kiraly, 1988). This increased synthesis of the cholesterol component is thought to appear at peak levels in the sebum excretion after 3 to 4 weeks of anabolic steroid administration (Kiraly, Alen, Rahkila, & Horsmanheimo, 1987).

Gynecomastia

Gynecomastia, the development of abnormal breast tissue in males, is another benign cosmetic disorder that is a well-recognized but poorly understood consequence of anabolic steroid use in athletes (Aiache, 1989;

Friedl & Yesalis, 1989). Transient gynecomastia or some of the early symptoms have also been occasionally reported in male contraceptive studies (Swerdloff et al., 1978). This disorder occurs in men when estrogen levels increase or androgen levels decrease relative to the amount of estrogen present (Wilson, Aiman, & MacDonald, 1980). Estradiol is a potent hormone that causes this effect, and once established the gynecomastia may persist, even after the initial stimulus is gone; thus, the effect may not be directly traceable to an elevated estradiol level. In rare cases, gynecomastia may be a direct consequence of the use of potent estrogens by male bodybuilders who apparently will add anything labeled "steroid" to their polypharmacy repertoire (Rozenek et al., 1990). Gynecomastia has been reported in men with various liver diseases, including alcoholic cirrhosis and hepatocellular carcinoma, and it is a common occurrence during male pubertal maturation. Gynecomastia has been occasionally reported in clinical applications of anabolic steroids, but it has always been observed as a mild and transient phenomenon that eventually ceases even with continued steroid treatment. Bodybuilders have tried to prevent or treat gynecomastia with estrogen blockers and by using other anabolic steroids that may be less likely to convert to potent estrogens (Friedl & Yesalis, 1989; Spano & Ryan, 1984), but these solutions usually do not provide clear relief; for the most severe cases, surgical removal of the excess breast tissue is cosmetically necessary (Reyes et al., 1995).

Heart Disease

Heart disease is a much discussed risk of anabolic steroid use, but as an outcome it remains to be demonstrated. There are good reasons to believe that use of anabolic steroids will increase the risk of heart disease, but there is no epidemiological data to demonstrate that this is the case. As previously discussed in connection with the case reports of stroke, anabolic steroids may affect clotting factors and platelets, leading to blood clots that can occlude critical vessels in the brain (Akhter, Hyder, & Ahmed, 1994; Frankle et al., 1988; Laroche, 1990), lungs (Montine & Gaede, 1992), or heart (Fisher et al., 1996; Huie, 1994; Nieminen et al., 1996). Several case reports have included individuals with atherosclerosis (McNutt et al., 1988; Lyngberg, 1991) and other predisposing factors for infarction, such as myocarditis, possibly associated with recent illness (Kennedy & Lawrence, 1993). However, some of the case reports of sudden death in steroid-using athletes suggest the possibility of a direct adverse effect on the heart, possibly including vasospasm of coronary vessels (Luke et al., 1990) and increased risks associated with hypertrophic cardiomyopathy (Dickerman et al., 1995; Mochizuki & Richter, 1988), where there was no sign of atheroma or coronary thrombosis. In the absence of a reliable denominator representing steroid users, it cannot be determined if these cases even represent a greater than expected prevalence in the young athlete population, and many case reports lack critical information. Use of other drugs such as amphetamines and diuretics (Appleby, Fisher, & Martin, 1994) must be considered. One case that was carefully investigated demonstrated a familial risk: the father of a 27-year-old steroid user who died of heart disease had died at age 32 of heart disease (Cowart, 1987). If there is an increased incidence of heart disease in athletes using anabolic steroids, it is likely to be detected only in a properly designed epidemiological study with careful control of the potential confounders.

Serum Lipids

One of the best established adverse effects of anabolic steroid self-administration by athletes is the reduction in serum HDLC (figure 6.1). However, even though this finding seems incontrovertible, reduced HDLC is not a necessary consequence of anabolic steroid use because not all anabolic steroids consistently produce this effect (Friedl et al., 1990; Thompson et al., 1989). Nevertheless, many athletes use the orally

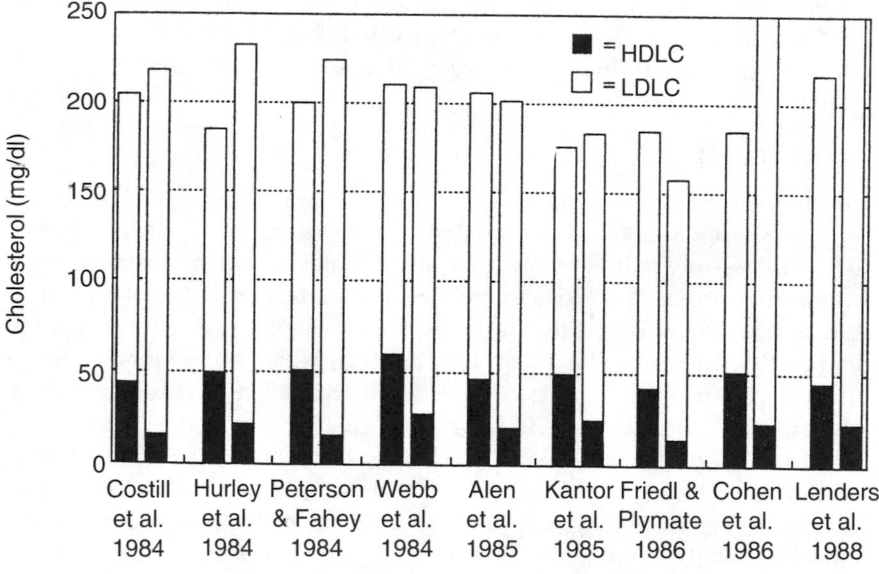

Figure 6.1 Serum lipid measurements without and with androgen self-administration in athletes. The decline in HDLC with androgen administration is consistent across studies, whereas total cholesterol increased significantly in two of the studies. All the studies used 17-alkylated androgens with or without injectable androgens.
Adapted from Friedl 1990.

active compounds that produce this effect, either by themselves or in addition to injectable steroids, and no study of self-administration by athletes has failed to report a significant decline in HDLC. HDLC levels begin to decline within a few days after the start of use and can recover within approximately a month after cessation, although this probably depends on the rate of steroid elimination.

This reduction in HDLC is due to a stimulation of a liver enzyme that regulates serum lipids, hepatic triglyceride lipase (Applebaum, Haffner, & Hazzard, 1987; Kantor, Bianchini, Bernier, Sady, & Thompson, 1985; Lenders et al., 1988). Stimulation of this enzyme leads to a reduction primarily in the HDL-2 cholesterol subfraction and its accompanying apolipoprotein-A1 (Cohen, Faber, Benade, & Noakes, 1986; Friedl et al., 1990; Thompson et al., 1989). This reduction can be profound, and in several of the lipid surveys, HDLC concentrations in the single-digit milligram-per-deciliter range have been observed for some of the athletes (Costill, Pearson, & Fink, 1984; Hurley et al., 1984). By itself, this reduction in HDLC is considered a risk factor for coronary artery disease (National Cholesterol Education Program Expert Panel, 1988). For middle-aged men studied in the Framingham Heart Study who had levels of 25 mg/dl compared to men with initial levels of 50 mg/dl, the risk of developing heart disease was tripled (Heller, Miller, Wheeler, & Kind, 1983).

Although a few studies have also reported increases in total cholesterol (Cohen, Faber, Benade, & Noakes, 1986; Hurley et al., 1984), this has not usually been observed. Instead, the decrease in circulating HDLC appears to be generally offset by the same magnitude of increase in low-density lipoprotein cholesterol (LDLC), with no net alteration in total cholesterol.

The HDLC depression observed so consistently in self-medicating athletes is not an obligatory consequence of anabolic steroid use. The substantial HDLC reduction produced by methyltestosterone in early anabolic steroid studies was actually proposed for use as an index of androgenic potency (Furman, Howard, Smith, & Norcia, 1957); however, subsequent studies in normolipid subjects have failed to demonstrate a clinically significant reduction in HDLC with anabolic steroid ester administration in doses that are markedly androgenic. One longterm study with testosterone enanthate administration (200 mg/wk) in normal men showed a 20% decrease in HDLC after 3 months, with gradual recovery to baseline in the group by 12 months of continuous use (Meriggiola et al. 1995). Thus, although 17-alkylated anabolic steroids reduce HDLC by approximately half, the administration of nandrolone and testosterone esters has little or no effect (Friedl, Dettori, Hannan, Patience, & Plymate, 1991; Friedl et al., 1990; Thompson et al., 1989). This difference is explained by the observation that methyltestosterone and stanozolol induced hepatic triglyceride lipase activity (HTGLA), whereas testosterone enanthate did not (Friedl et al., 1990; Thompson et al., 1989). Induction of HTGLA may be specific to the 17-alkyl-substituted anabolic steroids and may not be due to an androgenic effect at all, but a simpler explanation is that induction of HTGLA reflects an alteration in the androgen/estrogen balance in the presence of an anabolic steroid that is not readily aromatized to estrogen, because estrogen has an opposite effect, suppressing HTGLA and increasing HDLC (Applebaum, Goldberg, Pykalisto, Brunzell, & Hazzard, 1977; Furman, Howard, Norcia, & Keaty, 1958; Tikkanen, Nikkila, Kussi, & Sipinen, 1982). Testosterone enanthate administration results in a large increase in estrogen; and this can counteract the induction of HTGLA, whereas some other anabolic steroids, such as methyltestosterone, are aromatized to a lesser extent and only to 17α-methylestradiol, which appears to be a weak estrogen (Friedl et al., 1990). Further evidence for this modifying role of estrogen comes from one of our studies with co-administration of the aromatase inhibitor testolactone with testosterone enanthate. This suppressed the normally observed increase in estradiol following administration of the enanthate and produced a modest but significant reduction in HDLC that did not occur with testosterone enanthate alone (Friedl et al., 1990). This means that the estrogen inhibitors that some bodybuilders use along with their anabolic steroids in an attempt to prevent gynecomastia may enhance the suppression of HDLC.

Glucose Tolerance

Hyperinsulinemia and impaired glucose tolerance have been reported with use of methandienone (Landon, Wynn, Cooke, & Kennedy, 1962) and oxymetholone (Woodard, Burghen, Kitabchi, & Wilimas, 1981) and for athletes self-administering several other anabolic steroids (Cohen & Hickman, 1987). Such an effect may adversely affect serum HDLC (Stalder, Pometta, & Suenram, 1981), and researchers have suggested from epidemiological observations that testosterone increases risk of heart disease through an effect on insulin (Lichtenstein et al., 1987). Alternatively, glucose intolerance may count as an additional independent risk factor, additive to the risk associated with HDLC reduction. This effect has not been duplicated with anabolic steroid esters (Friedl, Jones, Hannan, & Plymate, 1989; Swerdloff et al., 1978; Landon, Wynn, & Samols, 1963) or with injected methenolone acetate, a 1-methylated anabolic steroid (Landon et al., 1963). In fact, anabolic steroid administration to normal men has been demonstrated to improve glucose disposal (Hobbs, Plymate, Bell, & Patience, 1991).

Hypertension

Hypertension is perhaps one of the most exaggerated health risks associated with anabolic steroid use. This claim appears to have originated in a position statement (American College of Sports Medicine [ACSM], 1987), which has since been quoted to athletes around the country. This position paper referenced a review article on high blood pressure (Messerli & Frohlich, 1979) that was based on a single study of weightlifters. In that study, athletes given methandienone (10 to 25 mg/d for 6 wk) were reported to show slight increases in systolic blood pressure, and one of the men "tended to be hypertensive on the drug" (Freed et al., 1975, p. 472). However, this observation has never been confirmed. Subjects given a substantially higher dose of methandienone (100 mg/d for 6 wk) demonstrated no changes in blood pressure (Hervey et al., 1976), and none of the half-dozen or more strength studies that have involved administration of 5 to 20 mg/d of methandienone to men have found such an effect. In a study that also reported an increase in blood pressure, the average systolic pressure was 118 mm Hg before and 121 mm Hg after 8 weeks of steroid self-administration by a group of amateur bodybuilders (Lenders et al., 1988); this was reported as statistically significant, although clinically this difference is minimal. No other studies have reported a change in blood pressure, even though some have specifically tested it in athletes who self-administer steroids (Alen, 1985) and in controlled studies with high-dose anabolic steroid administration (Friedl et al., 1990; Mauss et al., 1975; World Health Organization Task Force, 1990). Thus, although anabolic steroids can theoretically affect blood pressure in some susceptible individuals through a mechanism analogous to that observed with oral contraceptives (Vessey, Doll, Peto, Johnson, & Wiggins, 1976), it is not a well-established action.

Cardiovascular Risk

Anabolic steroid-induced alteration may actually reduce other health risk factors. For example, stanozolol administration has been shown to reduce the serum lipoprotein-(a) (Albers et al., 1984), which may signify a reduction in risk of ischemic heart disease (Schriewer, Assmann, Sandkamp, & Schulte, 1984) and cerebrovascular disease (Jurgens & Koltringer, 1987). Other characteristics of steroid-using male athletes tend to put them in a low-risk group for heart disease. While they are engaged in athletics, these men tend to exercise intensively, maintain relatively low body fat, and avoid smoking. Thus, it remains to be established whether or not the temporary serum lipid changes produced by 17-alkylated anabolic steroids produce a real difference in an eventual heart disease outcome in these athletes.

Cardiomyopathies

At least one study has suggested that injected methandienone can cause myocardial damage in guinea pigs, although exercising these animals produced similar changes (Appell, Heller-Umpfenbach, Feraudi, &

Weicker, 1983). Case reports have also suggested that anabolic steroids increase left ventricular mass beyond that which can be attributed to hypertrophic responses in strength athletes not using steroids. McKillop, Todd, and Ballantyne (1986) reported an extraordinarily large but not necessarily pathological heart in a 23-year-old bodybuilder who had used steroids intermittently for 8 years. His ventricular wall thickness of 27 mm far exceeded the upper limits measured in 947 elite athletes (Pelliccia, Maron, Spataro, Proschan, & Spirito, 1991). However, the role of anabolic steroid use in this hypertrophy cannot be determined, and several studies comparing strength athletes who use steroids with those who do not have failed to detect a difference in left-ventricular size (Salke, Rowland, & Burke, 1985; Yeater, Reed, Ullrich, Morise, & Borsch, 1996; Zuliani et al., 1989) or concluded that the larger heart mass was proportional to the greater skeletal muscle (Deligiannis & Mandroukas, 1993). There have also been a number of case reports of dilated cardiomyopathy occurring in association with anabolic steroid use by athletes (Ferrera et al., 1997; Melchert & Welder, 1995; Schollert & Bendixen, 1993); more have been reported only in the lay press, including a public case involving the National Football League lineman Steve Courson. These cases, defined by an enlarged left ventricle and a reduced cardiac output, can be associated with inflammation of the heart muscle (myocarditis), but a specific role of anabolic steroids in such cases has not been distinguished from other coincidental causes, such as infectious agents.

Liver Toxicity

Many pharmacological actions of steroids center on the liver. This is a target tissue for androgens and also a principal site of steroid clearance. If the main route of drug delivery is by ingestion, then the liver will also be exposed to the full dose arriving via the portal vein before it is further distributed in the circulation. The actions range from effects on specific proteins such as hepatic triglyceride lipase and sex hormone-binding globulin, to stimulation of hepatocyte hypertrophy and even the formation of benign tumors. At least in patients with already compromised hepatic function, the imposition of high doses of some orally active anabolic steroids has been demonstrated to produce cholestasis and may produce other forms of liver damage.

Liver Enzymes

Most clinical reviews on anabolic steroids have highlighted the alteration of liver function frequently observed following clinical administration of 17-alkylated anabolic steroids; however, this effect appears to be much overrated. Moderate increases in serum activity levels of these enzymes have also been observed in athletes using anabolic steroids (Alen, 1985); however, even with higher values than control subjects or increases over individual baseline values, serum activity levels tend to remain in the normal range. When enzyme levels such as serum glutamate oxaloacetate transaminase (SGOT) exceed the normal range in steroid-using athletes, this may be a reflection of skeletal muscle damage from intense training (and from steroid injections) rather than a reflection of specific liver tissue damage. The elevation in patients has been reported to be a transient phenomenon even with continued use. Petera, Bobek, and Lahn (1962) found that methyltestosterone (30 mg/d) produced a peak rise in both SGOT and glutamate pyruvate transaminase levels after approximately 10 to 12 days of administration to 40 patients, and with continued therapy, the levels declined again. This is consistent with the observation that there was no change in liver function tests at 1, 2, or 3 months of administration of oral methyltestosterone (40 mg/d) to normal men (Friedl et al., 1990). Furthermore, Petera, Bobek, and Lahn (1962) found that the transient enzyme elevation was associated with 17-alkylation; no change occurred if patients were treated with testosterone propionate (25 mg/d), either by oral or parenteral routes of administration. Oral testosterone given to normal men in four 100 mg doses per day also did not change any liver function tests over 21 days (Johnsen, Kampmann, Bennett, & Jorgensen, 1976). Kruskemper (1968) also found increased serum transaminase levels only with 17-alkylated anabolic steroids and no increase with testosterone propionate or even with an orally administered 1-methylated anabolic steroid. The pathological significance of this transient increase remains unknown.

Cholestatic Jaundice

Cholestatic jaundice has been noted in some patients treated with 17-alkylated anabolic steroids; usually this has involved individuals who are being treated for very serious diseases. This has not been an important complaint reported for athletes using anabolic steroids—only one case of cholestatic jaundice has been reported in association with testosterone propionate; there have been no reports in athletes associated with 17-alkylated steroid use. This may be because athletes usually do not use the androgens associated with this effect, stopping use of androgens on their own when they become icteric, or because jaundice is dismissed as a well-known consequence of anabolic steroid use and is not reported by treating physicians.

The first suggestion that some anabolic steroids might cause liver problems came when physicians tried to treat patients with methyltestosterone for the severe itching associated with obstructive jaundice; the jaundice worsened in most of the treated patients (Lloyd-Thomas & Sherlock, 1952). This, and several cases of jaundice in hypogonadal men treated with replacement doses of methyltestosterone (Werner, 1947; Werner, Hanger, & Kritzler, 1950), led to the association of cholestatic jaundice with 17-alkylated anabolic steroid administration. Nearly every report has been of patients treated orally with 17-alkylated anabolic steroids, usually involving methyltestosterone (Bonner & Homburger, 1952) or norethandrolone (Dunning, 1958; Schaffner, Popper, & Chesrow, 1959), but also including stanozolol (Evely, Triger, Milnes, Low-Beer, & Williams, 1987), methylnortestosterone (Peters et al., 1958), and methandienone (Wynn, Landon, & Kawerau, 1961). A case report of jaundice with testosterone enanthate administration (Gil, Lapuerta, Garcia, & Martin, 1986) was described for a pregnant woman, but this cannot be distinguished from pregnancy-related jaundice that occurs in some women (Svanborg & Ohlsson, 1959). A case of severe cholestasis and jaundice was reported in a young bodybuilder who claimed to have discontinued steroid use (testosterone propionate, 400 mg/wk for 4 wk) 3 months before his illness (Yoshida, Erb, Scudamore, & Owen, 1994).

The frequency of cholestasis in patients treated with high doses of anabolic steroids ranges in reports from a few patients demonstrating some histological evidence of disease (Westaby, Ogle, Paradinas, Randell, & Murray-Lyon, 1977) to 17.3% of patients developing an overt jaundice (Pecking, Lejolly, & Najean, 1980). This form of cholestatic drug reaction generally lacks histological features of inflammation and necrosis and is characterized by an accumulation of bile in cells and canaliculi (Foss & Simpson, 1959). Recovery typically occurs within several weeks after drug cessation, and jaundice does not necessarily recur in these patients with reinstitution of treatment (Pecking et al., 1980; Werner et al., 1950). Death is a highly unlikely consequence. The reported deaths caused by cholestatic jaundice have all occurred in elderly or very ill patients (Gilbert, DaSilva, & Queen, 1963), including two patients with metastatic carcinomas and at least one suspected of suffering from severe viral hepatitis (Gordon, Wolf, Krause, & Shai, 1960) (table 6.2). In four of these cases, the medication was continued until the death of the patient because it was not recognized as (nor was it necessarily) the cause of the cholestasis.

Intrahepatic cholestasis can be produced with norethandrolone infusion in rats. The primary defect appears to be a disruption of microfilaments similar to the action produced with cytochalasin B (Phillips, Oda, & Funatsu, 1978). This suggests that reduced bile transport and hepatocyte structural changes that lead to cholestasis are mediated through this single mechanism. Reduced transport may be an early marker of hepatic dysfunction because it appears to precede cholestasis and jaundice. In a large study with anemia patients given one of four oral anabolic steroids (norethandrolone, methandienone, oxymetholone, and the 6-methylated methenolone), 35% of patients had signs of abnormal liver function, including reduced bromosulfophthalein (BSP) uptake, and half of these had overt jaundice (Pecking et al., 1980). In another study, abnormal BSP retention was noted in 35 (74%) of 47 patients treated with

Table 6.2 Case Reports of Deaths Attributed to Androgen-Induced Cholestatic Jaundice by the Reporting Authors or Later Reviewers

Reference	Age/sex	Disorder treated	Androgen/dose/exposure	Cause of death
Koszalka, 1957	60 M	"To improve healing and protein anabolism" (metastatic disease)	Methyltestosterone (sublingual) 30 mg/d, 10 wk	"Obstructive jaundice"
Peters et al., 1958	62 M	"Therapeutic trial" (metastatic disease and angina, treated with 1^{131}-induced myxedema)	Methylnortestosterone 6–25 mg/d, 18 wk	Unknown (histology–"resolving jaundice")
Gordon et al., 1960	43 M	Corticosteroid-induced osteoporosis	Norethandrolone 30 mg/d, 23 wk	Cholestasis and peliosis
Gordon et al., 1960	57 F	Anorexia (result of "pancreatic insufficiency")	Norethandrolone 20 mg/d, 42 wk	"Severe viral hepatitis" with cholestasis and peliosis
Gilbert et al., 1963	74 M	Osteoporosis and hemiplegia	Norethandrolone 30 mg/d, 30 wk	Sepsis and intrahepatic cholestasis

Reprinted from Friedl 1990.

norethandrolone (25 or 50 mg/d), but liver biopsies from 7 of the patients with poor BSP retention times yielded normal tissue, with only one demonstrating a minimal bile stasis and focal necrosis (Kory, Bradley, Watson, Callahan, & Peters, 1959). Hypercholesterolemia is also a marker of cholestasis, and the reportedly high cholesterol levels in one study of athletes using anabolic steroids (Cohen et al., 1988) are conceivably related to such liver dysfunction.

Peliosis Hepatis

Peliosis hepatis is a potentially life-threatening hepatic lesion characterized by a spectrum of microscopic to grossly visible blood-filled cysts in the liver. Although peliosis hepatis was originally recognized as a very rare disease associated almost exclusively with pulmonary tuberculosis, a relationship between peliosis hepatis and anabolic steroid treatment was proposed in 1952 (Burger & Marcuse, 1952). Since then, more than 70 cases of hepatic and splenic peliosis have been reported in association with anabolic steroid administration (Friedl, 1990). In autopsies of Japanese patients with aplastic anemia, 7 of 19 patients who had been treated with oxymetholone or methenolone had peliosis, compared to only 1 of 28 patients not treated with anabolic steroids (Wakabayashi, Onda, Tada, Iijima, & Itoh, 1984). In an American series, 5 out of 9 patients treated with anabolic steroids for wasting diseases had peliosis at autopsy (Karasawa, Shikata, & Smith, 1979). In healthy patients, peliosis may not be as prevalent. Out of 60 transsexual women and impotent men treated with methyltestosterone (150 mg/d) for up to 5 years, 9 patients had sinusoidal dilatation and 3 patients had cyst formation, suggestive of potential prepeliotic lesions (Westaby et al., 1977). Although the patients in this series were free of symptoms, a later case report described peliosis hepatis and liver tumor rupture requiring emergency surgery in one of the transsexuals following 7 years of continuous anabolic steroid treatment. In a 3- to 5-year follow-up of many of the patients from this series and others who were administered various anabolic steroids, Lowdell and Murray-Lyon (1985) found hepatic abnormalities (based on liver scans and colloid uptake) only in the patients still using methyltestosterone, with resolution of abnormalities in those who had stopped using methyltestosterone, and essentially normal livers in those administering their steroids lingually or parenterally.

Most of these reported peliosis cases involve patients treated with 17-alkylated anabolic steroids, including fluoxymesterone (Kintzen & Sliny, 1960), norethandrolone (Gordon et al., 1960), oxymetholone (Groos, Arnold, & Brittinger, 1974), methenolone (Wakabayashi et al., 1984), and methyltestosterone (Bird, Vowles, & Anthony, 1979). Peliosis is not frequently associated with anabolic steroid esters, although one case of peliosis has been reported for a young bodybuilder who had injected 200 mg/wk of nandrolone decanoate for 5 weeks at the time of medical admission (Cabasso, 1994). He recovered from a hematocrit of 20% following repeated transfusions. Postmortem examinations of 52 dialysis patients treated with testosterone enanthate (up to 250 mg/wk for 5 months) revealed no peliosis (Saheb, 1980); however, another postmortem study revealed peliotic lesions in 6 chronic renal failure patients who had received only anabolic steroid esters for an average of more than 3 years (Turani, Levi, Zevin, & Kessler, 1983). Peliosis has also been observed in a woman treated with tamoxifen (Loomus, Aneja, & Bota, 1983), a drug that is also used by some athletes abusing anabolic steroids in an attempt to prevent gynecomastia. Although only a single case, it is unusual because peliosis is such a rare disorder, and this case may indicate a role of an androgenic/estrogenic component in this disorder.

Peliosis may not be readily diagnosed by standard laboratory studies, and it is usually discovered either as occult disease in postmortem examination or, rarely, as a result of symptomatic hemorrhage. At least five patients have died from internal hemorrhage resulting from their peliosis (Bagheri & Boyer, 1974; Nadell & Kosek, 1977; Taxy, 1978), but internal hemorrhage is also a frequent cause of death in severe anemias. Several cases of death from hepatic failure have also been attributed to an existing peliosis, although in some of these cases metastatic disease and severe cholestasis may have been more directly responsible for patient death. One case of histologically diagnosed peliosis hepatis was followed after anabolic steroid withdrawal, and complete recovery was observed (Nadell & Kosek, 1977).

Mechanism of Cholestasis and Peliosis Hepatis

A single mechanism has been proposed to explain the occurrence of both cholestasis and peliosis hepatis (Paradinas, Bull, Westaby, & Murray-Lyon, 1977). Based on microscopic evaluation of biopsy material from the Westaby series of patients treated with methyltestosterone, it has been proposed that 17-alkylated anabolic steroids specifically produce hepatocyte hyperplasia; the enlarged hepatocytes then encroach on the hepatic venous system, occluding vessels and perhaps also blocking bile canaliculi to produce cholestasis, peliotic sinusoids, and perhaps even esophageal varices (Paradinas et al., 1977).

Liver Tumors

Several diseases, including heart disease and hepatocellular carcinoma (HCC), occur with higher frequency in males than in females. Thus, androgen links to heart disease and HCC have been extensively investigated. Animal studies with castration and androgen replacement support a connection with HCC (Vesselinovitch & Mihailovich, 1967). However, anabolic steroids are not mutagenic in the Ames test (Ingerowski, Scheutwinkel-Reich, & Stan, 1981); instead, they appear to promote tumor formation by enhancing the effects of carcinogens (Lesna

& Taylor, 1986). Anabolic steroid doses that are 400 to 600 times the human clinical dose, given over the life span of a rodent, usually cause liver growth (hypertrophy and hyperplasia) but without tumors. In mice, 6 weeks of treatment with nandrolone decanoate (600 mg/kg/wk) did not produce liver tumors, but following exposure to dimethylnitrosamine, which is known to produce liver cancer in this model, the expected tumor formation was further enhanced (Lesna & Taylor, 1986).

Characteristics of Anabolic Steroid-Associated Liver Tumors

There is little question that administering anabolic steroid to men increases their risk of liver tumors. The type of tumor that is promoted appears to act more like a benign hepatocellular adenoma (HCA), which rarely occurs in men, than like the malignant HCC, with which it shares some diagnostic features (Craig, Peters, & Edmondson, 1989) (figure 6.2).

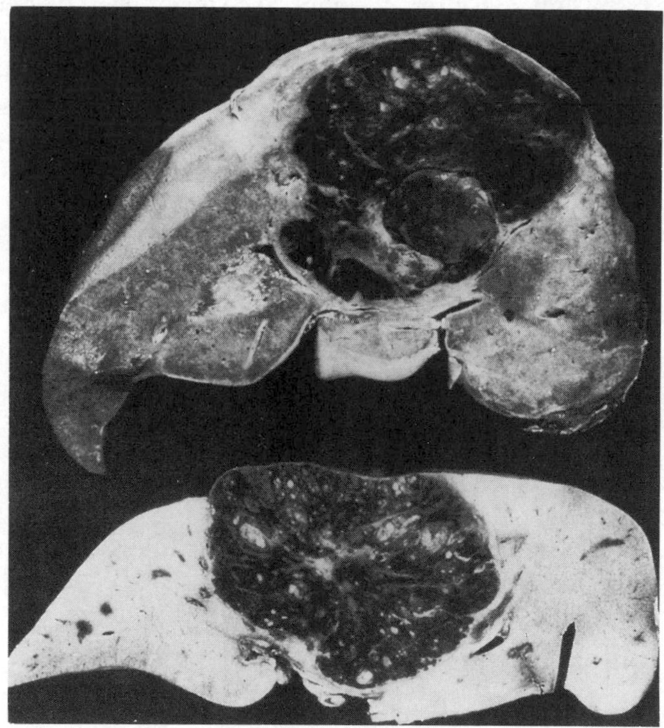

Figure 6.2 Anabolic steroid–associated hepatocellular adenoma, now recognized as a diagnostic category of benign epithelial tumors. The top view shows a hepatocellular adenoma with a diameter of 9 cm from a patient with Fanconi's anemia who was treated with methyltestosterone for 4 years; the bottom view shows a cross section of the tumor.

Reprinted from Craig, Peters, and Edmondson 1989.

The principal distinction between the diseases is reflected in the aggressive behavior of the typical HCC. The median survival time for patients with HCC may be as short as 1 month, with very few patients expected to live beyond 1 year (Peters, 1976), whereas the anabolic steroid–related tumors in some individuals have regressed following anabolic steroid withdrawal (Cocks, 1981; Drew, 1984; Goodman & Laden, 1977; McCaughan, Bilous, & Gallagher, 1985; Treuner, Niethammer, Flach, Fischbach, & Schenck, 1980) and even have regressed in some individuals without any other treatment (Johnson et al., 1972; McCaughan et al., 1985; Westaby, Portmann, & Williams, 1983). Nevertheless, benign should not be interpreted to mean non–life threatening, because at least several of the anabolic steroid–related cases have been diagnosed as a result of tumor rupture and serious internal bleeding, even culminating in the death of one bodybuilder.

Since a relation between anabolic steroid treatment and hepatic tumors was first suggested (Bernstein, Hunter, & Yachnin, 1971), at least 91 cases of anabolic steroid-associated tumors have been reported in the medical literature (Friedl, 1990). Nearly half of these have been diagnosed in patients with an inherited form of severe anemia (Fanconi's anemia) who were treated with anabolic steroids. Hereditary anemias such as Fanconi's syndrome carry an increased incidence of malignant neoplasia (Schaison, Leverger, & Yildez, 1983), and patients with such anemias may be predisposed to the development of hepatic tumors (Cattan, Kalifat, et al., 1974; Cattan, Vesin, Wautier, Kalifat, & Meignan, 1974), with such tumors emerging more frequently when lives are extended by anabolic steroid therapy. However, at least 43 of these cases are not Fanconi's patients and include definitive diagnoses based on microscopic evaluation of tumor material obtained from the patients. After we eliminate cases in which hepatic tumors were not the cause of death and were detected only at autopsy, and several diverse diagnoses involving hepatic angiosarcoma and focal nodular hyperplasia, a large set of cases that are variously diagnosed as HCA or HCC remains. These cases collectively exhibit characteristics that can be described as very unusual for tumors that look histologically malignant; with the common connection of anabolic steroid use, they suggest a peculiar androgen-specific form of liver tumor (Anthony, 1975). This is now recognized as a distinct form of liver tumor (Craig, Peters, & Edmonson, 1989).

The earliest known case with an androgen association (Drew, 1984) typifies the liver tumors that this section has described. In 1961, hepatocellular carcinoma was diagnosed in a 44-year-old man presenting with a right upper quadrant abdominal mass. Part of the tumor was removed, and he was given chemotherapy. Twenty-two years later, this patient was still alive with no complaints of liver dysfunction. The unusual characteristics of this HCC include the long survival following diagnosis, the absence of metastases, and the absence of elevated α-fetoprotein production. Nearly all of the reported cases are also negative for serum hepatitis surface antigen and lack evidence of an associated cirrhosis, which is found with many of the more typical HCC cases, in the absence of known exogenous androgen exposure (Peters, 1976). That these cases are androgen related is supported by the follow-up observation that tumor regression occurred in more than half of the cases after androgen withdrawal, with no other treatment (or only partial tumor excision). Most of these cases involved patients who were being treated for androgen deficiency (usually with methyltestosterone, at a typical dose of 50 mg/d) or for a severe anemia (usually with oxymetholone, at a typical dose of at least 100 mg/d). Only two cases were associated with exclusive use of anabolic steroid esters (Carrasco et al., 1985; Turani et al., 1983).

Liver Tumors in Athletes

At least three case reports involve liver tumors in athletes using anabolic steroids. These include one patient who died from a metastatic carcinoma (Overly et al., 1984), one who died from internal hemorrhage following the rupture of an adenoma (Creagh, Rubin, & Evans, 1988), and another who apparently survived following surgical removal of an adenoma (Goldman, 1985). In the case reported by Overly and colleagues (1984), the features are typical of the better-known malignant hepatocellular carcinoma, including high serum levels of α-fetoprotein synthesized by the carcinoma, and the aggressive biological behavior of the tumor, with metastasis and short time to death. This case also included cholangiole involvement, seen in only two other patients in these cases (one of which also metastasized). Thus, this cancer case does not bear the characteristics typical of the anabolic steroid-associated tumors.

Vascularization of the Tumors

The apparent likelihood of tumor rupture in the case reports of anabolic steroid–associated tumors is independent of the tendency to develop peliosis. In these patients, peliosis was not consistently present with the tumors (it was described in half of the cases), and it has been suggested that necrotic lesions described as peliosis may be more accurately represented as vascular ectasia, frequently seen with tumors (Peters, 1976). As an example, in the case of the athlete who died following tumor rupture (Creagh et al., 1988), the liver surrounding the adenomas was described as hyperplastic with ectactic sinusoids but was apparently devoid of peliotic cysts.

Certainly, the case reports emphasize symptomatic patients who were brought to medical attention, and the reports are submitted for publication because of the severity of the problems; 24 out of 28 anabolic steroid–related HCA or HCC case reports involved acute abdominal pain or internal hemorrhage. The majority of anabolic steroid–associated tumors may remain undetected because they do not rupture and the patients remain asymptomatic, such as the cases of occult diseases that have been described from careful postmortem examinations of anabolic steroid–treated patients (Chandra, Kapur, Kelleher, Luban, & Patterson, 1984; Sale & Lerner, 1977; Turani et al., 1983). On the other hand, in 31 cases of hepatocellular adenoma in males collected from the literature, all three tumors associated with anabolic steroid use ruptured (Pelletier, Frija, Szekely, & Clauvel, 1984). We can also hypothesize that 17-alkylation does not produce more tumors than the anabolic steroid esters but simply increases the likelihood of discovery through rupture; Turani and colleagues (1983) described tumors and peliosis associated with nonalkylated anabolic steroids in a mostly postmortem series. Anabolic steroids are likely to increase the risk of hemorrhage in individuals with liver tumors through an effect of increased fibrinolytic activity; this has been reported in patients receiving either oral anabolic steroids (Fearnley & Chakrabarti, 1962) or testosterone propionate (Fearnley & Chakrabarti, 1964), but only some 17-alkylated anabolic steroids (including oxymetholone) have been found to decrease fibrinogen (Barbosa et al., 1971). The high rate of adenoma rupture and hemorrhage in women using oral contraceptives, compared to women with HCA not using oral contraceptives, is particularly associated with the use of 17-alkyl-substituted progestagens (Klatskin, 1977). These data suggest a structural specificity; although this too can reflect selective reporting.

Incidence of Anabolic Steroid–Associated Liver Tumors

The occurrence of anabolic steroid–related tumors appears to be considerably higher than the rate of hepatic tumors associated with female oral contraceptive steroids. At least 117 cases had been documented in the literature within 5 years of the first case report associating oral contraceptives with liver tumors. Most of these cases (92%) involved benign tumors. Since fewer than 400 cases had been reported in women since 1937 this strongly suggested an oral contraceptive connection (Klatskin, 1977). Oral contraceptive–related tumors are rare relative to the size of the population at risk; at least 30 million women in the United States alone are estimated to be currently using contraceptive steroids. The prevalence of anabolic steroid use, even including use by anabolic steroid abusers, is not reasonably expected to come close to this, nor is exposure during the past 30 years likely to rival oral contraceptive exposures, yet the literature already documents nearly 100 cases of anabolic steroid–associated liver tumors. In patients with severe anemia who survived 2 years with anabolic steroid treatment, the incidence was 2 benign tumors in 137 patients (Joint Group, 1981; Pecking et al., 1980); previously, a case with tumor rupture was reported (Hernandez-Nieto, Bruguera, Bombi, Camacho, & Rozman, 1977) for a patient from the larger sample of 429 patients originally enrolled in the same series (in which 3 of the 429 patients had tumors), although many of these additional patients had a shorter exposure to anabolic steroids. In a series of 60 female-to-male transsexuals and impotent men treated with high-dose methyltestosterone (Coombes, Reiser, Paradinas, & Burn, 1977; Westaby et al., 1977), only one HCA was detected, although another case with tumor rupture was later reported (Bird et al., 1979) for a transsexual from the same series (in which 2 of the 60 patients had tumors). Thus, the incidence of hepatic tumors may be estimated to be 1 to 3% within 2 to 8 years of exposure of greater than replacement doses of 17-alkylated anabolic steroid; occult disease is likely to also be present and makes this incidence higher.

Another rare form of liver cancer, hepatic angiosarcoma, was also associated with anabolic steroid use in a retrospective epidemiological study. In a review of 168 cases of histologically confirmed cases of hepatic angiosarcoma, researchers identified four cases with some previous anabolic steroid exposure (3.1%) from a review of medical records (Falk, Thomas, Popper, & Ishak, 1979). The connection with anabolic steroid exposure remains unconfirmed, with no new anabolic steroid–associated cases reported since the latest of the four case deaths in 1974, and at least one of those four patients was exposed to isoniazid, another proposed agent of hepatic angiosarcoma (Daneshmend & Bradfield, 1979). Three cases of focal nodular hyperplasia (Alberti-Flor et al., 1974; Kessler, Bar-Meir, & Pinkhas, 1976; Sweeney & Evans, 1976) have been reported in patients with anabolic steroid exposure, in two cases with only 3 and 6 months of anabolic steroid exposure, also leaving open the possible role of anabolic steroid.

Infertility

Male athletes who self-administer high doses of anabolic steroid are likely to be infertile during their period of use and for some time after cessation of use, perhaps as long as 6 months after. This effect cannot be reliably produced in all males, and not all anabolic steroids are equally effective in this action. No cases of irreversible infertility as a result of anabolic steroid administration have ever been reliably documented, although athletes using these anabolic steroids are naturally concerned when they notice a shrinking testicular volume, which usually accompanies the temporary reduction in testicular stimulation by trophic hormones and the depletion of developing germ cells.

Spermatogenesis is markedly suppressed in athletes using a wide assortment of anabolic steroids. In a study of bodybuilders, the average sperm count of the men who had used steroids within the past 3 months was less than 20 million/ml, whereas those who had stopped their use for 4 to 24 months prior to the count averaged 84 million/ml (Knuth,

Maniera, & Nieschlag, 1989). The researchers observed no difference between fertile control subjects and these steroid users regarding the proportion of sperm motility or abnormal morphology, suggesting that these other characteristics may be unaffected.

Controlled Trials of Reversible Male Contraception

Many controlled studies have examined the effect of high-dose anabolic steroid administration to fertile males to test the suitability of male steroidal contraception. The oral anabolic steroids, such as methyltestosterone and testosterone undecanoate, have not proven effective (Paulsen, Bremner, & Leonard, 1982), whereas various testosterone esters (Matsumoto, 1990; Mauss et al., 1975; Steinberger, Smith, & Rodriguez-Rigau, 1978) and nandrolone decanoate (Schurmeyer, Knuth, Belkien, & Nieschlag, 1984) produce oligo- or azoospermia in normal men within weeks or months of continuous high-dose exposure. This has been most extensively studied with testosterone enanthate. A clear decline in sperm concentration is observable for normal men receiving at least 50 mg/wk (figure 6.3); 300 mg/wk does not further reduce the count in men who do not suppress at 100 mg/wk (Matsumoto, 1990), but fertilizing capacity is also reduced in these men at very low sperm counts (Matsumoto, 1988). Because the major portion of the testis is composed of seminiferous

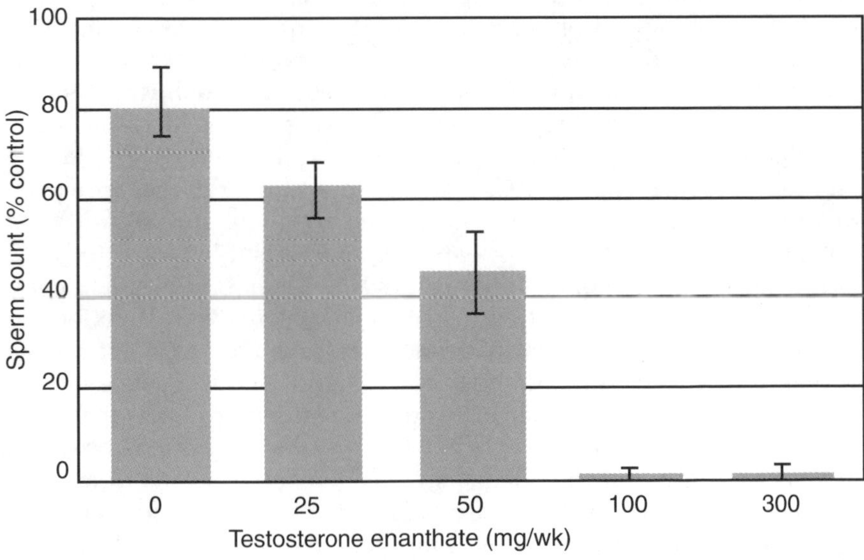

Figure 6.3 Sperm counts, expressed as a proportion of individual baseline values, at different doses of testosterone enanthate administered weekly by intramuscular injection for 6 months.

Adapted from Matsumoto and Bremner 1988.

tubules and developing germ cells, this reduction in the population of developing germ cells decreases testicular size by a measurable 15 to 35% from baseline (Friedl et al., 1991; Kiraly et al., 1987; Palacios, McClure, Campfield, & Swedloff, 1981; World Health Organization Task Force, 1990). Because the normal cycle of sperm development from spermatogonia to mature spermatid in the testis is about 2 months, it is not surprising that the repopulation of the germinal epithelium to pretreatment sperm counts following cessation of steroid administration may take 6 months or even nearly 1 year for some men (Paulsen et al., 1982); there is hope that some anabolic steroids with long halftimes will have an even more extended effect (Weinbauer, Marshall, & Nieschlag, 1986). A large multicenter trial sponsored by the World Health Organization has now demonstrated that long-term testosterone enanthate administration is effective as a male contraceptive in carefully screened males (World Health Organization Task Force, 1990). The mean time for individual subjects to recover to their baseline geometric mean from azoospermia following more than 1 year of weekly 200 mg injections of testosterone enanthate in this study was 6.7 months (range: 6.2 to 8.7 months) (World Health Organization Task Force, 1990).

The popular press has caused confusion about the reversibility of anabolic steroid–induced sterility, and like the confusion about the effects of steroids on blood pressure, this confusion appears to originate from the ACSM (1987) position statement on steroids. This statement refers to an early study in which prisoners were given estrogens and progestagens developed for female contraception, and in which sperm counts and testicular biopsy specimens were reported to be below baseline values after several months of recovery time (Heller, Moore, Paulsen, Nelson, & Laidley, 1959). There are several problems with using this report to suggest the possibility of a permanent sterility with anabolic steroid use. First, there was enough uncertainty in the interpretation of these data that one of the authors added a dissenting comment in the same journal (Nelson, 1959, p. 1065), stating his view that some of the changes reported for testicular biopsies "failed to reveal any change of real consequence" and doubting the accuracy of the semen analyses. Andrologists who have undertaken subsequent studies have been careful to take into account the wide day-to-day variability that is observed in semen quality, and this includes using geometric means of multiple samples. Second, the anabolic steroids tested by Heller and colleagues (1959) are not those that athletes are generally known to be using; in fact, the closest relative tested was the anabolic steroidic progestogen norethandrolone, and this has not been reported to be used by athletes. Finally, none of the authors of this study suggested that the effects might be permanent, and none of the many controlled prospective studies since then have made such a suggestion.

Spermatogenic Rebound With Cessation of Steroid Administration

High-dose anabolic steroids have also been administered to restore fertility in men with low sperm counts, through a well-recognized but poorly understood rebound that occurs following several months of high-dose anabolic steroid sperm suppression (Charney & Gordon, 1978; Rowley & Heller, 1972). Up to 60% of patients with below-normal spermatogenic activity but otherwise normal seminiferous epithelia show at least temporary improvement in their sperm counts, and some patients show permanent improvement. Norethandrolone, testosterone esters, and mesterolone have all been used in rebound therapy, and some researchers claim that these drugs improve pregnancy success rates. Other approaches to treatment of male infertility have included administration of mesterolone (Aafjes, Van der Vijver, Brugman, & Schenck, 1983) or testosterone undecanoate (Kloer, Hoogen, & Nieschlag, 1980) to oligospermic men in an attempt to support spermatogenesis.

Effects on Gonadotropins

The reduction of sperm count is primarily mediated through the suppression of gonadotropins (LH and FSH), although there may be some direct effects on the testes as well. This gonadotropin suppression has been well demonstrated in many of the contraceptive studies as well as in at least one detailed assessment of self-administering athletes (Alen, Rahkila, Reinila, & Vihko, 1987). Earlier studies have suggested that orally active mesterolone does not suppress gonadotropins at doses that elicit androgenic effects (Aakvaag & Stromme, 1974; Petry, Rausch-Stroomann, Hienz, Senge, & Mauss, 1968) and that 17-alkylated anabolic steroids also may not suppress gonadotropins at moderate doses (Friedl et al., 1990). Some steroid-using athletes administer human chorionic gonadotropin (HCG) during or at the end of their steroid cycles with the intention of preventing the reduction in activity or restimulating the testes to a more rapid recovery. Some evidence indicates that this will maintain testicular function during steroid use (Wing, Ewing, Zegeye, & Zirkin, 1985), but this may require more careful dosing than self-medicating athletes are likely to achieve. The testes were not fully responsive to a single dose of HCG in athletes treated 3 weeks after the ends of their cycles of steroid use (Martikainen, Alen, Rahkila, & Vihko, 1986), whereas repeated HCG treatments actually desensitized the testes to LH stimulation (Glass & Vigersky, 1980). The main risk that athletes run in this use of HCG is an increased probability for the development of gynecomastia (Friedl & Yesalis, 1989).

Binding Protein Interactions

Sex hormone-binding globulin (SHBG) is reduced by both 17-alkylated anabolic steroids and the esters (Friedl et al., 1991), but the 17-alkylated anabolic steroids are more potent in this effect (Friedl et al., 1990), reflecting either the difference in androgen/estrogen balance produced with these two classes of anabolic steroids or the difference in direct hepatic actions of these pharmacological preparations. SHBG is also reduced in steroid-using athletes (Ruokonen, Alen, Bolton, & Vihko, 1985), which leads to an increase in free and albumin-bound testosterone. The significance of this change is uncertain because many of the synthetic anabolic steroids have a reduced binding affinity to begin with (Saartok, Dahlberg, & Gustafsson, 1984) and will be little affected by a change in the binding protein concentration; however, diminished SHBG levels will result in a higher clearance rate for testosterone and other steroids that are bound by SHBG.

Case Reports of Athlete Users

The orthopedic literature describes two cases of athletes who, the report claims, demonstrate sustained hypogonadism as a result of their steroid use (Jarow & Lipshultz, 1990). This report demonstrates some of the problems encountered with such uncontrolled "studies." One bodybuilder had used anabolic steroids off and on for 4 years and was using high doses of three different anabolic steroids until 6 weeks before his work-up for infertility, when he demonstrated a low sperm count, reduced testosterone concentration, and poor response to gonadotropin-releasing hormone (GnRH) stimulation. One year later he still demonstrated a poor response to GnRH stimulation; however, the report did not verify that he had discontinued his steroid use. This is important, because I have encountered a similar case in which the husband was willing to let his wife go through a complete series of infertility tests before he would admit that he was still using anabolic steroids (Friedl, 1987). The second case cited by Jarow and Lipshultz (1990) was a 39-year-old competitive weightlifter who had fathered three children and now complained of decreased libido; he also had a history of epididymitis. He was found to have a reduced testosterone concentration but normal gonadotropin levels, and one semen analysis was within normal ranges. The report provided no details about this patient's treatment, including whether or not he received a prescription for steroids. The authors reported these two cases to highlight "the potentially permanent deleterious effects of anabolic steroids to the hypothalamic-pituitary-gonadal axis" (p. 431). These case reports illustrate several key problems that recur in this case report literature. The cessation of steroid use was not verified, the presteroid-use fertility status was unknown, and the fertility testing was inadequate for any conclusive diagnosis.

Conclusions

From the evidence of studies of anabolic steroid administration, it is not readily apparent that we can attribute significant adverse health effects to anabolic steroids as a general class. However, the 17-alkyl-substituted anabolic steroids have certain established consequences, all involving the liver. The 17-alkylated anabolic steroids produce a consistent and substantial reduction in HDLC/LDLC fractions, possibly increasing the risk of heart disease, although this outcome remains to be demonstrated in anabolic steroid users. Cholestatic jaundice has been observed in frequencies ranging from none to 17% in various categories of patients treated with 17-alkylated anabolic steroid, but this condition is readily reversed when anabolic steroid treatment is stopped. Peliosis hepatis is clearly associated with use of 17-alkylated anabolic steroid but with unknown frequency. Hepatic tumors are rare in men but occur with a frequency as high as 1 to 3% with 17-alkylated anabolic steroid treatment, with a latency of 2 to 30 years. Nearly half of these discovered tumors rupture, although a larger proportion of benign disease may remain undetected. In two cases, including one of a self-medicating bodybuilder, rupture proved fatal.

In contrast to the orally active anabolic steroids, anabolic steroid esters produce few reports of adverse effects, even though the clinical use of these injected anabolic steroids appears to be widespread. This is the basis for their use in male contraceptive trials (World Health Organization Task Force, 1990). However, several case reports involving death or significant illness in athletes self-administering anabolic steroids suggest the possibility of other adverse effects that have not been commonly associated with anabolic steroid doses in the clinical range. Foremost among these reports are the three cases of stroke reported in bodybuilders and a fourth in a hypogonadal man, who self-administered high doses of anabolic steroid. Because there is no established steroid dosing that can be recommended to produce desired competitive advantages of increased strength or increased aggressiveness, athletes use doses and steroids with no defined upper limit. This is substantially different from the approach used in the development of male steroidal contraception, for which the lowest effective dose has been carefully determined (Matsumoto, 1990). We may speculate that more serious side effects such as thrombotic stroke occur at very high doses, even with anabolic steroid esters, through estrogenic metabolites or by crossover interactions with nonandrogenic receptors. Researchers have speculated that suppression of immune function is a possible consequence through crossover interaction with corticosteroid receptors, although the only study that has examined immune function in anabolic steroid–using athletes found an enhancement of immune function (primarily enhanced natural killer-cell activity) in the steroid users (Calabrese et al., 1989). These higher-dose effects may only become apparent with prospective study of anabolic steroid abusers, that group with no scientifically determined steroid-dosing rationale and, especially, with no dose upper limit. Based on case reports of adverse effects, this group may comprise primarily bodybuilders.

Clearly, 17-alkyl substitution in an anabolic steroid introduces properties producing health risks that should not be ascribed to androgenic actions, and other nonandrogenic health consequences will occur through the use of black-market preparations of uncertain quality and composition. Other distinctions are emerging even among anabolic steroid esters (Friedl et al., 1991; Hannan et al., 1991; Hobbs et al., 1991), which suggest that testosterone esters, indistinguishable from endogenous testosterone after the compounds are hydrolyzed in circulation, are potent anabolic steroids possessing the fewest short-term health risks at high doses of up to 300 mg/wk for at least several months. On the other hand, there is reasonable suspicion that prostatic carcinoma is linked to androgen excess (Ross et al., 1986; Schally & Comaru-Schally, 1987). The bottom line is that an athlete would be foolish to conclude that there is a safe way to use anabolic steroids; although no disease of androgen excess has ever been described for men, the long-term consequences of anabolic steroid supplementation have not been investigated and are simply unknown.

References

Aafjes, J.H., Van der Vijver, J.C.M., Brugman, F.W., & Schenck, P.E. (1983). Double-blind crossover treatment with mesterolone and placebo of subfertile oligozoospermic men. Value of testicular biopsy. *Andrologia, 15,* 531–535.

Aakvaag, A., & Stromme, S.B. (1974). The effect of mesterolone administration to normal men on the pituitary-testicular function. *Acta Endocrinologica, 77,* 380–386.

Adamson, J.W., & Vapnek, D. (1991). Recombinant erythropoietin to improve athletic performance. *New England Journal of Medicine, 324,* 698–699.

Aiache, A.E. (1989). Surgical treatment of gynecomastia in the body builder. *Plastic and Reconstructive Surgery, 83,* 61–66.

Akhter, J., Hyder, S., & Ahmed, M. (1994). Cerebrovascular accident associated with anabolic steroid use in a young man. *Neurology, 44,* 2405–2406.

Albers, J.J., Taggart, H.M., Applebaum-Bowden, D., Haffner, S., Chesnut, C.H., III, & Hazzard, W.R. (1984). Reduction of lecithin-cholesterol acyltransferase, apolipoprotein D and the Lp(a) lipoprotein with the anabolic steroid stanozolol. *Biochimica et Biophysica Acta, 795,* 293–296.

Alberti-Flor, C.C., Iskandarani, M., Jeffers, L., Zappa, R., & Schiff, E.R. (1984). Focal nodular hyperplasia associated with the use of a synthetic anabolic androgen. *American Journal of Gastroenterology, 79,* 150–151.

Alen, M. (1985). Androgenic steroid effects on liver and red cells. *British Journal of Sports Medicine, 19,* 15–20.

Alen, M., Rahkila, P., & Marniemi, J. (1985). Serum lipid in power athletes self-administering testosterone and anabolic steroids. *International Journal of Sports Medicine, 6,* 139–144.

Alen, M., Rahkila, P., Reinila, M., & Vihko, R. (1987). Androgenic-anabolic steroid effects on serum thyroid, pituitary and steroid hormones in athletes. *American Journal of Sports Medicine, 15,* 357–361.

American College of Sports Medicine. (1987). Position stand on the use of anabolic-androgenic steroids in sports. *Medicine and Science in Sports and Exercise, 19,* 534–539.

Anthony, P.P. (1975). Hepatoma associated with androgenic steroids. *Lancet, 1,* 685–686.

Appell, H.J., Heller-Umpfenbach, B., Feraudi, M., & Weicker, H. (1983). Ultrastructural and morphometric investigations on the effect of training and administration of anabolic steroids on the myocardium of guinea pigs. *International Journal of Sports Medicine, 4,* 268–274.

Applebaum, D.M., Goldberg, A.P., Pykalisto, O.J., Brunzell, J.D., & Hazzard, W.R. (1977). Effect of estrogens on postheparin plasma lipolytic activity: Selective decline in hepatic triglyceride lipase. *Journal of Clinical Investigation, 59,* 601–608.

Applebaum, D.M., Haffner, S., & Hazzard, W.R. (1987). The dyslipoproteinemia of anabolic steroid therapy: Increase in hepatic triglyceride lipase precedes the decrease in high density lipoprotein2 cholesterol. *Metabolism, 36,* 949–952.

Appleby, M., Fisher, M., & Martin, M., (1994). Myocardial infarction, hyperkalaemia and ventricular tachycardia in a young male body-builder. *International Journal of Cardiology, 44,* 171–4.

Bach, B.R., Warren, R.F., & Wickiewicz, T.L. (1987). Triceps rupture: A case report and literature review. *American Journal of Sports Medicine, 15,* 285–289.

Bagheri, S.A., & Boyer, J.L. (1974). Peliosis hepatis associated with androgenic-anabolic steroid therapy: A severe form of hepatic injury. *Annals of Internal Medicine, 81,* 610–618.

Bain, J., Rachlis, V., Robert, E., & Khait, Z. (1980). The combined use of oral medroxyprogesterone acetate and methyltestosterone in a male contraceptive trial programme. *Contraception, 21,* 365–379.

Barbosa, J., Seal, U.S., & Doe, R.P. (1971). Effects of anabolic steroids on haptoglobin, orosomucoid, plasminogen, fibrinogen, transferrin, ceruloplasmin, α1-antitrypsin, β-glucuronidase and total serum proteins. *Journal of Clinical Endocrinology, 33,* 388–398.

Bernstein, M.S., Hunter, R.L., & Yachnin, S. (1971). Hepatoma and peliosis hepatis developing in a patient with Fanconi's anemia. *New England Journal of Medicine, 284,* 1135–1136.

Bird, D., Vowles, K., & Anthony, P.P. (1979). Spontaneous rupture of a liver cell adenoma after long term methyltestosterone: Report of a case successfully treated by emergency right hepatic lobectomy. *British Journal of Surgery, 66,* 212–213.

Bonner, C.D., & Homburger, F. (1952). Jaundice of the hepatocellular type during methyltestosterone therapy: Report of two cases. *Bulletin of the New England Medical Centers, 14,* 87–89.

Bowman, S.J., Tanna, S., Fernando, S., Ayodeji, A., & Weatherstone, R.M. (1989). Anabolic steroids and infarction. *British Medical Journal, 299,* 632.

Bronson, F.H., & Matherne, C.M. (1997). Exposure to anabolic-androgenic steroids shortens life span of male mice. *Medicine and Science in Sports and Exercise, 29,* 615–619.

Bryden, A.A.G., Rothwell, P.J.N., & O'Reilly, P.H. (1995). Anabolic steroid abuse and renal-cell carcinoma. *Lancet, 346,* 1306–1307.

Burger, R.A., & Marcuse, P.M. (1952). Peliosis hepatis: Report of a case. *American Journal of Clinical Pathology, 22,* 569–573.

Burkett, L.N., & Falduto, M.T. (1984). Steroid use by athletes in a metropolitan area. *The Physician and Sportsmedicine, 12,* 69–74.

Cabasso, A. (1994). Peliosis hepatis in a young adult bodybuilder. *Medicine and Science in Sports and Exercise, 26,* 2–4.

Calabrese, L.H., Kleiner, S.M., Barna, B.P., Skibinski, C.I., Kirkendall, D.T., Lahita, R.G., & Lombardo, J.A. (1989). The effects of anabolic steroids and strength training on the human immune response. *Medicine and Science in Sports and Exercise, 21,* 386–392.

Campbell, S.E., Farb, A., & Weber, K.T. (1993). Pathologic remodeling of the myocardium in a weightlifter taking anabolic steroids: Case report. *Blood Pressure, 2,* 213–216.

Cancer of the prostate. (1954). *Journal of the American Medical Association, 156,* 292.

Carrasco, D., Prieto, M., Pallardo, L., Moll, J.L., Cruz, J.M., Munoz, C., & Berenguer, J. (1985). Multiple hepatic adenomas after long-term therapy with testosterone enanthate: Review of the literature. *Journal of Hepatology, 1,* 573–578.

Catlin, D.H., Kammerer, R.C., Hatton, C.K., Sekera, M.H., & Merdink, J.L. (1987). Analytical chemistry at the games of the XXIIIrd Olympiad in Los Angeles, 1984. *Clinical Chemistry, 33,* 319–327.

Cattan, D., Kalifat, R., Wautier, J.L., Meignan, S., Vesin, P., & Piet, R. (1974). Fanconi's anemia and primary carcinoma of the liver. *Archives Francaises des Maladies de l'Appareil Digestif, 63,* 41–48.

Cattan, D., Vesin, P., Wautier, J., Kalifat, P., & Meignan, S. (1974). Liver tumors and steroid hormones. *Lancet, 1,* 878.

Chandra, R.S., Kapur, S.P., Kelleher, J., Jr., Luban, J., & Patterson, K. (1984). Benign hepatocellular tumors in the young. A clinicopathologic spectrum. *Archives of Pathology and Laboratory Medicine, 108,* 168–171.

Charny, C.W., & Gordon, J.A. (1978). Testosterone rebound therapy: A neglected modality. *Fertility and Sterility, 29,* 64–68.

Cocks, J.R. (1981). Methyltestosterone-induced liver-cell tumours. *Medical Journal of Australia, 2,* 617–619.

Cohen, J.C., Faber, W.M., Benade, A.J., & Noakes, T.D. (1986). Altered serum lipoprotein profiles in male and female power lifters ingesting anabolic steroids. *The Physician and Sportsmedicine, 14,* 131–136.

Cohen, J.C., & Hickman, R. (1987). Insulin resistance and diminished glucose tolerance in powerlifters ingesting anabolic steroids. *Journal of Clinical Endocrinology and Metabolism, 64,* 960–963.

Cohen, J.C., Noakes, T.D., & Benade, A.J. (1988). Hypercholesteremia in male power lifters using anabolic-androgenic steroids. *The Physician and Sportsmedicine, 16,* 49–56.

Collaborative Group for the Study of Stroke in Young Women. (1975). Oral contraceptives and stroke in young women. *Journal of the American Medical Association, 231,* 718–722.

Coombes, G.B., Reiser, J., Paradinas, F., & Burn, I. (1977). An androgenic-associated hepatic adenoma in a trans-sexual. *British Journal of Surgery, 65,* 869–870.

Cooper, C.S., Perry, P.J., Sparks, A.E., MacIndoe, J.H., Yates, W.R., & Williams, R.D. (1998). Effect of exogenous testosterone on prostate volume, serum and semen prostate specific antigen levels in healthy young men. *Journal of Urology, 159,* 441–3.

Coronary Drug Project Research Group. (1973). The coronary drug project: Findings leading to discontinuation of the 2.5-mg/day estrogen group. *Journal of the American Medical Association, 226,* 652–657.

Costill, D.L., Pearson, D.R., & Fink, W.J. (1984). Anabolic steroid use among athletes: Changes in HDL-C levels. *The Physician and Sportsmedicine, 12,* 113–117.

Cowart, V. (1987). Steroids in sports: After four decades, time to return these genies to bottle? *Journal of the American Medical Association, 257,* 421–427.

Craig, J.R., Peters, R.L., & Edmondson, H.A. (1989). *Atlas of tumor pathology, second series, Fascicle 26: Tumors of the liver and intrahepatic bile ducts* (pp. 36–41). Washington DC: Armed Forces Institute of Pathology.

Creagh, T.M., Rubin, A., & Evans, D.J. (1988). Hepatic tumours induced by anabolic steroids in an athlete. *Journal of Clinical Pathology, 41,* 441–443.

Daneshmend, T.K., & Bradfield, J.W. (1979). Hepatic angiosarcoma associated with androgenic-anabolic steroids. *Lancet, 2,* 1249.

David, H.G., Green, J.T., Grant, A.J., & Wilson, C.A. (1995). Simultaneous bilateral quadriceps rupture: A complication of anabolic steroid abuse. *Journal of Bone and Joint Surgery, 77,* 159–160.

Deligiannis, A.P., & Mandroukas, K. (1993). Noninvasive cardiac evaluation of weight-lifters using anabolic steroids. *Scandanavian Journal of Medicine and Science in Sports, 3,* 37–40.

Dickerman, R.D., Schaller F., Prather I., & McConathy, W.J. (1995). Sudden cardiac death in a 20-year-old bodybuilder using anabolic steroids. *Cardiology, 86,* 172–173.

Drew, E.J. (1984). Androgen related primary hepatic carcinoma in a patient on long term methyltestosterone therapy. *Journal of Abdominal Surgery, 26,* 103–106.

Dunning, M.F. (1958). Jaundice associated with norethandrolone (Nilevar) administration. *Journal of the American Medical Association, 167,* 1242–1243.

Edis, A.J., & Levitt, M. (1985). Anabolic steroids and colonic cancer. *Medical Journal of Australia, 142,* 426–427.

Evely, R.S., Triger, D.R., Milnes, J.P., Low-Beer, T.S., & Williams, R. (1987). Severe cholestasis associated with stanozolol. *British Medical Journal, 294,* 612–613.

Falk, H., Thomas, L.B., Popper, H., & Ishak, K.G. (1979). Hepatic angiosarcoma associated with androgenic-anabolic steroids. *Lancet, 2,* 1120–1123.

Fearnley, G.R., & Chakrabarti, R. (1962). Increase of blood fibrinolytic activity by testosterone. *Lancet, 2,* 128–132.

Fearnley, G.R., & Chakrabarti, R. (1964). The pharmacological enhancement of blood fibrinolytic activity with special reference to phenoformin. *Acta Cardiologica, 19,* 1–13.

Ferenchick, G.S., & Adelman, S. (1992). Myocardial infarction associated with anabolic steroid use in a previously healthy 37-year-old weight lifter. *American Heart Journal, 124,* 507–508.

Ferenchick, G.S., Hirokawa, S., Mammen, E.F., & Schwartz, K.A. (1995). Anabolic-androgenic steroid abuse in weight lifters: Evidence for activation of the hemostatic system. *American Journal of Hematology, 49,* 282–288.

Ferrera, P.S., Putnam, D.L., & Verdile, V.P. (1997). Anabolic steroid use as the possible precipitant of dilated cardiomyopathy. *Cardiology, 88,* 218–220.

Fisher, M., Appleby, M., Rittoo, D., & Cotter, L. (1996). Myodardial infarction with extensive intracoronary thrombus induced by anabolic steroids. *British Journal of Clinical Practice, 50,* 222–3.

Foss, G.L., & Simpson, S.L. (1959). Oral methyltestosterone and jaundice. *British Medical Journal, 1,* 259–263.

Franklc, M.A., Cicero, G.J., & Payne, J. (1984). Use of androgenic anabolic steroids by athletes. *Journal of the American Medical Association, 252,* 482.

Frankle, M.A., Eichberg, R., & Zachariah, S.B. (1988). Anabolic androgenic steroids and a stroke in an athlete: Case report. *Archives of Physical Medicine and Rehabilitation, 69,* 632–633.

Freed, D.L.J., Banks, A.J., Longson, D., & Burley, D.M. (1975). Anabolic steroids in athletics: Crossover double-blind trial on weightlifters. *British Medical Journal, 2,* 471–473.

Freeman, B.J.C., & Rooker, G.D. (1995). Spontaneous rupture of the anterior cruciate ligament after anabolic steroids. *British Journal of Sports Medicine, 29,* 274–275.

Friedl, K.E. (1987). Interview with anabolic steroid user seeking advice after purported cessation of use. Unpublished observations.

Friedl, K.E. (1990). Reappraisal of the health risks associated with the use of high doses of oral and injectable androgenic steroids. In G.C. Lin & L. Erinoff (Eds.), *Anabolic steroid abuse* (pp. 142–177). Washington DC: U.S. Government Printing Office.

Friedl, K.E., Dettori, J.R., Hannan, C.J., Patience, T.H., & Plymate, S.R. (1991). Comparison of the effects of high dose testosterone and 19-nortestosterone to a replacement dose of testosterone on strength and body composition in normal men. *Journal of Steroid Biochemistry & Molecular Biology, 40,* 607–612.

Friedl, K.E., Hannan, C.J., Jr., Jones, R.E., & Plymate, S.R. (1990). High-density lipoprotein cholesterol is not decreased if an aromatizable androgen is administered. *Metabolism, 39,* 69–74.

Friedl, K.E., Jones, R.E., Hannan, C.J., Jr., & Plymate, S.R. (1989). The administration of pharmacological doses of testosterone or 19-nortestosterone to normal men is not associated with increased insulin secretion or impaired glucose tolerance. *Journal of Clinical Endocrinology and Metabolism, 68,* 971–975.

Friedl, K.E., & Plymate, S.R. (1986). Parallel profound decrease in HDL-cholesterol and testosterone binding globulin during anabolic steroid self-administration in bodybuilders. Unpublished raw data.

Friedl, K.E., & Yesalis, C.E. (1989). Self-treatment of gynecomastia in bodybuilders who use anabolic steroids. *The Physician and Sportsmedicine, 17,* 67–79.

Furman, R.H., Howard, R.P., Norcia, L.N., & Keaty, E.C. (1958). The influence of androgens, estrogens and related steroids on serum lipids and lipoproteins: Observations in hypogonadal and normal human subjects. *American Journal of Medicine, 24,* 80–97.

Furman, R.H., Howard, R.P., Smith, C.W., & Norcia, L.N. (1957). Comparative androgenicity of oral androgens, determined by steroid-induced decrements in high density (alpha) lipoproteins: Studies utilizing testosterone, methyltestosterone, 19-nortestosterone, 17-methyl nortestosterone and 17-ethyl nortestosterone. *American Journal of Medicine, 22,* 966.

Garn, S.M. (1951). Types and distribution of the hair in man. *Annals of the New York Academy of Sciences, 53,* 498–507.

Gil, V.G., Lapuerta, J.B., Garcia, J.P., & Martin, M.R. (1986). A non-C17-alkylated steroid and long-term cholestasis. *Annals of Internal Medicine, 104,* 135–136.

Gilbert, E.F., DaSilva, A.Q., & Queen, D.M. (1963). Intrahepatic cholestasis with fatal termination following norethandrolone therapy. *Journal of the American Medical Association, 185,* 538–539.

Gittes, R.F. (1991). Carcinoma of the prostate. *New England Journal of Medicine, 324,* 236–245.

Glass, A.R., & Vigersky, R.A. (1980). Resensitization of testosterone production in men after human chorionic gonadotropin-induced desensitization. *Journal of Clinical Endocrinology and Metabolism, 51,* 1395–1400.

Goldman, B. (1985). Liver carcinoma in an athlete taking anabolic steroids. *Journal of the American Osteopathic Association, 85,* 56.

Goodman, M.A., & Laden, A.M. (1977). Hepatocellular carcinoma in association with androgen therapy. *Medical Journal of Australia, 1,* 220–221.

Gordon, B.S., Wolf, J., Krause, T., & Shai, F. (1960). Peliosis hepatis and cholestasis following administration of norethandrolone. *American Journal of Clinical Pathology, 33,* 156–165.

Grasso, M., Buonaguidi, A., Mondina, R., Borsellino, G., Lania, C., Banfi, G., & Rigatti, P. (1990). Plasma sex hormone binding globulin in patients with prostatic carcinoma. *Cancer, 66,* 354–357.

Groos, G., Arnold, O.H., & Brittinger, G. (1974). Peliosis hepatis after long-term administration of oxymetholone. *Lancet, 1,* 874.

Hamilton, J.B. (1948). The role of testicular secretions as indicated by the effects of castration in man and by studies of pathological conditions and the short lifespan associated with maleness. *Recent Progress in Hormone Research, 3,* 257–322.

Hannan, C.J., Jr., Friedl, K.E., Zold, A., Kettler, T.M., & Plymate, S.R. (1991). Psychological and serum homovanillic acid changes in men administered androgenic steroids. *Psychoneuroendocrinology, 16,* 335–343.

Haupt, H.A., & Rovere, G.D. (1984). Anabolic steroids: A review of the literature. *American Journal of Sports Medicine, 12,* 469–484.

Heller, C.G., Moore, D.J., Paulsen, C.A., Nelson, W.O., & Laidley, W.M. (1959). Progesterone and synthetic progestins: Effects of progesterone and synthetic progestins on the reproductive physiology of normal men. *Federation Proceedings, 18,* 1057–1064.

Heller, R.F., Miller, N.E., Wheeler, M.J., & Kind, P.R. (1983). Coronary heart disease in "low risk" men. *Atherosclerosis, 49,* 187–193.

Hernandez-Nieto, L., Bruguera, M., Bombi, J.A., Camacho, L., & Rozman, C. (1977). Benign liver-cell adenoma associated with long-term administration of an androgenic-anabolic steroid (methandienone). *Cancer, 40,* 1761–1764.

Herrick, R.T., & Herrick, S. (1987). Ruptured triceps in a powerlifter presenting as cubital syndrome: A case report. *American Journal of Sports Medicine, 11,* 269–271.

Hervey, G.R. (1975). Are athletes wrong about anabolic steroids? *British Journal of Sports Medicine, 9,* 74–7.

Hervey, G.R., Hutchinson, I., Knibbs, A.V., Burkinshaw, L., Jones, P.R., Nolan, N.G., & Levell, M.J. (1976). "Anabolic" effects of methandienone in men undergoing athletic training. *Lancet, 2,* 699–702.

Hill, J.A., Suker, J.R., Sachs, K., & Brigham, C. (1983). The athletic polydrug abuse phenomenon. *American Journal of Sports Medicine, 11,* 269–271.

Hobbs, C.J., Plymate, S.R., Bell, B.K., & Patience, T.H. (1991). The effect of androgens on glucose tolerance. *Clinical Research, 39,* 384A.

Hobbs, C.J., Plymate, S.R., Jones, R.E., Andress, D.L., & Patience, T.H. (1991). The effect of androgens on insulin-like growth factor-I levels in normal men. *Clinical Research, 39,* 55A.

Hughes, T.K., Fulep, E., Juelich, T., Smith, E.M., & Stanton, G.J. (1995). Modulation of immune responses by anabolic androgenic steroids. *International Journal of Immunopharmacology, 17,* 857–863.

Huie, M.J. (1994). An acute myocardial infarction occurring in an anabolic steroid user. *Medicine and Science in Sports and Exercise, 26,* 408–413.

Hurley, B.F., Seals, D.R., Hagberg, J.M., Goldberg, A.C., Ostrove, S.M., Holloszy, J.O., Wiest, W.G., & Goldberg, A.P. (1984). High-density-lipoprotein cholesterol in bodybuilders v. powerlifters: Negative effects of androgen use. *Journal of the American Medical Association, 252,* 507–513.

Ingerowski, G.H., Scheutwinkel-Reich, M., & Stan, H.J. (1981). Mutagenicity studies on veterinary anabolic drugs with the salmonella/microsome test. *Mutation Research, 91,* 93–98.

Janne, O.A. (1990). Androgen interaction through multiple steroid receptors. *NIDA Research Monograph, 102,* 178–86.

Jarow, J.P., & Lipshultz, L.I. (1990). Anabolic steroid-induced hypogonadotropic hypogonadism. *American Journal of Sports Medicine, 18,* 429–431.

Johnsen, S.G., Kampmann, J.P., Bennett, E.P., & Jorgensen, F.S. (1976). Enzyme induction by oral testosterone. *Clinical Pharmacology and Therapeutics, 20,* 233–237.

Johnson, A.S., Jones, M., Morgan-Capner, P., Wright, P.A., Wheldon, D.B., Flatt, N., & Bunting, P. (1995). Severe chickenpox in anabolic steroid user. *Lancet, 345,* 1447–1448.

Johnson, F.L., Lerner, K.G., Siegel, M., Faegler, J.R., Majerus, P.W., Hartmann, J.R., & Thomas, E.D. (1972). Association of androgenic-anabolic steroid therapy with development of hepatocellular carcinoma. *Lancet, 2,* 1273–1276.

Joint Group for the Study of Aplastic and Refractory Anemias. (1981). Long-term follow-up of patients with medullary aplasia. *Annales de Medicine Interne, 132,* 530–534.

Jurgens, G., & Koltringer, P. (1987). Lipoprotein(a) in ischemic cerebrovascular disease: A new approach to the assessment of risk for stroke. *Neurology, 37,* 513–515.

Kantor, M.A., Bianchini, A., Bernier, D., Sady, S.P., & Thompson, P.D. (1985). Androgens reduce HDL2-cholesterol and increase hepatic triglyceride lipase activity. *Medicine and Science in Sports and Exercise, 17,* 462–465.

Karasawa, T., Shikata, T., & Smith, R.D. (1979). Peliosis hepatis: Report of nine cases. *Acta Pathologica Japonica, 29,* 457–469.

Kennedy, M.C., Corrigan, A.B., & Pilbeam, S.T. (1993). Myocardial infarction and cerebral haemorrhage in a young body builder taking anabolic steroids. *Australian and New Zealand Journal of Medicine, 23,* 713.

Kennedy, M.C., & Lawrence, C. (1993). Anabolic steroid abuse and cardiac death. *Medical Journal of Australia, 158,* 346–348.

Kessler, E., Bar-Meir, S., & Pinkhas, J. (1976). Focal nodular hyperplasia and spontaneous hepatic rupture in aplastic anemia treated with oxymetholone. *Harefuah, 90,* 521–524.

Khankhanian, N.K., Hammers, Y.A., & Kowalski, P. (1992). Exuberant local tissue reaction to intramuscular injection of nandrolone decanoate (Deca-Durabolin), a steroid compound in a sesame seed oil base, mimicking soft tissue malignant tumors: A case report and review of the literature. *Military Medicine, 157,* 670–674.

Kintzen, W., & Silny, J. (1960). Peliosis hepatis after administration of fluoxymesterone. *Canadian Medical Association Journal, 83,* 860–862.

Kiraly, C.L. (1988). Androgenic-anabolic steroid effects on serum and skin surface lipids, on red cells, and on liver enzymes. *International Journal of Sports Medicine, 9,* 249–252.

Kiraly, C.L., Alen, M., Rahkila, P., & Horsmanheimo, M. (1987). Effect of androgenic and anabolic steroids on the sebaceous gland in power athletes. *Acta Dermatologica et Venereologica, 67,* 36–40.

Klatskin, G. (1977). Hepatic tumors: Possible relationship to use of oral contraceptives. *Gastroenterology, 73,* 386–394.

Kloer, H., Hoogen, H., & Nieschlag, E. (1980). Trial of high-dose testosterone undecanoate in treatment of male infertility. *International Journal of Andrology, 3,* 121–129.

Knuth, U.A., Maniera, H., & Nieschlag, E. (1989). Anabolic steroids and semen parameters in bodybuilders. *Acta Endocrinologica, 120*(Suppl.), 121–122.

Kory, R.C., Bradley, M.H., Watson, R.N., Callahan, R., & Peters, B.J. (1959). A six-month evaluation of an anabolic drug, norethandrolone, in underweight persons: 2. Bromosulfophthalein (BSP) retention and liver function. *American Journal of Medicine, 26,* 243–248.

Koszalka, M.F. (1957). Medical obstructive jaundice: Report of death due to methyltestosterone. *Lancet, 77,* 51–54.

Kramhoft, M., & Solgaard, S. (1986). Spontaneous rupture of the extensor pollicis longus tendon after anabolic steroids. *Journal of Hand Surgery, 11,* 87.

Kruskemper, H.L. (1968). *Anabolic steroids* (p. 176). New York: Academic Press.

Landon, J., Wynn, V., Cooke, J.N., & Kennedy, A. (1962). Effects of anabolic steroid methandienone, on carbohydrate metabolism in man. *Metabolism, 11,* 501–512.

Landon, J., Wynn, V., & Samols, E. (1963). The effect of anabolic steroids on blood sugar and plasma insulin levels in man. *Metabolism, 12,* 924–935.

Laroche, G.P. (1990). Steroid anabolic drugs and arterial complications in an athlete—a case history. *Angiology, 41,* 964–969.

Lenders, J.W., Demacker, P.N., Vos, J.A., Jansen, P.L., Hoitsma, A.J., van't Laar, A., & Thien, T. (1988). Deleterious effects of anabolic steroids on serum lipoproteins, blood pressure, and liver function in amateur body builders. *International Journal of Sports Medicine, 9,* 19–23.

Lesna, M., & Taylor, W. (1986). Liver lesions in BALB/C mice induced by an anabolic androgen (Decadurabolin), with and without pretreatment with diethylnitrosamine. *Journal of Steroid Biochemistry, 24,* 449–453.

Lichtenstein, M.J., Yarnell, J.W., Elwood, P.C., Beswick, A.D., Sweetnam, P.M., Marks, V., Teale, D., & Riad-Fahmy, D. (1987). Sex hormones, insulin, lipids, and prevalent ischemic heart disease. *American Journal of Epidemiology, 126,* 647–657.

Liddle, G.W., & Burke, H.A. (1960). Anabolic steroids in clinical medicine. *Helvetica Medica Acta, 27,* 504–513.

Liow, R.Y., & Tavares, S. (1995). Bilateral rupture of the quadriceps tendon associated with anabolic steroids. *British Journal of Sports Medicine, 29,* 77–79.

Lloyd-Thomas, H.G., & Sherlock, S. (1952). Testosterone therapy for the pruritis of obstructive jaundice. *British Medical Journal, 2,* 1289.

Lommi, J., & Harkonen, M. (1991). Temporary paralysis in a 17-year-old bodybuilder [Finnish]. *Duodecim, 107,* 1723–1725.

Loomus, G.N., Aneja, P., & Bota, R.A. (1983). A case of peliosis hepatis in association with tamoxifen therapy. *American Journal of Clinical Pathology, 80,* 881–883.

Lowdell, C.P., & Murray–Lyon, I.M. (1985). Reversal of liver damage due to long term methyltestosterone and safety of non-17α-alkylated androgens. *British Medical Journal, 291,* 637.

Luke, J.L., Farb, A., Virmani, R., & Sample, R.H. (1990). Sudden cardiac death during exercise in a weight lifter using anabolic androgenic steroids: Pathological and toxicology findings. *Journal of Forensic Sciences, 35,* 1441–1447.

Lyngberg, K.K. (1991). Myocardial infarction and death of a body builder after using anabolic steroids [Danish, with English summary]. *Ugeskraft for Laeger., 153,* 587–588.

Martikainen, H., Alen, M., Rahkila, P., & Vihko, R. (1986). Testicular responsiveness to human chorionic gonadotrophin during transient hypogonadotrophic hypogonadism induced by androgenic/anabolic steroids in power athletes. *Journal of Steroid Biochemistry, 25,* 109–112.

Matsumoto, A.M. (1988). Is high dosage testosterone an effective male contraceptive agent? *Fertility and Sterility, 50,* 324–328.

Matsumoto, A.M. (1990). Effects of chronic testosterone administration in normal men: Safety and efficacy of high dosage testosterone and parallel dose-dependent suppression of luteinizing hormone, follicle-stimulating hormone, and sperm production. *Journal of Clinical Endocrinology and Metabolism, 70,* 282–287.

Matsumoto, A.M., & Bremner, W.J. (1988). Parallel dose-dependent suppression of LH, FSH and sperm production by testosterone in normal men [Abstract No. 570]. *Proceedings of the 70th Annual Meeting of the Endocrine Society* (p. 163). Bethesda, MD: The Endocrine Society.

Mauss, J., Borsch, G., Bormacher, K., Richter, E., Leyendecker, G., & Nocke, W. (1975). Effect of long-term testosterone enanthate administration on male reproduction function: Clinical evaluation, serum FSH, LH, testosterone, and seminal fluid analyses in normal men. *Acta Endocrinologica, 78,* 373–384.

McCaughan, G.W., Bilous, M.J., & Gallagher, N.D. (1985). Long-term survival with tumor regression in androgen-induced liver tumors. *Cancer, 56,* 2622–2626.

McKillop, G., Todd, I.C., & Ballantyne, D. (1986). Increased left ventricular mass in a bodybuilder using anabolic steroids. *British Journal of Sports Medicine, 20,* 151–152.

McNutt, R.A., Ferenchick, G.S., Kirlin, P.C., & Hamlin, N.J. (1988). Acute myocardial infarction in a 22-year-old world class weight lifter using anabolic steroids. *American Journal of Cardiology, 62,* 164.

Melchert, R.B., & Welder, A.A. (1995). Cardiovascular effects of androgenic-anabolic steroids. *Medicine and Science in Sports and Exercise, 27,* 1252–1262.

Meriggiola, M.C., Marcovina, S., Paulsen, C.A., & Bremner, W.J. (1995). Testosterone enanthate at a dose of 200 mg/week decreases HDL-cholesterol levels in healthy men. *International Journal of Andrology, 18,* 237–242.

Messerli, F.H., & Frohlich, E.D. (1979). High blood pressure: A side effect of drugs, poisons, and food. *Archives of Internal Medicine, 139,* 682–687.

Michna, H. (1987). Tendon injuries induced by exercise and anabolic steroids in experimental mice. *International Orthopaedics, 11,* 157–162.

Miles, J.W., Grana, W.A., Egle, D., Min, K.W., & Chitwood, J. (1992). The effect of anabolic steroids on the biomechanical and histological properties of rat tendon. *Journal of Bone and Joint Surgery, 74,* 411–22.

Mochizuki, R.M., & Richter, K.J. (1988). Cardiomyopathy and cerebrovascular accident associated with anabolic-androgenic steroid use. *The Physician and Sportsmedicine, 16,* 109–114.

Montine, T.J., & Gaede, J.T. (1992). Massive pulmonary embolus and anabolic steroid abuse. *Journal of the American Medical Association, 267,* 2328.

Moss-Newport, J. (1993). Anabolic steroid use and cerebellar haemorrhage. *Medical Journal of Australia, 158,* 794.

Nadell, J., & Kosek, J. (1977). Peliosis hepatis. Twelve cases associated with oral androgen therapy. *Archives of Pathology and Laboratory Medicine, 101,* 405–410.

Nagelberg, S.B., Laue, L., Loriaux, D.L., Liu, L., & Sherins, R.J. (1986). Cerebrovascular accident associated with testosterone therapy in a 21-year-old hypogonadal man. *New England Journal of Medicine, 314,* 649–650.

National Cholesterol Education Program Expert Panel. (1988). Report of the National Cholesterol Education Program Expert Panel on detection, evaluation, and treatment of high blood cholesterol in adults. *Archives of Internal Medicine, 148,* 36–69.

Neff, M.S., Goldberg, J., Slifkin, R.F., Eiser, A.R., Calamia, V., Kaplan, M., Baez, A., Gupta, S., & Mattoo, N. (1981). A comparison of androgens for anemia in patients on hemodialysis. *New England Journal of Medicine, 304,* 871–875.

Nelson, W.O. (1959). Progesterone and synthetic progestins: Discussion. *Federation Proceedings, 18,* 1065.

Nieminen, M.S., Raemoe, M.P., Viitasalo, M., Heikkilae, P., Karjalainen, J., Maentysaari, M., & Heikkilae, J. (1996). Serious cardiovascular side effects of larger doses of anabolic steroids in weight lifters. *European Heart Journal, 17,* 1576–1583.

Noble, R.L. (1984). Androgen use by athletes: A possible cancer risk. *Canadian Medical Association Journal, 130,* 549–550.

Overly, W.L., Dankoff, J.A., Wang, B.K., & Singh, U.D. (1984). Androgens and hepatocellular carcinoma in an athlete. *Annals of Internal Medicine, 100,* 158–159.

Palacios, A., McClure, R.D., Campfield, A., & Swerdloff, R.S. (1981). Effect of testosterone enanthate on testis size. *Journal of Urology, 126,* 46–48.

Paradinas, F.J., Bull, T.B., Westaby, D., & Murray-Lyon, I.M. (1977). Hyperplasia and prolapse of hepatocytes into hepatic veins during long term methyltestosterone therapy: Possible relationships of these changes to the development of peliosis hepatis and liver tumors. *Histopathology, 1,* 225–226.

Paulsen, C.A., Bremner, W.J., & Leonard, J.M. (1982). Male contraception: Clinical trials. In D.R. Mishell (Ed.), *Advances in fertility research* (pp. 157–170). New York: Raven Press.

Pecking, A., Lejolly, J.M., & Najean, Y. (1980). Hepatic toxicity of androgen therapy in aplastic anemia. *Nouvelle Revue Française d'Hematologie, 22,* 257–265.

Pelletier, G., Frija, J., Szekely, A.M., & Clauvel, J.P. (1984). Adenoma of the liver in man. *Gastroenterologie Clinique et Biologique, 8,* 269–272.

Pelliccia, A., Maron, B.J., Spataro, A., Proschan, M.A., & Spirito, P. (1991). The upper limit of physiologic cardiac hypertrophy in highly trained elite athletes. *New England Journal of Medicine, 324,* 295–301.

Perry, H.M. (1994). An unusual cause of abnormal gait. *British Journal of Sports Medicine, 28,* 60.

Petera, V., Bobek, K., & Lahn, V. (1962). Serum transaminase (GOT, GPT) and lactic dehydrogenase activity during treatment with methyl testosterone. *Clinica Chimica Acta, 7,* 604–606.

Peters, J.H., Randall, A.H., Mendeloff, J., Peace, R., Coberly, J.C., & Hurley, M.B. (1958). Jaundice during administration of methylestrenolone. *Journal of Clinical Endocrinology and Metabolism, 18,* 114–115.

Peters, R.L. (1976). Pathology of hepatocellular carcinoma. In K. Okuda & R.L. Peters (Eds.), *Hepatocellular carcinoma* (pp. 107–168). New York: Wiley.

Peterson, G.E., & Fahey, T.D. (1984). HDL-C in five elite athletes using anabolic-androgenic steroids. *The Physician and Sportsmedicine, 12,* 120–130.

Petry, R., Rausch-Stroomann, J.G., Hienz, H.A., Senge, T., & Mauss, J. (1968). Androgen treatment without inhibiting effect on hypophysis and male gonads. *Acta Endocrinologica, 59,* 497–507.

Phillips, M.J., Oda, M., & Funatsu, K. (1978). Evidence for microfilament involvement in norethandrolone-induced intrahepatic cholestasis. *American Journal of Pathology, 93,* 729–744.

Pochi, P.E., & Strauss, J.S. (1974). Endocrinologic control of the development and activity of the human sebaceous gland. *Journal of Investigative Dermatology, 62,* 191–201.

Prat, J., Gray, G.F., Stolley, P.D., & Coleman, J.W. (1977). Wilms tumor in an adult associated with androgen abuse. *Journal of the American Medical Association, 237,* 2322–2323.

Rastad, J., Joborn, H., Ljunghall, S., & Akerstrom, G. (1985). Gluteal infection in weight lifters after injection of anabolic steroids. *Lakartidningen, 82,* 3407. (DIALOG b 155 8639139)

Reyes, R.J., Zicchi, S., Hamed, H., Chaudary, M.A., & Fentiman, I.S. (1995). Surgical correction of gynecomastia in bodybuilders. *British Journal of Clinical Practice, 49,* 177–179.

Roberts, J.T., & Essenhigh, D.M. (1986). Adenocarcinoma of prostate in 40-year-old body-builder. *Lancet, 2,* 742.

Ross, R., Bernstein, L., Judd, H., Hanisch, R., Pike, M., & Henderson, B. (1986). Serum testosterone levels in healthy young black and white men. *Journal of the National Cancer Institute, 76,* 45–48.

Rowley, M.J., & Heller, C.G. (1972). The testosterone rebound phenomenon in the treatment of male infertility. *Fertility and Sterility, 23,* 498–504.

Rozenek, R., Rahe, C.H., Kohl, H.H., Marple, D.N., Wilson, G.D., & Stone, M.H. (1990). Physiological responses to resistance-exercise in athletes self-administering anabolic steroids. *The Journal of Sports Medicine and Physical Fitness, 30,* 354–360.

Ruokonen, A., Alen, M., Bolton, N., & Vihko, R. (1985). Response of serum testosterone and its precursor steroids, SHBG and CBG to anabolic steroid and testosterone self-administration in man. *Journal of Steroid Biochemistry, 23,* 33–38.

Saartok, T., Dahlberg, E., & Gustafsson, J.A. (1984). Relative binding affinity of anabolic-androgenic steroids: Comparison of the binding to the androgen receptors in skeletal muscle and in prostate, as well as to sex hormone-binding globulin. *Endocrinology, 114,* 2100–2106.

Saheb, F. (1980). Absence of peliosis hepatis in patients receiving testosterone enanthate. *Hepato-Gastroenterology, 27,* 432–434.

Sale, G.E., & Lerner, K.G. (1977). Multiple tumors after androgen therapy. *Archives of Pathology and Laboratory Medicine, 101,* 600–603.

Salke, R.C., Rowland, T.W., & Burke, E.J. (1985). Left ventricular size and function in body builders using anabolic steroids. *Medicine and Science in Sports and Exercise, 17,* 701–704.

Schaffner, F., Popper, H., & Chesrow, E. (1959). Cholestasis produced by the administration of norethandrolone. *American Journal of Medicine, 26,* 249–254.

Schaison, G., Leverger, G., & Yildez, C. (1983). Fanconi's anemia: Frequency of leukemic transformation. *La Presse Medicale, 12,* 1269–1274.

Schally, A.V., & Comaru-Schally, A.M. (1987). Male contraception involving testosterone supplementation: Possible increased risks of prostate cancer? *Lancet, 1,* 448–449.

Schollert, P.V., & Bendixen, P.M. (1993). Dilated cardiomyopathy in a user of anabolic steroids. [Danish, with English summary]. *Ugeskraft for Laeger., 155,* 1217–1218.

Schriewer, H., Assmann, G., Sandkamp, M., & Schulte, H. (1984). The relationship of lipoprotein(a) (Lp(a)) to risk factors of coronary heart disease: Initial results of the prospective epidemiological study on company employees in Westfalia. *Journal of Clinical Chemistry and Clinical Biochemistry, 22,* 591–596.

Schurmeyer, T., Knuth, U.A., Belkien, L., & Nieschlag, E. (1984). Reversible azoospermia induced by the anabolic steroid 19-nortestosterone. *Lancet, 1,* 417–420.

Scott, M.J., & Scott, M.J., Jr. (1989). HIV infection associated with injections of anabolic steroids. *Journal of the American Medical Association, 262,* 207–298.

Scully, R.E., Mark, E.J., & McNeely, B.U. (1981). Weekly clinico-pathological exercises: Case 32-1981. *New England Journal of Medicine, 305,* 331–336.

Shiozawa, Z., Tsunoda, S., Noda, A., Saito, M., & Yamada, H. (1986). Cerebral hemorrhagic infarction associated with anabolic steroid therapy for hypoplastic anemia. *Angiology, 37,* 725–730.

Shiozawa, Z., Yamada, H., Mabuchi, C., Hotta, T., Saito, M., Sobue, I., & Huang, Y.P. (1982). Superior sagittal sinus thrombosis associated with androgen therapy for hypoplastic anemia. *Annals of Neurology, 12,* 578–580.

Simon, M., Jouet, J.P., Demory, J.L., Pollet, J.P., & Bauters, F. (1986). An unrecognized cause of polycythemia: Prolonged anabolic drug treatment. *Presse Medicale, 15,* 396.

Sklarek, H.M., Mantovani, R.P., Erens, E., Heisler, D., Niederman, M.S., & Fein, A.M. (1984). AIDS in a bodybuilder using anabolic steroids. *New England Journal of Medicine, 311,* 1701.

Spano, F., & Ryan, W.G. (1984). Tamoxifen for gynecomastia induced by anabolic steroids? *New England Journal of Medicine, 311,* 861–862.

Stalder, M., Pometta, D., & Suenram, A. (1981). Relationship between plasma insulin levels and high density lipoprotein cholesterol levels in healthy men. *Diabetologia, 21,* 544–548.

Steinberger, E., Smith, K.D., & Rodriguez-Rigau, L.J. (1978). Suppression and recovery of sperm production in men treated with testosterone enanthate for one year. A study of a possible reversible male contraceptive. *International Journal of Andrology, 2*(Suppl.), 748–760.

Strauss, J.S., & Pochi, P.E. (1963). III. Hormones and cellular metabolism: The human sebaceous gland: Its regulation by steroidal hormones and its use as an end organ for assaying androgenicity in vivo. *Recent Progress in Hormone Research, 19,* 385–444.

Strauss, R.H., Wright, J.E., Finerman, G.A., & Catlin, D.H. (1983). Side effects of anabolic steroids in weight-trained men. *The Physician and Sportsmedicine, 11,* 87–96.

Svanborg, A., & Ohlsson, S. (1959). Recurrent jaundice of pregnancy: A clinical study of twenty-two cases. *American Journal of Medicine, 27,* 40–49.

Sweeney, E.C., & Evans, D.J. (1976). Hepatic lesions in patients treated with synthetic anabolic steroids. *Journal of Clinical Pathology, 29,* 623–626.

Swerdloff, R.S., Palacios, A., McClure, R.D., Campfield, L.A., & Brosman, S.A. (1978). Male contraception: Clinical assessment of chronic administration of testosterone enanthate. *International Journal of Andrology, 2*(Suppl.), 731–747.

Taxy, J.B. (1978). Peliosis: A morphologic curiosity becomes an iatrogenic problem. *Human Pathology, 9,* 331–340.

Thompson, P.D., Culinane, E.M., Sady, S.P., Chenevert, C., Saritelli, A.L., Sady, M.A., & Herbert, P.N. (1989). Contrasting effects of testosterone and stanozolol on serum lipoprotein levels. *Journal of the American Medical Association, 261,* 1165–1168.

Thompson, P.D., Sadaniantz, A., Cullinane, E.M., Bodziony, K.S., Catlin, D.H., Torek-Both, G., & Douglas, P.S. (1992). Left ventricular function is not impaired in weight-lifters who use anabolic steroids. *Journal of American College of Cardiology, 19,* 278–282.

Tikkanen, M.J., Nikkila, E.A., Kussi, T., & Sipinen, S. (1982). High density lipoprotein-2 and hepatic lipase: Reciprocal changes produced by estrogen and norgestrel. *Journal of Clinical Endocrinology and Metabolism, 54,* 1113–1117.

Treuner, J., Niethammer, D., Flach, A., Fischbach, H., & Schenck, W. (1980). Hepatocellular carcinoma after oxymetholone treatment. *Medizinische Welt, 31,* 952–955.

Turani, H., Levi, J., Zevin, D., & Kessler, E. (1983). Hepatic lesions in patients on anabolic androgenic therapy. *Israel Journal of Medical Sciences, 19,* 332–337.

Verwilghen, R., Louwagie, A., Waes, J., & Vandenbroucke, J. (1966). Anabolic agents and relative polycythemia. *British Journal of Haematology, 12,* 712–716.

Vesselinovitch, S.D., & Mihailovich, N. (1967). The effect of gonadectomy on the development of hepatomas induced by urethane. *Cancer Research, 27,* 1788–1791.

Vessey, M., Doll, R., Peto, R., Johnson, B., & Wiggins, P. (1976). A long-term follow-up study of women using different methods of contraception—an interim report. *Journal of Biosocial Science, 8,* 373–427.

Visuri, T., & Lindholm, H. (1994). Bilateral distal biceps tendon avulsions with use of anabolic steroids. *Medicine and Science in Sports and Exercise, 26,* 941–944.

Wakabayashi, T., Onda, H., Tada, T., Iijima, M., & Itoh, Y. (1984). High incidence of peliosis hepatis in autopsy cases of aplastic anemia with special reference to anabolic steroid therapy. *Acta Pathologica Japonica, 34,* 1079–1086.

Webb, O.L., Laskarzewski, P.M., & Glueck, C.J. (1984). Severe depression of high-density lipoprotein cholesterol levels in weight lifters and body builders by self-administered exogenous testosterone and anabolic-androgenic steroids. *Metabolism, 33,* 971–975.

Weider, J. (1987). How drugs affect peaking. *Muscle & Fitness, 49,* 150–153, 232–233.

Weinbauer, G.F., Marshall, G.R., & Nieschlag, E. (1986). New injectable testosterone ester maintains serum testosterone of castrated monkeys in the normal range for four months. *Acta Endocrinologica, 113,* 128–132.

Werner, S.C. (1947). Clinical syndromes associated with gonadal failure in men. *American Journal of Medicine, 3,* 52–66.

Werner, S.C., Hanger, F.M., & Kritzler, R. (1950). Jaundice during methyl testosterone therapy. *American Journal of Medicine, 8,* 325–331.

Westaby, D., Ogle, S.J., Paradinas, F.J., Randell, J.B., & Murray-Lyon, I.M. (1977). Liver damage from long-term methyltestosterone. *Lancet, 1,* 261–263.

Westaby, D., Portmann, B., & Williams, R. (1983). Androgen related primary hepatic tumors in non-Fanconi patients. *Cancer, 51,* 1947–1952.

Widder, R.A., Bartz-Schmidt, K.U., Geyer, H., Brunner, R., Kirchhof, B., Donike, M., & Heinmann, K. (1995). *Candida albicans* endophthalmitis after anabolic steroid abuse. *Lancet, 345,* 330–331.

Wilson, J.D., Aiman, J., & MacDonald, P.C. (1980). Pathogenesis of gynecomastia. *Advances in Internal Medicine, 25,* 1–32.

Wing, T.Y., Ewing, L.L., Zegeye, B., & Zirkin, B.R. (1985). Restoration effects of exogenous luteinizing hormone on the testicular steroidogenesis and Leydig cell ultrastructure. *Endocrinology, 117,* 1779–1787.

Winwood, P.J., Robertson, D.A.F., & Wright, R. (1990). Bleeding oesophageal varices associated with anabolic steroid use in an athlete. *Postgraduate Medicine, 66,* 864–865.

Wood, T.O., Cooke, P.H., & Goodship, A.E. (1988). The effect of exercise and anabolic steroids on the mechanical properties and crimp morphology of the rat tendon. *American Journal of Sports Medicine, 16,* 153–8.

Woodard, T.L., Burghen, G.A., Kitabchi, A.E., & Wilimas, J.A. (1981). Glucose intolerance and insulin resistance in aplastic anemia treated with oxymetholone. *Journal of Clinical Endocrinology and Metabolism, 53,* 905–908.

World Health Organization Task Force on Methods for the Regulation of Male Fertility. (1990). Contraceptive efficacy of testosterone-induced azoospermia in normal men. *Lancet, 336,* 955–959.

Wynn, V., Landon, J., & Kawerau, E. (1961). Studies on hepatic function during methandienone therapy. *Lancet, 1,* 69–75.

Yeater, R., Reed, C., Ullrich, I., Morise, A., & Borsch, M. (1996). Resistance trained athletes using or not using anabolic steroids compared to runners: Effects on cardiorespiratory variables, body composition, and plasma lipids. *British Journal of Sports Medicine, 30,* 11–14.

Yesalis, C.E., Herrick, R.T., Buckley, W.E., Friedl, K.E., Brannon, D., & Wright, J.E. (1988). Self-reported use of anabolic-androgenic steroids by elite power lifters. *The Physician and Sportsmedicine, 16,* 91–100.

Yesalis, C.E., Kennedy, N.J., Kopstein, A.N., and Bahrke, M.S. (1993). Anabolic-androgenic steroid use in the United States. *Journal of the American Medical Association, 270,* 1217–1221.

Yoshida, E.M., Erb, S.R., Scudamore, C.H., & Owen, D.A. (1994). Severe cholestasis and jaundice secondary to an esterified testosterone, a non-C17 alkylated anabolic steroid. *Journal of Clinical Gastroenterology, 18,* 268–270.

Yoshida, E.M., Karim, M.A., Shaikh, J.F., Soos, J.G., & Erb, S.R. (1994). At what price, glory? Severe cholestasis and acute renal failure in an athlete abusing stanozolol. *Canadian Medical Association Journal, 151,* 791–793.

Zuliani, U., Bernardini, B., Catapano, A., Campana, M., Cerioli, G., & Spattini, G. (1989). Effects of anabolic steroids, testosterone, and HGH on blood lipids and echocardiographic parameters in body builders. *International Journal of Sports Medicine, 10,* 62–66.

CHAPTER

7

Women and Anabolic Steroids

Diane L. Elliot, MD, and Linn Goldberg, MD

Whatever muscles I have are the product of my own hard work and nothing else.

Evelyn Ashford
Olympic Champion 100 m, 1984

Supported in part by NIDA Grants #5R01 DA07356 and #5R01 DA11748.

Since enactment of the Title IX provision of the Education Amendments of 1972, we have seen a marked expansion in women's participation in sports (Boutillier & SanGiovanni, 1994). Coincident with that growth is an increase in the prevalence of young and adult women's substance abuse, including use of ergogenic and physique-altering agents. Today, a 15-year-old woman is 15 times more likely to be using illegal drugs than was her mother at the same age (Center on Addiction and Substance Abuse, 1996). Although sports participation has many benefits, young men and women athletes are not (contrary to public perceptions) protected from using drugs or engaging in other unhealthy behaviors (DuRant, Escobedo, & Heath, 1995; Faulkner & Slattery, 1990; Kokotailo et al., 1996; Mottram, 1996), and they may be at increased risk of using physique-altering/performance-enhancing agents (Kreipe et al., 1995; Whitaker et al., 1989).

In this chapter, we present information on the prevalence and consequences of women's use of anabolic steroids (AS). We address the psychological and social factors that influence women's androgenic drug use, and discuss these in the context of variables that motivate disordered eating habits and use of other physique-altering agents.

Normal Physiological Effects of Testosterone in Women and Men

Reviewing sex-specific changes during development and maturation is important in understanding the effects of AS use in women. Estrogen and testosterone are the major sex hormones, primarily produced in the ovaries and testes, respectively. Both sexes have the potential to respond in the same way to hormonal stimulation, as receptors specific for each type of hormone are present in tissues of women and men. Accordingly, the circulating levels of estrogen and testosterone have critical roles in the expressed differences between women and men (Conte & Grumbach, 1997).

Sex-specific differentiation begins at 7 weeks of gestation, when the testes-determining portion of the Y chromosome causes the embryonic male gonad to begin to synthesize testosterone (Conte & Grumbach, 1997). Testosterone causes the bipotential fetal urogenital tissue to form male structures. Unlike the testes, the fetal ovary does not produce any hormones at this developmental stage. Without the influence of testosterone (and other glycoprotein hormones), the urogenital tissue forms female structures, and at approximately 3 months of gestation, the female gonad begins producing oocytes.

Because urogenital structures are bipotential, a female fetus exposed to testosterone in the first trimester will experience virilization of the genitalia. This occurs with certain inherited metabolic disorders of the female fetus, such as the enzymatic blocks causing congenital adrenal hyperplasia (Sultan et al., 1997). Maternal androgens are aromatized and inactivated as they cross the placenta; so a marked increase in maternal level is needed to induce virilization of the female fetus. However, such an increase has been observed in pregnant women with androgen-secreting neoplasms (Sultan et al., 1997) and could result from a woman's use of anabolic steroids early in gestation. The potential of such steroid use to cause masculinization of a female fetus led to mandatory oral contraceptive use by the German Democratic Republic's female athletes who were given anabolic steroids, and any unexpected pregnancies were terminated (Franke & Berendonk, 1997).

Hormone levels in both sexes remain low until puberty, when the second component of sex-specific differentiation occurs. At that time, gonadotropin-releasing hormone stimulates increased release of the pituitary gonadotropic hormones LH (luteinizing hormone) and FSH (follicle-stimulating hormone). In males, LH stimulates testicular Leydig cells to secrete testosterone. During adolescence, a male's circulating testosterone increases from a prepubertal level of less than 10 ng/ml to the normal adult male values of approximately 600 ng/ml (Schiff & Walsh, 1995).

Only a small percentage of testosterone circulates freely in plasma; more than 95% is bound to plasm proteins. Testosterone binds most avidly to sex hormone–binding globulin (SHBG), and 60 to 70% is SHBG-bound (Petra, 1991). The remainder is bound to albumin, α_1-acid glycoprotein, and transcortin (Handelsman, 1996). The absolute increase in serum testosterone in males is augmented by their lower level of SHBG; so adult males have up to 40 times the circulating free testosterone of adult females. Adult males also have low levels of circulating estrogens and progesterone. A small amount of these hormones is synthesized in the testes, with the majority formed from the peripheral conversion of androgens to weak estrogens.

In teenage males, the increasing testosterone level results in the secondary sexual characteristics. Those changes include an increase in lean body mass and fourfold strength gain during adolescence (independent of physical activity level) (Forbes, 1985; Lee, 1995). Among pubertal females, the increased FSH causes the ovaries to produce estrogen and mature oocytes. Ovulation results in a menstrual cycle's normal sequence of estrogen and progesterone secretion. A female's estrogen level increases approximately 10-fold from prepubertal to adult levels, which causes feminization. Females also have low levels of circulating testosterone, due to synthesis by the normal adrenal gland and ovary. A slight increase in testosterone level in females also occurs during puberty. Body hair is stimulated only by androgens, and during maturation, a female's higher testosterone level is responsible for developing body hair. Normal levels of hormones for adult women and men are presented in table 7.1.

Table 7.1 Normal Hormone Levels in Women and Men

	Premenopausal adult woman	Postmenopausal woman	Adult man
Estradiol (pg/ml)	50–350*	0.16 ng/ml	25
Estrone (pg/ml)	80–200*	35	45
Testosterone (ng/ml)	0.35 (free 5 pg/ml)	0.25	600 (free 50–210 pg/ml)
Androstenedione (ng/ml)	0.15	0.6	1.5

*Levels vary with stage of the menstrual cycle. Pico- is 10^{-12} and nano- is 10^{-9}.

Data from Lee 1995 and Schiff & Walsh 1995.

Prevalence of Anabolic Steroid Use in Females

Two large U.S. cross-sectional studies indicate that, currently, young women are the demographic group with the most rapid growth in AS use. In the 1990s, studies sponsored by Centers for Disease Control and the National Institute on Drug Abuse found a doubling in the prevalence of AS use among adolescent females (Kann et al., 1995; Kann et al., 1996; U.S. Department of Health and Human Services [USDHHS], 1992; USDHHS, 1993–1995). AS use among young females is concentrated among those participating in sports (Kreipe et al., 1995; Whitaker et al., 1989). This increased use extends to collegiate women athletes, who estimated that 5.9% of women competitors use anabolic steroids (Yesalis et al., 1990).

Reports concerning elite women athletes—for example, Chinese distance runners (Medvedev, Edberg out at Monte Carlo, 1995) and U.S. swimming and track athletes (Track Body, 1997; IAAF Suspensions, 1997)—suggest that international women athletes are using anabolic steroids. Franke and Berendonk (1997) presented information from the German Democratic Republic, before its 1990 collapse, which indicated that AS use was widespread among its women athletes in all women's Olympic sports except sailing and gymnastics. Prevalence studies concerning AS use among young women are reviewed in chapter 3.

Physical Effects of Anabolic Steroids on Women

For both sexes, testosterone is the primary masculinizing hormone. It is activated further in certain tissues (e.g., scalp hair follicles and prostate gland) to the more potent androgen, dihydrotestosterone. Testosterone's effects in reproductive and nonreproductive tissue are mediated by a single androgen receptor, which activates DNA transcription and indirectly affects protein synthesis (Wu, 1997). Testosterone's effects among males and females are listed in table 7.2. The androgenic (producing male secondary sexual characteristics) and anabolic (causing tissue growth) effects are mediated by the same receptor (Harlan et al., 1979; Bagatell & Bremner, 1996), and it has not been possible to synthesize a hormone that is specific to only one of those two effects. Accordingly, testosterone and its synthetic analogues are all anabolic-androgenic hormones.

Most hormones produce their effects across a range of normal levels. Concentrations above that range may have benefits, but usually adverse consequences also occur. Hormones rarely are used in supraphysiologic doses without attendant side effects. With the androgen levels found among normal males from prepubescence to adulthood, there is a steep linear dose-response curve between testosterone concentration and its physiological effects (Forbes, 1985). However, in adult males, the androgen

Table 7.2 Testosterone Effects

	Among males	Among females
Androgenic		
	Increase in length and diameter of penis (during puberty)	Increase in length and diameter of clitoris
	Development/enlargement of prostate	May cause anovulation and development of polycystic ovaries
	Growth of pubic, axillary, body, and facial hair	Growth of pubic, axillary, body, and facial hair
	Loss of scalp hair (male pattern baldness)	Loss of scalp hair (may be diffuse loss)
	Increase in libido	Increase in libido
Anabolic		
	Increased muscle mass and strength	Increased muscle mass and strength
	Decrease in body fat	Decrease in body fat
	Enlargement of larynx and vocal cord thickening	Vocal cord thickening
	Long bone growth and epiphyseal closure (in puberty)	Long bone growth and epiphyseal closure (in puberty)
	Increase in RBC mass	Increase in RBC mass

receptor is almost fully saturated, and the response appears to plateau (Wu, 1997). Despite that, supraphysiologic androgen levels among men can further increase muscle mass and strength (Bhasin et al., 1996), perhaps from nonreceptor-mediated anticatabolic effects (Byerley et al., 1993).

As do men's, women's tissues have testosterone receptors and the ability to respond to androgens. However, in contrast to men, women are on the steep portion of the dose-response curve. The low testosterone level in women allows exogenous anabolic steroids to have a marked direct effect on muscle mass and strength. Even among healthy women not taking androgens, strength correlates with testosterone level (Hakkinen & Pakarinen, 1993).

Women's responsiveness to androgens is consistent with reports concerning AS use among athletes from the German Democratic Republic. Performance-enhancing effects were most marked among young women (Franke & Berendonk, 1997). Additional information concerning the effects of exogenous anabolic steroids among women athletes can be drawn from hormonal treatment of female-to-male transsexuals, comparison of normal women with different testosterone levels, and reports by women admitting to AS use.

Hormonal Effects in Female-to-Male Transsexuals

Before sexual reassignment surgery, female transsexuals are treated with androgens, with the usual dose being 200 mg of testosterone cypionate (DEPO-Testosterone) or enanthate (Delatestryl) every 2 weeks. This is comparable to the replacement dosage for a hypogonadal male. These genetic females, treated with testosterone, experience a series of changes: including altered body fat distribution; increased muscle mass, which is augmented by exercise; a deepened voice (which occurs within a few weeks and is irreversible [Gerritsma et al., 1994]); an increase in clitoral length (also an early and consistent finding); and acne (Blanchard & Steiner, 1990). Approximately 50 percent of patients note an increase in body hair and loss of scalp hair (Futterweit & Deligdisch, 1986). Women's androgenic hair loss can result in more diffuse alopecia, rather than the patterned loss that occurs among males (Callan & Montalto, 1995). For any individual, the precise timing and magnitude of changes vary. Those differences probably reflect genetic susceptibility and variability in testosterone administration, as centers caring for transsexual patients do not administer anabolic steroids in the same manner (Meyer, Walker, & Suplee, 1981).

Despite the virilization, many androgen-treated transsexual women continue to have regular menses while on testosterone therapy. In one series, 14 of the 19 women continued to have regular menses (Futterweit & Deligdisch, 1986), while other centers reported that most individuals' menses ceased after approximately 4 months of testosterone treatment (Blanchard & Steiner, 1990). When testosterone was administered to normally ovulating women (as therapy for premenstrual syndrome or loss of libido), a fivefold increase in circulating testosterone level did not disrupt the normal cyclic variation in LH, FSH, estrogen, and progesterone (Dewis, Newman, Ratcliffe, & Anderson, 1986). Normal ovarian function suggests that a woman's AS use would not be a reliable contraceptive, and that pregnancy could occur during its use (with the potential of virilizing a female fetus [Sultan et al., 1997]).

Effects in Women Using Anabolic Steroids

The changes observed among transsexual genetic females treated with testosterone can be compared with effects reported by women using illicit anabolic steroids. As with male AS users, women employ a variety of oral and parenteral preparations, and dose and cycle length vary. While androgen-treated female transsexuals have blood testosterone levels comparable to adult males, women abusing anabolic steroids can have testosterone levels 30 times that of normal women and twice that of normal men (Malarkey et al., 1991).

In one of the few assessments of female AS users, Strauss, Liggett, and Lanese (1985) interviewed 10 female bodybuilders who had used cyclic androgens for at least 2 years. All women reported an increase in muscle strength. The most consistent additional consequences were deepening of voice, increased facial hair, and clitoral lengthening. A decrease in body fat and an increase in aggressiveness occurred in 8 of the 10 women. Approximately half of the women also experienced an increase in libido, a decrease in breast size, and more severe acne. Two of the 10 women reported loss of scalp hair. In a similar study, 9 female athletes who had used androgens reported that it resulted in increased muscle size, acne, a deepened voice, increased body hair, and clitoral lengthening (Malarkey et al., 1991). A more recent investigation of 15 women AS users found a comparable spectrum and prevalence of side effects (Korkia, Lenehan, & McVeigh, 1996). These women's most frequent adverse effects, from an average use of 4 years, included psychological changes, voice deepening, menstrual disorders, and clitoral enlargement. Acne was reported by one woman, and none complained about loss of scalp hair. The findings from these three case series are compared in table 7.3.

Androgens also cause nonvisible adverse effects. Circulating estrogens favorably alter lipid levels and account for the higher levels of high-density lipoprotein cholesterol (HDLC) and lower levels of low-density lipoprotein cholesterol (LDLC) found in premenopausal women than is observed among males and postmenopausal women. Female transsexuals treated with testosterone have significantly higher levels of triglycerides, total cholesterol, and LDLC, while HDLC is reduced (compared to

Table 7.3 Series of Female Anabolic Steroid Users and the Reported Effects

	Malarkey et al., 1991	**Strauss, Liggett, & Lanese, 1985**	**Korkia, Lenehan, & McVeigh, 1996**
Subjects	9	10	15
Duration of anabolic steroid use	4 y (average)	At least 2 y	4 y (average)
Increased strength	100%*	100%	60%
Voice deepening	100%	100%	NP
Increased facial hair	NP	90%	47%
Clitoral lengthening	100%	80%	NP
Decreased body fat	NP	80%	NP
Increased aggressiveness	100%	80%	NP
Increased body hair	100%	50%	33%
Increased libido	100%	60%	NP
Decreased breast size	NP	50%	20%
Severe acne	NP	60%	7%
Loss of scalp hair	NP	20%	NP
Menstrual irregularities	NP	80%	53%

*Percentage of subjects with effect.

NP indicates data not provided.

control women and to their own values when not taking androgens) (Goh, Loke, & Ratnam, 1995; Meyer et al., 1986). Female athletes using high-dose anabolic steroids (especially alkylated forms that cannot be metabolized to estrogens [Friedl, Hannan, Jones, & Plymate, 1990]) reverse this benefit and can have HDLC levels lower than that of normal males (Cohen et al., 1986).

Due to the lipid changes, androgen use promotes atherosclerotic disease. Other androgen influences on cardiovascular disease have been assessed by comparing women's testosterone levels with the prevalence of cardiac risk factors and coronary heart disease. Even at the low testosterone levels observed among normal women, those with higher blood testosterone have an increase in hypertension, central obesity, diabetes, and cardiovascular disease (Modell, Goldstein, & Reyes, 1990; Bjorntorp, 1996).

Women using anabolic steroids would be susceptible to the adverse consequences observed among men—for example, hepatic dysfunction, and premature epiphyseal closure (see chapter 6). In addition, approximately one-quarter of adolescents using anabolic steroids have shared needles (DuRant et al., 1993). The prevalence of needle sharing is not established for women AS users, but if practiced, it would place users at risk for serious infectious complications, including HIV (Nemechek, 1991).

The many adverse effects of testosterone are especially worrisome, as young female athletes and their coaches are not familiar with these consequences; nor are they knowledgeable about potential outcomes of disordered eating and use of other physique-altering drugs (Elliot et al., 1998). In addition, coaches greatly underestimate the frequency with which female athletes engage in these unhealthy actions. Despite their underestimations of drug use, coaches strongly agree that female student-athletes need programs that help prevent use of performance-enhancing and physique-altering drugs as well as disordered eating habits, while promoting healthy sport nutrition and effective strength-training methods (Elliot, Goldberg, Wolf, & Moe, 1998).

Psychological Effects of Anabolic Steroids on Females

The central nervous system has receptors for both estrogens and testosterone (Sands & Studd, 1994). Researchers have assessed testosterone's effect on women's mood, cognitive function, and sexual behavior. As mentioned, initial male differentiation is controlled genetically, but subsequent development depends on exposure to testosterone early in utero and at puberty. Accordingly, sex-specific variation could reflect genetic differences, testosterone effects on the fetus, or consequences of hormonal stimulation during adolescence and adulthood.

Testosterone's primary putative psychological effect is increased aggressiveness. Animal studies assessing hormone effects were reviewed by Bahrke, Yesalis, and Wright (1996), with the authors concluding that a positive relationship exists between testosterone level and aggressive behavior. At puberty, an increase in testosterone level in male adolescents is associated with aggressiveness and loss of impulse control (Warren & Brooks-Gunn, 1989). In addition, several cross-sectional studies and anecdotal case reports of male AS users have suggested that testosterone increases aggression and hostile behavior (Bahrke, Yesalis, & Wright, 1996).

When studied prospectively, high-dose methyltestosterone administered for 3 days to normal men resulted in increased sexual arousal, irritability, and hostility (Su et al., 1993). However, individual responses varied, and 2 of the 20 men developed significant psychiatric illness, despite it being only a brief period of high-dose AS use. The observation is consistent with case reports of males using anabolic steroids and experiencing mania or psychosis (Pope & Katz, 1994). These adverse effects may require preconditioning by testosterone exposure during development, as reports of psychiatric illness consequent to androgen use involve males exclusively.

Psychological effects among women using anabolic steroid have varied. Unlike muscular strength (Hakkinen & Pakarinen, 1993), normal women's testosterone level is not correlated with consistent psychological differences (Modell, Goldstein, & Reyes, 1990). Female transsexuals treated with testosterone are predisposed toward anger and aggressiveness, while their overall mood is unchanged (Van Goozen et al., 1995). Female athletes using anabolic steroids also report an increase in aggressiveness (Strauss, Liggett, & Lanese, 1985; Malarkey et al., 1991). Bahrke and Strauss (1992) compared psychometrics among control women, female AS users, and those same users approximately 3 months after cessation of AS use. The three groups were similar in their Profile of Mood State dimensions. When hostility was assessed, paradoxically, females using anabolic steroids had decreased hostility, which remained low when androgens were stopped.

Cognition

Studies of transsexuals before and during testosterone therapy indicate that sex-specific cognition is affected by androgen levels. As a group, males have greater spatial abilities, and females excel in verbal fluency (Gouchie & Kimura, 1991). Following 3 months of testosterone treatment, genetic females experienced enhanced spatial abilities (the "male" pattern) and a decrement in verbal fluency (the "female" pattern) (Van Goozen et al., 1994, 1995).

Libido

Androgens also affect libido. Normal women's midcycle testosterone level correlates with sexual desire, behaviors, and responsiveness (Morris, Udry, Khan-Dawood, & Dawood, 1987). Women who have their ovaries removed experience a reduction in both estrogen and testosterone levels (Sands & Studd, 1994). For these women, hormone replacement with a combination of estrogen and testosterone more effectively restores libido than estrogens alone (Myers et al., 1990). Androgens used therapeutically by female transsexuals (Van Goozen et al., 1995) and illicitly by female bodybuilders (Strauss, Liggett, & Lanese, 1985) resulted in an increase in libido and sexual arousability .

Unhealthy Behaviors

Finally, AS use clusters with abuse of other drugs and may predispose to additional unhealthy behaviors. Meilman, Crace, Presley, and Lyerla

(1995) assessed college-aged AS users, 16% of whom were female, and compared them to matched controls. Users had significantly greater use of alcohol, tobacco, cocaine, amphetamines, and marijuana. Survey of high school students also revealed that AS use was independently associated with use of cocaine, marijuana, alcohol, and cigarettes (DuRant et al., 1993; DuRant, Escobedo, & Heath, 1995).

Several other cross-sectional studies of young women indicate that use of physique-altering drugs clusters with abuse of other drugs and unhealthy behaviors (e.g., disordered eating habits and multiple sexual partners) (Fisher, Schneider, Pegler, & Napolitano, 1991; Holderness, Brooks-Gunn, & Warren 1994; Killen et al., 1987; Neumark-Sztainer, Story, & French, 1996; Striegel-Moore & Huydic, 1993). Although prospective studies are needed to establish relationships among unhealthy behaviors and drug use, assessment of female adolescents suggests that use of physique-altering drugs and disordered eating are precursors to abuse of other illicit substances among female adolescents (Elliot, Goldberg, Moe, Clarke, & Witherrite, 1997).

DHEA: A Weak Androgen

Dehydroepiandrosterone (DHEA) is a steroid hormone produced in the adrenal, and it is a precursor to both estrogens and testosterone. Among normal women and men, DHEA's peak blood concentration is reached at approximately age 20. Thereafter, its level progressively decreases, so that at age 65, circulating DHEA is reduced by approximately 50%. Rates of DHEA decline vary, and the decrement in DHEA correlates with certain pathologic processes, such as development of cardiovascular disease (Barrett-Connor, Khaw, & Yen, 1986), weight gain (Cleary & Fisk 1986), insulin resistance (Coleman, Schwizer, & Leiter, 1984) and reduced immunity (Loria & Padgett, 1993). Recently, DHEA has become a popular supplement, advocated for its benefits in combating aging, restoring sexual potency, and improving mental function.

The effects of DHEA use are influenced by an individual's hormone milieu, alterations in hormone synthesis, and competitive inhibition of hormone-receptor binding. DHEA administration among women results in androgenic effects, due to DHEA's direct action and metabolism to more active androgens. This differs from its consequences in men, for whom DHEA acts like a weak estrogen (Ebeling & Koivisto, 1994). In addition, for both sexes, DHEA may have an antiglucocorticoid effect (Herbert, 1995).

Administration of DHEA to older men and women can restore serum DHEA to its peak level. However, most described benefits are based on cross-sectional studies that correlated DHEA level and pathological outcomes, and prospective controlled trials are limited. In one of the few prospective studies, DHEA (50 mg/day) was administered for 6 months to 13 men and 17 women (age range, 40 to 70 years). Women's androgen levels doubled, and subjects reported an almost uniform increase in their sense of well-being (Morales, Nolan, Nelson, & Yen, 1994). Use of DHEA can cause virilization. Women's continuous use of 100 mg/day of DHEA has been reported to cause acne, hirsutism, lowered voice, and hair loss ("Dehydroepiandrosterone," 1996; Yen, Morales, & Khorram, 1995). DHEA also appears to have an androgenic effect among adolescent women. Vogiatzi and colleagues (1996) administered DHEA at 80 mg/day for 8 weeks to overweight teenagers, in a controlled trial of its effects. Although body weight and composition were not changed, serum testosterone was elevated significantly among the female subjects.

Females using DHEA might be expected to experience anabolic-androgenic effects comparable to women with the polycystic ovary (PCO) syndrome. The PCO syndrome is characterized by hirsutism, anovulation, obesity, and insulin resistance (Franks, 1995). It is an idiopathic disorder that usually begins in adolescence. These women's DHEA levels are elevated, and their circulating testosterone levels may be normal or slightly above the normal limits for a woman. The diagnosis is established by a compatible clinical picture and an elevated DHEA level. DHEA ingestion by normal females could lead to an elevation in androgen level and masculinizing effects similar to those experienced by women with the PCO syndrome.

The Drug Enforcement Administration and Food and Drug Administration do not regard DHEA as an anabolic steroid. It is considered a dietary supplement, rather than a drug, and its sale is not regulated. Despite DHEA potentially having significant anabolic-androgenic effects in women, prior surveys of drug use among female athletes have not assessed its prevalence. Although DHEA is on the list of drugs banned by the International Olympic Committee (IOC) (Fuentes, Rosenberg, & Davis, 1995), DHEA use is not detectable by current methods of drug testing in sport.

Physique-Altering Drug Use

Eating disorders have become a major problem in the United States and are the third most common chronic illness among adolescent females (Kreipe et al., 1995; Sundgot-Borgen, 1994). AS use may be considered a subset of disordered eating habits and physique-altering drug use. Female adolescent athletes, in addition to having a higher prevalence of AS use, are at greater risk for disordered eating and use of other physique-altering agents (e.g., diuretics, laxatives, tobacco, diet pills, amphetamines, and cocaine). These problems are present among all female sports and not confined to those sports that encourage pursuit of a slender, immature body type, (e.g., gymnastics, dance, and cross country running) (Taub & Blinde, 1992).

The reported absolute rate of eating disorders among young female athletes varies from 25% to 74% (American College of Sports Medicine [ACSM], 1997; Holderness, Brooks-Gunn, & Warren, 1994). This broad range is due to variability in defining a threshold for diagnosing the condition, as the behaviors progress from the poor food choices and inconsistent nutrition that are typical in teens (Bull, 1992) to a more intense focus on dieting and *disrupted eating habits*. *Disordered eating* occurs when there is ongoing use of pathologic means to modify nutrient balance, such as self-induced vomiting, fasting, bingeing, purging, and food restriction and/or use of anabolic steroids, laxatives, diuretics, tobacco, diet pills, amphetamines, and cocaine to control body weight. Some individuals progress further and meet diagnostic criteria for an *eating disorder*. The prevalence of anorexia nervosa and bulimia nervosa is approximately 1% and 8%, respectively, among young women (Katz, 1990; Taub & Blinde, 1992).

Eating disorders, and their associated adverse sequelae, are so prevalent among female athletes that in 1997 the ACSM published a position stand on the "female athlete triad" (ACSM, 1997). Women athletes can develop a stereotyped syndrome, with three components. The triad's first feature is disordered eating and the use of physique-altering drugs (amphetamines, tobacco, diet pills, laxatives, diuretics, and anabolic steroids), which can result in amenorrhea (the second triad component). Athletic amenorrhea is associated with reduced estrogen levels and a predisposition to osteoporosis (third aspect). Osteoporosis can lead to an increase in musculoskeletal injuries (Lloyd et al., 1986; Putukian, 1994), scoliosis, and skeletal fractures (Drinkwater, Bruemner, & Chesnut, 1990). Eating disorders have other adverse physical and psychologic consequences, including metabolic abnormalities, reduced immunity, hypokalemia, muscle weakness, cardiac arrhythmias, renal dysfunction, and direct cardiotoxicity (Roberts & Elliot, 1991). In extreme forms, eating disorders have the highest mortality rates among all psychiatric diagnoses (Herzog & Copeland, 1985).

Many factors influence women's use of performance-enhancing and physique-altering drugs, and an analysis of these factors provides the potential means to deter these unhealthy behaviors. Combining information from several studies (summarized below), the primary factors predisposing toward use of anabolic steroids and other physique-altering behaviors appear to be the following:

1. Pressure to achieve a lean muscular physique
2. Drive for success in athletics
3. Reinforcing physical and psychological consequences

The cultural bias supporting extreme thinness affects women's drug use and weight loss practices (Rodin, 1993). Almost half of U.S. women are trying to lose weight (Serdula et al., 1993), and female teens often are obsessed with their weight (Camp, Klesges, & Relyea, 1993). The young female adolescent is bombarded by images promoting excessively thin women as a standard of both beauty and optimum sport performance. These pressures can lead to drug use. For example, a majority of females believe that smoking helps control weight (Charlton, 1984), and prospective studies document that weight concerns are related to initiation of smoking (French, Perry, Leon, & Fulkerson, 1994). Recognizing the potency of this factor, tobacco companies (e.g., Virginia Slims) have exploited the power of body image and tailored their advertising to women's weight concerns (Pentz, 1994).

Female images in advertising and the media have been categorized as three types (Brubach, 1996). One is a lean, androgynous, nonmuscular physique (Holmlund, 1989). This immature feminine body type may promote socialization to a stereotyped subordinate female gender role (Signorielli, 1993). Second is a more feminine body that is voluptuous and exudes female sexuality. In recent years, a third more muscular feminine representation has emerged. Although these women have physiques that are more fit, they usually, as with the first body type, have a body fat percentage less than physiologically normal for females (Cohen, 1993). Female athletes also have the pressure to achieve low body fat to excel in their sport. Maintaining the culturally defined desirable body composition usually is neither healthy nor feasible, and the unrelenting pressure to lower body weight is a factor that leads to disordered eating behaviors and use of performance-enhancing/physique-altering drugs (Garner, Garfinkel, Schwartz, & Thompson, 1980).

Anabolic steroids are made to order for a female wanting to attain a lean muscular physique. While most drug abuse has outcomes that tend to discourage use (e.g., reduced academic performance or the consequences of antisocial behavior), females who use anabolic steroids may experience loss of body fat, increased muscle size and strength, and enhanced sport performance. The resulting social rewards (e.g., scholarships, prize winnings), and approval by parents, coaches, peers, and society, may reinforce AS use.

Along with physical effects, the psychological consequences of AS use may help alleviate the disorders that predispose persons to developing disordered eating and substance abuse (Emery et al., 1993; Fisher et al., 1991; French et al., 1995; Lau, Quandrel, & Hartman, 1990; Patton et al., 1996). Female adolescents at higher risk for disordered eating have lower self-esteem and a more depressed mood than peers less likely to engage in these actions. Thus, the increased aggressiveness associated with AS use could "treat" a lowered self-esteem and be an additional positively reinforcing factor. The ACSM's review of the female athlete triad found that women predisposed to develop this disorder had a greater "win-at-all-costs" attitude, which also could predispose toward AS use (ACSM, 1997) .

In the near future, the influences promoting AS use among women are not expected to change, and women's use would be predicted to continue to increase. An effective program to deter AS use (using healthy sport nutrition and effective strength training as alternatives to AS use) is available for young male athletes (Goldberg et al., 1996) (see chapter 4). However, a comparable intervention has not been tested among adolescent female athletes. Extrapolating from the findings among males, successful programs to deter AS use among women should include alternative means to achieve a young woman's appearance and performance goals.

Summary

The social pressures to achieve a certain physique and level of sport performance, an increase in the monetary rewards for successful elite women athletes, and positive physical and psychological consequences can motivate women to use anabolic steroids. The potential benefits of anabolic steroids for females are an increased muscle mass and strength, a more confident and aggressive performance, and faster muscle recovery during intense training. Androgenic side effects are observed, even from brief use (such as voice deepening). The more cosmetic adverse effects (e.g., increased acne, loss of scalp hair) do not occur uniformly (Strauss, Liggett, & Lanese, 1985; Malarkey et al., 1991; Korkia, Lenehan, & McVeigh, 1996). The enhanced strength and muscle mass, a lack of understanding of potential adverse consequences, and the prominence of anabolic steroid abuse among international class female athletes all may contribute to young women being the U.S. population group with the greatest growth in AS use (Kann et al., 1995; Kann et al., 1996; USDHHS, 1992; USDHHS, 1993–1995).

References

American College of Sports Medicine. (1997). Position stand on the female athlete triad. *Medicine and Science in Sports and Exercise, 29,* i–ix.

Bagatell, C.J., & Bremner, W.J. (1996). Androgens in men—uses and abuses. *Drug Therapy, 334,* 707–713.

Bahrke, M.S., & Strauss, R.H. (1992). Selected psychological characteristics of female anabolic-androgenic (AAS) users. *Medicine and Science in Sports and Exercise, 24,* S136.

Bahrke, M.S., Yesalis, C.E., III, & Wright, J.E. (1996). Psychological and behavioural effects of endogenous testosterone and anabolic-androgenic steroids. *Sports Medicine, 6,* 367–390.

Barrett-Connor, E., Khaw, K.T., & Yen, S.S.C. (1986). A prospective study of dehydroepiandrosterone sulfate, mortality, and cardiovascular disease. *New England Journal of Medicine, 315,* 1519–1524.

Bhasin, S., Storer, T.W., Berman, N., Callgari, C., Clevenger, B., Phillips, J., Bunnell, T.J., Tricker, R., Shirazi, A., & Casaburi, R. (1996). The effects of supraphysiologic doses of testosterone on muscle size and strength in normal men. *New England Journal of Medicine, 335,* 1–7.

Bjorntorp, P. (1996). The android woman—a risky condition. *Journal of Internal Medicine, 239,* 105–110.

Blanchard, R., & Steiner, B.W. (1990). *Clinical management of 5 identity disorders in children and adults* (pp. 139–154). Washington, DC: American Psychiatric Press.

Boutillier, M.A., & SanGiovanni, L.F. (1994). Politics, public policy, and Title IX: Some limitations of liberal feminism. In S. Birrell & C.L. Cole (Eds.), *Women, sport, and culture* (pp. 97–109). Champaign, IL: Human Kinetics.

Brubach, H. (1996, June 23). The athletic esthetic. *New York Times Magazine.*

Bull, N.L. (1992). Dietary habits, food consumption, and nutrient intake during adolescence. *Journal of Adolescent Health, 13,* 384–388.

Byerley, L.O., Lee, W.P., Buena, F., et al. (1993). Effect of modulating serum testosterone in the normal male range on protein dynamics, carbohydrate and lipid metabolism. *Endocrinology Journal, 1,* 253–259.

Callan, A.W., & Montalto, J. (1995). Female androgenetic alopecia: An update. *Australasian Journal of Dermatology, 36,* 51–55.

Camp, D.E., Klesges, R.C., & Relyea, G. (1993). The relationship between body weight concerns and adolescent smoking. *Health Psychology, 12,* 24–32.

Center on Addiction and Substance Abuse, Columbia University. (1996). *Substance abuse and the American woman.* New York: Author.

Charlton, A. (1984). Smoking and weight control in teenagers. *Public Health, 98,* 277–281.

Cleary, M.P., & Fisk, J.F. (1986). Anti-obesity effect of two different levels of dehydroepiandrosterone in lean and obese middle-aged female Zucker rats. *International Journal of Obesity, 10,* 193–204.

Cohen, G.L. (1993). Media portrayal of the female athlete. In G.L. Cohen (Ed.), *Women in sports: Issues and controversies.* Newbury, CA: Sage.

Cohen, J.C., Faber, W.M., Benade, A.J.S., & Noakes, T.D. (1986). Altered serum lipoprotein profiles in male and female power lifters ingesting anabolic steroids. *The Physician and Sportsmedicine, 14,* 131–136.

Coleman, D.L., Schwizer, R.W., & Leiter, E.H. (1984). Effect of genetic background on the therapeutic effects of dehydroepiandrosterone (DHEA) in diabetes-obesity mutant and in aged normal mice. *Diabetes, 33,* 26–32.

Conte, F.A., & Grumbach, M.M. (1997). Abnormalities of sexual determination & differentiation. In F.S. Greenspan & G.J. Strewler (Eds.), *Basic and clinical endocrinology* (5th ed., pp. 487–520). Stamford, CT: Appleton & Lange.

Dehydroepiandrosterone (DHEA). (1996). *Medical Letter, 38,* 91–92.

Dewis, P., Newman, M., Ratcliffe, W.A., & Anderson, D.C. (1986). Does testosterone affect the normal menstrual cycle? *Clinical Endocrinology, 24,* 515–521.

Drinkwater, B.L., Bruemner, B., & Chesnut, C.G.H., III. (1990). Menstrual history as a determinant of current bone density in young athletes. *Journal of the American Medical Association, 263,* 545–548.

DuRant, R.H., Escobedo, L.G., & Heath, G.W. (1995). Anabolic-steroid use, strength training and multiple drug use among adolescents in the United States. *Pediatrics, 96,* 23–28.

DuRant, R.H., Rickert, V.I., Ashworth, C.S., Newman, C., & Slavens, G. (1993). Use of multiple drugs among adolescents who use anabolic steroids. *New England Journal of Medicine, 328,* 922–926.

Ebeling, P., & Koivisto, V.A. (1994). Physiological importance of dehydroepiandrosterone. *Lancet, 343,* 1479–1481.

Elliot, D., Goldberg, L., Moe, E., Clarke, G., Poole, L., & Witherrite, T. (1997). A validated etiologic model for adolescent girls' future disordered eating and drug use. *Medicine and Science in Sports and Exercise, 29*(Suppl.), S295.

Elliot, D.L., Goldberg, L., Wolf, S.L., & Moe, E.L. (1998). Coaches' estimates of drug use and eating disorders: A potential blind spot. *Strength and Conditioning, 20,* 31–34.

Emery, E.M., McDermott, R.J., Holcomb, D.R., & Marty, P.J. (1993). The relationship between youth substance use and area-specific self-esteem. *Journal of School Health, 63,* 224–228.

Faulkner, R.A., & Slattery, C.M. (1990). The relationship of physical activity to alcohol consumption in youth. *Canadian Journal of Public Health, 81,* 168–169.

Fisher, M., Schneider, M., Pegler, C., & Napolitano, B. (1991). Eating attitudes, health-risk behaviors, self-esteem, and anxiety among adolescent females in a suburban high school. *Journal of Adolescent Health, 12,* 377–384.

Forbes, G.B. (1985). The effect of anabolic steroids on lean body mass: The dose response curve. *Metabolism, 34,* 571–573.

Franke, W.W., & Berendonk, B. (1997). Hormonal doping and androgenization of athletes: A secret program of the German Democratic Republic government. *Clinical Chemistry, 43,* 1262–1279.

Franks, S. (1995). Polycystic ovary syndrome. *New England Journal of Medicine, 333,* 853–859.

French, S.A., Perry, C.L., Leon, G.R., & Fulkerson, J.A. (1994). Weight concerns, dieting behavior, and smoking initiation among adolescents: A prospective study. *American Journal of Public Health, 84,* 1818–1820.

French, S.A., Story, M., Downes, B., et al. (1995). Frequent dieting among adolescents: Psychosocial and health behavior correlates. *American Journal of Public Health, 85,* 695–701.

Friedl, K.E., Hannan, C.J., Jr., Jones, R.E., & Plymate, S.R. (1990). High-density lipoprotein is not decreased if an aromatizable androgen is administered. *Metabolism, 39,* 69–74.

Fuentes, R.J., Rosenberg, J.M., & Davis, A. *Athletic drug reference '95* (pp. 107–108). Research Triangle Park, NC: Clean Data.

Futterweit, W., & Deligdisch, L. (1986). Histopathological effects of exogenously administered testosterone in 19 female to male transsexuals. *Journal of Clinical Endocrinology and Metabolism, 62,* 16–21.

Garner, D.M., Garfinkel, P.E., Schwartz, D., & Thompson, M. (1980). Cultural expectations of thinness in women. *Psychological Reports, 47,* 483–491.

Gerritsma, E.J., Brocaar, M.P., Hakkesteegt, M.M., & Birkenhager, J.C. (1994). Virilization of the voice in post-menopausal women due to the anabolic steroid nandrolone decanoate (Decadurabolin). The effects of medication for one year. *Clinical Otolaryngology, 19,* 79–84.

Goh, H.H., Loke, D.F.M., & Ratnam, S.S. (1995). The impact of long-term testosterone replacement therapy on lipid and lipoprotein profiles in women. *Maturitas, 21,* 65–70.

Goldberg, L., Elliot, D., Clarke, G.N., MacKinnon, D.P., Moe, E., Zoref, L., Green, C., Wolf, S.L., Greffrath, E., Miller, D.J., Lapin, A. (1996). Effects of a multi-dimensional anabolic steroid prevention intervention. The Adolescents Training and Learning to Avoid Steroids (ATLAS) Program. *Journal of the American Medical Association, 276,* 1555–1562.

Gouchie, C., & Kimura, D. (1991). The relationship between testosterone levels and cognitive ability patterns. *Psychoneuroendocrinology, 16,* 323–346.

Hakkinen, K., & Pakarinen, A. (1993). Muscle strength and serum testosterone, cortisol and SHBG concentrations in middle-aged and elderly men and women. *Acta Physiologica Scandia, 148,* 199–207.

Handelsman, D.J. (1996). Testosterone and other androgens: Physiology, pharmacology, and therapeutic use. In M.A. Sperling (Ed.), *Pediatric endocrinology* (pp. 2351–2361). Philadelphia: Saunders.

Harlan, W.R., Grillo, G.P., Cornoni–Huntley, J., & Leaverton, P.E. (1979). Secondary sex characteristics of boys 12 to 17 years of age: the U.S. Health Examination Survey. *Journal of Pediatrics, 95*, 293.

Herbert J. (1995). The age of dehydroepiandrosterone. *Lancet, 345,* 1193–1194.

Herzog, D.B., & Copeland, P.M. (1985). Eating disorders. *New England Journal of Medicine, 313,* 295–303.

Holderness, C.C., Brooks-Gunn, J., & Warren, M.P. (1994). Co-morbidity of eating disorders and substance abuse. Review of the literature. *International Journal of Eating Disorders, 16,* 1–34.

Holmlund, C.A. (1989). The body, sex, sexuality and race. *Cinema Journal, 28,* 38–51.

IAAF suspensions. (1997, June 1). *Oregonian,* p. A16.

Kann, L., Warren, C.W., Harris, W.A., et al. (1995). Youth risk behavior surveillance. United States, 1993. *Morbidity and Mortality Weekly Report (MMWR), 44,* 1–56.

Kann, L., Warren, C.W., Harris, W.A., et al. (1996). Youth risk behavior surveillance. United States, 1995. *Morbidity and Mortality Weekly Report (MMWR), 45,* 1–85.

Katz, J.L. (1990). Eating disorders: A primer for the substance abuse specialist: 1. Clinical features. *Journal of Substance Abuse Treatment, 7,* 143–149.

Killen, J.D., Taylor, C.B., Telch, M.J., et al. (1987). Depressive symptoms and substance use among adolescent binge eaters and purgers: A defined population study. *American Journal of Public Health, 77,* 1539–1541.

Kokotailo, P.K., Henry, B.C., Koscik, R.E., Fleming, M.F., & Landry, G.L. (1996). Substance use and other health risk behaviors in collegiate athletes. *Clinical Journal of Sports Medicine, 6,* 183–189.

Korkia, P., Lenehan, P., & McVeigh, J. (1996). Non-medical uses of androgens among women. *Journal of Performance Enhancing Drugs, 1,* 71–76.

Kreipe, R.E., Golden, N.H., Katzman, D.K., Fisher, M., Rees, J., Tonkin, R.S., Silber, T.J., Sigman, G., Schebendach, J., Ammerman, S.D., et al. (1995). Eating disorders in adolescents: A position paper of the Society for Adolescent Medicine. *Journal of Adolescent Health, 16,* 476–479.

Lau, R.R., Quandrel, M.J., & Hartman, K.A. (1990). Development and change of young adults' preventive health beliefs and behavior: Influence from parents and peers. *Journal of Health and Social Behavior, 31,* 240–259.

Lee, P.A. (1995). Physiology of puberty. In K.L. Becker (Ed.), *Principles and practice of endocrinology and metabolism* (pp. 822–830). Philadelphia: Lippincott.

Lloyd, T., Triantafyllou, S.J., Baker, E.R., Houts, P.S., Whiteside, J.A., Kalenak, A., & Stumpf, P.G. (1986). Women athletes with menstrual irregularity have increased musculoskeletal injuries. *Medicine and Science in Sports and Exercise, 18,* 374–379.

Loria, R.M., & Padgett, D.A. (1993). Androstenediol regulates systemic resistance against lethal infections in mice. *Annals of the New York Academy of Science, 685,* 293–295.

Malarkey, W.B., Strauss, R.H., Leizman, D.J., Liggett, M.T., & Demers, L.M. (1991). Endocrine effects in female weight lifters who self-administer testosterone and anabolic steroids. *American Journal of Obstetrics and Gynecology, 165,* 1385–1390.

Medvedev, Edberg out at Monte Carlo. (1995, April 26). *USA Today,* p. 13C.

Meilman, P.W., Crace, R.K., Presley, C.A., & Lyerla, R. (1995). Beyond performance enhancement: Polypharmacy among collegiate users of steroids. *Journal of American College Health, 44,* 98–104.

Meyer, W.J., III, Walker, P.A., & Suplee, Z.R. (1981). A survey of transsexual hormonal treatment in twenty gender-treatment centers. *Journal of Sex Research, 17,* 344–349.

Meyer, W.J., III, Webb, A., Stuart, C.A., et al. (1986). Physical and hormonal evaluation of transsexual patients: A longitudinal study. *Archives of Sexual Behavior, 15,* 121–138.

Modell, E., Goldstein, D., & Reyes, F. (1990). Endocrine and behavioral responses to psychological stress in hyperandrogenic women. *Fertility and Sterility, 53,* 454–459.

Morales, A.J., Nolan, J.J., Nelson, J.C., & Yen, S.S.C. (1994). Effects of replacement dose of dehydroepiandrosterone in men and women of advancing age. *Journal of Clinical Endocrinology and Metabolism, 78,* 1360–1366.

Morris, N.M., Udry, J.R., Khan-Dawood, F., & Dawood, M.Y. (1987). Marital sex frequency and midcycle female testosterone. *Archives of Sexual Behavior, 16,* 27–32.

Mottram, D.R. (1996). *Drugs in sport* (2nd ed.). London, UK: Routledge, Chapman and Hall.

Myers, L.S., Dixen, J., Morrissette, D., et al. (1990). Effects of oestrogen, androgen, and progestin on sexual psychophysiology and behavior in postmenopausal women. *Journal of Clinical Endocrinology and Metabolism, 70,* 1124–1131.

Nemechek, P.M. (1991). Anabolic steroid users—another potential risk group for HIV infection. *New England Journal of Medicine, 325,* 357.

Neumark-Sztainer, D., Story, M., & French, S.A. (1996). Covariations of unhealthy weight loss behaviors and other high-risk behaviors among adolescents. *Archives of Pediatric and Adolescent Medicine, 150,* 304–308.

Patton, G.D., Hibbert, M., Rosier, M.J., et al. (1996). Is smoking associated with depression and anxiety in teenagers? *American Journal of Public Health, 86,* 225–230.

Pentz, M.A. (1994). Directions for future research in drug abuse prevention. *Preventive Medicine, 23,* 646–652.

Petra, P.H. (1991). The plasma sex steroid binding protein (SBP or SHBG): A critical review of recent developments on the structure, molecular biology and function. *Journal of Steroid Biochemistry and Molecular Biology, 40,* 735–753.

Pope, H.G., Jr., & Katz, D.L. (1994). Psychiatric and medical effects of anabolic-androgenic steroid use. *Archives of General Psychiatry, 51,* 375–382.

Putukian, M. (1994). The female triad: Eating disorders, amenorrhea and osteoporosis. *Medical Clinics of North America, 78,* 345–356.

Roberts, W.O., & Elliot, D.L. (1991). Malnutrition in a compulsive runner. *Medicine and Science in Sports and Exercise, 23,* 513–516.

Rodin J. (1993). Cultural and psychosocial determinants of weight concerns. *Annals of Internal Medicine, 119,* 643–645.

Sands, R., & Studd, J. (1994). Exogenous androgens in postmenopausal women. *American Journal of Medicine, 98*(Suppl. 1A), 76S–79S.

Schiff, I., & Walsh, B. (1995). Menopause. In K.L. Becker (Ed.), *Principles and practice of endocrinology and metabolism* (pp. 822–830). Philadelphia: Lippincott.

Serdula, M.K., Collins, M.E., Williamson, D.F., Anda, R.F., Pamuk, E., & Byers, T.E. (1993). Weight control practices of U.S. adolescents and adults. *Annals of Internal Medicine, 119,* 667–671.

Signorielli, N. (1993). Sex roles and stereotyping on television. *Adolescent Medicine, 4,* 551–561.

Strauss, R.H., Liggett, M.T., & Lanese, R.R. (1985). Anabolic steroid use and perceived effects in ten weight-trained women athletes. *Journal of the American Medical Association, 253,* 2871–2873.

Striegel-Moore, R.H., & Huydic, E.S. (1993). Problem drinking and symptoms of disordered eating in female high school students. *International Journal of Eating Disorders, 14,* 417–425.

Su, T-P., Pagliaro, M., Schmidt, P.J., Pickar, D., Wolkowitz, O., & Rubinow, D.R. (1993). Neuropsychiatric effects of anabolic steroids in male normal volunteers. *Journal of the American Medical Association, 269,* 2760–2764.

Sultan, C., Lumbroso, S., et al. (1997). Intrauterine virilization of the female fetus. In R. Azziz, J. Nestler, & D. Dewailly (Eds.), *Androgen excess disorders in women* (pp. 593–599). Philadelphia: Lippincott-Raven.

Sundgot-Borgen, J. (1994). Eating disorders in female athletes. *Sports Medicine, 17,* 176–188.

Taub, D.E., & Blinde, E.M. (1992). Eating disorders among adolescent female athletes: Influence of athletic participation and sport team membership. *Adolescence, 27,* 833–848.

Track body suspends Eugene Slaney. (1997, June 1). *Oregonian,* p. A1.

U.S. Department of Health and Human Services, National Institute on Drug Abuse. (1992). *National household survey on drug abuse: Population estimates, 1991* (USDHHS publication number [ADM]-92-1887). Washington, DC: USDHHS, Public Health Service and Alcohol, Drug Abuse, and Mental Health Administration.

U.S. Department of Health and Human Services, Substance Abuse and Mental Health Services Administration. (1993–1995). *National household survey on drug abuse: Population estimates, 1992, 1993, and 1994* (USDHHS publication numbers [SMA] 93-2053, [SMA] 94-3017, and [SMA] 95-3063, respectively). Rockville, MD: Author.

Van Goozen, S.H.M., Cohen-Kettenis, P.T., Gooren L.J.G., et al. (1994). Activating effects of androgens on cognitive performance: Causal evidence in a group of female-to-male transsexuals. *Neuropsychologia, 32,* 1153–1157.

Van Goozen, S.H.M., Cohen-Kettenis, P.T., Gooren, L.J.G., et al. (1995). Gender differences in behaviour: Activating effects of cross-sex hormones. *Psychoneuroendocrinology, 4,* 343–363.

Vogiatzi, M.G., Boeck, M.A., Vlachopapadopoulou, E., et al. (1996). Dehydroepiandrosterone in morbidly obese adolescents: Effects on weight, body composition, lipids, and insulin resistance. *Metabolism: Clinical and Experimental, 45,* 1011–1015.

Warren, M.P., & Brooks-Gunn, J. (1989). Mood and behavior of adolescence: Evidence for hormonal factors. *Journal of Clinical Endocrinology and Metabolism, 69,* 77–83.

Whitaker, A., Davies, M., Shaffer, D., et al. (1989). The struggle to be thin: A survey of anorexic and bulimic symptoms in a non-referred adolescent population. *Psychological Medicine, 19*(1), 143–163.

Wu, F.C.W. (1992). Testicular steroidogenesis and androgen use and abuse. *Clinical Endocrinol Metabolism, 6,* 373.

Yen, S.S.C., Morales, A.J., & Khorram O. (1995). Replacement of DHEA in aging men and women. *Annals of the New York Academy of Science, 774,* 128–142.

Yesalis, C.E., Buckley, W.A, Anderson, W.A., Wang, M.O., Norwig, I.A., Ott, G., Puffer, I.C., & Strauss, R.H. (1990). Athletes' projections of anabolic steroid use. *Clinical Sports Medicine, 2,* 155–171.

CHAPTER

8

Psychological Effects of Endogenous Testosterone and Anabolic-Androgenic Steroids

Michael S. Bahrke, PhD

I was driving and this [#$%&@!] fingered me. So without any regard for my brand new Jaguar, I pulled up right next to this guy in his little [#$%&@!] box Chevette and started whacking his [#$%&@!] box with an ice scraper. I just kept hanging out the window of my new Jaguar taking swings at his car.

From an interview with an anabolic steroid user, Chicago, December, 1993.

This chapter is adapted from *Sports Medicine* 1996; see credits page for more information.

Interest in the psychological and behavioral aspects of using anabolic-androgenic steroids was heightened during the late 1980s due to the interaction of several events: (1) use of anabolic-androgenic steroids by professional, Olympic, and collegiate athletes was increasingly reported by the media (Blackwell, 1991; Pearson & Hansen, 1990); (2) use among children and adolescents was documented (Buckley et al., 1988; Johnson, Jay, Shoup, & Rickert, 1989); (3) anecdotal reports and testimonials of violent behavior associated with anabolic-androgenic steroid use were presented by the media ("The Insanity of Steroid Abuse," 1988); and (4) studies examining the psychiatric effects of anabolic-androgenic steroid abuse began to appear in the scientific literature (Brower, Blow, Beresford, & Fuelling, 1989; Pope & Katz, 1988). Nearly 50 reports examining the psychological and behavioral effects of using endogenous testosterone and anabolic steroids have been published since this chapter was first published (Bahrke, 1993). This new chapter extends the analysis of the previous chapter to include studies published since 1993.

From the late 1930s to the late 1970s, anabolic steroids were used in clinical settings to successfully treat depression, melancholia, and involutional psychoses (Bahrke, Yesalis, & Wright, 1990). It is unclear why the use of anabolic steroids to treat certain psychiatric disorders diminished over time, but presumably it was due to the development of other, more efficacious drugs. Recently, however, in contrast to the previously successful use of these drugs to treat psychiatric disorders, a number of scientific and clinical reports have suggested that affective and psychotic syndromes, some of violent proportions and including suicide (Elofson & Elofson, 1990; "NHL Tough Guy Kordic," 1992), may be associated with the use of anabolic steroids in individuals seeking to enhance their performance or appearance (Bahrke et al., 1990). Citing an association between steroid abuse and violent behavior, Orchard and Best (1994) have recommended that violent offenders be tested for anabolic steroid use at the time of arrest in order to document the possible association between steroid abuse and violent acts, and that the information obtained be used to develop additional tactics to control steroid abuse.

The purpose of this chapter is to discuss the following: (1) the effects of anabolic steroids on aggressive behavior in animals; (2) the relationship between endogenous testosterone levels and moods and behavior in humans; (3) the effects of estrogen on aggression; (4) the effects of the clinical use of anabolic steroids on moods and behavior in human male contraceptive studies; (5) the relationship of anabolic steroid use and mental health in athletes, including issues of psychological dependence and withdrawal; and (6) selected methodological issues involved in assessing the psychological and behavioral effects of anabolic steroids.

Anabolic Steroids and Aggressive Behavior in Animals

Previous studies have documented significant positive relationships between testosterone levels, dominance, and aggressive behavior in various species of animals, including nonhuman primates (Bahrke et al., 1990).

Rejeski, Gregg, Kaplan, and Manuck (1990) examined the effects of anabolic steroids on behavior, baseline heart rate, and stress-induced heart rate responses in cynomolgus monkeys who were assigned to one of four mixed social groups of both steroid- and sham-injected control animals. Hormone administration resulted in increases in dominant behavior in dominant animals and increased submission in subordinate animals. Behavior returned to pretreatment levels 8 weeks after cessation of drug administration. Affiliative behaviors decreased in all steroid-treated animals and, with the exception of play behavior, failed to return to pretest levels after an 8-week recovery period. Testosterone appeared to have a relatively long lasting suppressive influence on most affiliative responses. Minkin, Meyer, and van Haaren (1993) administered an anabolic steroid, nandrolone decanoate, for 8 weeks to six groups of normal and castrated male rats and also found a decrease in spontaneous behavior.

To determine if long-term exposure to high doses of anabolic steroids increases aggression and sexual activity in gonadally intact male rats, Lumia, Thorner, and McGinnis (1994) administered testosterone propionate 3 times per week for 10 consecutive weeks. Long-term treatment did not alter any parameter of male copulation. However, testosterone propionate–treated males were significantly more dominant and less submissive toward gonadally intact opponents than were control males. Using a high-dose cocktail of anabolic steroids (testosterone cypionate, nandrolone deconate, and boldenone undecylenate), Melloni, Connor, Hang, Harrison, and Ferris (1997) have also demonstrated increased aggressive behavior in adolescent male hamsters. Clark and Barber (1994) utilized the resident-intruder paradigm of aggression to evaluate the aggression-inducing properties of two anabolic steroids (methyltestosterone and stanozolol) in castrated male rats. Castrated male rats treated with methyltestosterone displayed levels of aggression equivalent to the levels displayed by castrated males treated with testosterone propionate on most of the behavioral indices assessed. In contrast, treatment with stanozolol produced no changes in aggressive behavior. Nor were any effects observed with either steroid treatment on the levels of locomotor behavior. Likewise, Martinez-Sanchis, Brain, Salvador, and Simon (1996), using high, moderate, and low doses of stanozolol over 21 days, have reported no significant effects on aggression and motor activity in young and adult intact male mice. These findings highlight the heterogeneity of anabolic steroid effects on the nervous system and behavior and indicate that the psychological effects reported by human anabolic steroid users may likewise depend upon the distinct chemical structures of the anabolic steroids used.

With regard to the behavioral and neurochemical effects of anabolic steroids and the neural mechanisms that may mediate the adverse effects of anabolic steroids on mental health, Bitran, Kellog, and Hilvers (1993) have reported that 1 week of treatment with testosterone propionate in intact male rats resulted in anxiolytic behavior that was accompanied by an increase in the sensitivity of cortical gamma-aminobutyric acid (GABA) receptors. However, observed changes were no longer present in a second group after 2 weeks of testosterone propionate exposure, indicating that tolerance to this may have developed.

To study the short-term effect of an anabolic steroid on behavior, Agren, Thiblin, Tirassa, Lundeberg, and Stenfors (1999) administered Metenolon three times, at a low dose, to rats. The steroid-treated rats showed less fear or anticipatory anxiety when compared with control animals, leading the researchers to conclude that Metenolon produced an anxiolytic drug effect at a low dose in rats. Similarly, Salvador, Moya-Albiol, Martinez-Sanchis, and Simon (1999), using several different steroids (testosterone propionate, nandrolone decanoate, and a mixture of both steroids), and single or repeated injections, found no effect of the steroids on spontaneous locomotor activity in intact, male rats. These results emphasize the importance of duration of treatment, the interaction with endogenous androgen levels, and specific type of activity (spontaneous or forced). Previous investigation by Martinez-Sanchis, Salvador, Moya-Albiol, Gonzalez-Bono, and Simon (1998) also found 10 weeks of treatment with various doses of testosterone propionate had little effect on aggression levels in intact male mice.

Anabolic steroid effects on brain reward have been investigated by Clark, Lindenfeld, and Gibbons (1996) using the rate-frequency curve shift paradigm of brain stimulation reward in male rats with electrodes implanted in the lateral hypothalamus. In the first experiment, treatment for 2 weeks with methandrostenolone had no effect on either the reward or performance components of intracranial self-stimulation. In a second experiment, treatment for 15 weeks with an anabolic steroid "cocktail" (testosterone cypionate, nandrolone decanoate, boldenone undecylenate) did not alter brain reward, but did produce a significant change in bar-press rate. In addition to the steroid treatment in the second study, animals were administered a single injection of dexamphetamine before and after 15 weeks of steroid exposure. The rate-frequency curve shift was significantly greater in animals after 15 weeks of steroid cocktail treatment. Results indicate that anabolic steroids may influence the sensitivity of the brain reward system.

Research by Le Greves, Huang, Johansson, Thornwall, Zhou, and Nyber (1997) demonstrates that chronic high doses of nandrolone decanoate affect the mRNA expression of NMDA receptor units in certain areas of the brain. Some of these areas may relate to a mechanism involved in the recently suggested steroid-induced stimulation of the brain reward system.

Bronson, Nguyen, and de la Rosa (1996) exposed adult female mice to a combination of four anabolic steroids for 9 weeks at doses that were either the same or 5 times the level of the androgenic maintenance level for male mice, in an investigation designed to examine the effects of anabolic steroids on the behavior and physiological characteristics of female mice. Behaviorally, steroid exposure decreased activity in an open field, increased aggressiveness, and eliminated one type of sexual behavior. Overall, there was little or no difference in the effect of high and low steroid dose, suggesting a threshold effect. In a related study by Bronson (1996), adult male and female mice were treated with the same combination of four anabolic steroids at pharmacological doses for 6 months to determine the effects of prolonged exposure to steroids on behavior. Males were exposed to either 5 or 20 times androgenic maintenance levels, and females were exposed to either the same or 5 times the maintenance level for males. Steroids increased aggressiveness in females, but not in males. Results of this experiment suggest no enhancement of normal androgenic-mediated behavior in males, but significant effects on female behavior.

In summary, these recent investigations, demonstrating behavioral changes associated with the administration of exogenous testosterone, support previous reports documenting a relationship between endogenous testosterone levels and behavioral changes in animals (Bahrke, Yesalis, & Wright, 1990). However, conclusions drawn from animal models must be applied cautiously to humans. For example, it is difficult to show that animals experience emotional states that are qualitatively similar to human experiences, such as euphoria, depression, and anger. Also, humans cannot be subjected to many of the same stringent controls and manipulations used in animal research. Finally, the effects of sex hormones vary considerably among individuals as well as species.

Effect of Endogenous Testosterone Levels on Human Moods and Behaviors

Relative to the animal literature, fewer studies have assessed the relationship of endogenous or exogenous androgens to aggression or violent behavior in humans. Although a pattern of association between testosterone levels and both subjectively perceived and observed aggressive behavior in humans has been revealed in many earlier studies, the relationships between plasma testosterone and psychometric indices of aggression and hostility have been less consistent (Albert, Walsh, & Jonik, 1993; Archer, 1991, 1994; Bahrke, Yesalis, & Wright, 1990; Bahrke, Wright, Strauss, & Catlin, 1992; Gray, Jackson, & McKinlay, 1991; Rubinow & Schmidt, 1996).

Aggressive Behavior

Gladue (1991a) assessed aggressive behavioral characteristics in a large group of college men (*N* = 517) and women (*N* = 43) using a self-report instrument and found significant gender differences, with men reporting more physical and verbal aggression than women. Gladue (1991b) has also reported on the relationship of resting levels of testosterone and estradiol and self-reported aggressive behavior in men and women, including those who differed in sexual preferences. Adult men reported more physical and verbal aggression than did women. Men also had higher scores on measures of impulsivity and lack of frustration tolerance than did women, while women were more likely to avoid confrontation. Homosexual men were indistinguishable from heterosexual men on all measures of aggression. Homosexual women differed from heterosexual women on only physical aggression, in which homosexual women had lower scores. Total testosterone and estradiol were positively correlated with several indices of aggressive behavioral characteristics in men, but were negatively correlated with those same measures in women.

Data from a study designed to examine the relationship between testosterone and antisocial behavior in a sample of 4,462 U.S. male military veterans were reported by Dabbs and Morris (1990). They found that testosterone was correlated with a variety of antisocial behaviors among all individuals; however, socioeconomic status proved to be a moderating variable, with weaker testosterone-behavior relationships among individuals with high socioeconomic status. In another study, Booth and Dabbs (1993) found that men producing more testosterone are less likely to marry; once married, they are more likely to leave home because of troubled marital relations, extramarital sex, hitting or throwing things at their spouses, and experiencing a lower quality of marital interaction.

Dabbs, Jurkovic, and Frady (1991) have also examined the relationship of salivary testosterone and cortisol concentrations to personality, criminal violence, prison behavior, and parole decisions among 113 late-adolescent male offenders. Offenders high in testosterone had committed more violent crimes, were judged more harshly by the parole board, and violated prison rules more often than those low in testosterone. A significant interaction between testosterone and cortisol was found, in which cortisol moderated the correlation between testosterone and violence of crime. As cortisol concentrations increased, the correlation between testosterone and violent behavior dropped. Dabbs, Jurkovic, and Frady (1991) concluded that cortisol may be a biological indicator of psychological variables that moderate the testosterone-behavior relationship. Likewise, in a more recent study examining testosterone levels, crime, and prison misbehavior among 692 prison inmates, Dabbs, Carr, Frady, and Riad (1995) found that inmates who had committed personal crimes of sex and violence had higher testosterone levels than inmates who had committed property crimes of burglary, theft, and drugs. Inmates with higher testosterone levels also violated more prison rules, especially those involving confrontation.

Lindman, von der Pahlen, Ost, and Eriksson (1992), however, found no relationship between violent behavior and the serum concentrations of testosterone, cortisol, glucose, and ethanol obtained from 16 adult men taken into police custody after incidents of spouse abuse when concentrations were compared with sober state levels and data from equally intoxicated but nonviolent men. Similarly, measures of testosterone and concurrent self-ratings of aggression in 100 adolescent males over a 3-year period provide little evidence of a systematic relationship between aggression and concurrent or earlier measures of testosterone (Halpern, Udry, Campbell, & Suchindran, 1993).

Berman, Gladue, and Taylor (1993) found a significant positive relationship between endogenous testosterone levels in 38 male college students and direct aggression. Although individuals were also classified as either Type A or Type B behavior pattern, observations gave little evidence for the moderating effects of hormones on the level of aggression expressed by Type A behavior.

Responses to Winning and Losing

Gladue, Boechler, and McCaul (1989) have examined hormonal response to competition in men. Winners had higher testosterone levels than losers, with no significant difference between close and decisive contests. Cortisol levels did not differ between winners and losers, nor between close and decisive contests. Mood was depressed in decisive losers. The results indicate that the perception of winning or losing, regardless of actual performance, differentially influenced testosterone levels but not cortisol levels, and that changes are not simply general arousal effects but are related to mood and status change.

Findings from two experiments by McCaul, Gladue, and Joppa (1992) suggest that winning, even by luck or chance, can alter testosterone levels in men, and that mood may mediate such changes. In experiments in which male college students either won or lost money on a task controlled entirely by chance, winners reported more positive mood change than did losers. Winners also reported a more positive mood change and higher testosterone levels than did a neutral group that did not win or lose money. In both cases, winners exhibited significantly higher testosterone levels than losers. Likewise, Mazur, Booth, and Dabbs (1992) have observed that in nonphysical face-to-face competition, tournament winners show higher testosterone levels than losers. In addition, under certain circumstances such as closeness of competition, competitors show increases in testosterone before their games.

Conclusions

In summary, although several recent studies reveal a significant positive association between endogenous testosterone levels and aggressive behavior, other investigations do not. Additional research suggests that humans may undergo specific endocrine changes in response to victory or defeat and that mood may influence the degree of change.

Estrogen-Related Aggression

Research findings from animal studies have shown that aggressive behavior can be developed by estrogen as well as androgen administration (Simon & Whalen, 1986). In adolescent boys and girls, Susman, Dorn, and Chrousos (1991) have shown fewer emotional effects for gonadal hormones compared to adrenal androgens and other hormones. Although testosterone has been linked with aggression for many years, particularly in males, recent research indicates that estrogen, and not testosterone, may be partly responsible for increased aggression. Since testosterone, through the enzyme aromatase, can be converted in the brain to estrogen, higher levels of estrogen can act directly on brain cells.

Ogawa, Luban, Korach, and Pfaff (1995), in a study of the behavioral consequences of loss of functional estrogen receptors in male estrogen receptor knockout mice, have shown that a lack of estrogen receptors in the central nervous system modifies male emotional behavior in a manner not restricted to simple reproductive behaviors, demonstrating the relative importance of estrogen receptors in the regulation of male aggression.

In a study to assess the effects of sex steroids on aggressive behavior, Finkelstein and colleagues (1997) administered either depo-testosterone to hypogonadal boys or estrogen to girls at three physiological doses using a double-blind, placebo-controlled, 3-month, crossover design. Responses to placebo were compared with responses to hormones at specific doses. At the low dose, scores for aggressive impulses and physical aggression against peers significantly increased only for girls. At mid-dose, the scores for girls significantly increased for aggressive impulses, physical aggression against peers, and physical aggression against adults. The scores for boys significantly increased for physical aggression against adults. At the high dose, physical aggression against peers significantly increased only for boys. These results suggest that sex steroids affect aggressive behavior in adolescents. Girls showed larger and earlier increases than boys, suggesting that estrogen has a significant role in the change in aggression scores during puberty and that testosterone may exert its effect via conversion to estrogen.

The relationship between aggressive behavior and hormone levels appears to be more complex than just the result of elevated levels of testosterone. Taken together, these studies suggest an increased role for estrogen in aggressive behavior.

Male Contraceptive Studies and Moods

In addition to the above studies, which have examined the relationship between endogenous testosterone levels and aggression, others have been carried out over the past three decades to assess the contraceptive efficacy of testosterone-induced azoospermia.

In an investigation conducted by the World Health Organization Task Force on Methods for the Regulation of Male Fertility (1990), 157 of 271 men became azoospermic following weekly injections of testosterone enanthate (200 mg/wk), and were followed over a 1-year efficacy phase. Although many participants withdrew from the study, only 3 reported increased aggressiveness and libido resulting from the injections as the cause for their discontinuation. Problems of increased aggressiveness or libido, if there were any, for men who remained in the study were not reported by the authors. Wu, Farley, Peregoudov, and Waites (1996), in a recent follow-up report to the original study, confirm the low overall incidence of adverse reactions and other side effects leading to discontinuation from the study. Increased fatigue, aggression, and cyclical changes in mood were among the most common reasons for discontinuation given by the participants.

Of the 399 healthy, male participants in a similar, but more recent investigation conducted by the World Health Organization Task Force on Methods for the Regulation of Male Fertility (1996), only 10 participants discontinued due to mood, aggression, or libido change.

Anderson, Bancroft, and Wu (1992), using a single-blind, placebo-controlled design and daily mood ratings, found no alteration in any of the mood states studied, including those associated with increased aggression, in 31 healthy men injected with testosterone enanthate (200 mg/wk) for 8 weeks. Bagatell, Heiman, Matsumoto, Rivier, and Bremner (1994) also found no significant change in self-reported sexual and aggressive behaviors (although some individuals complained of increased irritability) in 19 healthy men given testosterone enanthate (200 mg/wk) for 20 weeks and followed for several months thereafter.

In a study examining the effect of testosterone replacement therapy on mood changes in 54 hypogonadal males, Wang and colleagues (1995) found significant decreases in anger, irritability, sadness, tiredness, and nervousness and significant improvement in energy level, friendliness, and well/good feelings.

These studies suggest that concerns about adverse effects of moderate doses (200 mg/wk) of exogenous testosterone on male sexual and aggressive behavior have perhaps been overstated, particularly by the media. This dose (200 mg/wk), while less than that used by most serious competitive bodybuilders and strength athletes, equals or exceeds that used by many athletes in other sports (Yesalis & Bahrke, 1995).

Effects of Anabolic Steroids on Athletes' Moods and Behavior

Psychological and behavioral changes, such as increased aggressiveness and irritability, have been reported on an anecdotal basis by anabolic steroid users as well as their families and friends for many years. However, a previous review had determined that objective evidence documenting the short-term psychological and behavioral changes accompanying and following anabolic steroid use by athletes was extremely limited and inconclusive (Bahrke et al., 1990). Since then, several case, survey, and research studies addressing these issues have been published.

Case Reports

Leckman and Scahill (1990) have described two male athletes whose Tourette's syndrome symptoms uncharacteristically acutely worsened rather than improved in young adult life. Both were abusing high doses of anabolic steroids when, two weeks into a course of increasing androgen dosage, they noted worsened tic symptoms, heightened irritability, and aggressiveness. Both improved after withdrawal of exogenous androgens. According to Leckman and Scahill, the association between abuse of anabolic steroids and increased tic symptoms in these two patients may have been a chance event or a nonspecific response.

Pope and Katz (1990) have described three men who impulsively committed violent crimes, including murder, while taking anabolic steroids. Structured psychiatric interviews of each man suggested that steroids played a role in the etiology of the violent behavior. Pope and Katz suggest that the aggressive behavior associated with the use of anabolic steroids may pose a significant public health problem. Several other cases of apparent steroid-induced crimes have also been reported by Pope and colleagues (1996), suggesting that steroid use may occasionally be a significant, although uncommon, factor in criminal behavior. Corrigan (1996) has commented on two recent violent murders in which anabolic steroid use was implicated. In one case, a 29-year-old male bodybuilder used a hammer to batter his wife to death, and then shot himself through the head. In the second case, a 22-year-old male bodybuilder murdered a female companion by repeatedly bashing her head against a wall and then kicking her. However, Byrne (1997) has pointed out the presence of other psychoactive drugs (benzodiazepines and alcohol), in addition to anabolic steroid use, in these two murder cases.

A case in which brief exposure to a low dose of anabolic steroid resulted in a significant detrimental change in behavior, culminating in armed robbery, has been reported by Dalby (1992). The patient, a 20-year-old man, reported irritability, depression, and violent rages following a 5-week cycle of anabolic steroids. A 1-year jail sentence was imposed by a judge who ruled that steroid use was a mitigating factor in the commission of the robbery.

Schulte, Hall, and Boyer (1993) have described the case of child abuse and spouse battery by a 19-year-old male college football player who had been using multiple anabolic steroids over a 4-month period. No previous steroid use or aggressive and violent behavior was reported. However, during steroid use, the man became increasingly irritable and "rough" with his wife, both physically and sexually, and more impatient and punitive with their 2-year-old son. In an effort to discipline the child, the child's buttocks were scalded with boiling water. Upon cessation of steroid use, the man's irritability and violent outbursts resolved within a 2-month period. There was no recurrence at follow-up 18 months later. Repeated child sexual abuse and hypomanic episodes associated with anabolic steroid use and moderate cannabis intake has been reported in a 25-year-old male bodybuilder by Driessen, Muessigbrodt, Dilling, and Driessen (1996). Choi (1993) has also described several cases of violent criminal behavior, including rape and murder, associated with the use of anabolic steroids.

Stanley and Ward (1994) have recently described a case that relates anabolic steroid abuse to the development of psychiatric illness and violent crime in a 27-year-old male bodybuilder. He was treated with an antipsychotic drug, ceased anabolic steroid use, and his psychotic symptoms and mood improved without further treatment. Increased self-reported aggression and libido has also been reported by Wemyss-Holden, Hamdy, and Hastie (1994) as an undesirable effect in a pilot study evaluating the effects of exogenous anabolic steroids on prostatic volume, reduction in urine flow rate, and alteration in voiding patterns in a 49-year-old male bodybuilder.

Cross-Sectional Studies

In addition to case reports, many cross-sectional studies documenting the psychological and behavioral effects of anabolic steroids have been published recently.

Lindstrom and colleagues (1990) surveyed 138 male bodybuilders from a local gym to determine the prevalence of anabolic steroid use, the relationship of health risks to use, medical knowledge of steroids, social background, and current socioeconomic status of users and found that

38% had used anabolic steroids and 81% had experienced undesired effects. Changes in mood (51%) and increased libido (34%) were two of the more frequently self-reported effects among steroid users.

Parrott, Choi, and Davies (1994) administered an aggression inventory and a mood questionnaire to 21 steroid-using male amateur athletes attending a needle-exchange clinic and found individuals reporting significantly higher levels of aggression, alertness, irritability, anxiety, suspiciousness, and negativism while using steroids compared with periods of nonuse.

Silvester (1995) interviewed 22 former elite male shot put and discus throw athletes to determine self-perceptions of the acute and long-range effects of anabolic steroids. Among other acute effects while on the drugs, an increase in aggressiveness and irritability was reported by 13 athletes, distinct feelings of well-being were reported by 10, and quicker recovery from workouts was reported by 5. Twenty athletes reported no long-range psychological effects attributed to steroid use, while 2 believed that their occasionally elevated level of aggressiveness or irritability stemmed from their past use of steroids.

In an investigation examining the effects of long-term, relatively high dose anabolic steroid use on hostility and aggression in 6 male strength athletes, Choi, Parrott, and Cowan (1990) reported significantly more self-rated aggression in the 3 steroid users during periods of use compared with periods of nonuse. Users, however, were also significantly more hostile and aggressive than nonusers during periods of nonuse. Violence toward women during periods of anabolic steroid use has also been reported by Choi and Pope (1994), who found significantly more verbal aggression and violence in steroid-using athletes toward their wives and girlfriends during periods of steroid use than in nonuser athletes.

In an investigation to determine psychiatric symptoms associated with anabolic steroid use, Perry, Yates, and Andersen (1990) compared 20 male weightlifters who were currently using anabolic steroids with 20 male weightlifters who had never used steroids. The steroid users reported significantly more somatic, depressive, anxiety, hostility, and paranoid complaints when using steroids than when they were not using the drugs and significantly more complaints of depression, anxiety, and hostility during cycles of steroid use than did nonusers. The absence of significant differences in the frequency of major mental disorders between the two groups led Perry, Yates, and Andersen to conclude that the organic affective changes associated with abuse of anabolic steroids usually present as a subsyndromal depressive disorder were not severe enough to be classified as a psychiatric disorder.

In another study, Perry, Andersen, and Yates (1990) used two self-report instruments and a verbal interview to examine mental status changes in 20 competitive and noncompetitive anabolic steroid–using weightlifters. Based on responses to the questionnaire, significant percentages of individuals admitted to increased hostility and aggression, depression, paranoid thoughts, and psychotic features during steroid use. The steroid users displayed more personality disturbances overall compared with a control group of 20 weightlifters who did not use anabolic steroids and with a sex- and age-matched control group from the local community. However, no individual personality disorder or trait differences were significant between steroid users and the weightlifter control group, and both the steroid-user and nonsteroid-user weightlifter groups exhibited more flamboyant features than the community controls. The verbal interview was unable to identify any psychiatric diagnoses that were occurring more frequently in either the weightlifter control group or the steroid group. No cases of panic disorder, major depressive episode, grief reaction, mania, or atypical bipolar disorder were found. Interestingly, there were two cases of major depression in the control group and one in the steroid users. Alcohol abuse was diagnosed in 65% of the weightlifter control group, while seven (35%) cases of abuse and two (10%) cases of dependence were recognized in the steroid users. Drug abuse was observed in one individual in the control group and in one steroid user, while drug dependence was seen in one of the steroid users.

Malone, Dimeff, Lombardo, and Sample (1995), using a demographic survey, psychological testing, and psychiatric diagnosis, examined the psychiatric effects of anabolic steroid use and the frequency of other psychoactive substance use in 164 participants. Current and past steroid users did not differ on psychological testing, but past steroid users had a significantly higher incidence of psychiatric diagnoses than nonuser and current user groups. Hypomania was associated with steroid use and major depression with steroid discontinuation. Past steroid dependence was observed in 13% of current users and 15% of past users. Current psychoactive substance abuse or dependence was relatively low in all user groups. Malone and colleagues concluded that anabolic steroid use may lead to psychiatric disorders in certain individuals, and the concurrent use of psychoactive drugs, other than steroids, does not appear to be common in weightlifters and bodybuilders who are training intensively.

Yates, Perry, and Andersen (1990) evaluated a series of illicit anabolic steroid users and compared them with a control group of age-matched alcoholics and two control groups. Using a self-report measure, anabolic steroid users were found to have increased risk for personality psychopathology compared with one of the control groups, although this risk appeared to be partially explained by a group membership effect, as weightlifter controls also had higher rates of psychopathology. Additionally, similar to the alcoholic groups, illicit anabolic steroid users demonstrated significant antisocial traits.

Lefavi, Reeve, and Newland (1990) used two questionnaires to compare present steroid users with nonusers and former users, and concluded that anabolic steroid use may be associated with more frequent episodes of anger that are of greater intensity and duration and are characterized by a more hostile attitude toward others.

In an investigation similar to the study by Lefavi and colleagues, Bahrke and colleagues (1992) examined the psychological characteristics and subjectively perceived behavioral and somatic changes accompanying steroid usage in current anabolic steroid users. The results were compared with those obtained from previous users and nonusers. Although both current and former users reported subjectively perceived changes in enthusiasm, aggression, irritability, insomnia, muscle size, and libido when using anabolic steroids, these changes were not confirmed in comparisons across groups using standardized psychological inventories. No relationship was found between steroid dose and psychological moods in steroid users. More recently, Galligani, Renck, and Hansen (1996) assessed personality traits in three groups of strength athletes who self-administered anabolic steroids at the time of testing, had stopped using steroids for at least 6 months, or had never used steroids. Current steroid users were significantly more verbally aggressive than past steroid users and nonusers. No other statistically significant group differences were found for the other 14 personality factors that included somatic anxiety, muscular tension, psychic anxiety, psychasthenia, inhibition of aggression, socialization, social desirability, impulsiveness, monotony avoidance, detachment, indirect aggression, irritability, suspicion, and guilt.

In one of the few investigations examining the psychological changes accompanying anabolic steroid use by female athletes, Bahrke and Strauss (1992) found lower hostility among female steroid users in comparison with nonuser female athletes. A significant decrease in hostility among steroid users following 14 weeks of steroid use was also reported. These findings both conflict with and confirm earlier research with male and female athletes and emphasize the need to further delineate the relationship between anabolic steroid use and psychological changes in female athletes.

Yates, Perry, and Murray (1992) compared the aggression and hostility levels of current and recent steroid-using weightlifters with a nonuser weightlifter control group. Significantly elevated scores were found for active steroid users compared with both former and nonusers. These researchers were unable to demonstrate a relationship between dosage and psychometric scores in users.

Moss, Panazak, and Tarter (1992) have examined the relationship between the use of anabolic steroids and specific personality dimensions in 50 male bodybuilders who were current or past users in comparison with a sample of 25 age-matched, “natural” bodybuilders who never used steroids. No personality differences were found. Current steroid users scored higher than nonusers only on psychometric scales measuring hostility, aggression, and somatization. No statistical differences were found for the numerous other scales, including, among others, anxiety, depression, confidence, vigor, confusion, obsessiveness, and sensitivity.

Two questionnaires were used by Burnett and Kleiman (1994) in a cross-sectional study to assess a broad range of psychological characteristics in adolescent athletes who reported anabolic steroid use. Similar data were obtained from adolescent athletes who did not use steroids and from non-athletic adolescents. Although some personality variables differentiated between athletes and nonathletes, no personality variables significantly differentiated between athletes who used steroids and athletes who did not use steroids. However, steroid users who were currently on a steroid-use cycle had significantly more depression, anger, psychic vigor, and total mood disturbance than those who were not on a cycle.

Using a structured interview, Pope and Katz (1994) compared athletes who were using steroids with nonusers and found 23% of the users experienced major mood syndromes in association with steroid use. In addition, steroid users displayed mood disorders during steroid exposure significantly more frequently than in the absence of steroid exposure, and significantly more frequently than nonusers. Significant positive relationships were found between total weekly dose of steroids used and the prevalence of mood disorders. Approximately 25% of the users appeared to show a syndrome of dependence on steroids.

Bond, Choi, and Pope (1995) used an aggression scale, three scales of current feelings (alertness, contentment, and calmness), and a color-word conflict task containing sets of neutral, verbally aggressive, and physically aggressive words to measure the effects of anabolic steroids on mood and attentional bias to aggressive cues in current users, former users, and nonusers. Attention bias did not significantly differ between groups, but current users took longer to name the colors of all three sets. Nonusers rated themselves as more affable on the only significantly different item of the aggression scale. There were no significant differences between the groups on the three scales of current feelings.

The relationship between anabolic steroids and psychiatric symptoms, including aggressiveness and violent behavior, among steroid users has been examined by Thiblin, Kristiansson, and Rajs (1997). Using retrospective evaluation based on information from forensic psychiatric evaluations, police reports, and court records, violent offenders were evaluated for current or previous use of steroids. Results suggest that steroids may produce violent behavior and other mental disturbances, including psychosis. According to Thiblin, Kristiansson, and Rajs, steroids may lead to violent acts in vulnerable persons not only during current use, but also after withdrawal. In a similar investigation, but with a considerably different outcome, Isacsson, Garle, Ljung, Asgard, and Bergman (1998) screened for anabolic steroids in the urine of individuals in a Stockholm jail who had been arrested for violent crimes. No steroids were detected in the urine samples of 50 prisoners who had volunteered to participate in the study. However, 2 of the participants admitted steroid abuse and 16 prisoners refused to participate. Consequently, no conclusions can be drawn regarding the relationship between steroid use and violent crime.

In summary, investigations reviewed in this section have been cross-sectional in design. Unfortunately, retrospective studies rely on recall, the accuracy of which depends upon the honesty and ability of the individual to provide information on both the frequency and type of psychological and behavioral disturbances as well as on the training and skills of the researchers responsible for the assessments. To recall psychological and behavioral problems, individuals must have specific memories about the disturbances and be able to retrieve the information. Some may lack the ability to recall incidents, some may have little awareness of what has happened, and others may tend to "blow" incidents out of proportion to the actual events. In addition, some events may be selectively forgotten or reported. Investigations reviewed in this section have not reported on the validity and reliability of an individual's ability to recall psychological and behavioral disturbances. While cross-sectional studies of the psychological and behavioral effects encountered by anabolic steroid users are generally easier to perform than longitudinal studies, they require considerable care in sampling so that the participants selected accurately reflect the population being studied. Methods of participant selection are significant limitations to many of the studies reviewed in this section. Cross-sectional studies are also limited in that the only information they provide is an indication of current status, with information regarding previous conditions generally missing.

Longitudinal Investigations

Although a considerable number of cross-sectional or retrospective studies have examined the psychological and behavioral effects of anabolic steroids, only a small number of longitudinal or prospective investigations have been conducted.

Hannan and colleagues (1991) found significant increases in hostility, resentment, and aggression after administering nandrolone decanoate and testosterone enanthate in a 6-week, double-blind study using healthy men. During the study, one participant reported an incident of unprovoked anger and another participant was treated in an outpatient clinic for a transient episode of confusion and uncontrolled crying. No other problems were reported by participants during this study. However, the failure to include control or placebo treatments and the small sample size were serious limitations in the design of this investigation. Note that these problems encountered by participants in this investigation have not been seen in the male contraceptive studies using similar doses and much larger participant groups (World Health Organization Task Force, 1990; Wu, Farley, Peregoudov, and Waites, 1996).

Su and colleagues (1993) used a 2-week, double-blind, fixed-order, placebo-control, crossover trial of methyltestosterone to evaluate the neuropsychiatric effects of an anabolic steroid in normal male volunteers. A sequential trial for 3 days each of placebo, lower dose, higher dose, and placebo was administered to participants. Significant increases in symptom scores were observed during higher-dose administration compared with baseline in positive mood, negative mood, and cognitive impairment. An acute manic episode was observed in one of the participants. Another participant became hypomanic. Based on these results, these researchers concluded that an anabolic steroid had a significant impact on mood and behavior in normal male volunteers during what they labeled as a "relatively low dose," short-term period of administration. The results of this study confirm anecdotal reports by steroid users of the aggressive effects of methyltestosterone (Duchaine, 1989). As Clark and Barber (1994) and Martinez-Sanchis and colleagues (1996) have pointed out, the psychological effects of steroids may depend upon the distinct chemical structure of the steroids used.

The personality traits of bodybuilders using high doses of anabolic steroids were observed over a period of 5 months and compared with a control group of nonusers by Cooper and Noakes (1994). Personality traits of users before the onset of steroid use, as assessed retrospectively, were not significantly different from those of the control group. However, users scored significantly higher than the control group on seven personality traits when using steroids. Also, users scored significantly higher on the same seven personality traits during periods of steroid use than during periods of nonuse. It is interesting to note that this study was able to document significant changes in personality traits that, by their very nature, are considered to be enduring and generally unchangeable characteristics.

Increased aggressive responding (button pressing) in male volunteers following experimenter-administered, gradually increasing doses of testosterone cypionate or placebo, using a double-blind, randomized, crossover design, has been recently reported by Kouri, Lukas, Pope, and Oliva (1995) in a prospective study examining the effects of anabolic steroids on level of aggression.

Bhasin and colleagues (1996) examined the effects of supraphysiologic doses of testosterone enanthate, administered for 10 weeks, on muscle size and strength. They randomly assigned healthy men to one of four groups: placebo with no exercise, testosterone with no exercise, placebo plus exercise, and testosterone plus exercise. Men in the exercise groups performed standardized weight training exercises 3 times per week. Standardized questionnaires were administered during the first week of a

4-week control period and after 6 and 10 weeks of treatment. For each man, a live-in partner, spouse, or parent answered the same questions about the man's mood and behavior. Neither mood nor behavior was altered in any group. In addition to increased fat-free mass and muscle size and strength in the strength-training men, the results of this prospective, double-blind, placebo-controlled study indicate that supraphysiologic doses of testosterone, with or without exercise, did not increase the occurrence of angry behavior. However, these researchers note, "the possibility exists that still higher doses of multiple steroids may provoke angry behavior in men with pre-existing psychiatric or behavioral problems." (p. 6)

In a long-term, 3-year, physician-managed, harm-reduction program for 169 anabolic steroid-using weight trainers, Millar (1996) reported that side effects were minimal, including aggression, which "was not a problem at any time." (p. 7)

The psychosexual effects of 3 doses of testosterone cycling in normal men have been studied by Yates, Perry, MacIndoe, Holman, and Ellingrod (1999). A sequential trial of 2 weeks of placebo injections, 14 weeks of 1 of 3 weekly doses of testosterone cypionate, and 12 weeks of placebo injections, was administered to the participants. All doses of testosterone demonstrated only minimal effects on measures of mood and behavior. There was no evidence of a dose-dependent effect on any measure and only 1 high-dose participant developed a brief syndrome with symptoms similar to an agitated and irritable mania. Ellingrod, Perry, Yates, MacIndoe, Watson, Arndt, and Holman (1997) have also reported that high doses of testosterone cypionate do not increase aggressive driving behavior, nor result in increased aggression among normal men.

Using a double-blind study design, Fingerhood, Sullivan, Testa, and Jasinski (1997) have evaluated the subjective and physiological effects of 3 single, increasing doses of testosterone; 1 dose of morphine; and placebo over 5 consecutive days. Testosterone produced no significant changes in self-reported or observed measures, unlike morphine, which produced significant changes in several measures, including "feel the drug," "like the drug," and "feel high." There were no adverse effects of administering high doses of testosterone, leading the researchers to conclude that single doses of testosterone do not result in the usual pharmacologic effects that are associated with abuse.

Finally, in a double-blind experiment, Bjorkqvist, Nygren, Bjorklund, and Bjorkqvist (1994) administered testosterone undecanoate, placebo, or no treatment to men over a 1-week period. Subjective and observer-assessed mood estimations were conducted before and after treatment. The results revealed a significant placebo effect. After treatment, the placebo group scored higher than both the testosterone and control groups on self-estimated anger, irritation, impulsivity, and frustration. Observer-estimated mood scores yielded similar results. The results suggest that androgen use causes expectations of, rather than an actual increase of, aggressiveness. As previously noted (Bahrke, Yesalis, & Wright, 1990), many of the psychological and behavioral changes reported by, and observed in, anabolic steroid users may be a direct result of expectancy, imitation, or role modeling. And, as Bjorkqvist and colleagues (1994) have so adroitly pointed out, "Dissemination of the myth of the steroid-aggressiveness connection may lead to anticipation (a placebo effect) of aggressiveness among steroid abusers and, in turn, to actual acts of violence. It may, in fact, work as an excuse for aggression." At least one investigation has noted the physiological and psychological placebo effects of anabolic steroids (Ariel & Saville, 1972).

In summary, while several recently published reports reveal a pattern of association between use of anabolic steroids by athletes and increased levels of irritability, aggression, personality disturbance, and psychiatric diagnoses, other reports do not. Several reports also document significant alterations in users' moods and, at times, violent behavior. One study indicates a relationship between total weekly steroid dose and the prevalence of mood disorders; several other studies do not.

Effects of Anabolic Steroids on Body Image

In addition to studies examining the psychological and behavioral effects of anabolic steroids, several investigations have examined the relationship between anabolic steroid use and body image (Wroblewska, 1997).

Using structured interviews with steroid-using bodybuilders and non-user controls, Pope, Katz, and Hudson (1993) found two disorders of body image. Three of the 108 participants reported a history of anorexia nervosa. Nine of the participants, 2 of whom were former anorexics, described a "reverse anorexia" syndrome, in which they believed that they appeared small and weak even though they were actually large and muscular. All 9 reverse anorexia cases occurred among steroid users. Four participants reported that their reverse anorexia symptoms contributed to their decision to begin using steroids.

Pope, Gruber, Choi, Olivardia, and Phillips (1997) also have presented preliminary observations, including several case studies, suggesting that a substantial number of men and women may have a particular subtype of body dysmorphic disorder which they have termed "muscle dysmorphia." This condition may cause severe subjective distress, impaired social and occupational functioning, and abuse of anabolic steroids and other substances.

Blouin and Goldfield (1995) also have examined the association between body image and steroid use among male bodybuilders, runners, and martial artists. The bodybuilders in the study self-reported the greatest use of steroids and had significantly greater body dissatisfaction, with a high drive for bulk, high drive for thinness, and greater bulimic tendencies than either of the other two athletic groups. Bodybuilders also reported significant elevations on measures of perfectionism, ineffectiveness, and lower self-esteem. The results suggest that male bodybuilders who use anabolic steroids may be at risk for body image disturbance. Conversely, male bodybuilders may be more susceptible to anabolic steroid use.

Contrary to the researchers' expectations, anabolic steroid use was rare (0.6%) and was not associated with a desire for weight gain in a cross-sectional survey by Drewnowski, Kurth, and Krahn (1995) that examined body image, dieting and exercise variables, and steroid use in 2,088 male high school graduates. Steroid users were more likely to engage in running and swimming than football.

In an effort to construct a psychological profile of anabolic steroid users, Porcerelli and Sandler (1995), in a cross-sectional study, compared weightlifters and bodybuilders who did or did not use anabolic steroids on an objective measure of narcissism and on clinical ratings of empathy. Steroid users had significantly higher scores on dimensions of pathological narcissism and significantly lower scores on clinical ratings of empathy.

Effects of Anabolic Steroids on Psychological Dependence and Withdrawal

Previous research concerning the withdrawal effects encountered by some anabolic steroid users has led to a hypothesis that anabolic steroid use may result in psychological dependence (Bahrke, Yesalis, & Wright, 1990). (See chapters 9 and 10.)

In 1991, Brower, Blow, Young, and Hill published their findings from the anonymous, self-administered questionnaire they used to investigate addiction patterns in male steroid-using weightlifters. At least one symptom of dependence was reported by 94% of the participants. Three or more symptoms, consistent with a diagnosis of dependence, were reported by 57%. Dependent users were distinguished from nondependent users by their use of large doses, more cycles of use, more dissatisfaction with body size, and more aggressive symptoms. Multiple regression analysis revealed that dosage and dissatisfaction with body size were the best predictors of dependent use. Patterns of other substance use, although not predictive of anabolic steroid dependence, revealed very low cigarette use but high alcohol consumption. Results from this study support the hypothesis that anabolic steroids can be addictive and suggest that dissatisfaction with body size may lead to dependent patterns of use.

The use of fluoxetine in treating depression associated with anabolic steroid withdrawal has been examined by Malone and Dimeff (1992). All four patients suffering from anabolic steroid withdrawal depression treated with fluoxetine responded in a time-course consistent with the response of major depression to antidepressant medications. Further study is needed to confirm these results.

In an investigation designed to determine factors undermining the success of prevention and harm-reduction strategies for anabolic steroid abuse, Cooper (1994) found that 10 of 12 steroid-using bodybuilders satisfied the diagnostic number of criteria for at least 1 of 11 standard personality disorders. All 12 users satisfied criteria for psychological substance abuse and 9 for psychoactive substance dependence on anabolic steroids.

Allnut and Chaimowitz (1994) have described the case of anabolic steroid withdrawal depression that was resistant to antidepressant therapy, but responded to electroconvulsive treatment. The patient had been using anabolic steroids for a period of approximately 2 years. During his steroid use, the patient noticed feelings of aggression and aggressive behavior. After reading about anabolic steroids, he became concerned and discontinued their use. Two months later he presented at the psychiatric emergency room with complaints of depression and suicidal ideation, which he related to the discontinuation of anabolic steroids 2 months earlier. He was treated with desipramine and haldol. A 4-week washout period followed an 8-week trial of fluoxetine. At this time, the patient received seven electroconvulsive treatments, after which he showed marked improvement in his depressive symptomatology and was discharged on desipramine.

Cowan (1994) has also reported a similar case of severe depression, in which a male bodybuilder that had been using steroids on and off for 2 years, as well as other drugs, presented to his physician with suicidal ideation following withdrawal from anabolic steroids. The patient also experienced loss of energy, deteriorated concentration, insomnia, and appetite impairment accompanied by weight loss. There was a family history of affective disorder. Following treatment and a partial recovery the man was discharged to an outpatient program. Cowan proposed that prolonged exposure to anabolic steroids and a biological vulnerability to affective disorder would explain the severity of the episode.

Previously only men have been reported as dependent on anabolic steroids. However, recently, the first case of steroid dependence in a woman has been reported by Copeland, Peters, and Dillon (1998). A 30-year-old woman was prescribed methenolone acetate and oxymetholone tablets by her general practitioner. This was followed by her purchase and use of another illicit steroid (stanozolol). The patient reported various adverse effects, including increased aggression, as a result of her steroid use. She also qualified for the diagnosis of substance dependence. Copeland and colleagues recommend advising all patients of the potential for dependence when using anabolic steroids.

Methodological Issues

Although a number of reports documenting the occurrence of behavior changes, mood swings, and depression following cessation of steroid use have been published, most of these reports are case studies or studies involving small numbers of participants (Bahrke, Yesalis, & Wright, 1990). Case studies are limited in their representativeness. They do not necessarily allow valid generalizations to the population from which they came, and they are vulnerable to subjective biases. Cases may be selected because of their dramatic, rather than typical, attributes, or because they neatly fit an observer's preconceptions.

Methodological shortcomings of previously reviewed investigations designed to examine the psychological and behavioral effects of anabolic steroids have included (Bahrke, Yesalis, & Wright, 1990) inappropriate sampling strategies; lack of adequate control and placebo groups; failure to report the types, dosage, and length of administration of anabolic steroids; use of several types, doses, and lengths of administration of anabolic steroids; failure to assess and report other drug use; not measuring free testosterone levels and not measuring testosterone at appropriate times; not confirming anabolic steroid use by urinalysis; limitations of drug testing; the veracity of self-reports of aggression and drug use (Ferenchick, 1996); and a variety of techniques used to assess the psychological and behavioral outcomes. Unfortunately, despite attempts to reduce and eliminate these methodological limitations over the past few years, many of the same problems persist (Bahrke, Yesalis, & Wright, 1996).

Only three prospective, blinded studies documenting aggressive or adverse overt behavior resulting from anabolic steroid use have been reported (Hannan et al., 1991; Kouri et al., 1995; Su et al., 1993), and these studies have limitations. Additional methodological problems that have arisen recently include

- the impurity and content of anabolic steroids, especially those available through the black market,
- not differentiating between anabolic steroids and corticosteroids in prevalence surveys with adolescent participants, and
- the failure to consider weight training as a confounding variable when examining the psychological and behavioral effects of anabolic steroids.

Weight Training as a Confounding Variable

The idea that weight training must be considered a confounding factor when examining the psychometric and behavioral effects of anabolic steroids has been raised by Bahrke and Yesalis (1994). While psychological and behavioral changes are reportedly associated with anabolic steroid use, changes in personality, moods, and self-esteem following weight training have also been documented. However, the fact that many steroid users are also dedicated weight trainers has been overlooked in most studies examining the relationship between steroid use and behavioral changes. A triad may exist between steroid use, weight training as part of a "lifestyle" or commitment, and behavioral change (including dependence). Weight training and related practices must be considered potential confounding factors in future studies designed to examine the psychological and behavioral effects of steroids.

It is also possible that changes frequently attributed to steroid use may also reflect changes resulting from the concurrent use of other substances, such as alcohol, cocaine, amphetamines, or other stimulants such as ephedrine and caffeine, and from dietary manipulations, including nutritional supplements (McBride, Williamson, & Petersen, 1996; Newton, Hunter, Bammon, & Roney, 1993). The long-term effects of alcohol abuse include depression, psychosis, and hallucinations. Insomnia, confusion, anxiety, and psychosis, characterized by paranoia and hallucinations, are some of the long-term consequences of cocaine use. Chronic, high-dose use of amphetamines also can produce hallucinations, delusions, and disorganized behavior (Donatelle & Davis, 1996).

Distinguishing Between Anabolic Steroids and Corticosteroids

Recently, scientists have become aware that it is necessary in their surveys to differentiate between anabolic steroids and corticosteroids (Edbauer, Levine, & Stapleton, 1992). As a result of widespread media coverage of the adverse effects of anabolic steroids, many people now confuse anabolic steroids with corticosteroids that are frequently used in the treatment of many common medical disorders, including acute inflammatory conditions. "Steroidophobia" has become a legitimate concern in asthma management, because asthma patients and the general public frequently confuse anabolic steroids with corticosteroids ("Steroidophobia," 1993).

In a related issue, Higgins (1993) has described the confusion of a bodybuilder over the use of prednisone (a corticosteroid) and anabolic steroids. Perry and Hughes (1992) have also described the problems encountered by a bodybuilder taking a substance (haldol decanoate) he mistakenly thought was an anabolic steroid (nandrolone decanoate).

Purity and Content of Anabolic Steroids

It has been estimated that as much as 50 to 80% or more of the anabolic steroids used by athletes may have been obtained from black-market sources (Office of Diversion Control, 1994). Many of the anabolic steroids found in the illegal market often do not contain the ingredients or dose indicated on the label.

Conclusions

Nearly fifty reports concerning the psychological and behavioral effects of endogenous testosterone levels and anabolic steroids have been published in the past few years. In addition to their traditional medical uses, anabolic steroids are now beginning to be used as male contraceptives and to supplement declining testosterone levels in aging males. Unfortunately, information concerning the legitimate adverse behavioral effects of anabolic steroids has often been inaccurate and wildly speculative. As a result, the frequent and often hysterical references by the media to the unsubstantiated adverse behavioral effects of anabolic steroids has resulted in the loss of both media and medical/scientific credibility, deterring research on beneficial and legitimate uses, and stimulating litigation against physicians (Kochakian, 1989). Significant positive effects resulting from anabolic steroid administration also may have been overlooked. Also, it is quite possible that the lack of accurate and balanced reporting by the media has hindered efforts to prevent and reduce the use of anabolic steroids. Despite enactment of legislation to restrict the use of anabolic steroids, use to promote muscular strength development and improve physical appearance continues among a diverse population.

Previous and current research documents an association between levels of endogenous testosterone and behavioral changes in animals. Although fewer studies have examined the relationship between endogenous androgens and aggressive and violent behavior in humans, a pattern of association between endogenous testosterone levels and aggressive behavior in males has been increasingly established. While studies using moderate doses of exogenous testosterone for contraceptive and clinical purposes reveal few adverse effects on male sexual and aggressive behavior, other investigations, and case reports of athletes using higher doses, suggest the possibility of affective and psychotic syndromes (some of violent proportions), psychological dependence, and withdrawal symptoms.

Aggression is defined on a broad spectrum. The fact that a steroid user feels more aggressive and self-reports more aggression does not necessarily indicate increased violent behavior or a psychiatric disorder.

The prevalence and symptomology of anabolic steroid dependence is difficult to reliably establish because of the small number of cases. In addition to small sample sizes, the variety of anabolic steroids used, and the diversity of techniques used to assess the psychological and behavioral changes associated with anabolic steroid use, other factors such as the purity and content of steroids and the concomitant use of other drugs further complicate an already complex area. Unfortunately, despite attempts to reduce and eliminate the number of methodological limitations associated with investigating the psychological and behavioral effects of anabolic steroids, these problems persist.

Although anabolic steroid dependency may be a problem, its prevalence and symptomology is difficult to reliably establish based upon the existing literature. With present estimates of 300,000 yearly anabolic steroid users in the United States (Yesalis, Kennedy, Kopstein, & Bahrke, 1993), an extremely small percentage of users appear to experience psychological dependence requiring clinical treatment. Additional research with larger and more heterogeneous samples will be needed.

Only three prospective, blinded studies documenting aggression and adverse overt behavior resulting from steroid use have been reported (Hannan et al., 1991; Kouri et al., 1995; Su et al., 1993). As Bjorkqvist and colleagues (1994) point out, much of the psychological and behavioral effect of steroid intake may be placebo. Anticipation of the aggressiveness related to steroid use may lead to actual violent acts and become, in effect, an excuse for aggression. Again, it is interesting to note that with a million or more steroid users in the United States (Yesalis et al., 1993), only an extremely small percentage of users appear to experience mental disturbances that result in clinical treatment. Also, of the small number of individuals who do experience significant changes, most apparently recover without additional problems when the use of steroids is terminated.

References

Agren, G., Thiblin, I., Tirassa, P., Lundeberg, T., & Stenfors, C. (1999). Behavioural anxiolytic effects of low-dose anabolic androgenic steroid treatment in rats. *Physiology and Behavior, 66*, 503–509.

Albert, D.J., Walsh, M.L., & Jonik, R.H. (1993). Aggression in humans: What is its biological foundation? *Neuroscience and Biobehavioral Reviews, 17,* 405–425.

Allnutt, S., & Chaimowitz, G. (1994). Anabolic steroid withdrawal depression: A case report. *Canadian Journal of Psychiatry, 39*, 317–318.

Anderson, R.A., Bancroft, J., & Wu, F.C.W. (1992). The effects of exogenous testosterone on sexuality and mood of normal men. *Journal of Clinical Endocrinology and Metabolism, 75*, 1503–1507.

Archer, J. (1991). The influence of testosterone on human aggression. *British Journal of Psychology, 82,* 1–28.

Archer, J. (1994). Testosterone and aggression. *Journal of Offender Rehabilitation, 21*(3/4), 3–39.

Ariel, G., & Saville, W. (1972). Anabolic steroids: The physiological effects of placebos. *Medicine and Science in Sports, 4*(2), 124–126.

Bagatell, C.J., Heiman, J.R., Matsumoto, A.M., Rivier, J.E., & Bremner, W.J. (1994). Metabolic and behavioral effects of high-dose exogenous testosterone in healthy men. *Journal of Clinical Endocrinology and Metabolism, 79*, 561–567.

Bahrke, M.S. (1993). Psychological effects of endogenous testosterone and anabolic-androgenic steroids. In C.E. Yesalis (Ed.), *Anabolic steroids in sport and exercise* (pp. 161–192). Champaign, IL: Human Kinetics.

Bahrke, M.S., & Strauss, R.H. (1992). Selected psychological characteristics of female anabolic-androgenic steroid (AAS) users. *Medicine and Science in Sports and Exercise, 24*, S136.

Bahrke, M.S., Wright, J.E., Strauss, R.H., & Catlin, D.H. (1992). Psychological moods and subjectively perceived behavioral and somatic changes accompanying anabolic-androgenic steroid usage. *American Journal of Sports Medicine, 20*, 717–724.

Bahrke, M.S., & Yesalis, C.E. (1994). Weight training: A potential confounding factor in examining the psychological and behavioral effects of anabolic-androgenic steroids. *Sports Medicine, 18*, 309–318.

Bahrke, M.S., Yesalis, C.E., and Wright, J.E. (1990). Psychological and behavioural effects of endogenous testosterone levels and anabolic-androgenic steroids among males: A review. *Sports Medicine, 10*, 303–337.

Bahrke, M.S., Yesalis, C.E., & Wright, J.E. (1996). Psychological and behavioural effects of endogenous testosterone levels and anabolic-androgenic steroids: An update. *Sports Medicine, 22*, 367–390.

Berman, M., Gladue, B., & Taylor, S. (1993). The effects of hormones, Type A behavior pattern, and provocation on aggression in men. *Motivation and Emotion, 17*(2), 125–138.

Bhasin, S., Storer, T.W., Berman, N., Callgari, C., Clevenger, B., Phillips, J., Bunnell, T.J., Tricker, R., Shirazi, A., & Casaburi, R. (1996). The effects of supraphysiologic doses of testosterone on muscle size and strength in normal men. *New England Journal of Medicine, 335*(1), 1–7.

Bitran, D., Kellog, C.K., & Hilvers, R.J. (1993). Treatment with an anabolic-androgenic steroid affects anxiety-related behavior and alters the sensitivity of cortical $GABA_A$ receptors in the rat. *Hormones and Behavior, 27*, 568–583.

Bjorkqvist, K., Nygren, T., Bjorklund, A-C., & Bjorkqvist, S-E. (1994). Testosterone intake and aggressiveness: Real effect or anticipation. *Aggressive Behavior, 20*, 17–26.

Blackwell, J. (1991). Discourses on drug use: The social construction of a steroid scandal. *Journal of Drug Issues, 21*(1), 147–164.

Blouin, A.G., & Goldfield, G.S. (1995). Body image and steroid use in male bodybuilders. *International Journal of Eating Disorders, 18*(2), 159–165.

Booth, A., & Dabbs, J.M. (1993). Testosterone and men's marriages. *Social Forces, 72*, 463–477.

Bond, A.J., Choi, P.Y.L., & Pope, H.G. (1995). Assessment of attentional bias and mood in users and non-users of anabolic-androgenic steroids. *Drug and Alcohol Dependence, 37*(3), 241–245.

Bronson, F.H. (1996). Effects of prolonged exposure to anabolic steroids on the behavior of male and female mice. *Pharmacology, Biochemistry and Behavior, 53*, 329–334.

Bronson, F.H., Nguyen, K.Q., & de la Rosa, J. (1996). Effect of anabolic steroids on behavior and physiological characteristics of female mice. *Physiology and Behavior, 59*(1), 49–55.

Brower, K.J., Blow, F.C., Beresford, T.P., & Fuelling, C. (1989). Anabolic-androgenic steroid dependence. *Journal of Clinical Psychiatry, 50*(1), 31–33.

Brower, K.J., Blow, F.C., Young, J.P., & Hill, E.M. (1991). Symptoms and correlates of anabolic-androgenic steroid dependence. *British Journal of Addiction, 86,* 759–768.

Buckley, W.E., Yesalis, C.E., Friedl, K.E., Anderson, W.A., Streit, A., & Wright, J. (1988). Estimated prevalence of anabolic steroid use among male high school seniors. *Journal of the American Medical Association, 260*, 3441–3445.

Burnett, K.F., & Kleiman, M.E. (1994). Psychological characteristics of adolescent steroid users. *Adolescence, 29*(113), 81–89.

Byrne, A.J. (1997). Anabolic steroids and the mind. *Medical Journal of Australia, 166,* 224.

Choi, P.Y.L. (1993, June). Alarming effects of anabolic steroids. *The Psychologist,* 258–260.

Choi, P.Y.L., Parrott, A.C., & Cowan, D. (1990). High-dose anabolic steroids in strength athletes: Effects upon hostility and aggression. *Human Psychopharmacology, 5,* 349–356.

Choi, P.Y.L., & Pope, H.G. (1994). Violence toward women and illicit androgenic-anabolic steroid use. *Annals of Clinical Psychiatry, 6*(1), 21–25.

Clark, A.S., & Barber, D.M. (1994). Anabolic-androgenic steroids and aggression in castrated male rats. *Physiology and Behavior, 56*, 1107–1113.

Clark, A.S., Lindenfeld, R.C., & Gibbons, C.H. (1996). Anabolic-androgenic steroids and brain reward. *Pharmacology, Biochemistry and Behavior, 53*, 741–745.

Cooper, C. (1994). Factors undermining the success of prevention and harm reduction strategies for anabolic-androgenic steroid abuse. In D. Adey, P. Steyn, N. Herman, et al. (Eds.), *State of the art in higher education* (Vol. 1, pp. 133–142). Pretoria, South Africa: University of South Africa.

Cooper, C.J., & Noakes, T.D. (1994). Psychiatric disturbances in users of anabolic steroids. *South African Medical Journal, 84*, 509–512.

Copeland, J., Peters, R., & Dillon, P. (1998). Anabolic-androgenic steroid dependence in a woman. *Australian New Zealand Journal of Psychiatry, 32*, 589.

Corrigan, B. (1996). Anabolic steroids and the mind. *Medical Journal of Australia, 165*(4), 222–226.

Cowan, C.B. (1994). Depression in anabolic steroid withdrawal. *Irish Journal of Psychological Medicine, 11*(1), 27–28.

Dabbs, J.M., Carr, T.S., Frady, R.L., & Riad, J.K. (1995). Testosterone, crime, and misbehavior among 692 male prison inmates. *Personal and Individual Differences, 18*, 627–633.

Dabbs, J.M., Jurkovic, G.J., & Frady, R.L. (1991). Salivary testosterone and cortisol among late adolescent male offenders. *Journal of Abnormal Child Psychology, 19*, 469–478.

Dabbs, J.M., & Morris, R. (1990). Testosterone, social class, and antisocial behavior in a sample of 4,462 men. *Psychological Science, 1*(3), 209–211.

Dalby, J.T. (1992). Brief anabolic steroid use and sustained behavioral reaction. *American Journal of Psychiatry, 149*(2), 271–272.

Donatelle, R.J., & Davis, L.G. (1996). *Access to health*. Boston: Allyn & Bacon.

Drewnowski, A., Kurth, C.L., &. Krahn, D.D. (1995). Effects of body image on dieting, exercise, and anabolic steroid use in adolescent males. *International Journal of Eating Disorders, 17*, 381–386.

Driessen, M., Muessigbrodt, H., Dilling, H., & Driessen, B. (1996). Child sexual abuse associated with anabolic androgenic steroid use. *American Journal of Psychiatry, 153*, 1369.

Duchaine, D. (1989). *Underground steroid handbook II*. Venice, CA: HLR Technical Books.

Edbauer, M.J., Levine, A.M., & Stapleton, F.B. (1992). The importance of differentiating between anabolic steroids and glucocorticoids. *New York State Journal of Medicine, 92*(8), 365.

Ellingrod, V.L., Perry, P.J., Yates, W.R., MacIndoe, J.H., Watson, G., Arndt, S., & Holman, T.L. (1997). The effects of anabolic steroids on driving performance as assessed by the Iowa Driver Simulator. *American Journal of Drug and Alcohol Abuse*, *23*, 623–636.

Elofson, G., & Elofson, S. (1990). Steroids claimed our son's life. *The Physician and Sportsmedicine, 18*(8), 15–16.

Ferenchick, G.S. (1996). Validity of self-report in identifying anabolic steroid use among weightlifters. *Journal of General Internal Medicine, 11*, 554–556.

Fingerhood, M.I., Sullivan, J.T., Testa, M., & Jasinski, D.R. (1997). Abuse liability of testosterone. *Journal of Psychopharmacology, 11*, 59–63.

Finkelstein, J.W., Susman, E.J., Chinchilli, V.M., Kunselman, S.J., D'arcangelo, M.R., Schwab, J., Demers, L.M., Liben, L.S. Lookingbill, G., & Kulin, H.E. (1997). Estrogen or testosterone increases self-reported aggressive behaviors in hypogonadal adolescents. *Journal of Clinical Endocrinology and Metabolism, 82*, 2423–2438.

Galligani, N., Renck, A., & Hansen, S. (1996). Personality profile of men using anabolic androgenic steroids. *Hormones and Behavior, 30,* 170–175.

Gladue, B.A. (1991a). Qualitative and quantitative sex differences in self-reported aggressive behavioral characteristics. *Psychological Reports, 68,* 675–684.

Gladue, B.A. (1991b). Aggressive behavioral characteristics, hormones, and sexual orientation in men and women. *Aggressive Behavior, 17*, 313–326.

Gladue, B.A., Boechler, M., & McCaul, K.D. (1989). Hormonal responses to competition in human males. *Aggressive Behavior, 15,* 409–422.

Gray, A., Jackson, D.N., & McKinlay, J.B. (1991). The relation between dominance, anger, and hormones in normally aging men: Results from the Massachusetts Male Aging Study. *Psychosomatic Medicine, 53,* 375–385.

Halpern, C.T., Udry, J.R., Campbell, B., & Suchindran, C. (1993). Relationship between aggression and pubertal increases in testosterone: A panel analysis of adolescent males. *Social Biology, 40*(1/2), 8–24.

Hannan, C.J., Friedl, K.E., Zold, A., Kettler, T.M., & Plymate, S.R. (1991). Psychological and serum homovanillic acid changes in men administered androgenic steroids. *Psychoneuroendocrinology, 16,* 335–342.

Higgins, G.L. (1993). Adonis meets Addison: Another potential cause of occult adrenal insufficiency. *Journal of Emergency Medicine, 11,* 761–762.

The insanity of steroid abuse. (1988, May 23). *Newsweek,* 75.

Isacsson, G., Garle, M., Ljung, E-B., Asgard, U., & Bergman, U. (1998). Anabolic steroids and violent crime—an epidemiological study at a jail in Stockholm, Sweden. *Comprehensive Psychiatry, 39*(4), 203–205.

Johnson, M.D., Jay, S., Shoup, B., and Rickert, V.I. (1989). Anabolic steroid use in adolescent males. *Pediatrics, 83,* 921–924.

Kochakian, C.D. (1989, July 30–31). *The steroids in sports problem.* Paper presented at the National Steroid Consensus Meeting.

Kouri, E.M., Lukas, S.E., Pope, H.G., & Oliva, P.S. (1995). Increased aggressive responding in male volunteers following the administration of gradually increasing doses of testosterone cypionate. *Drug and Alcohol Dependence, 40*(1), 73–79.

Leckman, J.F., & Scahill, L. (1990). Possible exacerbation of tics by androgenic steroids. *New England Journal of Medicine, 322,* 1674.

Lefavi, R.G., Reeve, T.G., & Newland, M.C. (1990). Relationship between anabolic steroid use and selected psychological parameters in male bodybuilders. *Journal of Sport Behavior, 13*(3), 157–166.

Le Greves, P., Huang, W., Johansson, P., Thornwall, M., Zhou, Q., & Nyberg, F. (1997). Effects of anabolic-androgenic steroid on the regulation of the NMDA receptor NR1, NR2A subunit mRNAs in brain regions of the male rat. *Neuroscience Letters, 226,* 61–64.

Lindman, R., von der Pahlen, B., Ost, B., & Eriksson, C.J.P. (1992). Serum testosterone, cortisol, glucose, and ethanol in males arrested for spouse abuse. *Aggressive Behavior, 18,* 393–400.

Lindstrom, M., Nilsson, A.L., Katzman, P.L., Janson, L., & Dymling, J-F. (1990). Use of anabolic-androgenic steroids among bodybuilders—frequency and attitudes. *Journal of Internal Medicine, 227,* 407–411.

Lumia, A.R., Thorner, K.M., & McGinnis, M.Y. (1994). Effects of chronically high doses of the anabolic androgenic steroid, testosterone, on intermale aggression and sexual behavior in male rats. *Physiology and Behavior, 55,* 331–335.

Malone, D.A., & Dimeff, R.J. (1992). The use of fluoxetine in depression associated with anabolic steroid withdrawal: A case series. *Journal of Clinical Psychiatry, 53*(4), 130–132.

Malone, D.A., Dimeff, R.J., Lombardo, J.A., & Sample, R.H.B. (1995). Psychiatric effects and psychoactive substance use in anabolic-androgenic steroid users. *Clinical Journal of Sports Medicine, 5*(1), 25–31.

Martinez-Sanchis, S., Brain, P.F., Salvador, A., & Simon, V.M. (1996). Long-term chronic treatment with stanozolol lacks significant effects on aggression and activity in young and adult male laboratory mice. *General Pharmacology, 27*(2), 293–298.

Martinez-Sanchis, S., Salvador, A., Moya-Albiol, L., Gonzalez-Bono, E., & Simon, V.M. (1998). Effects of chronic treatment with testosterone propionate on aggression and hormonal levels in intact male mice. *Psychoneuroendocrinology, 23*(3), 275–293.

Mazur, A., Booth, A., & Dabbs, J.M. (1992). Testosterone and chess competition. *Social Psychology Quarterly, 55*(1), 70–77.

McBride, A.J., Williamson, K., & Petersen, T. (1996). Three cases of nalbuphine hydrochloride dependence associated with anabolic steroids use. *British Journal of Sports Medicine, 30,* 69–70.

McCaul, K.D., Gladue, B.A., & Joppa, M. (1992). Winning, losing, mood, and testosterone. *Hormones and Behavior, 26*(4), 486–504.

Melloni, R.H., Connor, D.F., Hang, P.T.X., Harrison, R.J., & Ferris, C.F. (1997). Anabolic-androgenic steroid exposure during adolescence and aggressive behavior in golden hamsters. *Physiology and Behavior, 61*, 359–364.

Millar, A.P. (1996). Anabolic steroids—a personal pilgrimage. *Journal of Performance Enhancing Drugs, 1*(1), 4–9.

Minkin, D.M., Meyer, M.E., & van Haaren, F. (1993). Behavioral effects of long-term administration of an anabolic steroid in intact and castrated male Wistar rats. *Pharmacology, Biochemistry and Behavior, 44*, 959–963.

Moss, H.B., Panazak, G.L., & Tarter, R.E. (1992). Personality, mood, and psychiatric symptoms among anabolic steroid users. *American Journal on Addictions, 1*(4), 315–324.

Newton, L.E., Hunter, G., Bammon, M., & Roney, R. (1993). Changes in psychological state and self-reported diet during various phases of training in competitive bodybuilders. *Journal of Strength and Conditioning Research, 7*(3), 153–158.

NHL tough guy Kordic dies of lung failure at 27. (1992, August 10). *USA Today,* p. 15C.

Office of Diversion Control. (1994). *Report of the International Conference on the Abuse and Trafficking of Anabolic Steroids.* Washington, DC: United States Drug Enforcement Administration Conference Report.

Ogawa, S., Luban, D.B., Korach, K.S., & Pfaff, D.W. (1995, June 14–17). *Behavioral characteristics of transgenic estrogen receptor knockout male mice: Sexual aggressive and open-field behaviors.* Paper presented at the Seventy-Seventh Annual Meeting of the Endocrine Society, Washington, DC.

Orchard, J.W., & Best, J.P. (1994). Test violent offenders for anabolic steroid use. *Medical Journal of Australia, 161*(3), 232.

Parrott, A.C., Choi, P.Y.L., & Davies, M. (1994). Anabolic steroid use by amateur athletes: Effects upon psychological mood states. *Journal of Sports Medicine and Physical Fitness, 34*(3), 292–298.

Pearson, B., & Hansen, B. (1990, February 5). Survey of U.S. Olympians. *USA Today,* p. C10.

Perry, H.M., & Hughes, G.W. (1992). A case of affective disorder associated with the misuse of "anabolic steroids." *British Journal of Sports Medicine, 26*(4), 219–220.

Perry, P.J., Andersen, K.H., & Yates, W.R. (1990). Illicit anabolic steroid use in athletes: A case series analysis. *American Journal of Sports Medicine, 18*, 422–428.

Perry, P.J., Yates, W.R., & Andersen, K.H. (1990). Psychiatric symptoms associated with anabolic steroids: A controlled, retrospective study. *Annals of Clinical Psychiatry, 2*(1), 11–17.

Pope, H.G., Gruber, A.J., Choi, P., Olivardia, B.A., & Phillips, K.A. (1997). Muscle dysmorphia: an unrecognized form of body dysmorphic disorder. *Psychosomatics, 38,* 548–557.

Pope, H.G., & Katz, D.L. (1988). Affective and psychotic symptoms associated with anabolic steroid use. *American Journal of Psychiatry, 145*, 487–490.

Pope, H.G., & Katz, D.L. (1990). Homicide and near-homicide by anabolic steroid users. *Journal of Clinical Psychiatry, 51*(1), 28–31.

Pope, H.G., & Katz, D.L. (1994). Psychiatric and medical effects of anabolic-androgenic steroid use. *Archives of General Psychiatry, 51*(5), 373–382.

Pope, H.G., Katz, D.L., & Hudson, J.I. (1993). Anorexia nervosa and "reverse anorexia" among 108 male bodybuilders. *Comprehensive Psychiatry, 34*, 406–409.

Pope, H.G., Kouri, E.M., Powell, K.F., Campbell, C., & Katz, D.L. (1996). Anabolic-androgenic steroid use among 133 prisoners. *Comprehensive Psychiatry, 37*, 322–327.

Porcerelli, J.H., & Sandler, B.A. (1995). Narcissism and empathy in steroid users. *American Journal of Psychiatry, 152*, 1672–1674.

Rejeski, W.J., Gregg, E., Kaplan, J.R., & Manuck, S.B. (1990). Anabolic steroids: Effects on social behavior and baseline heart rate. *Health Psychology, 9*, 774–791.

Rubinow, D.R., & Schmidt, P.J. (1996). Androgens, brain, and behavior. *American Journal of Psychiatry, 153*, 974–984.

Salvador, A., Moya-Albiol, L., Martinez-Sanchis, S., & Simon, V.M. (1999). Lack of effects of anabolic-androgenic steroids on locomotor activity in intact male mice. *Perceptual and Motor Skills, 88,* 319–328.

Schulte, H.M., Hall, M.J., & Boyer, M. (1993). Domestic violence associated with anabolic steroid abuse. *American Journal of Psychiatry, 150*, 348.

Silvester, L.J. (1995). Self-perceptions of the acute and long-range effects of anabolic-androgenic steroids. *Journal of Strength and Conditioning Research, 9*(2), 95–98.

Simon, N.G., & Whalen, R.E. (1986). Hormonal regulation of aggression: Evidence for a relationship among genotype, receptor binding, and behavioral sensitivity to androgen and estrogen. *Aggressive Behavior, 12,* 255–267.

Stanley, A., & Ward, M. (1994). Anabolic steroids—the drugs that give and take away manhood. A case with an unusual physical sign. *Medicine, Science and the Law, 34*(1), 82–83.

Steroidophobia: Public misperceptions of steroid medications. (1993). *Pharmacy Times, 59,* 42, 44.

Su, T-P., Pagliaro, M., Schmidt, P.J., Pickar, D., Wolkowitz, O., & Rubinow, D.R. (1993). Neuropsychiatric effects of anabolic steroids in male normal volunteers. *Journal of the American Medical Association, 269*, 2760–2764.

Susman, E.J., Dorn, L.D., & Chrousos, G.P. (1991). Negative affect and hormone levels in young adolescents: Concurrent and predictive perspectives. *Journal of Youth and Adolescence, 20*(2), 167–190.

Thiblin, I., Kristiansson, M., & Rajs, J. (1997). Anabolic androgenic steroids and behavioural patterns among violent offenders. *Journal of Forensic Psychiatry, 8*(2), 299–310.

Wang, C., Alexander, G., Berman, N., Salahain, B., Davidson, T., McDonald, V., Callegori, C., & Swerdloff, R.S. (1995, June 14–17). Effect of testosterone replacement therapy on mood changes in hypogonadal men. Paper presented at the Seventy-Seventh Annual Meeting of the Endocrine Society, Washington, DC.

Wemyss-Holden, S.A., Hamdy, F.C., & Hastie, K.J. (1994). Steroid abuse in athletes, prostatic enlargement and bladder outflow obstruction—is there a relationship? *British Journal of Urology, 74*, 476–478.

World Health Organization Task Force on Methods for the Regulation of Male Fertility. (1990). Contraceptive efficacy of testosterone-induced azoospermia in normal men. *Lancet, 36,* 955–959.

World Health Organization Task Force on Methods for the Regulation of Male Fertility. (1996). Contraceptive efficacy of testosterone-induced azoospermia and oligozoospermia in normal men. *Fertility and Sterility, 65*, 821–829.

Wroblewska, A-M. (1997). Androgenic-anabolic steroids and body dysmorphia in young men. *Journal of Psychosomatic Research, 42*(3), 225–234.

Wu, F.C., Farley, T.M.M., Peregoudov, A., & Waites, G.M.H. (1996). Effects of testosterone enanthate in normal men: Experience from a multicenter contraceptive efficacy study. *Fertility and Sterility, 65*, 626–636.

Yates, W.R., Perry, P.J., & Andersen, K.H. (1990). Illicit anabolic steroid use: A controlled personality study. *Acta Psychiatrica Scandinavica, 81,* 548–550.

Yates, W.R., Perry, P.J., MacIndoe, J., Holman, T., & Ellingrod, V.L. (1999). Psychosexual effects of three doses of testosterone cycling in normal men. *Biological Psychiatry, 45,* 254–260.

Yates, W.R., Perry, P., & Murray, S. (1992). Aggression and hostility in anabolic steroid users. *Biological Psychiatry, 31*, 1232–1234.

Yesalis, C.E., & Bahrke, M.S. (1995). Anabolic-androgenic steroids: Current issues. *Sports Medicine, 19*, 326–340.

Yesalis, C.E., Kennedy, N.J., Kopstein, A.N., & Bahrke, M.S. (1993). Anabolic-androgenic steroid use in the United States. *Journal of the American Medical Association, 270*, 1217–1221.

CHAPTER

9

Anabolic Steroids: Potential for Physical and Psychological Dependence

Kirk J. Brower, MD

When faced with the syringe, even my own worst fears didn't matter, I couldn't stop. Seventeen-inch arms were not enough, I wanted 20. And when I got to 20, I was sure that I'd want 22. My retreat to the weight room was a retreat into the simple world of numbers. Numerical gradations were the only thing left in my life that made sense. Twenty was better than 17, but worse than 22. Bench pressing 315 was better than bench pressing 275, but worse than 365. I was reduced to a world where such thinking ruled, and it was only by embracing it that I could sleep at night.

Samuel Wilson Fussell
Muscle: Confessions of an Unlikely Bodybuilder, 1991

It is commonly accepted that anabolic steroids are abused substances (ACSM, 1987; American Medical Association [AMA], 1988; Wilson, 1988). What is generally meant by *abuse*, however, is that some people use anabolic steroids in ways that other people disapprove of. When we view abuse in terms of social disapproval, then the ethical and sociological implications of the problem are most apparent. Indeed, there are strong ethical reasons for disapproving of the use of anabolic steroids for nonmedical purposes (Murray, 1987). Moreover, when a society is "addicted" to values such as winning, competition, and physical attractiveness, then its individuals may be more likely to use drugs like anabolic steroids (Yesalis, 1990).

What is less clear, however, is whether anabolic steroids are drugs of abuse in the sense that they can lead to physical and psychological dependence. The question is important for a variety of reasons. If taking anabolic steroids can lead to dependence, then users, potential users, and other concerned individuals need to be informed. Also, drug-dependent persons may be unable to stop using drugs simply in response to education or sanctions and may require specialized treatment (Brower, 1989, 1997; Malone, 1995). Therefore, solutions to the problem of illicit anabolic steroid use may require that we expand our thinking beyond ethical and sociological concerns to include psychological and medical concepts of drug dependence. Finally, in 1990 the U.S. Congress passed legislation that added anabolic steroids to Schedule III among controlled substances (Nightingale, 1991), despite opposition from the American Medical Association (Dreyfus, 1990) and despite the lack of scientific consensus (Cicero & O'Connor, 1990; Uzych, 1990). Thus, by legal decree anabolic steroids are recognized to have a potential for abuse that may lead to either low to moderate physical dependence or high psychological dependence. An important question is whether the scientific evidence supports the current legal classification of anabolic steroids.

The purpose of this chapter is to review what we know about the potential of anabolic steroids to produce dependence, while highlighting areas for further study. The chapter discusses the nature of drug dependence, paying particular attention to how this term is defined both clinically and scientifically. The chapter reviews the evidence that anabolic steroids can lead to dependence and discusses mechanisms, predictors, and the course of anabolic steroid dependence. Finally, the implications of the data for prevention and treatment efforts are explored.

The Nature of Drug Abuse and Dependence

Drug abuse and *dependence* have been variably defined. Terms such as *abuse*, *misuse*, *dependence*, and *addiction* are commonly confused and frequently employed without regard to their clinical and scientific definitions. Indeed, our society has so broadly applied the term *addiction* as to include addictions to television, food, work, love, and sex. Some authors have commented on the misuse and abuse of the terms themselves and on our "addiction" to addiction terminology (Gomberg, 1989). In this climate, it is prudent to question whether anabolic steroids are truly addicting.

Classification Systems

From a clinical and medical perspective, *dependence* and *abuse* are diagnostic terms. Definitions of these two diagnoses appear in both the World Health Organization's *International Classification of Diseases* (*ICD-10*) (1993) and the American Psychiatric Association's (APA) *Diagnostic and Statistical Manual of Mental Disorders* (*DSM*) (1987, 1994). Collectively, these books constitute the American and worldwide standards for defining, classifying, and diagnosing drug abuse and dependence. Although these diagnostic systems are not entirely free from controversy and are subject to future change, they do provide the most widely accepted criteria for determining if dependence has resulted from drug use.

The *DSM* is currently in its fourth edition (*DSM-IV*) (APA, 1994), but most if not all of the research on anabolic steroid dependence published to date (1999) utilized an earlier edition known as the *DSM-III-R* (APA, 1987). Therefore, this section will focus primarily on the *DSM-III-R* criteria, but will compare these criteria to *DSM-IV* for completeness. One comparison is worth noting from the start. Anabolic steroids as a class of substances were not mentioned at all in *DSM-III-R,* whereas they are described in *DSM-IV* in a section labeled "Other Substance-Related Disorders" (APA, 1994, p. 270):

> *Anabolic steroids sometimes produce an initial sense of well-being (or even euphoria), which is replaced after repeated use by lack of energy, irritability, and other forms of dysphoria. Continued use of these substances may lead to more severe symptoms (e.g., depressive symptomatology) and general medical conditions (liver disease).*

The inclusion of anabolic steroids in *DSM-IV* reflected a growing awareness in the scientific literature that anabolic steroids are associated with mental or behavioral changes that could come to the attention of practicing psychiatrists and other health professionals. Although the *DSM-IV* does not specifically state that anabolic steroids can cause dependence (as it does for drugs such as alcohol and cocaine), it does allow for this possibility in its diagnostic code and classification, *304.90—Other*

Substance Dependence. On the other hand, *ICD-10* defines all steroids under the category of "non-dependence-producing substances."

The term *addiction* is generally, although not always, used interchangeably with *dependence*, but *addiction* does not appear in either *ICD-10* or *DSM-III-R/IV*. Likewise, terms such as *addictive disease*, *addictive behaviors*, and *chemical dependency* do not appear in these systems of classification either. Therefore, the discussion that follows uses the terms *abuse* and *dependence* and for the most part avoids the other terms.

Dependence

The *DSM-III-R* category of dependence is more specifically called "psychoactive substance dependence." *Psychoactive* means the ability of a drug or substance to alter mood, thinking, perceptions, or behavior. *ICD-10* also stipulates that a diagnosis of "dependence syndrome" (F1χ.2) must involve a psychoactive substance. *ICD-10* does not recognize that dependence on a substance without psychoactive properties, such as laxatives, can occur. In general, anabolic steroids are taken for their "muscle-active" properties rather than their psychoactive properties. Perhaps it should come as no surprise, therefore, that *ICD-10* classifies the harmful self-use of steroids along with laxatives under the category of "abuse of non-dependence-producing substances." Nevertheless, evidence will be presented later to illustrate that anabolic steroids do have psychoactive effects and that some users specifically take anabolic steroids for their psychoactive effects.

The criteria for diagnosing dependence according to *DSM-III-R* are presented in table 9.1. The user must evidence three of nine criteria for at least 1 month to be diagnosed as dependent. The essential features of dependence in *DSM-III-R* are that the person has impaired control over the substance use (criteria 1-3) and that the person continues to take the substance despite adverse consequences resulting from the substance use (criteria 4-6). Tolerance and withdrawal symptoms (criteria 7-9) may be more or less present, depending on the particular class of substance used or on the severity of the dependence (APA, 1987). In *DSM-IV*, only seven criteria for dependence are listed. No new criteria were added in *DSM-IV*, but *DSM-III-R* criterion 4 was deleted, and criteria 8 and 9 were combined (table 9.1). In *DSM-IV*, three of seven criteria are required for diagnosis. The other major change in *DSM-IV* is that all three criteria need not occur in the same month, as long as they all occurred within the same 1-year period.

Physical Versus Psychological Dependence

Physical dependence, also referred to as physiological or pharmacological dependence, is characterized by symptoms of withdrawal. *Withdrawal* refers to newly experienced physical or psychological symptoms of

Table 9.1 Self-Reported Symptoms of Dependence

DSM-III-R criterion symptom	Percent (%)[a]
1. More substance taken than intended[b]	51
2. Desire yet unable to cut down or control use[b]	16
3. Large time expenditure on substance-related activity[b]	40
4. Frequent intoxication or withdrawal symptoms when expected to function or when physically hazardous	9
5. Social, work, or leisure activities replaced by drug use[b]	29
6. Continued drug use despite problems caused or worsened by use[b]	37
7. Tolerance[b]	18
8. Withdrawal symptoms[b]	84
9. Substance used to relieve or avoid withdrawal symptoms[c]	4

[a] *N* = 49, but group size was smaller for some symptoms due to incomplete responses.

[b] Criteria retained in *DSM-IV* (APA, 1994).

[c] Combined with criterion 8 in *DSM-IV*.

Adapted from *British Journal of Addiction* 1991.

distress that occur when the user stops using a drug. Physical dependence is often associated with *tolerance*, which is established when a user needs larger amounts of a substance to obtain the same effects previously experienced with smaller amounts, or when the user experiences diminished effects over time with the same amount of drug use. Tolerance and withdrawal are thought to be indicators of a physiological adaptation of the body to a particular drug, and they can result in the user increasing drug use both to continue experiencing the drug's effects and to avoid withdrawal symptoms.

Psychological dependence is characterized by a *compulsion* to take a drug for its psychological effects, despite the adverse consequences that result from the drug use. The psychologically dependent person has impaired ability to control the use of the drug and tends to resume drug use even after withdrawal symptoms have subsided. Physical and psychological dependence may, and often do, occur together, but they may also occur independently. Nevertheless, physical dependence that occurs in the absence of psychological dependence is probably a simpler problem to manage than vice versa.

In the *DSM-III-R* diagnosis of dependence, criteria 1 through 6 refer to psychological aspects of dependence, whereas criteria 7 through 9 refer to physical aspects of dependence (table 9.1). Moreover, the symptoms of psychological dependence are considered the essential features of the diagnosis. In *DSM-IV,* for example, where three of seven criteria are required for diagnosis, dependency criteria cannot be met if only physical dependence is observed, because tolerance and withdrawal count for only two criteria. However, dependency criteria can be met in the absence of physical dependence by meeting three of the remaining five criteria.

Dependence Versus Abuse

Both *DSM* and *ICD-10* make a distinction between abuse and dependence; *abuse* is considered a residual category for cases of maladaptive drug-taking that do not meet full criteria for dependence. Thus, *DSM-III-R* contains a diagnosis called *psychoactive substance abuse* that is described as follows:

> *A residual category for noting maladaptive patterns of psychoactive substance use that have never met the criteria for dependence for that particular class of substance. The maladaptive pattern of use is indicated by either (1) continued use of the psychoactive substance despite knowledge of having a persistent or recurrent social, occupational, psychological, or physical problem that is caused or exacerbated by use of the substance or (2) recurrent use of the substance in situations when use is physically hazardous (e.g., driving while intoxicated). The diagnosis is made only if some symptoms of the disturbance have persisted for at least one month or have occurred repeatedly over a longer period of time. (APA, 1987, p. 169)*

In *DSM-IV,* substance abuse is diagnosed by repeated use resulting in harmful consequences in the absence of tolerance, withdrawal, or compulsive use. The symptom list was expanded from two to four items by adding (1) recurrent legal problems from use and (2) failure to function at work, home, or school because of repeated use.

In *ICD-10,* psychoactive substance abuse is defined most simply as *harmful use* (F1χ.1) or "a pattern of psychoactive substance use that is causing damage to health." As mentioned above, *ICD-10* distinguishes between psychoactive substance abuse and *abuse of non-dependence producing substances* (F55); the latter diagnosis is reserved for substances that are not considered by *ICD-10* to be psychoactive, including steroids (F55.5).

According to these definitions, abuse might be considered a less severe form of drug problem that could eventually, although not necessarily, lead to dependence. As stated, the focus of this chapter is the potential of anabolic steroids to produce dependence. If dependence on anabolic steroids occurs, then we can readily assume that abuse, as either a preceding event or a less severe problem, occurs as well. Thus, the discussion that follows will consider the possibility of dependence on anabolic steroids as the primary phenomenon of interest.

Evidence for Dependence on Anabolic Steroids

The opinion that using anabolic steroids could lead to dependence was noted in the scientific literature as early as 1980 (Wright, 1980). Others involved in the treatment of anabolic steroid users later echoed this opinion (Taylor, 1985; Goldman, 1987; Whitehead [cited in Cowart, 1987]). Unfortunately, these early observers did not provide systematic data to support their opinions. In the absence of data, some have questioned the idea that using anabolic steroids can lead to dependence (see Dreyfuss, 1990; Cicero & O'Connor, 1990).

Since 1988, at least four case reports of anabolic steroid dependence have appeared in the medical literature. Tennant, Black, and Voy (1988) reported a case of a 23-year-old bodybuilder who felt "addicted" because he could not stop taking anabolic steroids without experiencing disabling withdrawal symptoms, including depression, fatigue, and craving. Brower, Blow, Beresford, and Fuelling (1989) reported the case of a 24-year-old noncompetitive weightlifter who felt unable to stop taking anabolic steroids without professional help, because he experienced suicidal depression when he tried to stop on his own. The patient met six out of nine *DSM-III-R* criteria for dependence and manifested severe social impairment as a result, indicating that the dependence was severe. Hays, Littleton, and Stillner (1990) described a 22-year-old noncompetitive weightlifter who also admitted that he could not stop taking anabolic steroids despite feeling depressed. When he tried to stop, he experienced low self-esteem and craving and felt he was not big enough. Most recently, Copeland, Peters, and Dillon (1998) described the first published case of anabolic steroid dependence in a woman. The 30-year-old woman used steroids for about four years, including two years of an injectable form. She met five of seven DSM-IV criteria for dependence.

Three of these cases involved young male weightlifters who reported inabilities to stop taking anabolic steroids, partly because of the withdrawal symptoms that ensued. These withdrawal symptoms were depressive in nature and were accompanied by cravings for more drugs. All three subjects also took multiple steroid drugs simultaneously, including both injectable and oral preparations, for durations ranging from

9 months to 3 years. Two of the reports noted that subjects had no histories of either pre-existing psychiatric illness or prior substance abuse with another drug (Brower, Blow, Beresford, & Fuelling, 1989; Hays, Littleton, & Stillner, 1990), but the third report did not mention these factors (Tennant, Black, & Voy, 1988). Nevertheless, this third report did note a negative urine drug screen for other drugs of abuse. In all three cases, subjects initially used the anabolic steroids to enhance weightlifting activity, but the subjects eventually used the drugs to combat depression. In other words, it is clear that as these subjects became dependent, they took the anabolic steroids for their psychic effects, a finding consistent with the definitions for dependence discussed previously. Other case reports (Allnutt & Chaimowitz, 1994; Cowan, 1994; Malone & Dimeff, 1992) have described depressive syndromes requiring treatment that followed cessation of anabolic steroids; but the authors did not provide enough information to determine if these patients met full criteria for substance dependence.

Survey research has provided additional evidence of dependence on anabolic steroids. In a survey of 3,403 male high school seniors, Buckley, Yesalis, Friedl, Anderson, Streit, and Wright (1988) reported that 226 (6.6%) students admitted to using anabolic steroids. A further analysis of these users revealed that approximately one-fourth indicated they would not stop using anabolic steroids even if it was proven beyond doubt that the drugs lead to permanent sterility, increase the risk of liver cancer, or greatly influence the risk of early heart attacks (Yesalis, Vicary, Buckley, Streit, Katz, & Wright, 1990). Among "heavy users," defined as those reporting five or more cycles (or episodes) of use, 40 to 50% indicated that they would not stop using steroids despite the potential risks of sterility, liver cancer, and heart attacks. The responses of these users were consistent with the *DSM-III-R* criterion symptom of continued drug use despite adverse consequences (see table 9.1, criterion 6). Nevertheless, these responses were only an indirect measure of the dependency symptom, because the users did not necessarily or actually experience the adverse consequences. Because the study did not use the full *DSM-III-R* criteria, the authors could not determine if these heavy users were dependent on anabolic steroids in a diagnostic sense.

In a survey of community weightlifters, our research group at the University of Michigan distributed a self-administered questionnaire that contained questions designed to elicit *DSM-III-R* criteria for dependence (Brower, Blow, Young, & Hill, 1991; Brower, Eliopulos, Blow, Catlin, & Beresford, 1990). Of the first 8 subjects to complete the questionnaire, all 8 met *DSM-III-R* criteria for abuse and 6 met criteria for dependence. All 8 subjects reported withdrawal symptoms on cessation of use or on completing cycles of use. Withdrawal symptoms were primarily depressive in nature and included depressed mood, fatigue, decreased sex drive, insomnia, anorexia, and dissatisfaction with body image. We then extended our findings to 49 anabolic steroid users, of whom 57% met *DSM-III-R* criteria for dependence (Brower et al., 1991). We noted the full spectrum of dependency symptoms, including symptoms of both psychological and physical dependence (table 9.1). Interestingly, the least commonly reported symptoms (criteria 4 and 9) by our sample of steroid users were deleted or reclassified in *DSM-IV* (table 9.1). The most frequently reported withdrawal symptoms are presented in table 9.2. Unfortunately, these data were limited by selection bias and by a lack of methods to corroborate self-report. Therefore, the statistic of 57% may not apply to other samples of anabolic steroid users and may overestimate the prevalence of anabolic steroid dependence. Nevertheless, Gridley and Hanrahan (1994), who employed the same questionnaire in an Australian sample of 21 steroid users, corroborated our 57% prevalence rate of steroid dependence.

At least three other studies have employed the *DSM-III-R* criteria for substance dependence to diagnose steroid dependence among illicit steroid users. Rates of dependence across these studies ranged from 14% to 69%, reflecting differences in sampling and differences in interview methods. Malone, Dimeff, Lombardo, and Sample (1995) administered, at the Cleveland Clinic, a structured diagnostic instrument to 77 anabolic steroid users recruited from community gyms and found that 14.3% met *DSM-III-R* criteria for dependence. Pope and Katz (1994) reported that approximately 25% of 88 steroid users recruited from the community appeared to manifest

Table 9.2 Self-Reported Withdrawal Symptoms

Symptom	Percent reporting (%)[a]
Desire to take more steroids ("craving")	52
Fatigue	43
Body image dissatisfaction	42
Depressed mood	41
Restlessness	29
Anorexia	24
Insomnia	20
Decreased libido	20
Headaches	20

[a] *N* = 49

Adapted from *British Journal of Addiction* 1991.

dependence on steroids based on extensive clinical research interviews and psychiatric assessments. Finally, Clancy and Yates (1992) surveyed 91 inpatient substance abuse treatment programs and identified 68 steroid users of whom 69% were judged to meet *DSM-III-R* criteria for steroid dependence.

Interestingly, Kochakian in 1950 reported a phenomenon he dubbed the "wearing-off effect," in which rats treated with an anabolic steroid initially manifested a protein anabolic response that disappeared with continued doses unless the doses were increased. Our study revealed a wearing-off effect or tolerance in 18% of anabolic steroid users (table 9.1) but did not distinguish between tolerance to psychoactive effects and tolerance to anabolic effects (Brower et al., 1991). Whether users develop tolerance to the psychological effects of anabolic steroids, therefore, is not known. Nevertheless, the phenomenon of tolerance to anabolic steroids has been appreciated for over 40 years. Finally, many anabolic steroid users intentionally take higher than therapeutic doses of anabolic steroids in order to maximize the desired effects. Indeed, studies suggest that one must take 3 to 10 times the therapeutic replacement dose in order to observe appreciable differences in male characteristics (Bardin, Catterall, & Janne, 1990). Therefore, high dosage by itself does not signify tolerance or dependence. Rather, tolerance occurs when even higher doses are used, because previous high doses no longer produce the desired effect that they once did.

More recently, Bonson, Garrick, and Murphy (1994) reported a withdrawal syndrome in rats after 10 (but not after 3) weeks of daily injections of testosterone propionate. The withdrawal syndrome lasted up to 2 weeks after cessation of steroid administration and consisted of facial tremor, head weaving, full-body lurches, and ptosis. Thus, both tolerance and withdrawal have been demonstrated experimentally in animals exposed to anabolic steroids. However, animals have not been shown to self-administer anabolic steroids as they will other drugs of abuse such as cocaine and opioids (Foltin, 1992). Traditional animal models of drug self-administration may need to be modified to demonstrate a reinforcing effect for anabolic steroids. For example, animals made physically dependent on anabolic steroids (see Bonson, Garrick, & Murphy, 1994) might be more likely to self-administer them than steroid-naive animals.

In 1989, Kashkin and Kleber published a review of the "anabolic steroid addiction hypothesis" and concluded both that "a proportion of anabolic steroid abusers may develop a previously unrecognized sex steroid hormone-dependence disorder" (p. 3,166) and that the "addiction hypothesis is speculative and needs to be confirmed by scientific investigation" (p. 3,169). Presently, however, the medical literature supports dependence on anabolic steroids as a clinical phenomenon that has been observed for many years in various settings by multiple professionals. In other words, the existing case studies and survey data clearly describe dependence from both clinical and phenomenological perspectives. The task of future research, therefore, is to explore further the phenomenology of anabolic steroid dependence and withdrawal, and to reveal the mechanisms, predictors, and course of anabolic steroid dependence in order to optimize prevention and treatment efforts.

Mechanisms of Anabolic Steroid Dependence

If we accept the phenomenon of anabolic steroid dependence, then we must understand how anabolic steroids produce dependence if we are to prevent and treat it. Not surprisingly, the mechanism by which anabolic steroids may produce symptoms of dependence is unknown. One area of controversy is whether or not anabolic steroids can produce dependence by the mechanism of "primary reinforcement." Cocaine, for example, is thought to operate through a primary reinforcement mechanism. After administering cocaine, a user may experience an immediate feeling of pleasure or euphoria that results from cocaine's stimulation of those parts of the brain involved with reward (Wise, 1984). Although it is generally accepted that using anabolic steroids does not result in immediate pleasure or reinforcement (as does cocaine or opioid use) (Fingerhood, Sullivan, Testa, & Jasinski, 1997; Yesalis, 1990), up to 43% of anabolic steroid users reported feeling "high" or feeling extreme pleasure from using anabolic steroids over extended periods of time (Brower et al., 1991). Similarly, many other uncontrolled studies have noted euphoric effects among athletes who took anabolic steroids for relatively long periods of time (see review by Taylor, 1987).

What is debatable is whether anabolic steroids produce this delayed euphoria via a direct stimulatory effect on the brain (primary reinforcement) or whether the euphoric effect is secondary to the social reinforcement and pleasure the athlete feels from experiencing improved performance or having a big muscular body (figure 9.1). A theoretical way to separate primary from secondary reinforcing effects of anabolic steroids—which helps to conceptualize the primary-secondary distinction—is to conceive of an anabolic steroid drug that is "muscle-active" (providing secondary reinforcement) but not cerebrally active (providing primary reinforcement) because it does not cross the blood-brain barrier (i.e., it does not enter into the brain). If taking the theoretical anabolic steroid drug, which is solely muscle-active, produces the same degree of euphoria and pleasure over time, then support for the secondary reinforcement mechanism would be bolstered.

However, we know that anabolic steroids do enter the brain, that multiple sites exist in the brain to which anabolic steroids selectively and specifically bind (McEwen, 1981; Sheridan, 1983, 1984), that anabolic steroids can alter the structure of the brain (DeVoogd, 1987), and that complex

Positive reinforcement mechanisms

Primary reinforcement from brain reward systems, including

- endogenous opioid systems,
- monoaminergic systems (e.g., dopamine),
- brain centers that mediate sexual function and pleasure.

Secondary reinforcement from muscular development, including

- psychological benefits (e.g., increased self-esteem),
- social benefits (e.g., admiration from others),
- vocational benefits (e.g., "making the team," winning competitions).

Negative reinforcement mechanisms

Avoidance of depressive and other withdrawal symptoms. Withdrawal symptoms may be both

- biologically mediated, by, for example,
  - testosterone deficiency,
  - endogenous opioid systems,
  - monoaminergic systems, and
- psychosocially mediated, as a
  - psychological response to loss of muscular development or physical capacities and/or
  - psychological response to loss of social and vocational rewards.

Avoidance of feeling not big enough.

Figure 9.1 Hypothetical mechanisms of dependence on anabolic steroids.

systems of enzymes exist in the brain for metabolizing and mediating the behavioral effects of anabolic steroids (Hutchison & Steimer, 1984; McEwen, 1981). Other evidence indicates that anabolic steroids can modulate opioid activity in the brain (Kashkin & Kleber, 1989; Limonta, Maggi, Dondi, Martini, & Piva, 1987; Menard, Hebert, Dohanich, & Harlan, 1995; Tennant, Black, & Voy, 1988), can mimic the brain wave activity produced by psychostimulants (Itil, 1976; Itil, Cora, Akpinar, Herrmann, & Patterson, 1974; Stenn, Klaiber, Vogel, & Broverman, 1972), and can affect the same neurotransmitters that are involved in the action of cocaine and other stimulants (Alderson & Baum, 1981; Goudsmit, Feenstra, & Swaab, 1990; Jalilian-Tehrani, Karakiulakis, Le Blond, Powell, & Thomas, 1982; Mitchell & Stewart, 1989; Kashkin & Kleber, 1989; Vermes, Varszegi, Toth, & Telegdy, 1979).

Of particular interest are the effects of anabolic steroids and their estrogen metabolites on dopamine and reward systems. Many addiction researchers believe that the mesolimbic dopamine system in the brain is involved in the reinforcing action of drugs of abuse and constitutes a final common pathway for many dependence-producing drugs (Koob & Le Moal, 1997; Koob, 1992). Two research groups have reported that castration of rats causes a decrease in dopamine levels in the mesolimbic system, whereas administration of either testosterone or estradiol restores mesolimbic dopamine levels in castrated rats (Alderson & Baum, 1981; Mitchell & Stewart, 1989). Unfortunately, the effects of supraphysiologic doses of androgen or estrogen administered to noncastrated animals, which more closely approximate illicit steroid use in humans, were not studied. Another line of animal research utilized a conditioned–place-preference paradigm (Alexander, Packard, & Hines, 1994). Male rats were injected with supraphysiologic doses of testosterone every other day for six injections and then immediately placed in either a black or white compartment for 30 minutes. On alternate days, rats were injected with placebo and placed in the oppositely colored compartment for 30 minutes. On day 14, they were not injected, but allowed to roam freely between compartments. Rats spent more time in the compartment that was paired with testosterone than with placebo injections. Similar results have been obtained when natural rewards such as food or highly reinforcing drugs such as cocaine are used. The authors concluded that testosterone has rewarding properties when given in supraphysiologic doses (Alexander, Packard, & Hines, 1994). Interestingly, another research group found a positive conditioned place preference in male, but not female, rats in response to testosterone injections (De Beun, Jansen, Slangen, & Van de Poll, 1992)

Intracranial brain stimulation provides another paradigm for studying the rewarding properties of anabolic steroids. When an electrode is inserted into certain brain regions, including the mesolimbic system, animals will readily press a bar to deliver an electrical current to that area. Many drugs of abuse will increase rates of bar-pressing for electrical brain stimulation, which is generally regarded as an indication of a drug's rewarding effects (Kornetsky, 1995). Some studies (Caggiula & Hoebel, 1966; Caggiula, 1970; Campbell, 1970; Herberg, 1963; Olds, 1958) but not all (Clark, Lindenfeld, & Gibbons, 1996) reported that anabolic-androgenic steroids increased rates of bar-pressing for electrical brain stimulation. Nevertheless, even the negative study found that anabolic-androgenic steroids enhanced the rewarding effect of amphetamine (Clark, Lindenfeld, & Gibbons, 1996). Therefore, studies of electrical brain stimulation are generally consistent with the notion that anabolic steroids have a positive effect on brain reward systems.

Some effects of testosterone may result from its metabolism to estrogen. Indeed, gynecomastia (enlarged breast tissue) in male anabolic steroid users is generally considered a consequence of supraphysiologic estrogen levels (Wilson, 1988). The psychoactive effects of testosterone may also result in part from estrogen metabolites. Like androgens, estrogens bind receptors in the brain, appear to influence the limbic system (Fink & Sumner, 1996), and have been suggested to cause drug dependence (Bewley & Bewley, 1992). Nevertheless, the evidence that estrogens produce drug dependence is less substantial than for androgens.

Numerous psychiatric effects have been associated with, if not attributed to, anabolic steroid use (Bahrke, Yesalis, & Wright, 1996; Brower, 1992; see also chapter 8). Among the purported psychiatric effects are manic and hypomanic syndromes, during which a euphoric mood can occur (Pope & Katz, 1988, 1994), and elevations of mood in depressed patients, who were not reportedly engaged in activities of muscle development (reviewed by Bahrke, Yesalis, & Wright, 1990). Finally, some users of anabolic steroids report enhancement of sexual desire and pleasure (Greenblatt & Karpas, 1983; Taylor, 1987), effects that are mediated cerebrally and that may reinforce use.

Taken together, animal studies of neurochemistry, reward pathways, and electrical brain stimulation, and human studies of psychiatric effects suggest that a primary reinforcement mechanism is certainly possible, although far from confirmed.

Whether by primary or secondary reinforcement, and whether by brain or muscle action, both these mechanisms imply that either the psychic or social rewards of taking anabolic steroids lead to a dependence on them. When drug-taking behavior is increased by consequences the user perceives as positive (rewards), the mechanism is called *positive reinforcement*. Two lines of evidence, however, suggest that a different mechanism of reinforcement may operate among dependent anabolic steroid users. First is the observation from the cases previously reviewed that subjects took anabolic steroids to avoid symptoms of depression (Brower, Blow, Beresford, & Fuelling, 1989; Hays, Littleton, & Stillner, 1990; Tennant, Black, & Voy, 1988). When drug users continue to take drugs in order to avoid consequences that are perceived as negative, as in these three cases, then the mechanism is called *negative reinforcement* (figure 9.1).

A second line of evidence derives from our study of 49 anabolic steroid users, of whom 28 (57%) met *DSM-III-R* criteria for dependence (Brower et al., 1991). When we compared the dependent and nondependent groups of anabolic steroid users, we found no significant differences in terms of the reported physical or psychological benefits of taking anabolic steroids. By contrast, the dependent anabolic steroid users were significantly more likely to report “feeling not big enough,” despite reporting physical gains equivalent to those of nondependent users. In other words, dependent anabolic steroid users in our sample appeared to be driven more by attempts to avoid feeling not big enough (negative reinforcement) than by experiences of positive benefits (positive reinforcement). Interestingly, both these lines of evidence in support of a mechanism of negative reinforcement are consistent with a self-medication hypothesis of addictive disorders (Khantzian, 1985), which views dependent users as trying to overcome negative moods or deficits in themselves.

It is possible that users may become dependent on anabolic steroids by either one or several of these mechanisms. In fact, a clinically important typology of dependent anabolic steroid users, if substantiated by further research, might be based on the particular mechanism of dependence operating in a particular individual. For example, those who exhibit dependence based on a social reinforcement mechanism might best be treated by changing their social environments, whereas those whose dependence results in part either from stimulation of brain reward systems or from avoidance of withdrawal symptoms might require pharmacological treatment. Other users may be affected by complex patterns of reinforcement. For example, an athlete may have experienced performance improvements after initiating steroids and obtained further improvements with continued use (positive reinforcement). When the athlete tried to quit taking steroids, athletic performance decreased, which reinforced resumption of drug use. Although these mechanisms are speculative, the important point is that an understanding of mechanisms can have substantial treatment implications.

Predictors of Anabolic Steroid Dependence

Not all users of anabolic steroids necessarily become dependent on them. Summarizing the studies cited above, the prevalence rates of steroid dependence among illicit users range from 14% to 69%, depending on sample selection and interview methods. Only one case involved a woman (Copeland, Peters, & Dillon, 1998), so female dependence on male hormones is apparently rare. However, few female steroid users have been studied.

One set of factors may predict the initial use of anabolic steroids, and a different, if not overlapping, set of factors may predict dependent use (Brower, 1989; Brower, Blow, & Hill, 1994). This section explores the user characteristics and patterns of use that appear to be associated with dependent use of anabolic steroids.

Yesalis and colleagues (1990) identified a group of heavy users of anabolic steroids who "reported behaviors, perceptions, and opinions that are consistent with psychological dependence, in terms of their unwillingness to stop use, their perceptions of risks and benefits of use and their rationalizations of use" (p. 207). Compared to other anabolic steroid users, these heavy users were more likely to have initiated use before age 16, to have completed both more and longer cycles of use, to have combined multiple anabolic steroid drugs simultaneously, and to have used injectable anabolic steroids. They were also more likely to perceive their peers as using anabolic steroids. Interestingly, they were more likely to perceive their strength as less than average (7.1% for heavy users vs. 2.6% for the lightest users). On the basis of these data, age of onset, intensive patterns of use, and certain perceptions of self and others appear to be associated with heavy use, which resembles dependence.

Likewise, we found that both pharmacological factors and self-perceptions were predictive of dependent use in men (Brower et al., 1991). More specifically, dependent users took larger doses of anabolic steroids and were significantly more likely to perceive themselves as not big enough when compared to nondependent users. We did not find differences between dependent and nondependent users in either age of onset or other substances used.

These studies suggest that a perception of oneself as not big enough or not strong enough may represent a psychological vulnerability to dependency on anabolic steroids. In addition, those who take larger than therapeutic doses over long periods of time appear more likely to manifest dependence. By contrast, the literature has not reported dependence resulting from an individual taking therapeutic doses of anabolic steroids to treat medical conditions such as testosterone deficiency, anemia, hereditary angioedema (a rare skin condition), and advanced breast cancer. Likewise, cases of dependence have not been reported among subjects in experimental trials taking anabolic steroids as contraceptives.

Course of Dependence on Anabolic Steroids

Little is known about the course of dependence on anabolic steroids. The following are among the questions to be answered:

- How rapidly may dependence on anabolic steroids develop after initial use?
- How severe can the dependence become?
- What is the course of withdrawal symptoms following cessation of anabolic steroid use?
- How readily does remission of the dependence occur either with or without treatment?

Unfortunately, no longitudinal studies of anabolic steroid users exist to help resolve these questions (Yesalis & Bahrke, 1995). Nevertheless, some tentative answers to guide future research can be surmised from existing data.

Based on two of the case reports described previously, it appears that dependence on anabolic steroids can occur within 9 to 12 months after use is initiated (Brower, Blow, Beresford, & Fuelling, 1989; Hays, Littleton, & Stillner, 1990). Both patients in these reports combined multiple anabolic steroid drugs, leading to higher than therapeutic doses and combined oral and injectable forms of anabolic steroids as well. However, we have described another anabolic steroid user whose responses to a questionnaire were consistent with a diagnosis of dependence and who took only one drug orally but for nearly 9 years at 3 times the therapeutic dose (Brower et al., 1990). We concluded that "dependence may develop more rapidly in users who combine high doses of oral and injectable forms of steroids, but taking only one drug by mouth does not necessarily protect against dependence" (Brower et al., 1990, p. 512). Other unstudied factors that may affect the rapidity of a user's developing dependence on anabolic steroids include psychological vulnerability, genetics, and a prior history of other substance dependence (Brower, 1989).

Severe dependence, as defined in *DSM-III-R,* requires both an excess of dependency symptoms and marked social dysfunction that results from the dependence (APA, 1987, p. 168). The male weightlifter described in Brower, Blow, Beresford, and Fuelling (1989) exemplifies severe dependence: He had six of nine *DSM-III-R* dependency symptoms; he separated from his wife because of anabolic steroid–associated temper outbursts; and he had suicidal thoughts during withdrawal. Moreover, in our survey of 49 anabolic steroid users in the community, 8.2% of the sample reported six or more *DSM-III-R* symptoms of dependence, which suggested severe dependence (Brower et al., 1991). Therefore, at least some anabolic steroid users develop severe dependence.

Some authors have speculated that withdrawal from anabolic steroids follows a two-phase course (Kashkin & Kleber, 1989). The initial phase is apparently characterized by symptoms that resemble opioid withdrawal, such as increased pulse and blood pressure, sweats, chills, piloerection ("goose pimples"), nausea, headache, and dizziness (Tennant, Black, & Voy, 1988). The mood during this first phase may be more anxious and irritable than depressed. By contrast, the second phase is marked predominantly by depressive symptoms and craving (table 9.2). Neither the duration nor the validity of these phases has been established. Roughly estimated, phase 1 may begin and end during the first week of cessation, whereas phase 2 may begin in the first week and last for several months (Brower, 1997). Consistent with the estimated duration for phase 2, Pope and Katz (1988) found that 5 (12.2%) of 41 anabolic steroid users developed symptoms of major depression during the first 3 months of withdrawal from anabolic steroids. If further research substantiates the two-phase course, then the treatment of anabolic steroid withdrawal may need to be biphasic as well (Brower, 1997). Nevertheless, the possibility of an opioidlike withdrawal syndrome after an individual stops using anabolic steroids is suggested only by an uncontrolled, single case study that has yet to be replicated (Tennant, Black, & Voy, 1988).

Remission from dependence on anabolic steroids may depend not only on the severity of dependence and the characteristics of the individual user but also on the mechanism of dependence. For example, if the dependence is maintained mostly by social reinforcement for having a well-developed body (rather than by direct stimulation of the brain or by avoidance of either withdrawal symptoms or a negative self-perception), then remission may occur somewhat readily when the social environment changes. Anecdotally, some researchers have asserted that most athletes who use anabolic steroids to enhance competitive performance experience no difficulty stopping use after they retire from competition (Malone, 1995; Yesalis, personal communication, 1990). This can mean that none of these users were dependent on anabolic steroids or that many dependent users can stop using with relative ease when their social circumstances change. To the extent that any of these athletes were dependent on anabolic steroids, they were nonetheless able to stop using them when their retirement eliminated their social need for larger, stronger bodies.

Prevention and Treatment

A program of prevention must first define its target population, its goals, and the stage of problem development at which to direct itself. A program of *primary prevention*, for example, might direct itself toward young or potential weightlifters and athletes who have never used anabolic steroids, with the goal of preventing any initial, nonmedical use of anabolic steroids. A program of *secondary prevention* might direct itself toward those who have already experimented with anabolic steroids, with the goal of preventing continued use that could lead to dependence and other adverse health effects. Finally, a program of *tertiary prevention* would consist of treatment for dependent anabolic steroid users who are unable to stop taking drugs safely on their own. Each of these types of prevention program is likely to require somewhat different and specific strategies to optimize effectiveness.

Perhaps the most critical task of prevention programs is to target the predictors of anabolic steroid use and dependence (Brower et al., 1991; Brower, Blow, & Hill, 1994). Programs that do not address predictors (or risk factors) are likely to fail. For example, one research group found that a prevention program that provided information only about the anabolic and harmful effects of anabolic steroids paradoxically increased student athletes' interest in trying anabolic steroids (Bents, Trevisan, Bosworth, Boysea, Elliot, & Goldberg, 1989; Bosworth, Bents, Trevisan,

& Goldberg, 1988). The negative results probably occurred because lack of information is not the strongest predictor of future use and because the information-only program did not address psychosocial factors that do favor use. Therefore, research into the predictors of anabolic steroid use and dependence is crucial for successful prevention efforts.

The preceding review of existing research points to the importance of targeting both the psychological vulnerabilities related to body image and the social environments that may reinforce anabolic steroid use. Prevention programs must also address the broader cultural context that places high values on physical attractiveness and on winning competitions (Yesalis, 1990). Programs that address these influences, by providing alternatives for managing them, are most likely to be effective and should be tested.

Treatment is indicated when the severity of dependence precludes the user from stopping safely on his or her own. Treatment should be based on an individualized assessment of the dependent user's characteristics and needs and of the mechanisms or forces that underlie and perpetuate the drug taking. The major goals of treatment are abstinence from anabolic steroids and the restoration of health. In cases in which withdrawal symptoms and the avoidance of withdrawal symptoms are either occurring or likely to occur, professional monitoring and supportive therapy are necessary, because the risk of suicidal depression and relapse appears to be highest during the withdrawal period (Brower, 1989, 1997; Brower, Blow, Eliopulos, & Beresford, 1989). Pharmacological treatments for anabolic steroid withdrawal are mostly unstudied, but suggested approaches have been reviewed elsewhere (Brower, 1997; Malone, 1995). Clinical issues to consider during rehabilitation have also been reviewed previously (Brower, 1989, 1992; Corcoran & Longo, 1992; Frankle & Leffers, 1992).

Given the estimated prevalence of anabolic steroid use and dependence, it is surprising that treatment settings for drug dependence do not see more steroid users. An estimated 300,000 Americans use steroids illicitly each year (Yesalis, Kennedy, Kopstein, & Bahrke, 1993), of which 14% to 69% are considered at risk for dependence (see above). Yet one study estimated that less than 0.1% of patients entering substance abuse treatment programs from 1989 to 1990 even used steroids; and only 1 of 41 identified steroid users in treatment actually sought help for steroids as opposed to concurrent substance abuse (Clancy & Yates, 1992). There are many possible reasons for this. A similar lag time occurred with the cocaine epidemic, in which treatment settings did not register an increase in cocaine-related admissions until about 4 years after the prevalence of cocaine use increased in the general population (Adams & Durell, 1984). Experts speculated that 4 years was the lag time between initial use and problematic use of cocaine (Adams & Durell, 1984). Thus, the rapidity with which dependency symptoms and other adverse consequences occur may be one factor affecting the number of anabolic steroid users who seek treatment. (Unfortunately, during the lag time in the cocaine epidemic, experts were lulled into thinking that cocaine was a comparatively benign drug.)

A second factor that affects treatment seeking may be the ease with which some dependent users stop taking anabolic steroids without treatment. Elite athletes, for example, are reportedly able to quit using anabolic steroids quite readily when the social reinforcers of use are no longer operative (Yesalis, personal communication, 1990). Other dependent users may be able to stop on their own, because their dependence is not severe. Only 4 (14.3%) of our community sample of 28 dependent users, for example, had evidence of severe anabolic steroid dependence (Brower et al., 1991). Likewise, only 8 (16%) of 49 users reported an inability to cut down their use despite a desire to do so (Brower et al., 1991). Thus, both the mechanism and severity of dependence may influence the ability to stop using anabolic steroids without treatment.

Other factors might include users' negative perceptions of the need for treatment and the unavailability of informed treatment programs. Most anabolic steroid users do not consider anabolic steroids harmful, and they may deny or minimize harmful effects when they do occur (U.S. Department of Health and Human Services [USDHHS], 1990). Anabolic steroid users may also distrust physicians and other treatment providers because of a long-standing "credibility gap" regarding the effects of anabolic steroids (Wade, 1972). Treatment programs espousing such views as (1) steroid users "ignore the paucity of objective support of performance claims" or (2) "steroid addiction is no different than any other addiction" (Giannini, Miller, & Kocjan, 1991, p. 541) will likely discourage steroid users from seeking treatment. For those who do desire help, there are few programs that offer specific treatment for anabolic steroid dependence.

Finally, it is possible that many anabolic steroid users are being seen in treatment settings but are not identified as such. The failure to detect anabolic steroid users in treatment settings, therefore, should not imply that anabolic steroids are benign drugs that do not lead to dependence. Rather, the treatment community needs to develop programs that address the specific needs of anabolic steroid users, and we need to train treatment providers to identify anabolic steroid users in clinical practice.

Summary

Drug dependence can best be viewed as a clinical diagnosis that is defined in terms of widely accepted criteria. The essential features of the diagnosis are impaired control over the drug-taking and continued drug use despite adverse consequences, features that are often referred to as psychological dependence. Other pertinent features are tolerance and withdrawal, which are indicators of a physiological adaptation to a drug. When we apply these criteria to case reports and existing survey data, we conclude that dependence occurs in some individuals who take anabolic steroids. Future research should investigate the prevalence, mechanisms, predictors, and course of anabolic steroid dependence in order to optimize prevention and treatment efforts.

References

Adams, E.H., & Durell, J. (1984). Cocaine: A growing public health problem. *National Institute on Drug Abuse Research Monograph Series, 50,* 9–14.

Alderson, L.M., & Baum, M.J. (1981). Differential effects of gonadal steroids on dopamine metabolism in mesolimbic and nigro-striatal pathways of male rat brain. *Brain Research, 218,* 189–206.

Alexander, G.M., Packard, M.G., & Hines, M. (1994). Testosterone has rewarding affective properties in male rats: Implications for the biological basis of sexual motivation. *Behavioral Neuroscience, 108,* 424–428.

Allnutt, S., & Chaimowitz, G. (1994). Anabolic steroid withdrawal depression: A case report. *Canadian Journal of Psychiatry, 39,* 317–318.

American College of Sports Medicine. (1987). Position stand on the use and abuse of anabolic-androgenic steroids in sports. *Medicine and Science in Sports and Exercise, 19,* 534–539.

American Medical Association, Council on Scientific Affairs. (1988). Drug abuse in athletes: Anabolic steroids and human growth hormone. *Journal of the American Medical Association, 259,* 1703–1705.

American Psychiatric Association. (1987). *Diagnostic and statistical manual of mental disorders* (3rd ed., rev. [*DSM-III-R*]). Washington, DC: Author.

American Psychiatric Association. (1994). *Diagnostic and statistical manual of mental disorders* (4th ed. [*DSM-IV*]). Washington, DC: Author.

Bahrke, M.S., Yesalis, C.E., & Wright, J.E. (1990). Psychological and behavioral effects of endogenous testosterone levels and anabolic-androgenic steroids among males: A review. *Sports Medicine, 10,* 303–337.

Bahrke, M.S., Yesalis, C.E., & Wright, J.E. (1996). Psychological and behavioural effects of endogenous testosterone levels and anabolic-androgenic steroids among males: An update. *Sports Medicine, 22,* 367–390.

Bardin, C.W., Catterall, J.F., & Janne, O.A. (1990). The androgen-induced phenotype. *National Institute on Drug Abuse Research Monograph Series, 102,* 131–141.

Bents, R., Trevisan, L., Bosworth, E., Boysea, S., Elliot, D., & Goldberg, L. (1989). The effect of teaching interventions on knowledge and attitudes of anabolic steroids among high school athletes. *Medicine and Science in Sports and Exercise, 21*(Suppl. 2), S26.

Bewley, S., & Bewley, T.H. (1992). Drug dependence with oestrogen replacement therapy. *Lancet, 339*, 290–291.

Bonson, K.R., Garrick, N.A., & Murphy, D.L. (1994). Evidence for a withdrawal syndrome following chronic administration of an anabolic steroid to rats. *Society for Neuroscience Abstracts, 20,* 1527.

Bosworth, E., Bents, R., Trevisan, L., & Goldberg, L. (1988). Anabolic steroids and high school athletes. *Medicine and Science in Sports and Exercise, 20*(Suppl. X), S3.

Brower, K.J. (1989). Rehabilitation for anabolic-androgenic steroid dependence. *Clinical Sports Medicine, 1,* 171–181.

Brower, K.J. (1992). Anabolic steroids: Addictive, psychiatric, and medical consequences. *American Journal on Addictions, 1,* 100–114.

Brower, K.J. (1997). Withdrawal from anabolic steroids. In C.W. Bardin (Ed.), *Current therapy in endocrinology and metabolism* (pp. 338–343). St. Louis: Mosby.

Brower, K.J., Blow, F.C., Beresford, T.P., & Fuelling, C. (1989). Anabolic-androgenic steroid dependence. *Journal of Clinical Psychiatry, 50,* 31–33.

Brower, K.J., Blow, F.C., Eliopulos, G.A., & Beresford, T.P. (1989). Anabolic-androgenic steroids and suicide [Letter to the editor]. *American Journal of Psychiatry, 146,* 1075.

Brower, K.J., Blow, F.C., & Hill, E.M. (1994). Risk factors for anabolic-androgenic steroid use in men. *Journal of Psychiatric Research, 28*(4), 369–380.

Brower, K.J., Blow, F.C., Young, J.P., & Hill, E.M. (1991). Symptoms and correlates of anabolic-androgenic steroid dependence. *British Journal of Addiction, 86,* 759–768.

Brower, K.J., Eliopulos, G.A., Blow, F.C., Catlin, D.H., & Beresford, T.P. (1990). Evidence for physical and psychological dependence on anabolic androgenic steroids in eight weight lifters. *American Journal of Psychiatry, 147,* 510–512.

Buckley, W.E., Yesalis, C.E., Friedl, K., Anderson, W.A., Streit, A.L., & Wright, J.E. (1988). Estimated prevalence of anabolic steroid use among male high school seniors. *Journal of the American Medical Association, 260,* 3441–3445.

Caggiula, A. R. (1970). Analysis of the copulation-reward properties of posterior hypothalamic stimulation in male rats. *Journal of Comparative and Physiological Psychology, 70,* 399–412.

Caggiula, A.R., & Hoebel, B.G. (1966). "Copulation reward site" in the posterior hypothalamus. *Science, 153,* 1284–1285.

Campbell, H.J. (1970). The effect of steroid hormones on self-stimulation, central and peripheral. *Steroidologia, 1*(1), 8–24.

Cicero, T.J., & O'Connor, L.H. (1990). Abuse liability of anabolic steroids and their possible role in the abuse of alcohol, morphine, and other substances. *National Institute on Drug Abuse Research Monograph Series, 102,* 548–550.

Clancy, G.P., & Yates, W.R. (1992). Anabolic steroid use among substance abusers in treatment. *Journal of Clinical Psychiatry, 53*(3), 97–100.

Clark, A.S., Lindenfeld, R.C., & Gibbons, C.H. (1996). Anabolic-androgenic steroids and brain reward. *Pharmacology, Biochemistry and Behavior, 53,* 741–745.

Copeland, J., Peters, R., & Dillon, P. (1998). Anabolic-androgenic steroid dependence in a woman. *Australian and New Zealand Journal of Psychiatry, 32,* 589.

Corcoran, J.P., & Longo, E.L. (1992). Psychological treatment of anabolic-androgenic steroid-dependent individuals. *Journal of Substance Abuse Treatment, 9,* 229–235.

Cowan, C.B. (1994). Depression in anabolic steroid withdrawal. *Irish Journal of Psychological Medicine, 11,* 27–28.

Cowart, V. (1987). Steroids in sports: After four decades, time to return these genies to bottle? *Journal of the American Medical Association, 257,* 421–427.

De Beun, R., Jansen, E., Slangen, J.L., & Van de Poll, N.E. (1992). Testosterone as appetitive and discriminative stimulus in rats: Sex- and dose-dependent effects. *Physiology and Behavior, 52,* 629–634.

DeVoogd, T.J. (1987). Androgens can affect the morphology of mammalian CNS neurons in adulthood. *Trends in Neuroscience, 10,* 341–342.

Dreyfuss, I.J. (1990). Congress considers restricting steroids. *The Physician and Sportsmedicine, 18*(3), 38.

Fingerhood, M.I., Sullivan, J.T., Testa, M., & Jasinski, D.R. (1997). Abuse liability of testosterone. *Journal of Psychopharmacology, 11,* 59–63.

Fink, G., & Sumner, B.E. (1996). Oestrogen and mental state [Letter to the editor]. *Nature, 383*, 306.

Foltin, R.W. (1992). The importance of drug self-administration studies in the analysis of abuse liability: An analysis of caffeine, nicotine, anabolic steroids, and designer drugs. *American Journal on Addictions, 1,* 139–149.

Frankle, M., & Leffers, D. (1992). Athletes on anabolic-adrogenic steroids. *The Physician and Sportsmedicine, 20*(6), 75–87.

Fussell, S.W. (1991). *Muscle: Confessions of an unlikely bodybuilder.* New York: Avon.

Giannini, A.J., Miller, N., & Kocjan, D.K. (1991). Treating steroid abuse: A psychiatric perspective. *Clinical Pediatrics, 30,* 538–542.

Goldman, B. (1987). *Death in the locker room* (2nd ed.). Tucson, AZ: Body Press.

Gomberg, E. (1989). On terms used and abused: The concept of "codependency." *Drugs and Society, 3*(3/4), 113–132.

Goudsmit, E., Feenstra, M.G.P., & Swaab, D.F. (1990). Central monoamine metabolism in the male Brown-Norway rat in relation to aging and testosterone. *Brain Research Bulletin, 25,* 755–763.

Greenblatt, R.B., & Karpas, A. (1983). Hormone therapy for sexual dysfunction. The only "true aphrodisiac." *Postgraduate Medicine, 74*(2), 78–80, 84–89.

Gridley, D.W., & Hanrahan, S.J. (1994). Anabolic-androgenic steroid use among male gymnasium participants: Dependence, knowledge, and motives. *Sport Health, 12(1),* 11–14.

Hays, L.R., Littleton, S., & Stillner, V. (1990). Anabolic steroid dependence [Letter to the editor]. *American Journal of Psychiatry, 147,* 122.

Herberg, L.J. (1963). Seminal ejaculation following positively reinforcing electrical stimulation of the rat hypothalamus. *Journal of Comparative and Physiological Psychology, 56,* 679–685.

Hutchison, J.B., & Steimer, T. (1984). Androgen metabolism in the brain: Behavioural correlates. *Progress in Brain Research, 61,* 23–51.

Itil, T.M. (1976). Neurophysiological effects of hormones in humans: Computer EEG profiles of sex and hypothalamic hormones. In E.J. Sachar (Ed.), *Hormones, behavior, and psychopathology* (pp. 31–40). New York: Raven Press.

Itil, T.M., Cora, R., Akpinar, S., Herrmann, W.M., & Patterson, C.J. (1974). "Psychotropic" action of sex hormones: Computerized EEG in establishing the immediate CNS effects of steroid hormones. *Current Therapeutic Research, 16,* 1147–1170.

Jalilian-Tehrani, M.H., Karakiulakis, G., Le Blond, C.B., Powell, R., & Thomas, P.J. (1982). Androgen-induced sexual dimorphism in high affinity dopamine binding in the brain transcends the hypothalamic-limbic region. *British Journal of Pharmacology, 75,* 37–48.

Kashkin, K.B., & Kleber, H.D. (1989). Hooked on hormones? An anabolic steroid addiction hypothesis. *Journal of the American Medical Association, 262,* 3166–3170.

Khantzian, E.J. (1985). The self-medication hypothesis of addictive disorders: Focus on heroin and cocaine dependence. *American Journal of Psychiatry, 142,* 1259–1264.

Kochakian, C.D. (1950). Comparison of protein anabolic property of various androgens in the castrated rat. *American Journal of Physiology, 160,* 53–61.

Koob, G. F. (1992). Drugs of abuse: Anatomy, pharmacology and function of reward pathways. *Trends in Pharmacological Sciences, 13,* 177–184.

Koob, G.F., & Le Moal, M. (1997). Drug abuse: Hedonic homeostatic dysregulation. *Science, 278,* 52–58.

Kornetsky, C. (1995). Reward pathways and drugs. In J.H. Jaffe (Ed.), *The encyclopedia of drugs and alcohol* (pp. 117–122). New York: Macmillan.

Limonta, P., Maggi, R., Dondi, D., Martini, L., & Piva, F. (1987). Gonadal steroid modulation of brain opioid systems. *Journal of Steroid Biochemistry, 27,* 691–698.

Malone, D.A., Jr. (1995). Pharmacological therapies of anabolic androgenic steroid addiction. In N.S. Miller & M.S. Gold (Eds.), *Pharmacological therapies for drug and alcohol addictions* (pp. 227–237). New York: Marcel Dekker.

Malone, D.A., Jr., & Dimeff, R.J. (1992). The use of fluoxetine in depression associated with anabolic steroid withdrawal: A case series. *Journal of Clinical Psychiatry, 53,* 130–132.

Malone, D.A., Dimeff, R.J., Lombardo, J.A., & Sample, R.H.B. (1995). Psychiatric effects and psychoactive substance use in anabolic-androgenic steroid users. *Clinical Journal of Sport Medicine, 5,* 25–31.

McEwen, B.S. (1981). Neural gonadal steroid actions. *Science, 211,* 1303–1311.

Menard, C.S., Hebert, T.J., Dohanich, G.P., & Harlan, R.E. (1995). Androgenic-anabolic steroids modify beta-endorphin immunoreactivity in the rat brain. *Brain Research, 669,* 255–262.

Mitchell, J.B., & Stewart, J. (1989). Effects of castration, steroid replacement, and sexual experience on mesolimbic dopamine and sexual behaviors in the male rat. *Brain Research, 491,* 116–127.

Murray, T.H. (1987). The ethics of drugs in sports. In R.H. Strauss (Ed.), *Drugs and performance in sports* (pp. 11–21). Philadelphia: Saunders.

Nightingale, S.L. (1991). Anabolic steroids as controlled substances. *Journal of the American Medical Association, 265,* 1229.

Olds, J. (1958). Effects of hunger and male sex hormone on self-stimulation of the brain. *Journal of Comparative and Physiological Psychology, 51,* 320–324.

Pope, H.G., Jr., & Katz, D.L. (1988). Affective and psychotic symptoms associated with anabolic steroid use. *American Journal of Psychiatry, 145,* 487–490.

Pope, H.G., Jr., & Katz, D.L. (1994). Psychiatric and medical effects of anabolic-androgenic steroid use. *Archives of General Psychiatry, 51,* 375–382.

Sheridan, P.J. (1983). Androgen receptors in the brain: What are we measuring? *Endocrine Reviews, 4,* 171–178.

Sheridan, P.J. (1984). Autoradiographic localization of steroid receptors in the brain. *Clinical Neuropharmacology, 7*(4), 281–295.

Stenn, P.G., Klaiber, E.L., Vogel, W., & Broverman, D.M. (1972). Testosterone effects upon photic stimulation of the electroencephalogram (EEG) and mental performance of humans. *Perceptual and Motor Skills, 34,* 371–378.

Taylor, W.N. (1985). *Hormonal manipulation.* Jefferson, NC: McFarland.

Taylor, W.N. (1987). Synthetic anabolic-androgenic steroids: A plea for controlled substance status. *The Physician and Sportsmedicine, 15,* 140–150.

Tennant, F., Black, D.L., & Voy, R.O. (1988). Anabolic steroid dependence with opioid-type features [Letter to the editor]. *New England Journal of Medicine, 319,* 578.

U.S. Department of Health and Human Services, Office of Inspector General. (1990). *Adolescents and steroids: A user perspective* (OEI-06-90-01081). Washington, DC: Author.

Uzych, L. (1990). Steroids and the Controlled Substances Act. *Biological Psychiatry, 27,* 561–562.

Vermes, I., Varszegi, M., Toth, E.K., & Telegdy, G. (1979). Action of androgenic steroids on brain neurotransmitters in rats. *Neuroendocrinology, 28,* 386–393.

Wade, N. (1972). Anabolic steroids: Doctors denounce them, but athletes aren't listening. *Science, 176,* 1399–1403.

Wilson, J.D. (1988). Androgen abuse by athletes. *Endocrine Reviews, 9,* 181–199.

Wise, R.A. (1984). Neural mechanisms of the reinforcing action of cocaine. *National Institute on Drug Abuse Research Monograph Series, 50,* 15–33.

World Health Organization. (1993). *ICD-10, the ICD-10 classification of mental and behavioural disorders: Diagnostic criteria for research.* Geneva: Author.

Wright, J.E. (1980). Anabolic steroids and athletics. *Exercise and Sport Sciences Reviews, 8,* 149–202.

Yesalis, C.E. (1990). Winning and performance-enhancing drugs—our dual addiction. *The Physician and Sportsmedicine, 18,* 161–167.

Yesalis, C.E., & Bahrke, M.S. (1995). Anabolic-androgenic steroids. Current issues. *Sports Medicine, 19*(5), 326–340.

Yesalis, C.E., Kennedy, N.J., Kopstein, A.N., & Bahrke, M.S. (1993). Anabolic-androgenic steroid use in the United States. *Journal of the American Medical Association, 270,* 1217–1221.

Yesalis, C.E., Vicary, J.R., Buckley, W.E., Streit, A.L., Katz, D.L., & Wright, J.E. (1990). Indications of psychological dependence among anabolic-androgenic steroid abusers. *National Institute on Drug Abuse Research Monograph Series, 102,* 196–214.

CHAPTER

10

Assessment and Treatment of Anabolic Steroid Abuse, Dependence, and Withdrawal

Kirk J. Brower, MD

The (Chargers) continued to offer Dianabol to the team as long as I was in San Diego. Civilian casualties were acceptable.

Ron Mix
Former San Diego Charger
Member of the Football Hall of Fame
Sports Illustrated, October 19, 1987

Portions of this chapter are from Bardin 1997; see credits page for more information.

This chapter addresses three areas of concern for clinicians who treat anabolic steroid users. The first concern includes the identification and assessment of anabolic steroid users. For the purposes of the following discussion, *identification* refers to the detection of new cases, and *assessment* refers to the evaluation of known cases. Although the sports community has paid widespread attention to the identification of drug-using athletes via drug testing, little has been written about identifying anabolic steroid users in clinical practice via a careful search for the signs and symptoms associated with anabolic steroid use. Thus, this chapter will review the clinical manifestations of anabolic steroid use as might be evident during a history, physical examination, mental status examination, and laboratory examination. The second area of concern is a clinical approach to identified steroid users who are not motivated to stop using drugs. Both harm-reduction strategies and motivational techniques will be discussed as potentially useful in these cases. The third area of concern is the clinical management of anabolic steroid users who agree to stop using these drugs. Withdrawal from anabolic steroids may be problematic for some users, necessitating informed clinical care. Accordingly, this chapter will provide guidelines for the treatment of anabolic steroid withdrawal. Although the use of anabolic steroids has both sociocultural and biomedical implications, the major intent of this chapter is to place the problems associated with anabolic steroid use in a clinical context so they are subject to clinical interventions.

Identification and Assessment

Anabolic steroid users only rarely present for substance abuse treatment (Clancy & Yates, 1992). Instead, they may present for treatment of the various side effects of their drug-taking, with or without divulging their drug use. Surgeons may see bodybuilders who want treatment for gynecomastia (Aide, 1989), and dermatologists may see anabolic steroid users who want treatment for acne (Scott, 1989). Even when patients do admit to anabolic steroid use, a thorough assessment is necessary to guide the proper course of treatment (Brower, Catlin, Blow, Eliopulos, & Beresford, 1991; Frankle & Leffers, 1992).

Clinical identification, assessment, and treatment occur in the context of a confidential relationship. The clinician is not as interested in any punitive sanctions to which the patient may be subject, as in the health and well-being of the patient. Although some physicians have dual responsibilities to both sports organizations and patients, the emphasis here is on identification for clinical, not punitive, purposes. When the clinical examination is conducted in the context of a confidential relationship, the patient can view the clinician as an ally rather than an adversary. This context should attenuate the tendency to deny drug use.

Epidemiologic studies indicate that young males who are recreational weightlifters, bodybuilders, or participants in sports that require strength or power are at highest risk for using anabolic steroids (Yesalis, Wright, & Lombardo, 1989). Thus, a high index of clinical suspicion for these patients is warranted, especially if the physical, mental status, or laboratory examinations reveal pertinent findings, as outlined in the following discussion.

History

The clinician may first ask the patient about his or her use of legal substances, such as alcohol and tobacco, then about nutrition and legal performance aids, such as protein supplements and amino acids. The clinician may then ask if the patient knows other people who have used or are using anabolic steroids. Finally, the clinician may ask if the patient has ever used anabolic steroids. If not, the patient should be asked if he or she has considered using anabolic steroids or if others have suggested it. The clinician and patient can then discuss the patient's reasons for not using or for considering use. Questions such as these can be useful for initiating a dialogue about anabolic steroids, for providing education, and for understanding both the personal goals of patients and the pressures they may experience to use anabolic steroids. The astute clinician will derive information from both the content of the patient's answers and the manner in which the patient responds. Nervousness, defensiveness, or evasiveness may be clues that the patient requires extra attention, even if anabolic steroid use is overtly denied. Corroborating history from a family member or a significant other can be extremely helpful in cases in which the patient appears to be in denial.

The clinician is interested in identifying not only patients who use steroids but also ones who may be thinking about using them. Some research suggests that peer influences (knowing other steroid users) and dissatisfaction with body size (feeling not big enough) may contribute to the risk of using steroids among young males who train with weights in community gymnasiums (Brower, Blow, & Hill, 1994). Other potential risk factors include training for a bodybuilding competition, spending more than 10 hours a week lifting weights, and using four or more nonsteroidal substances for performance enhancement (Brower, Blow, & Hill, 1994) Thus, the clinician should pay particular attention to these items when taking a history.

The review of systems, a standard part of history taking when interviewing patients, should inquire about subjective complaints that have been associated with anabolic steroid use and withdrawal, such as headaches, dizziness, nausea, muscle spasms and aches, urinary frequency, and menstrual abnormalities (Haupt, 1993; Haupt & Rovere, 1984). In addition, the clinician should look for psychiatric symptoms such as mood swings, depression, irritability, aggressiveness, increased or decreased energy level, disturbance in appetite, insomnia, dissatisfaction with one's physical appearance, and changes in libido (Brower, Catlin, et al., 1991). Finally, social dysfunction should be evaluated, such as arguments with or estrangement from family and friends, and decrements in performance on the job, at school, or on the playing field.

When patients do admit to using anabolic steroids, the clinician should determine the specific drugs used, source (licit or illicit), dosages, time of last use, duration of use, frequency of use, and routes of administration. A comprehensive inventory of other possibly used substances should be obtained, including opioids, aspirin, other nonsteroidal anti-inflammatory drugs, sedative-hypnotics, marijuana, alcohol, and tobacco (Wadler & Hainline, 1989). The clinician should determine use of substances that are taken to treat the side effects of anabolic steroids (e.g., estrogen blockers), to augment effects (e.g., human chorionic gonadotropin, growth hormone, erythropoietin, stimulants), and to mask use of anabolic steroids (e.g., diuretics, probenecid). Finally, the clinician should ascertain the degree of dependence on anabolic steroids by asking about efforts to stop or cut down, using more anabolic steroids than intended, continuing use despite adverse consequences, withdrawal symptoms, and tolerance (Brower, Blow, Young, & Hill, 1991) (see chapter 9).

Physical Examination

The following signs, arranged by system, may be associated with anabolic steroid use (Brower, Catlin, et al., 1991; Haupt & Rovere, 1984; Hickson, Ball, & Falduto, 1989; Kibble & Ross, 1987; Wilson, 1988). Some signs, such as high blood pressure, are not commonly seen (Palatini et al., 1996); so they have little value for identification or screening but are important for assessment and monitoring of known cases. The absence of many signs, therefore, does not rule out anabolic steroid use, because some anabolic steroid users manifest relatively few side effects. Moreover, none of the following signs are specific for anabolic steroid use. Nevertheless, the presence of one or more of these signs in a high-risk patient should signal the possibility of anabolic steroid use.

- *Vital signs and physical dimensions*—High blood pressure (Freed, Banks, Longson, & Burley, 1975; Lenders et al., 1988); marked, rapid weight gain with maintenance of, or increase in, lean body mass.
- *Skin*—Acne; needle marks in large muscle groups (deltoids, gluteals); male pattern baldness; hirsutism in females; jaundice.
- *Head and neck*—Jaundiced eyes; deepened voice in females.
- *Chest*—Gynecomastia in males; atrophied breasts in females.
- *Abdominal*—Right upper quadrant tenderness; hepatomegaly (Ishak & Zimmerman, 1987; Soe, Soe, & Gluud, 1992).

- *Genitourinary*—Testicular atrophy and prostatic hypertrophy in males; clitoral hypertrophy in females.
- *Musculoskeletal*—Marked muscular hypertrophy; disproportionate development of the upper torso, especially the neck, shoulders, and chest.
- *Extremities*—Edema.

Mental Status Exam

There is hardly a psychiatric symptom for which anabolic steroids have not been implicated in either causing or exacerbating (Bahrke, Yesalis, & Wright, 1996; Malone, Dimeff, Lombardo, & Sample, 1995; Pope & Brower, 1999; Pope & Katz, 1988, 1994). The mental status exam is performed to obtain objective or observer-rated information about a patient's psychiatric condition. Although there may be scientific debate about the exact role of anabolic steroids in causing psychiatric disturbance (Bahrke & Yesalis, 1994), few would disagree that anabolic steroid users who exhibit one or more of the following signs require therapeutic attention. Therefore, the clinician should assess the following indicators of psychiatric disturbance.

- *Behavior*—Psychomotor agitation or retardation, consistent with either manic or depressive disorders.
- *Mood*—Euphoria; irritability; depression; marked anxiety.
- *Affect*—Lability with abrupt shifts in moods.
- *Thought process*—Slowed with depressive states; rapid or disorganized with manic states.
- *Thought content*—Suicidal or homicidal thoughts; grandiose or persecutory thoughts that may progress to delusions.
- *Hallucinations*

Laboratory Examination

Anabolic steroid users may show abnormalities of the following laboratory tests; thus, these tests should be ordered for those suspected of using anabolic steroids. Although urine testing for anabolic steroids should also be ordered (Brower, Catlin, et al., 1991), the following tests are usually more readily available and have a faster turnaround time. A urine drug screen for other drugs of abuse should also be included. Importantly, the clinician can use laboratory abnormalities to alert the user of adverse consequences that require monitoring and intervention. Because normal reference values for the following tests may vary from laboratory to laboratory, clinicians should follow the normal reference range provided by their laboratories of use.

• *Liver function tests*—Elevations in bilirubin, lactate dehydrogenase (LDH), alkaline phosphatase, aspartate amino transferase (AST, or SGOT [serum glutamic oxaloacetic transaminase]), and alanine amino transferase (ALT, or SGPT [serum glutamic pyruvic transaminase]) can be found (O'Connor, Skinner, Baldini, & Einstein, 1990). Serum levels of gamma-glutamyltransferase are usually not affected (Kiraly, 1988; Lenders et al., 1988; Morrison, 1994; Pope & Katz, 1994). Elevations in ALT and AST can be due to intensive weightlifting even without anabolic steroid use and to intramuscular injections, due to the presence of these enzymes in skeletal muscle. Thus, liver-specific enzymes (e.g., the LDH isoenzyme) may be needed to rule out liver dysfunction (Haupt & Rovere, 1984).

• *Muscle enzymes*—In addition to elevations in ALT and AST, elevations in creatine phosphokinase (CPK) have been observed in both steroid-using and nonusing weightlifters after a training session (Hakkinen & Alen, 1989). Anabolic steroid users, however, have even greater elevations than nonusers after exercising (Hakkinen & Alen, 1989), and they can have abnormal elevations in CPK before exercising (McKillop, Ballantyne, Borland, & Ballantyne, 1989). Serum creatinine may be elevated in both users and nonusers simply due to increased muscle bulk.

• *Cholesterol profile*—Although total cholesterol may be elevated (O'Connor et al., 1990), the most consistent findings with 17-alkylated oral anabolic steroid administration are significantly decreased levels of high-density lipoprotein cholesterol (HDLC) (Sachtleben, Berg, Cheatham, Felix, & Hofschire, 1997) and increased levels of low-density lipoprotein cholesterol (LDLC) (Kiraly, 1988; Lenders et al., 1988; O'Connor, Skinner, Baldini, & Einstein, 1990). Triglycerides may also be elevated (O'Connor et al., 1990).

• *Hematocrit and hemoglobin*—Due to the erythropoietic effect of anabolic steroids, the hematocrit and hemoglobin levels may be elevated relative to the patient's usual baseline level (Kiraly, 1988), although the hematocrit is rarely abnormally elevated (O'Connor et al., 1990). However, when athletes combine anabolic steroids with erythropoietin, as some endurance athletes have done, abnormal elevations are even more likely.

• *Endocrine tests of the pituitary-gonadal axis*—Serum levels of luteinizing hormone (LH) and follicle-stimulating hormone (FSH) are reduced in response to the feedback inhibition of exogenously administered anabolic steroids on the hypothalamus and pituitary gland (Alen & Rahkila, 1988). Serum testosterone levels may be increased with the use of testosterone esters (that are metabolized to testosterone) but decreased with the exclusive use of other anabolic steroids or following cessation of anabolic steroid use (Alen, Reinila, & Vihko, 1985). Similarly, serum estradiol levels may be either increased or decreased, depending on the use of testosterone esters (which are also metabolized to estradiol) and depending on whether the user is on a cycle or between cycles of use.

• *Semen analysis*—Sperm count and motility may be decreased, and sperm morphology may be abnormal (Knuth, Maniera, & Nieschlag, 1989).

• *Glucose tolerance test*—Although fasting serum glucose levels are not affected, one study revealed that anabolic steroid users had diminished 2-hour glucose tolerance tests when compared to controls (Cohen & Hickman, 1987). Nevertheless, none of the anabolic steroid users had abnormal tests indicative of diabetes. Thus, the value of the glucose tolerance test as a marker of anabolic steroid use is unproven.

• *Cardiac function tests*—There are a few case reports in the medical literature of myocardial infarction (MI) and dilated cardiomyopathy in anabolic steroid users (Ferrera, Putman, & Verdile, 1997; Melchert & Welder, 1995). Although the value of an electrocardiogram (EKG) to screen for occult MIs in anabolic steroid users is unknown, a baseline EKG is recommended for known or suspected users. Electrocardiographic evidence of left ventricular hypertrophy (LVH) is likely in bodybuilders and strength athletes who use anabolic steroids (Urhausen, Holpes, & Kindermann, 1989), although this finding may be seen in nonusing strength athletes as well (Alpert, Pape, Ward, & Rippe, 1989). Nevertheless, some (Urhausen, Holpes, & Kindermann, 1989), but not all (Zuliani, Bernardini, Catapano, Campana, Cerioli, & Spattini, 1988), studies reveal that the LVH in anabolic steroid users is associated with impaired diastolic function, and so a clinician should consider an echocardiogram for a patient with EKG evidence of LVH.

Treatment Goals and Strategies

Apparently few steroid users seek substance abuse treatment (Clancy & Yates, 1992). Perhaps most steroid users are able to stop on their own without formal treatment, or perhaps many current steroid users are not ready to stop using. This section will discuss the treatment of patients who have little to no interest in abstaining from steroids. Such steroid users may request treatment for steroid side effects such as gynecomastia or acne, or they may be brought to treatment by relatives and friends who are concerned about mood or behavioral changes. Once a steroid-using patient is identified and properly assessed, the health professional should inquire about the patient's motivation to quit using steroids. In assessing motivation (Brower & Rootenberg, 1999; Miller & Rollnick, 1991), the clinician can ask: "How do you feel about your steroid use?" "Do you have any concerns we have not talked about?" "Are you interested in stopping altogether?"

Most authors consider abstinence to be the primary goal of treatment (Brower, 1989; Frankle & Leffers, 1992; Friedl & Yesalis, 1989; Malone,

1995), but physicians also have a role in monitoring and treating adverse symptoms among patients who persist in using steroids (Frankle & Leffers, 1992). *In this author's opinion, abstinence from nonmedical steroid use is always the preferred goal of treatment*, both because abstinence is the surest way to reduce the risk of harm as much as possible and because nonmedical steroid use is illegal. Littlepage and Perry (1993) have argued that a comprehensive approach to steroid problems should include both abstinence and harm-reduction strategies. Harm reduction is an alternative goal to abstinence in patients who refuse to quit using steroids. Ideally, an initial goal of harm reduction will lead eventually to abstinence (Frankle & Leffers, 1992), because a patient's motivation to discontinue drug use can be increased over time through a therapeutic relationship in which the user comes to trust the credibility and advice of the physician or other health professional (Brower & Rootenberg, 1999; Miller & Rollnick, 1991). Therefore, combining an initial goal of harm reduction with motivational techniques to encourage abstinence can be an alternative but powerful treatment strategy. This alternative approach is exemplified by the treatment model developed by Frankle and Leffers (1992).

Frankle and Leffers (1992) outlined a problem-oriented treatment approach to steroid users that has striking similarities to effective motivational techniques described by Miller and Rollnick (1991). These techniques include providing feedback, decreasing desirability of drug use, giving advice, emphasizing personal responsibility for decision-making while clarifying options, employing empathy, and supporting self-efficacy. After completing a comprehensive medical assessment, patients received feedback about any physical or laboratory findings that were attributable to steroid use (Frankle & Leffers, 1992). This helped patients to make the connection between their steroid use and harmful consequences in a way that was immediately real and personalized, as opposed to receiving lists of theoretical adverse consequences. By balancing the positive steroid effects that patients sought with the objective, harmful consequences they actually incurred, the authors aimed to decrease the perceived desirability of steroid use. Importantly, the authors gave patients the advice that their safest choice was to stop using steroids. Yet they educated patients about other options as well, and they encouraged patients to decide for themselves. For example, if a patient with cholesterol abnormalities did not choose abstinence, then the patient was advised to make dietary modifications and to change the dose or type of steroid. The authors also emphasized a trusting, doctor-patient relationship, which was encouraged by an empathic understanding of the patient's reasons for and concerns about using steroids. Finally, the authors believed in their patients' self-efficacy, the idea that their patients could and would stop using steroids if provided with therapeutic support and good care. Frankle & Leffers (1992) presented preliminary outcome data. Of 15 steroid users who entered their program, 10 were followed up 3 to 8 months after their first visit. Of these 10 patients, 8 stopped using steroids altogether, and 2 patients decreased their use by half. If the 5 patients lost to follow-up were assumed to have continued using steroids at equivalent amounts or more, then 33% of patients did not change, 53% stopped using altogether, and 13% cut down their use by half. An additional 3 nonusers who considered using steroids at their initial visit remained steroid-free for 3 to 6 months.

Although negotiating treatment goals and making patients partners in the decision-making can facilitate the therapeutic relationship between doctors and patients, compromising abstinence is not always possible or advisable. For example, some users should be advised to abstain immediately, because of severe adverse consequences such as myocardial infarction, liver tumors, or violence to self or others. Whenever the patient's health is imminently and seriously jeopardized, then abstinence must be advised. Nevertheless, Barker (1987) reported a case of severe aggression in a young man who was prescribed therapeutic doses of oxymethalone for aplastic anemia. Because steroid treatment was indicated at the same dose for another 1 month, the patient was treated with cognitive-behavioral psychotherapy, which successfully diminished his aggressiveness.

Some professionals believe that harm reduction is most effectively executed by having physicians prescribe steroids to weightlifters and other athletes (Millar, 1994). The rationale for the Australian "steroid prescription programme" is that drug use and side effects can be diminished by putting the physician in control of the types, dosages, and duration of steroids used (Millar, 1994). Advantages of this approach include (1) an avoidance of illicit "street" drugs that could be harmfully contaminated or falsely labeled, (2) initial screening of patients who should not take steroids because of health problems such as hepatitis, and (3) regular monitoring by physicians who should be better informed about the risks and benefits of particular steroid regimens than illicit users who rely on unscientific literature and advice from dealers and peer users. In contrast to the approach by Frankle & Leffers (1992), the steroid prescription program places responsibility for controlling use with the physician rather than the patient, because the patient is dependent on the physician's prescription. Another difference between the two approaches is the assumption each program makes about patients' choices and values. Millar (1994) assumes that reasonable weightlifters and other athletes will and should want to take steroids after considering the options. Consequently, physician prescribing is preferable to an illicit market. By contrast, Frankle & Leffers (1992) assume that reasonable athletes and other users will ultimately decide to discontinue use after exposure to good medical care, accurate information, and therapeutic support.

This author believes that patients should take responsibility for their own use, recognizing that such use is illegal (at least in the United States) and potentially harmful. From their physicians, patients should expect and seek advice about, and monitoring for, their health; they should not expect and seek prescriptions for anabolic steroids. However, a randomized, comparative trial of these two approaches to harm reduction might prove more interesting than competing opinions.

Another reported approach to steroid harm reduction included a needle exchange program (Williamson, Davies, & McBride, 1992). Dubbed by its authors in Wales the "Well-Steroid Users Clinic," its services included needle exchange, steroid information, injection advice, and health assessment and feedback. A goal of the program was to reduce adverse medical consequences, including HIV infection among steroid users who shared needles. Outcome data were not reported. Similarly, Morrison (1994) reported that increasing numbers of steroid users were making use of a needle and syringe exchange program in England.

Treatment of Withdrawal

Patients who agree to stop using steroids may develop withdrawal symptoms and endocrine dysfunction. The clinical management of withdrawal from high-dose, illicit anabolic steroid use is mostly unstudied (Brower, 1997; Malone, 1995). At the time of this writing, there were no publications of controlled studies that evaluated treatment protocols for withdrawal from anabolic steroids. A few case reports of treated, steroid-related depression have described favorable outcomes (Allnutt & Chaimowitz, 1994; Cowan, 1994; Malone & Dimeff, 1992). Among the few case reports of anabolic steroid dependence in the literature (Brower, Blow, Beresford, & Fuelling, 1989; Hays, Littleton, & Stillner, 1990; Tennant, Black, & Voy, 1988), however, the treatment outcomes were invariably characterized by "lost to follow-up." As such, the following approaches are based on limited numbers of patients reviewed in the literature, seen in the author's clinical practice, or seen by other physicians who treat illicit steroid users.

Symptoms of withdrawal from anabolic steroids include depressed mood, fatigue, muscle and joint pain, restlessness, anorexia, insomnia, decreased libido, headache, and the desire to take more steroids (craving) (Brower, Blow, et al., 1991; Brower, Eliopulos, Blow, Catlin, & Beresford, 1990; Kashkin & Kleber, 1989; see also table 9.2). The most life-threatening complication of withdrawal from anabolic steroids that has been reported to date is suicidal depression (Brower, Blow, Eliopulos, & Beresford, 1989; Elofson & Elofson, 1990). Obviously, therefore, withdrawal symptoms may be severe enough to warrant treatment. Some authors hypothesize that withdrawal from anabolic steroids is biphasic in nature, with an initial phase marked by hyperadrenergic symptoms resembling opioid withdrawal and a later phase marked predominantly by depressive symptoms and craving (Kashkin & Kleber, 1989). Unfortunately, the validity and durations of these phases have not been adequately studied or described. Nevertheless, the depressive phase of steroid withdrawal is better documented (Allnutt & Chaimowitz, 1994; Brower, Blow, et al., 1991; Cowan, 1994; Malone & Dimeff, 1992; Pope & Katz, 1988) than a phase of opioidlike withdrawal; the evidence for the latter is based on only one case report from over 10 years ago (Tennant, Black, & Voy, 1988). Roughly estimated, the depressive withdrawal syndrome usually begins within the first week of steroid discontinuation and can last for several months. Depressive symptoms of steroid withdrawal may also develop into a major depressive episode (see American Psychiatric Association [APA], 1994, pp. 320–327) within the first 3 months of discontinuation (Pope & Katz, 1988). Depressive symptoms that begin more than a month after steroid discontinuation are unlikely to be related to steroid withdrawal.

The goals of treatment are

- to alleviate distressing withdrawal symptoms and prevent complications,
- to facilitate and initiate abstinence from illicit anabolic steroids,
- to prevent relapse to further use of anabolic steroids, and
- to restore the functioning of the hypothalamic-pituitary-gonadal (HPG) axis.

The treatment of withdrawal from anabolic steroids may be thought of as detoxification. As with other drugs of abuse, steroid detoxification consists of supportive therapy with or without pharmacotherapy (see figure 10.1). (Steroid abusers may be concomitantly dependent on other substances, such as alcohol, for which other specific detoxification measures are indicated [Brower & Severin, 1997]. Assessment, therefore, needs to include a history of the full range of addictive substance use.)

Supportive Therapy

Supportive therapy refers to psychological measures such as reassurance, education, and counseling. Patients are most reassured when the clinician is nonjudgmental, understanding, and knowledgeable about anabolic steroids and withdrawal. The need to establish a therapeutic alliance with the patient cannot be overstated. For both pharmacological and psychological reasons, a patient may initially be aggressive and

Supportive therapy

Pharmacotherapy

For hypothalamic-pituitary-gonadal dysfunction:

- Testosterone esters
- Human chorionic gonadotropin (HCG)
- Antiestrogens (clomiphene, tamoxifen)
- Short-acting LHRH agonists

For symptomatic relief and/or treatment of coexisting disorders:

- Antidepressants
- Clonidine
- Nonsteroidal anti-inflammatory drugs (NSAIDs)
- Tranquilizers
    - Neuroleptics (with or without lithium)
    - Benzodiazepines

Figure 10.1 Treatment alternatives for anabolic steroid withdrawal.[1]

[1]Please see text for specific recommendations.

Reprinted from Bardin 1997.

combative and may thus perceive the clinician as an opponent (B. Goldman, personal communication, 1990). If the clinician is also an athlete, he or she may use this to advantage for establishing rapport. If not, then the patient needs other evidence that the clinician understands his or her condition from both a medical and nonmedical perspective. More specifically, the clinician needs to understand the patient's point of view, because patients perceive their reasons for taking anabolic steroids as good ones. Almost invariably, the illicit steroid user is extremely invested in his or her physical attributes and body image (Blouin & Goldfield, 1995). When the clinician understands these and other reasons for drug-taking, he or she can counsel the patient about finding acceptable alternatives.

Acceptable alternatives for a bodybuilder, for example, may include nutritional counseling and consultation with an exercise physiologist or other fitness expert, who can both assist the patient with setting realistic training goals and provide safe regimens to achieve them. Although these substitutes probably will not provide the same physical gains that anabolic steroids can, the psychological benefits of substitutes can be powerful both for engaging patients in treatment and for preventing relapse. Moreover, the selection of appropriate substitutes conveys to patients that their needs have been understood.

Clinicians should educate patients about what they may experience during withdrawal, including depressed mood. By anticipating possible symptoms, the patient is reassured by the clinician's knowledge if such symptoms should occur. If symptoms have already occurred, the patient is reassured by the explanation that these are withdrawal symptoms rather than something intrinsically wrong with the patient or his or her character.

Although the clinician neither condones nor facilitates the drug-taking, persuasion to discontinue anabolic steroids should be based on health concerns rather than moralistic ones. In this regard, education about the health effects of anabolic steroids is important. The clinician can reinforce and personalize education by giving feedback to the patient about his or her own abnormal clinical findings or laboratory values. During abstinence, the clinician and patient can follow reversible abnormalities—such as testicular atrophy or abnormal cholesterol profiles—that provide concrete and reassuring evidence of improvement. Steroid users invariably believe that these drugs improve physical attributes in a variety of ways. Although some experts previously disputed the efficacy of anabolic steroids for these uses (Wilson, 1988), attempts to dissuade steroid users are fruitless and serve no clinical purpose. Moreover, despite some earlier negative studies (see review by Haupt & Rovere, 1984), recent studies indicate that anabolic steroids do produce increases in lean body mass, muscle size, and muscle strength (Bhasin et al., 1996; Forbes, Porta, Herr, & Griggs, 1992). Therefore, the clinician should agree that these are very potent drugs, and then raise concerns about their potential for causing adverse consequences.

Supportive therapy is always indicated during withdrawal, because the risks of suicidal depression and relapse are especially high during this period (Brower, Blow, Eliopulos, & Beresford, 1989; Elofson & Elofson, 1990; Malone et al., 1995). Clinicians should ask patients if they feel depressed and if they have ever felt so depressed that they thought about killing themselves. Patients should be encouraged to discuss these feelings if they occur. When the patient is suicidal, prompt consultation with a psychiatrist is strongly recommended and a plan for safety should be implemented.

Pharmacotherapy

Pharmacotherapy is considered adjunctive to supportive therapy. Pharmacotherapy is indicated when the clinical symptoms, with or without laboratory evidence of HPG dysfunction, are persistently severe. Persistently severe is not precisely defined, because each patient's treatment plan should be decided individually. As long as the patient can tolerate the withdrawal symptoms and responds to supportive therapy, however, watchful waiting is the prudent strategy. Pharmacotherapy is generally contraindicated when the patient cannot make a commitment to abstinence, because the physician may then be facilitating drug-taking behavior as well as the likelihood of an adverse drug interaction between the physician's prescribed drug and the patient's illicit drugs. Contraindications and precautions for specific agents are noted as follows. Pharmacotherapy can be divided into two major types: endocrine medications that are targeted specifically at the HPG axis to restore HPG functioning, and other medications that are targeted at withdrawal symptoms or psychiatric symptoms to provide symptomatic relief, regardless of HPG axis functioning. The first group includes testosterone esters, human chorionic gonadotropin (HCG), estrogen blockers such as clomiphene, and synthetic forms of gonadotropin-releasing hormone (GnRH) such as leuprolide. The second group includes antidepressants, nonnarcotic analgesics, clonidine, and tranquilizers.

Pharmacotherapy for HPG Axis Functioning

The prolonged use of high-dose anabolic steroids results in hypogonadotropic hypogonadism (Alen & Rahkila, 1988; Jarow & Lipshultz, 1990). Before initiating pharmacotherapy of this type, therefore, a physician should determine baseline levels of serum testosterone, estradiol, luteinizing hormone (LH), and follicle-stimulating hormone (FSH). Sperm counts may also be useful in some cases. Most hormonal abnormalities will return to normal without treatment within 12 weeks (Alen, Reinila, & Vihko, 1985; Frankle & Leffers, 1992), although cases have been reported in which endogenous testosterone production required more than a year to normalize (Bickelman, Ferries, & Eaton, 1995; Malone, 1995). Pharmacotherapy for HPG axis functioning is indicated only in the presence of clinically significant symptoms and severe or persistent abnormalities of these laboratory parameters. *Endocrine pharmacotherapy of nonmedical anabolic steroid users is not routinely recommended.* Because of the dearth of clinical experience with these drugs for the treatment of anabolic steroid withdrawal, combined in some cases (i.e., clomiphene and leuprolide) with the lack of approval by the Food and Drug Administration (FDA) for treating hypogonadotropic hypogonadism, these approaches are recommended mainly as an impetus for designing research protocols. Furthermore, these pharmacotherapies are based on the rationale of restoring HPG axis functioning in men. Case descriptions of anabolic steroid withdrawal in women are lacking, although some agents are used in women to treat infertility (HCG, clomiphene, gonadorelin), breast cancer (tamoxifen), and endometriosis (nafarelin). In addition, notwithstanding the use of HCG to treat boys with cryptorchidism and hypogonadotropic hypogonadism, and the use of testosterone esters to treat boys with hypogonadism, micropenis, and delayed puberty, these agents are infrequently used in children. Thus, the benefits and dangers of endocrine pharmacotherapy for female and pediatric steroid users must be carefully weighed. Nonspecialists in endocrinology should consult with gynecologic and pediatric endocrinologists before initiating endocrine therapies in women and children, respectively. Consultation with an endocrinologist is also advisable when treating adult males.

Testosterone Esters A common approach to detoxification for other drugs of abuse is to substitute a long-acting drug with cross-tolerance and then taper the substituted drug. For example, chlordiazepoxide, a long-acting benzodiazepine with cross-tolerance to ethanol, is a drug of choice for alcohol detoxification (Brower & Severin, 1997). Likewise, high therapeutic doses of a testosterone ester can be substituted for the illicit steroid regimen and then tapered at 1- to 2-week intervals. For example, an initial injection of 200 to 400 mg of testosterone enanthate can be decreased by 50 to 100 mg every 1 to 2 weeks. A single injection of testosterone enanthate (200 mg) has been reported to alleviate withdrawal symptoms in 1 to 2 days in patients whose serum testosterone levels are low (D. Coleman, personal communication, 1990). Prolonged tapers beyond 2 to 3 months are not recommended, and they suggest an iatrogenic prolongation of steroid dependence. However, Malone (1995) points out that heavy users may require starting doses of 500 mg or more of testosterone enanthate.

Inasmuch as withdrawal symptoms are correlated with persistent depression of the HPG axis, a tapering course of testosterone enanthate shares an analogous rationale to a tapering course of corticosteroids following chronic use of those drugs. Although theoretically plausible, this approach presents a number of difficulties. First, prescription of an abused substance to a substance abuser can be problematic unless closely supervised. Thus, the medical administration of anabolic steroids for detoxification should occur only in the physician's office or clinic, and self-administration of take-home prescriptions should be avoided. Unfortunately, steroid abusers might readily agree to medically administered injections as a means to bolster their illicit, self-administered steroid regimens. In these cases, urine testing for the illicit use of anabolic steroids may prove valuable. Also, the physician should guard against courses of testosterone treatment in which the dosage is increased or maintained for prolonged periods.

Second, the initial dose for taper can be difficult to determine, because illicit steroid users typically consume between 10 and 100 times the therapeutic dosage (Wilson, 1988), and their regimens often include both falsely labeled and veterinary preparations for which the human dose is incalculable. Thus, the physician may need to titrate the medically administered dose against the severity of withdrawal symptoms on an empirical basis. Third, the substitution of testosterone esters may provide symptomatic relief but actually prolong the recovery time of the HPG axis by continuing to suppress hypothalamic-pituitary function. Thus, other medication for symptomatic relief may be preferable. Finally, before treating men with testosterone, prostate and breast cancer should be ruled out as well as other symptoms of prostatism, because testosterone can exacerbate these conditions (Wang & Swerdloff, 1997). Prostatism (Wemyss, Hamdy, & Hastie, 1994) and, rarely, cases of prostate cancer (Larkin, 1991; Roberts & Essenhigh, 1986) have been reported in anabolic steroid users, although breast cancer has not.

Human Chorionic Gonadotropin During withdrawal, steroid abusers have abnormally low serum testosterone and LH values (Alen, Reinila, & Vihko, 1985), and they resemble prepubertal boys in their responses to HCG (Martikainen, Alen, Rahkila, & Vihko, 1986). During withdrawal, a single dose of 50 IU/kg can double serum testosterone levels at 3 to 4 days after HCG administration (Martikainen, Alen, Rahkila, & Vihko, 1986). For treatment of steroid withdrawal, the dosage of HCG need not exceed that recommended by the manufacturer for treatment of male hypogonadism. Therapy can be continued for 4 to 6 weeks or until serum LH values return to normal. Malone (1995) proposed a 6-week protocol of administering 500 to 1,000 USP units 3 times weekly for the first 3 weeks followed by the same dose twice weekly for the next 3 weeks. However, systematic data to support this approach are lacking, even though steroid users sometimes self-administer HCG in equivalent or higher doses (Galloway, 1997). Physicians need to be aware that HCG is sold illicitly to stimulate endogenous testosterone production and to prevent testicular atrophy in steroid users; thus, prescription-seeking for HCG can occur for diversion to the black market. Administration of HCG is typically by intramuscular injection.

Antiestrogens: Clomiphene and Tamoxifen Estradiol levels can increase during illicit androgen administration due to peripheral aromatization. Indeed, male steroid abusers sometimes self-administer antiestrogenic agents (such as tamoxifen or clomiphene) to prevent bothersome, feminizing side effects such as gynecomastia (Friedl & Yesalis, 1989). Once again, therefore, the physician must be alert to prescription-seeking for illegal diversion. As with exogenous anabolic steroids, high estradiol levels may suppress gonadotropin (including LH) secretion via feedback inhibition at the hypothalamic-pituitary level. Clomiphene and tamoxifen may increase secretion of LH by blocking estrogen receptors and preventing this feedback inhibition (Willis, London, Bevis, Butt, Lynch, & Holder, 1977). Although estradiol levels can be expected to return to physiological values within 3 weeks of discontinued use of androgens, serum testosterone may take 12 or more weeks to return to normal (Alen, Reinila, & Vihko, 1985). Clomiphene may be useful not only when serum estradiol levels are high but also when serum estradiol has returned to normal while the serum testosterone level remains depressed. During this latter hormonal configuration, clomiphene may result both in a more favorable ratio of testosterone-to-estradiol activity and in diminished feedback inhibition of LH secretion. One approach in men is to prescribe 50 mg twice daily for 10 to 14 days, which can be repeated according to symptomatic response and serial measures of serum testosterone and LH (D. Coleman, personal communication, 1990). Bickelman and colleagues (1995) reported a successful HPG response to clomiphene in a male patient with symptoms that persisted for 1 year after stopping anabolic steroids. The patient had only a partial response to 50 mg of clomiphene daily for the first month, and then responded fully to 100 mg daily for the next month. However, clomiphene is FDA-approved only for the treatment of female infertility. Whether tamoxifen (approved only for the treatment of breast cancer) might have any advantages over clomiphene for the treatment of anabolic steroid withdrawal is unknown, although some authors consider tamoxifen more effective than clomiphene for treating gynecomastia (Braunstein & Glassman, 1997). Millar (1994) reported that three cases of steroid-induced gynecomastia responded to 20 mg of tamoxifen daily for 4 weeks.

Synthetic Forms of Luteinizing Hormone–Releasing Hormone (LHRH) LHRH, also referred to as gonadotropin releasing hormone (GnRH), is the natural hypothalamic hormone that stimulates the pituitary gland to release LH. LH in turn stimulates the testes to produce testosterone. During steroid withdrawal, LHRH, LH, and testosterone levels are all decreased, which may contribute to withdrawal symptoms. The use of synthetic LHRH for treating anabolic steroid withdrawal was probably first suggested by Di Pasquale (1987).

Synthetic LHRH is currently available in several different forms and delivery systems. Pulsatile intravenous injection of GnRH is administered to women to treat infertility caused by primary hypothalamic amenorrhea. Because a physiologic dose of GnRH is delivered into the vein by a special pump device every 90 to 120 minutes, approximating the pulsatile rate of the natural hormone, LH is stimulated for the duration of the treatment period. Although its use in men is investigational at this time, pulsatile GnRH therapy via a subcutaneous infusion pump has been used successfully to treat infertility in men with hypogonadotropic hypogonadism (Butcher, Behre, Kliesch, & Nieschlag, 1998; Whitcomb & Crowley, 1997). Di Pasquale (1990) reported that pulsatile LHRH therapy was effective in treating HPG dysfunction after discontinuation of prolonged anabolic steroid use by athletes.

Leuprolide acetate is a synthetic analog of LHRH that is FDA-approved for the treatment of prostate cancer. Daily administration of LHRH (1 mg subcutaneously) for 1 week leads to an increase in serum LH and testosterone levels, whereas daily administration for more than 1 week leads to a decrease in these levels. Therefore, long-term administration (>1 wk) of leuprolide could exacerbate symptoms of withdrawal and HPG dysfunction. Nafarelin nasal spray is a short-acting LHRH analog that is approved for the treatment of endometriosis and central precocious puberty. Like leuprolide, nafarelin nasal spray leads to initial stimulation of LH and FSH, followed by a decrease in these hormones after 1 week of daily administration. Theoretically, then, brief treatment (<1 wk) with either leuprolide acetate or nafarelin nasal spray could have a place in the pharmacological armamentarium for treating anabolic steroid withdrawal. However, treatment of anabolic steroid withdrawal with leuprolide or nafarelin cannot be recommended without extreme caution and medical expertise in endocrinology, because no research supports its use for this purpose.

Finally, a long-acting LHRH analog, the goserelin acetate implant, is contraindicated in the treatment of anabolic steroid withdrawal. Because each implant delivers LHRH for 28 days in a nonpulsatile manner, it leads to a decrease in LH and testosterone. The goserelin acetate implant is indicated to treat prostate cancer, endometriosis, and advanced breast cancer. A three-month implant form is indicated to treat prostate cancer.

Pharmacotherapy for Symptomatic Relief of Withdrawal or Psychiatric Symptoms

This group of medications includes antidepressants, clonidine, nonnarcotic analgesics, and tranquilizers.

Antidepressants Because the majority of withdrawal symptoms are depressive in nature, antidepressant treatment may be indicated (Cowan, 1994; Malone & Dimeff, 1992). One uncontrolled study revealed that 5 (12%) of 41 steroid users suffered from a "clinical" or major depression during the first 3 months after stopping the use of anabolic steroids (Pope & Katz, 1988). A more recent and controlled study found that 5 (6.5%) of 77 users suffered a major depression after discontinuing steroids, all of whom experienced suicidal thoughts (Malone et al., 1995). Antidepressant therapy has been effective in treating several cases of major depression associated with steroid withdrawal (Cowan, 1994; Malone & Dimeff, 1992). In another case of steroid-related depression, electroconvulsive therapy was required after several antidepressants failed to produce a remission (Allnutt & Chaimowitz, 1994). Thus, the full range of biological treatments for major depression may be utilized in cases associated with anabolic steroids.

Although one study failed to find higher rates of major depression in steroid users than in controls, it did find increased rates of "subsyndromal" depressive symptoms (Perry, Yates, & Andersen, 1990). Likewise, Brower, Blow, and colleagues (1991) found that 20 (41%) of 49 steroid users reported the symptom of depressed mood during steroid withdrawal. Whether antidepressants will prove effective in treating depressive withdrawal symptoms (and perhaps craving) in the absence of major depression is unknown. Malone (1995) recommends antidepressant therapy only when the steroid user meets criteria for major depression (APA, 1994). Clearly, the indication for antidepressant therapy is bolstered when a coexisting reason for its use exists, such as major depression, panic disorder, obsessive-compulsive disorder, migraine headaches, or chronic pain. Unlike the agents previously discussed (e.g., testosterone, HCG, clomiphene), antidepressants are not likely to be abused or diverted for illicit sales.

The therapeutic action of the antidepressants is generally attributed to their effects on various neurotransmitter systems, particularly serotonergic and noradrenergic systems. When the interactions of anabolic steroids with these neurotransmitter systems are better understood, the selection of antidepressants based on their relative specificities for certain neurotransmitters might be possible. At this time, however, there is no reason to expect that any particular antidepressant is more effective than any other for the treatment of steroid withdrawal. Antidepressants do differ in terms of their side-effect profiles and in the availability of established therapeutic blood levels. Moreover, certain disorders that may coexist (as cited previously) have responded differentially to specific antidepressants. These differences can influence the selection of a particular agent for a particular patient.

Some antidepressants, especially the tricyclic antidepressants, have considerable overdose potential and may potentiate the adverse cardiac effects reported in steroid users. The physician must carefully assess the potentials for cardiotoxicity and suicide, therefore, before starting tricyclic antidepressants. Patients should have baseline and serial EKGs, orthostatic pulse and blood pressure measurements, and close monitoring of any cardiac symptoms. Antidepressants with high anticholinergic activity should either be avoided or used with caution in patients with steroid-induced (or steroid-exacerbated) prostatic hypertrophy, in order to prevent urinary retention. To avoid these potential problems of overdose, cardiotoxicity, and anticholinergic activity, the serotonin selective re-uptake inhibitors (such as fluoxetine [Prozac], paroxetine [Paxil], and sertraline [Zoloft]) might be preferred, first-choice antidepressants for steroid-induced depression (Malone & Dimeff, 1992; Malone, 1995). On the other hand, the prominent sexual side effects of these antidepressant medications, including impotence, may make them poorly tolerated by some men.

The same doses that are recommended for the treatment of depression are recommended for anabolic steroid withdrawal. In general, the physician gradually raises the dose until either symptomatic relief is obtained or bothersome side effects are experienced. Unfortunately, optimal effects may not take place until 2 to 6 weeks after adequate dosing has been achieved. Thus, patience on the part of both the physician and patient is required to ensure an adequate trial of therapy. In the interim, other treatment measures may be needed. The duration of therapy will depend on the responsiveness of symptoms, the presence of coexisting disorders, and the potential for relapse. For treatment of major depression, therapy is usually continued for 6 to 12 months.

Clonidine One case report suggested that the initial stage of anabolic steroid withdrawal is marked by hyperadrenergic symptoms resembling opioid withdrawal (Tennant, Black, & Voy, 1988). These symptoms were precipitated by a naloxone challenge and included nausea, headache, diaphoresis, piloerection, chills, dizziness, and increased pulse and blood pressure. Clonidine, which ameliorates opioid withdrawal, was noted to suppress these symptoms as well. Although dosage was not specified, 0.1 mg of clonidine every 4 to 6 hours by mouth is generally given on the first day of treatment for opioid withdrawal, is increased daily as needed by 0.1 to 0.2 mg to a maximum of 1.2 mg/d, and is then gradually tapered by 0.1 to 0.2 mg/d (Brower & Severin, 1997). Major side effects are hypotension and sedation, which require careful monitoring and possible adjustment of dosage. Because sedation may be poorly tolerated by patients who are already feeling depressed and fatigued, and who generally strive to feel strong at all costs, clonidine is not recommended unless there is clear evidence of opioidlike withdrawal symptoms. Indeed, the presence of such symptoms has not been well documented during anabolic steroid withdrawal, and the use of opioid withdrawal rating scales may be useful in this regard for both clinical and research purposes (Handelsman, Cochrane, Aronson, Ness, Rubinstein, & Kanof, 1987).

Analgesics Steroid users maintain that anabolic steroids decrease their recovery time between workouts, allowing them to train for longer hours and more frequently without experiencing fatigue or pain. After steroid use is stopped, this effect is lost along with a concomitant decrease in strength. The exercise intensity places extra stress on tendons and ligaments, which can lead to injury or inflammation. During withdrawal, patients commonly experience muscle and joint pains that partly reflect the extreme, exertional effects of intensive training but without the attenuation of pain that anabolic steroids might possibly provide. Headaches are also frequently reported. Whether the musculoskeletal pains and headaches bear any resemblance to the discomforts of opioid withdrawal is unknown. In either case, nonsteroidal anti-inflammatory drugs (NSAIDs), such as ibuprofen or naproxen, may represent the analgesic drugs of choice for the headaches and musculoskeletal pains of anabolic steroid withdrawal. NSAIDS are not addictive (an important consideration in someone who is abusing anabolic steroids and perhaps other drugs), provide effective analgesia, and counter the inflammation resulting from overstressed ligaments and tendons.

Certain side effects of the NSAIDs, albeit rare (less than 3% of patients), are of particular concern in steroid abusers. For example, NSAIDs can cause elevations in liver function tests, which may already be elevated due to the patient's anabolic steroid use. Thus, monitoring of liver function tests is important. These agents may also result in edema and fluid retention, as can anabolic steroids; this is especially important if cardiac function has been affected by the use of anabolic steroids. In addition, NSAIDs have been associated with psychiatric symptoms such as nervousness, depression, and emotional lability. In actual practice, however, the likelihood of these effects is small. Nevertheless, the physician must be alert to the possibility of these side effects when initiating and monitoring the course of treatment. Finally, these agents are contraindicated in the presence of angioedema, a condition for which anabolic steroids are legitimately prescribed.

Tranquilizers Major tranquilizers, or neuroleptics, are indicated in the presence of psychotic symptoms or acute mania. Physicians should also consider these drugs for treating marked irritability, aggressiveness, or agitation. As with corticosteroid-induced psychosis or mania, the addition of lithium may be considered. Long-term treatment with neuroleptics and lithium will probably be unwarranted in most cases, and these drugs can be tapered over a period of days to weeks after symptoms have subsided. Although minor tranquilizers, of which benzodiazepines are the drugs of choice, can alleviate short-term anxiety symptoms associated with withdrawal, the physician must carefully weigh their potential for paradoxically causing aggressiveness, although rare, in a patient who may already exhibit signs of aggressiveness. Moreover, the minor tranquilizers have their own potential for abuse. Nevertheless, some authors have suggested that benzodiazepines may be useful in the treatment of anabolic steroid withdrawal that is characterized by hyperadrenergic symptoms (Rosse & Deutsch, 1990).

Indications for Hospitalization

When the patient is suicidal, hospitalization may be needed. Other patients may manifest irritability and hostility during the initial withdrawal period. If the patient has been violent or presents a danger to others, then hospitalization is usually required. A third indication for hospitalization is when the patient has been unable to initiate abstinence as an outpatient.

Preferred Approach

The preferred approach is rapid discontinuation of anabolic steroids accompanied by supportive therapy and watchful waiting. If symptoms are prolonged or severe, pharmacotherapy and/or hospitalization may be needed. All patients require an evaluation for suicidal thoughts.

Endocrine pharmacotherapies directed at the HPG axis are not routinely recommended, because of the absence of studies demonstrating their efficacy in illicit steroid users. Endocrinologists should be consulted prior to endocrine pharmacotherapy. HCG may have some advantages compared to other endocrine pharmacotherapies. First, there is research evidence that steroid abusers during withdrawal respond to HCG with increased testosterone levels (Martikainen et al., 1986). Second, the injections can be administered in the physician's office; this periodic contact between physician and patient allows monitoring and support as well as prevents illegal diversion of prescription drugs. Third, HCG has FDA approval in the treatment of hypogonadotropic hypogonadism, a condition that characterizes withdrawal from anabolic steroids. Fourth, HCG stimulates the testes and should not lead to further suppression of the HPG axis, as might occur with the administration of testosterone esters.

In terms of pharmacotherapy for symptomatic relief, each of the agents deserves consideration depending on which symptoms dominate the clinical picture. However, antidepressants and NSAIDs will likely be the most commonly used agents, because depressive symptoms and musculoskeletal pains are frequently reported and can easily lead to resumed use of anabolic steroids. Antidepressants have been reported to successfully treat major depression associated with anabolic steroid withdrawal (Cowan, 1994; Malone & Dimeff, 1992), although one case of medication-resistant depression has also been reported (Allnutt & Chaimowitz, 1994).

Pros and Cons of Treatment

Supportive therapy is necessary but requires a psychological orientation and can be time-intensive. Patients may require referrals to clinicians who provide this type of care, if the treating physician is not so inclined. Pharmacotherapy offers the hope of more rapid relief of symptoms and restoration of HPG functioning. It is essential for the treatment of coexisting diagnoses such as major depression or psychosis but is considered adjunctive in the treatment of anabolic steroid withdrawal. Unfortunately, pharmacotherapy is completely unstudied for the treatment of anabolic steroid withdrawal, and each of the agents has its own side effects that the physician must consider. Moreover, patients may abuse some of the drugs given to them or divert them for illicit sales.

Although providing supportive therapy and pharmacological relief of symptoms may facilitate both initial abstinence and trust in the physician, the treatment of withdrawal symptoms (detoxification) is only the first step in managing steroid dependence. Patients may require rehabilitation to rebuild their lives without the use of anabolic steroids and other drugs (Brower, 1989; Corcoran & Longo, 1992). Further clinical research is needed to determine the optimal combinations of treatment for anabolic-androgenic steroid withdrawal and dependence.

Conclusions

Knowledge of the clinical manifestations of anabolic steroid use will help clinicians identify and assess anabolic steroid users. The highest risk patients are young males who lift weights for the purposes of enhancing either athletic performance or physical appearance. Dissatisfaction with body size and knowing other steroid users are potential risk factors for steroid use among nonusing male weightlifters. The physician should take a complete history and conduct both a physical and mental status examination as well as pertinent laboratory tests. Among steroid users, clinicians should assess the user's motivation in seeking treatment and ascertain signs and symptoms of dependence. Abstinence is the preferred goal of treatment, but harm-reduction approaches may be useful for some steroid users who refuse to discontinue steroid use. Although optimal treatment strategies must await further research, attention to both pharmacological and psychosocial factors is crucial in treating anabolic steroid users.

References

Aide, A.E. (1989). Surgical treatment of gynecomastia in the body builder. *Plastic and Reconstructive Surgery, 83,* 61–66.

Alen, M., & Rahkila, P. (1988). Anabolic-androgenic steroid effects on endocrinology and lipid metabolism in athletes. *Sports Medicine, 6,* 327–332.

Alen, M., Reinila, M., & Vihko, R. (1985). Response of serum hormones to androgen administration in power athletes. *Medicine and Science in Sports and Exercise, 17,* 354–359.

Allnutt, S., & Chaimowitz, G. (1994). Anabolic steroid withdrawal depression: A case report. *Canadian Journal of Psychiatry, 39,* 317–318.

Alpert, J.S., Pape, L.A., Ward, A., & Rippe, J.M. (1989). Athletic heart syndrome. *The Physician and Sportsmedicine, 17*(7), 103–107.

American Psychiatric Association. (1994). *Diagnostic and statistical manual of mental disorders* (4th ed. [*DSM-IV*]). Washington, DC: Author.

Bahrke, M.S., & Yesalis, C.E. (1994). Weight training: A potential confounding factor in examining the psychological and behavioural effects of anabolic-androgenic steroids. *Sports Medicine, 18,* 309–318.

Bahrke, M.S., Yesalis, C.E., & Wright, J.E. (1996). Psychological and behavioural effects of endogenous testosterone levels and anabolic-androgenic steroids among males: An update. *Sports Medicine, 22,* 367–390.

Barker, S. (1987). Oxymethalone and aggression (Letter to the editor). *British Journal of Psychiatry, 151,* 564.

Bhasin, S., Storer, T.W., Berman, N., Callegari, C., Clevenger, B., Phillips, J., Bunnell, T.J., Tricker, R., Shirazi, A., & Casaburi, R. (1996). The effects of supraphysiologic doses of testosterone on muscle size and strength in normal men. *New England Journal of Medicine, 335,* 1–7.

Bickelman, C., Ferries, L., & Eaton, R.P. (1995). Impotence related to anabolic steroid use in a body builder. Response to clomiphene citrate. *Western Journal of Medicine, 162,* 158–160.

Blouin, A.G., & Goldfield, G.S. (1995). Body image and steroid use in male bodybuilders. *International Journal of Eating Disorders, 18,* 159–165.

Braunstein, G.D., & Glassman, H.A. (1997). Gynecomastia. In C.W. Bardin (Ed.), *Current therapy in endocrinology and metabolism* (6th ed., pp. 401–404). St. Louis: Mosby.

Brower, K.J. (1989). Rehabilitation for anabolic-androgenic steroid dependence. *Clinical Sports Medicine, 1,* 171–181.

Brower, K.J. (1997). Withdrawal from anabolic steroids. In C.W. Bardin (Ed.), *Current therapy in endocrinology and metabolism* (6th ed., pp. 338–343). St. Louis: Mosby.

Brower, K.J., Blow, F.C., Beresford, T.P., & Fuelling, C. (1989). Anabolic-androgenic steroid dependence. *Journal of Clinical Psychiatry, 50,* 31–33.

Brower, K.J., Blow, F.C., Eliopulos, G.A., & Beresford, T.P. (1989). Anabolic-androgenic steroids and suicide [Letter to the editor]. *American Journal of Psychiatry, 146,* 1075.

Brower, K.J., Blow, F.C., & Hill, E.M. (1994). Risk factors for anabolic-androgenic steroid use in men. *Journal of Psychiatric Research, 28*(4), 369–380.

Brower, K.J., Blow, F.C., Young, J.A., & Hill, E.M. (1991). Symptoms and correlates of anabolic-androgenic steroid dependence. *British Journal of Addiction, 86,* 759–768.

Brower, K.J., Catlin, D.H., Blow, F.C., Eliopulos, G.A., & Beresford, T.P. (1991). Clinical assessment and urine testing for anabolic-androgenic steroid abuse and dependence. *American Journal of Drug and Alcohol Abuse, 17,* 161–171.

Brower, K.J., Eliopulos, G.A., Blow, F.C., Catlin, D.H., & Beresford, T.P. (1990). Evidence for physical and psychological dependence on anabolic androgenic steroids in eight weight lifters. *American Journal of Psychiatry, 147,* 510–512.

Brower, K.J., & Rootenberg, J.H. (1999). Counseling for substance abuse problems. In R. Ray, D.M. Wiese-Bjornstal (Eds.), *Counseling in Sports Medicine* (pp. 179–204). Champaign, IL: Human Kinetics.

Brower, K.J., & Severin, J.D. (1997). Alcohol and other drug-related problems. In D. Knesper, M. Riba, T. Schwenk (Eds.), *Primary care psychiatry.* Philadelphia: Saunders.

Butcher, D., Behre, H.M., Kliesch, S., & Nieschlag, E. (1998). Pulsatile GnRH or human chorionic gonadotropin/human menopausal gonadotropin as effective treatment for men with hypogonadotropic hypogonadism: A review of 42 cases. *European Journal of Endocrinology, 139,* 298–303.

Clancy, G.P., & Yates, W.R. (1992). Anabolic steroid use among substance abusers in treatment. *Journal of Clinical Psychiatry, 53*(3), 97–100.

Cohen, J.C., & Hickman, R. (1987). Insulin resistance and diminished glucose tolerance in powerlifters ingesting anabolic steroids. *Journal of Clinical Endocrinology and Metabolism, 64,* 960–963.

Corcoran, J.P., & Longo, E.L. (1992). Psychological treatment of anabolic-androgenic steroid-dependent individuals. *Journal of Substance Abuse Treatment, 9,* 229–235.

Cowan, C.B. (1994). Depression in anabolic steroid withdrawal. *Irish Journal of Psychological Medicine, 11,* 27–28.

Di Pasquale, M.G. (1987). *Drug use and detection in amateur sports (updates one and two).* Warkworth, ON, Canada: M.G.D. Press.

Di Pasquale, M.G. (1990). *Anabolic steroid side effects: Facts, fiction and treatment.* Warkworth, ON, Canada: M.G.D. Press.

Elofson, G., & Elofson, S. (1990). Steroids claimed our son's life. *The Physician and Sportsmedicine, 18,* 15–16.

Ferrera, P.C., Putman, D.L., & Verdile, V.P. (1997). Anabolic steroid use as the possible precipitant of dilated cardiomyopathy. *Cardiology, 88,* 218–220.

Forbes, G.B., Porta, C.R., Herr, B.E., & Griggs, R.C. (1992). Sequence of changes in body composition induced by testosterone and reversal of changes after drug is stopped. *Journal of the American Medical Association, 267,* 397–399.

Frankle, M., & Leffers, D. (1992). Athletes on anabolic-androgenic steroids: New approach diminishes health problems. *The Physician and Sportsmedicine, 20*(6), 75–87.

Freed, D.L., Banks, A.J., Longson, D., & Burley, D.M. (1975). Anabolic steroids in athletics: Crossover double-blind trial on weightlifters. *British Medical Journal, 2,* 471–473.

Friedl, K.E., & Yesalis, C.E. (1989). Self-treatment of gynecomastia in bodybuilders who use anabolic steroids. *The Physician and Sportsmedicine, 17,* 67–79.

Galloway, G.P. (1997). Anabolic-androgenic steroids. In J.H. Lowinson, P. Ruiz, R.P. Millman, & J.G. Langrod (Eds.), *Substance abuse: A comprehensive textbook* (3rd ed., pp. 308–318). Baltimore: Williams & Wilkins.

Hakkinen, K., & Alen, M. (1989). Training volume, androgen use and serum creatine kinase activity. *British Journal of Sports Medicine, 23,* 188–189.

Handelsman, L., Cochrane, K.J., Aronson, M.J., Ness, R., Rubinstein, K.J., & Kanof, P.D. (1987). Two new rating scales for opiate withdrawal. *American Journal of Drug and Alcohol Abuse, 13,* 293–308.

Haupt, H.A. (1993). Anabolic steroids and growth hormone. *American Journal of Sports Medicine, 21*(3), 468–474.

Haupt, H.A., & Rovere, G.D. (1984). Anabolic steroids: A review of the literature. *American Journal of Sports Medicine, 12,* 469–484.

Hays, L.R., Littleton, S., & Stillner, V. (1990). Anabolic steroid dependence [Letter to the editor]. *American Journal of Psychiatry, 147,* 122.

Hickson, R.C., Ball, K.L., & Falduto, M.T. (1989). Adverse effects of anabolic steroids. *Medical Toxicology and Adverse Drug Experience, 4,* 254–271.

Ishak, K.G., & Zimmerman, H.J. (1987). Hepatotoxic effects of the anabolic/androgenic steroids. *Seminars in Liver Disease, 7,* 230–236.

Jarow, J.P., & Lipshultz, L.I. (1990). Anabolic steroid-induced hypogonadotropic hypogonadism. *American Journal of Sports Medicine, 18,* 429–431.

Kashkin, K.B., & Kleber, H.D. (1989). Hooked on hormones? An anabolic steroid addiction hypothesis. *Journal of the American Medical Association, 262,* 3166–3170.

Kibble, M.W., & Ross, M.B. (1987). Adverse effects of anabolic steroids in athletes. *Clinical Pharmacy, 6,* 686–692.

Kiraly, C.L. (1988). Androgenic-anabolic steroid effects on serum and skin surface lipids, on red cells, and on liver enzymes. *International Journal of Sports Medicine, 9,* 249–252.

Knuth, U.A., Maniera, H., & Nieschlag, E. (1989). Anabolic steroids and semen parameters in bodybuilders. *Fertility and Sterility, 52,* 1041–1047.

Larkin, G.L. (1991). Carcinoma of the prostate (Letter to the editor). *New England Journal of Medicine, 324,* 1892.

Lenders, J.W.M., Demacker, P.N.M., Vos, J.A., Jansen, P.L.M., Hoitsma, A.J., van't Lar, A., & Thien, T. (1988). Deleterious effects of anabolic steroids on serum lipoproteins, blood pressure, and liver function in amateur body builders. *International Journal of Sports Medicine, 9,* 19–23.

Littlepage, B.N.C., & Perry, H.M. (1993). Misusing anabolic drugs: Possibilities for future policies. *Addiction, 88,* 1469–1471.

Malone, D.A., Jr. (1995). Pharmacological therapies of anabolic androgenic steroid addiction. In N.S. Miller & M.S. Gold (Eds.), *Pharmacological therapies for drug and alcohol addictions* (pp. 227–237). New York: Marcel Dekker.

Malone, D.A., Jr., & Dimeff, R.J. (1992). The use of fluoxetine in depression associated with anabolic steroid withdrawal: A case series. *Journal of Clinical Psychiatry, 53,* 130–132.

Malone, D.A., Jr., Dimeff, R.J., Lombardo, J.A., & Sample, R.H.B. (1995). Psychiatric effects and psychoactive substance use in anabolic-androgenic steroid users. *Clinical Journal of Sport Medicine, 5,* 25–31.

Martikainen, H., Alen, M., Rahkila, P., & Vihko, R. (1986). Testicular responsiveness to human chorionic gonadotropin during transient hypogonadotropic hypogonadism induced by androgenic/anabolic steroids in power athletes. *Journal of Steroid Biochemistry, 25,* 109–112.

McKillop, G., Ballantyne, F.C., Borland, W., & Ballantyne, D. (1989). Acute metabolic effects of exercise in bodybuilders using anabolic steroids. *British Journal of Sports Medicine, 23,* 186–187.

Melchert, R.B., & Welder, A.A. (1995). Cardiovascular effects of androgenic-anabolic steroids. *Medicine and Science in Sports and Exercise, 27*(9), 1252–1262.

Millar, A.P. (1994). Licit steroid use—hope for the future. *British Journal of Sports Medicine, 28*(2), 79–83.

Miller, W.R., & Rollnick, S. (1991). *Motivational interviewing: Preparing people to change addictive behavior.* New York: Guilford Press.

Morrison, C.L. (1994). Anabolic steroid users identified by needle and syringe exchange contact. *Drug and Alcohol Dependence, 36,* 153–155.

O'Connor, J.S., Skinner, J.S., Baldini, F.D., & Einstein, M. (1990). Blood chemistry of current and previous anabolic steroid users. *Military Medicine, 155,* 72–75.

Palatini, P., Giada, F., Garavelli, G., Sinisi, F., Mario, L., Michieletto, M., & Baldo-Enzi, G. (1996). Cardiovascular effects of anabolic steroids in weight trained subjects. *Journal of Clinical Pharmacology, 36,* 1132–1140.

Perry, P.J., Yates, W.R., & Andersen, K.H. (1990). Psychiatric symptoms associated with anabolic steroids: A controlled, retrospective study. *Annals of Clinical Psychiatry, 2,* 11–17.

Pope, H.G., Jr., & Brower, K.J. (1999). Anabolic steroids. In H.I. Kaplan & B.J. Sadock (Eds.), *Comprehensive textbook of psychiatry/VII.* Baltimore: Williams & Wilkins.

Pope, H.G., Jr., & Katz, D.L. (1988). Affective and psychotic symptoms associated with anabolic steroid abuse. *American Journal of Psychiatry, 145,* 487–490.

Pope, H.G., Jr., & Katz, D.L. (1994). Psychiatric and medical effects of anabolic-androgenic steroid use. *Archives of General Psychiatry, 51,* 375–382.

Roberts, J.T., & Essenhigh, D.M. (1986). Adenocarcinoma of prostate in 40-year-old bodybuilder. *Lancet, 2,* 742.

Rosse, R.B., & Deutsch, S.I. (1990). Hooked on hormones [Letter to the editor]. *Journal of the American Medical Association, 263,* 2048–2049.

Sachtleben, T.R., Berg, K.E., Cheatham, J.P., Felix, G.L., & Hofschire, P.J. (1997). Serum lipoproteins in long-term anabolic steroid users. *Research Quarterly for Exercise and Sport, 68*(1), 110–115.

Scott, M.J. (1989). Cutaneous side effects of anabolic-androgenic steroid use. *Clinical Sports Medicine, 1,* 5–16.

Soe, K.L., Soe, M., & Gluud, C. (1992). Liver pathology associated with the use of anabolic-androgenic steroids. *Liver, 12,* 73–79.

Tennant, F., Black, D.L., & Voy, R.O. (1988). Anabolic steroid dependence with opioid-type features [Letter to the editor]. *New England Journal of Medicine, 319,* 578–579.

Urhausen, A., Holpes, R., & Kindermann, W. (1989). One- and two-dimensional echocardiography in bodybuilders using anabolic steroids. *European Journal of Applied Physiology, 58,* 633–640.

Wadler, G.I., & Hainline, B. (1989). *Drugs and the athlete.* Philadelphia: Davis.

Wang, C., & Swerdloff, R.S. (1997). Androgen replacement therapy. In C.W. Bardin (Ed.), *Current therapy in endocrinology and metabolism* (6th ed., pp. 331–337). St. Louis: Mosby.

Wemyss, H.S., Hamdy, F.C., & Hastie, K.J. (1994). Steroid abuse in athletes, prostatic enlargement and bladder outflow obstruction—is there a relationship? *British Journal of Urology, 74,* 476–478.

Whitcomb, R.W., & Crowley, W.F., Jr. (1997). Hypogonadotropic hypogonadism: Gonadotropin-releasing hormone therapy. In C.W. Bardin (Ed.), *Current therapy in endocrinology and metabolism* (6th ed., pp. 353–355). St. Louis: Mosby.

Williamson, K., Davies, M., & McBride, A. (1992, September/October). A well-steroid user clinic. *Druglink,* 15.

Willis, K.J., London, D.R., Bevis, M.A., Butt, W.R., Lynch, S.S., & Holder, G. (1977). Hormonal effects of tamoxifen in oligospermic men. *Journal of Endocrinology, 73,* 171–178.

Wilson, J.D., (1988). Androgen abuse by athletes. *Endocrine Reviews, 9,* 181–199.

Yesalis, C.E., Wright, J., & Lombardo, J.A. (1989). Anabolic-androgenic steroids: A synthesis of existing data and recommendations for future research. *Clinical Sports Medicine, 1,* 109–134.

Zuliani, U., Bernardini, B., Catapano, A., Campana, M., Cerioli, G., & Spattini, M. (1988). Effects of anabolic steroids, testosterone, and HGH on blood lipids and echocardiographic parameters in body builders. *International Journal of Sports Medicine, 10,* 62–66.

CHAPTER

11

Legal Aspects of Anabolic Steroid Use and Abuse

Carol Cole Kleinman, MD, JD, and C.E. Petit, JD

But at the very least, [athletes using bodybuilding supplements] must test positive for stupidity...

John Bryant
The Times (London), February 10, 2000

Despite evidence of adverse physical effects, anabolic steroid use was largely ignored by state and federal laws until Canadian sprinter Ben Johnson tested positive at the Seoul Olympics in October 1988, after winning the gold medal in the men's 100 m. The stripping of Ben Johnson's gold medal dramatically increased the level of national and international attention focused on the problem. In the months following, there was a great deal of media attention about the possible epidemic use of these drugs among high-level athletes. A well-publicized study in the December 1988 issue of the *Journal of the American Medical Association* suggested that as many as half a million American adolescents could be using anabolic steroids (Buckley et al., 1988). These factors led to congressional interest in the problem of steroid use, resulting in the classification of anabolic steroids as a controlled substance on November 29, 1990.

Discussion of anabolic steroid abuse has been generally limited to the context of professional sports and major international sporting events such as the Olympics. The situation involving Michelle Smith de Bruin, the Irish swimmer, has grabbed worldwide headlines (Lord, 1998a). Anabolic steroid abuse is not limited to professional athletes, nor only to athletes. It has spread to amateur and lower-level athletes as well as to the general public. It is now an issue of great concern because of the significant and increasing percentage of young people involved in steroid abuse (see chapter 3). The problem is international in scope, and the control actions taken by a few nations have been, to date, unsuccessful.

Aware of the growing steroid abuse problem, the Drug Enforcement Administration (DEA) arranged for an International Conference on the Abuse and Trafficking of Anabolic Steroids, which was held December 7–10, 1993, in Prague, Czech Republic, including 19 nations and several international organizations (Haislip, 1994). The purposes of this conference, the first of its kind, were

- to develop recognition of the consequences of steroid abuse,
- to examine steroid trafficking at the national and international levels, and
- to explore appropriate responses to the steroid abuse problem.

The DEA reported to the conference that most cases investigated since anabolic steroids were made a controlled drug have involved international trafficking, with steroids entering the United States from all over the world. The DEA also reported that many steroid traffickers are involved with drugs other than steroids, especially cocaine, and that at the highest level the traffickers are well organized, never coming in contact with the drugs (Bahrke, 1994).

Only a few countries, including the United States, Canada, and Sweden, have enacted legislation so far to control steroids (Bahrke, 1994).

The Prague Conference concluded that governments should examine their national legislation with a view to strengthening controls over anabolic agents so as to curb their diversion into illicit traffic, and also to identify manufacturers and quantities produced, imported, and exported. The conference also agreed that national authorities, consistent with their national legislation, should increase their cooperation concerning the international commerce and movement of anabolic agents with a view to combating the diversion of these substances.

Several other areas of the law also affect steroid use and abuse. An athlete who tests positive for steroids may be banned from competing in his or her sport by the sport's governing body for a first offense—for as little as several games in the National Football League to two years or more in international swimming and athletics, and may receive a lifetime ban in the United States (federal and state) and in foreign countries for a second positive test. Legislation now on the books can also confront a user with serious state, federal, and international criminal charges. The United States federal government and virtually all states have laws against the distribution, possession, or prescription of anabolic steroids for nonmedical use (Yesalis et al., 1997).

In addition to masculinization of females and a variety of potential adverse long-term health consequences, steroid use has been associated with psychotic symptoms, including hallucinations, paranoia, delusions of grandeur, and severe mood disorders (Pope & Katz, 1988). It goes without saying that crimes committed while taking steroids can and do lead to state prosecution. At the same time, the severity of legal consequences faced by a steroid user for such crimes as murder, robbery, arson, domestic violence, assault and battery, and other felonies and misdemeanors associated with loss of control can vary from jurisdiction to jurisdiction (Jancin, 1989).

Anabolic steroids are merely one example of the broader problem of performance-enhancing drugs (PEDs). Effective legal control of the use and trafficking of anabolic steroids could drive athletes to the use of other, possibly more dangerous PEDs. Thus, anabolic steroid abuse is part of a far broader public policy issue.

Direct Legal Consequences of Steroid Abuse

The law directly concerns itself with two aspects of steroid abuse. The first, and most publicly known, is testing for steroid abuse among competitive athletes. The law also regulates traffic in steroids, treating them as controlled substances.

Testing

In 1988, the Ben Johnson incident and the documentation of steroid use by adolescents placed the issue of steroid use firmly on the legislative agenda of many states. Within two years, 31 states had passed legislation to control steroid use (Blowman, 1992). In all this legislation, states used state laws, regulations, and/or mandated education programs. None of this legislation specifically addressed drug testing of world-class athletes. That was left to nongovernmental sport institutions, such as the professional sport leagues, the National Collegiate Athletic Association (NCAA), and, with respect to Olympic sports, the United States Olympic Committee and the national governing bodies in the United States that are responsible for those sports under the provisions of the Amateur Sports Act of 1978.

The rationale underlying drug testing for anabolic steroids is that testing allegedly deters anabolic steroid use in sports. Drug testing, therefore, attempts to reduce demand for anabolic steroids, as opposed to controlled substance scheduling and prohibition, which attempts to reduce supply. However, drug testing cannot address the problem of steroid use by nonathletes. About 30 to 45% of the anabolic steroid user group in high school and college do not participate in competitive sports (Buckley et al., 1988). They use steroids simply to enhance size, strength, appearance, and self-confidence, rather than to improve athletic performance.

Drug testing has been part of sports for more than thirty years. Participating in sports sponsored by private sport associations is not a right but a privilege, and most of the legal decisions upholding testing are based on that principle. This derives from the fact that sport organizations are, by and large, private associations, and such membership is an intangible property right. Traditionally, the courts have given private associations wide latitude to control and define those rights. When private organizations do propose testing athletes for drugs, a criterion of the testing program should be that clear evidence can be demonstrated of a relationship between use of the banned drugs and their adverse effects on performance, health, or quality of the competition.

In order to be at least somewhat effective, drug testing for anabolic steroids must be random, frequent, and unannounced (see chapters 12 and 13). Sanctions for positive tests must be significant enough to deter steroid use. A reduced incidence of positive tests may not imply reduced steroid use, but a switch to less detectable forms of PEDs. There are several forms of anabolic steroids on the market for which tests currently lack adequate sensitivity. For example, many athletes use esters of testosterone that are difficult to detect (see chapter 13).

The major financial cost of drug testing is the testing itself. Institutions incur costs of about $50 to $250 per test for collecting, storing, and shipping samples, and the laboratories charge about $100 more for analyzing the sample. The cost of drug testing at each of the last three Summer Olympic Games exceeded $2 million. If each of the approximately one million high school football players in the United States were tested just once yearly, the cost would be more than $150 million.

In 1986, the National Collegiate Athletic Association responded to allegations of college athletes' use of controlled substances and PEDs by enacting a mandatory drug-testing program. This program sparked much debate regarding the constitutionality of mandatory drug testing, generating challenges based on both federal and state constitutional protections (Scanlan, 1987; Locke & Jennings, 1986; Meloch, 1987; Ford, 1984; Martin, 1989).

Suspicionless Drug Testing and Privacy

The United States Supreme Court has considered drug testing in three different contexts. In *National Treasury Employees Union v. Von Raab* (1989), the Court considered whether the suspicionless drug testing of United States Customs employees who apply for promotions to positions involving the interdiction of drugs or requiring the handling of firearms was constitutional under the Fourth Amendment. The Fourth Amendment provides that "the right of the people to be secure in their persons, houses, papers, and effect, against unreasonable searches and seizures, shall not be violated. . . ." The Court held that under the Fourth Amendment, the drug testing, conducted without a warrant or individualized suspicion, was constitutional. The Court ruled that the drug testing was reasonable because the Customs officials' expectations of privacy were outweighed by compelling governmental interests.

Similarly, in *Skinner v. Railway Labor Executives' Association* (1989), the Supreme Court ruled that the random drug testing of certain railroad employees was constitutional. When the Court balanced the privacy interests of the employees against the governmental interests, it found that the otherwise valid expectations of privacy were diminished because the industry in which the employees worked was pervasively regulated to assure public safety. Although taking samples of bodily fluids does impinge on Fourth Amendment privacy interests, the Court found taking urine samples as prescribed in the regulation relatively unintrusive. The Court therefore concluded that public safety concerns outweighed the Fourth Amendment privacy interest of the employees.

Vernonia School District No. 47J v. Acton (1995) is the most recent decision in this line of cases, and directly concerns scholastic and collegiate athletics. The Supreme Court ruled that a school district's random drug testing of its athletes was constitutional under the Fourth Amendment of the U.S. Constitution. As in *Von Raab* and *Skinner*, the Court found that government-compelled urinalysis implicated an individual's privacy interests. The Court, relying on its earlier decision in *New Jersey v. T.L.O.* (1985), stated that because the urinalysis was conducted in the public school setting, it fell within the "special need" category of searches, eliminating the need for a warrant of probable cause. "Fourth . . . Amendment rights . . . are different in public school than elsewhere; the 'reasonableness' inquiry cannot disregard the schools' custodial and tutelary responsibility for children." The continual regulation of public school children, be it student vaccinations, physical exams, or implementation of rules of conduct, according to the Court, serves to diminish their expectations of privacy. The court found that student athletes have particularly diminished expectations of privacy because they subject themselves to a more regulated life, and they voluntarily expose themselves to the revealing circumstances of the locker room.

After considering the scope of the students' privacy interests, the Court focused on the intrusiveness of urinalysis. The court recognized that such an examination intruded upon a bodily function traditionally accorded great privacy. The seriousness of the intrusion, according to the Court, depended on how the monitoring was conducted. The Court concluded that the school district's policy was not significantly intrusive because the male athletes remained fully clothed and were monitored, if at all, from behind and the female athletes provided urine samples in enclosed stalls. The Court also briefly considered how the test intruded upon the private sphere of one's medical information. The Court found that the drug-testing program was not unnecessarily invasive of this aspect of the students' privacy because the test screened only for drugs. In addition, the kind of drugs tested for did not vary from individual to individual, and the results were available only to a limited number of school personnel.

The Court acknowledged the respondents' concern that, in order to prevent false positive readings, the student athlete had to reveal, in advance, medication he or she was taking. However, the court noted that this requirement has never been held per se unreasonable. It dismissed this concern by pointing out that the school policy did not prohibit the randomly chosen student from bypassing school officials and giving this information directly to the testing facility. In summary, the Court was satisfied that the interests of deterring drug use and protecting the health and safety of student athletes were important enough to overcome the student athletes' privacy rights.

These three Supreme Court cases are consistent with drug-testing law as it developed in the 1980s (LaFave & Israel, 1992). This particularly resulted in reduced expectations of privacy for students and athletes. For example, in *O'Halloran v. University of Washington* (1988), the United States District Court for the Western District of Washington upheld the validity of the NCAA drug-testing program under the Fourth Amendment. The Court found sufficient evidence of student athlete drug use to justify random urinalysis. Moreover, the court ruled that the diminished expectations of privacy in collegiate athletics were outweighed by the NCAA's countervailing interests in the health and safety of student athletes and in fair competition. Thus, under the reasonableness standard of the Fourth Amendment, the court held that the NCAA drug-testing program was constitutional.

Many athletes have argued that mandatory drug testing violates a student-athlete's privacy rights. Privacy as a right springs from several sources, both federal and state (Gormley, 1992). Because several state constitutions offer a greater level of protection than the federal constitution, students have attempted to challenge the NCAA program on state grounds. Recognizing the federal courts' inability to prohibit NCAA testing on federal constitutional grounds, opponents hoped that these state challenges would be successful.

Federal challenges to the NCAA program have little chance of succeeding. In order to prevail, plaintiffs must prove that the challenged conduct constituted state action and that the "conduct deprived [the athlete] of rights, privileges or immunities secured by the Constitution or laws of the United States." The United States Supreme Court has definitively stated that the NCAA is not a state actor. Currently, student athletes have been unable to establish that the drug-testing program has deprived them of a right guaranteed by the federal constitution. Therefore, challenges to NCAA drug testing will fail both prongs of a successful federal constitutional challenge. The right to privacy provided in the United States Constitution, then, does not offer student athletes sufficient protection to prohibit the NCAA from testing athletes.

For that reason, many commentators looked to *Hill v. National Collegiate Athletic Association* for a definitive statement that drug testing violates the right to privacy. In *Hill*, the California Supreme Court analyzed the Privacy Initiative of the California Constitution in light of the NCAA's policy of testing collegiate athletes for drug use. To determine whether the NCAA's policy violated the students' right to privacy, the court examined whether the right to privacy enumerated in the California Constitution governs nongovernmental entities. The court held that the right of privacy protects the citizenry against intrusions by private actors as well as governmental entities. Additionally, the court established the standards for determining when an invasion of privacy occurs. The court applied these findings to the facts of *Hill*, and determined that the NCAA's drug-testing program nonetheless did not violate the California Constitution. Other cases have upheld the right of private organizations such as the International Olympic Committee (IOC) and the National Football League (NFL) to conduct drug testing.

Finally, one must remember that this discussion applies only in the United States. With the increasing internationalization of sport, the laws of other regions and nations will become more and more relevant, even to American athletes. For example, Michelle Smith de Bruin, an Irish swimmer, submitted an out-of-competition sample in early 1998 that was contaminated with a high level of alcohol (Lord, 1998a). The contamination was alleged to have occurred after the sample was procured, since the level of alcohol in the urine sample was so high that had it come from her body, the dose would have been lethal. She lost her initial challenge to sanctions in front of FINA, the international swimming federation. The next step is the Court for Arbitration in Sport (CAS; see discussion below). However, should the CAS reject her position, she intends to appeal the entire testing procedure to the European Court of Human Rights (Lord, 1998b). Presuming that she overcomes several procedural hurdles to such review, recent decisions of that court on other privacy issues indicate that it is unlikely to agree with the sweeping scope of the U.S. Supreme Court's decisions, and may well completely contradict them.

Due Process

The IOC and other international sporting bodies are concerned about the ability of athletes to challenge drug-testing procedures, results, and sanctions in national courts. The intervention of national courts could wreak havoc on the whole idea of an international regime prohibiting PEDs. If a suspended athlete can obtain a court order reversing an IOC decision or injunction allowing him/her to continue competing while more procedures are exhausted, the whole enforcement system will collapse. Even if the athlete is ultimately unsuccessful, the delay may have in effect negated the sanction. Moreover, the cost to the sport governing body of defending such suits may be prohibitive and therefore become a major impediment to realizing the goals of the drug-testing project.

Some athletes have challenged drug testing on due process grounds. For example, in one case the plaintiff claimed that the procedures offered to challenge a positive result were insufficient on due process grounds (*Schaill v. Tippecanoe County School Corporation,* 1988). However, the court found that any liberty interest was not infringed because the stigma attached to being removed from an athletic team was minimal.

A recent trend in international sport competitions has been to restrict athletes' rights to sue by requiring them to sign an arbitration agreement before competing. For example, in order to compete in the 1996 Summer Olympics in Atlanta, athletes were required to agree to resolve any disputes through arbitration, except that they were allowed to use the courts in cases of "gross violation of due process, fundamental rights or public order." Commentators agree that there needs to be a way to discourage national courts and legislatures from interfering with drug testing. Although national courts have generally deferred to the law of international sport federations, international sporting organizations are particularly concerned about litigation in American courts (Downes, 1998;

Barnes v. International Amateur Athletic Federation, 1993; *Reynolds v. International Amateur Athletic Federation,* 1994).

On the other hand, arbitration presents a viable replacement for the courts in resolving doping accusations if, and only if, the arbitration procedure provides adequate protection for due process (Gorman, 1995; Federal Arbitration Act [FAA], 1994). The so-called Court for Arbitration in Sport (CAS), established for the Atlanta Games and continued since, does not appear to provide such protection.

- The arbitrators are under the influence and often control of the governing body bringing the charge—a potential conflict of interest, possibly sufficient to void the arbitration (FAA, § 10(a)(2); *Hooters v. Phillips*, 1998; *Rosenberg v. Merrill Lynch*, 1998; *Graham v. Scissor-Tail*, 1981).
- The various governing federations, and the CAS, have a history of inconsistently assessing penalties for positive test results. This raises further questions about the impartiality not of individual panels, but of the system itself. For example, dissatisfied after Mary Decker Slaney was cleared of doping charges by U.S. Track and Field, the international federation has decided to reopen its case against Decker Slaney—over two and a half years after the test that led to the initial charges (Downes, 1998).
- The time frame for in-competition testing is so short that an accused athlete has little or no opportunity to investigate, let alone controvert, the "fact" of the positive test result. Any defense must arise from a technical failure by the governing federation, such as Ross Rebagliati's escape after a positive test for marijuana at the Nagano Olympic Games. One U.S. court recently refused to require arbitration when an employer unilaterally imposed an arbitration plan that eliminated an employee's remedies, gave the employer the sole approval over arbitrators, and essentially eliminated discovery, witness disclosure, and judicial review (*Hooters v. Phillips,* 1998).
- Given the recent trend toward criminalization of steroids, the arbitral system appears to be moving dangerously close to the boundary of a potentially criminal proceeding. It is not difficult to imagine attempts to admit the result of the CAS's limited inquiry as evidence in a later criminal proceeding against an athlete. While Anglo-American rules of evidence *should* prevent admission of the evidence, the athlete will suffer obvious prejudice from the "verdict" itself and from the prosecution's attempts to admit the "verdict."

Every nation has its own view of due process and of athletes' substantive rights; inevitably, there will be conflict between one or more nations' laws and IAAF and IOC rules. Ultimately, an international Performance Enhancing Drug Elimination Treaty signed by all nations may be necessary to keep drug-testing cases out of national courts. Such an agreement will need to establish a single dispute-resolution mechanism. Any appeal of sanctions must be to a body independent of the organization imposing the sanctions. The CAS is probably not sufficiently independent to serve this appellate function.

Other due process concerns involve basic principles of fairness, such as timely notification of a positive test, an opportunity for the athlete to appear and refute the findings, and an appeals process for correction of any errors. Much concern has been expressed that some sport organizations are inconsistent or uneven in their publication and sanctions regarding positive tests (Lord, 1998a, 1998b). Organizations are vulnerable to law suits for selective application of standards. These questions are sure to come up as the drug-testing rules face future legal challenges.

Trafficking in Steroids

Historically the FDA and state agencies have regulated anabolic steroids (*Legislation to Amend,* 1988; Taylor, 1991). The passage of the Federal Food, Drug, and Cosmetic Act (FDCA) in 1938 established criteria for the classification of prescription drugs. This action was intended to restrict access to certain drugs to people with legitimate medical needs. For example, synthetic testosterone was classified as a prescription drug by the FDA in the same year. Later, as different chemical derivatives and some of the precursors of testosterone entered the market, they too were classified as prescription drugs.

The FDA determines whether a substance falls within the over-the-counter (OTC) or prescription category; each state then has the legal power to determine who can legally prescribe and dispense OTC and prescription substances. By 1973, growing awareness that anabolic steroids, with other drugs, were being used by healthy athletes to enhance athletic performance brought the issue to the attention of policy makers. Hearings were held before the Senate Subcommittee to Investigate Juvenile Delinquency in June and July of 1973 (*Proper and Improper Use,* 1973). However, despite general acceptance of the opinion that nonmedical use of anabolic steroids should be stopped, no legislation was passed to regulate such use for 15 years.

By 1987, a gradual increase in the awareness of anabolic steroid use in sports again led to public congressional hearings. In May 1987, hearings before the House Subcommittee on Health and the Environment considered a bill to make human growth hormone a controlled substance. In July of that year, a bill strengthening the penalties for the distribution of anabolic steroids was referred to the House Committee on Energy and Commerce. In July 1988, hearings were held before the House Subcommittee on Crime on a bill to make one anabolic steroid, methandrosterolone, a controlled substance.

Finally, in 1988, legislation covering anabolic steroids was passed as sections 2401 and 2403 of the broader federal Anti-Drug Abuse Act of 1988 (also called the Omnibus Drug Abuse Initiative). It placed a special category of anabolic steroids within the prescription class, and all violations involving the sale or possession with intent to distribute anabolic steroids became felonies. Section 2401 provides for the "forfeiture of property of an individual convicted of a violation of the FDCA involving steroids or human growth hormone if such a violation is punishable for more than one year." Section 2403 imposes criminal liability upon "any person who distributes or possesses with the intent to distribute any anabolic steroid for any use in humans other than the treatment of disease pursuant to the order of a physician. . . ."

Even before the passage of the Anti-Drug Abuse Act, it was illegal to possess anabolic steroids without a prescription in all 50 states, whether the steroids were intended for human or animal use. The Anti-Drug Abuse Act added teeth to the state control. Many states have since adopted legislative or regulatory versions of the Act (Yesalis et al., 1997).

However, not all steroids and precursors have been treated consistently. For example, dehydroepiandrosterone (DHEA) is a steroidal hormone produced by the adrenal glands. It is the natural precursor to testosterone. It is heavily marketed as a "food supplement" in health food stores and is also available through AIDS buyers' clubs. It is advertised as a "fat fighter" for weight control, cancer prevention, and life extension. Health food stores state that DHEA "may have a profound influence on positive body composition alteration favoring lean muscle tissue accrual." DHEA has not been approved for any indication by the FDA. According to *The Medical Letter* ("Preliminary Draft," 1996), it may prevent catabolism, cardiovascular disease, and aging with no adverse effects.

Until 1994, DHEA was regarded as a "drug" within the meaning of section 201(g) of the Federal Food, Drug, and Cosmetic Act. Since it was not generally recognized as safe and effective, it was a "new drug" within the meaning of sections 201(p) and 505(a) of the act. The FDA was able to seize the products or issue an injunction against the manufacturer or distributor of these illegal products. In 1984, the FDA instituted a class action to remove these products from the market (Chastonay, 1984). Since the passage of the Dietary Supplement Health and Education Act of 1994 (DSHEA), DHEA, a steroid that in the presence of certain enzymes could be translated to testosterone in the body, is considered a dietary supplement. Under the DSHEA, dietary supplement manufacturers can make statements of nutritional support ("structure" or "function" claims), without preclearance and without subjecting the product to regulation as a drug. Only when the manufacturers make statements claiming to diagnose, treat, cure, or prevent disease are they subject to regulation as a drug. Before 1994, the FDA was effective in removing steroid alternatives, like DHEA, from the market. Now the burden of proof is on the FDA to show that the dietary supplement is unsafe and is causing harm, before it can be removed from the marketplace. Hence DHEA, which was formerly regulated by the FDA, is now widely available without the controls that existed in the past. On the other hand, testosterone is still treated as a drug, requires a prescription to obtain, and is strictly controlled by the FDA. Androstendione's availability as an over-the-counter "supplement" continues for the same reason—the FDA has not yet conducted the years-long process necessary to show that it is unsafe and causing harm.

Enforcement Efforts

Anabolic steroids became a Schedule III controlled substance when President George Bush signed the Anabolic Steroid Control Act of 1990 on November 28 of that year. The act further criminalized illegal drug trafficking of anabolic steroids. Controlled substance status transferred primary responsibility for the control and enforcement of steroids from the Food and Drug Administration (FDA) to the Drug Enforcement Administration (DEA). The DEA now controls the manufacture, importation, exportation, distribution and dispensing of anabolic steroids.

While Congress has the authority to place any substance on any controlled substance schedule, the scheduling of anabolic steroids by Congress marked the first bypassing of the regular scheduling process. The regular scheduling process involves the Attorney General, acting on findings from the Secretary of the U.S. Department of Health and Human Services (USDHHS), placing a drug on a controlled substance schedule (*Legislation to Amend,* 1988).

Classification of controlled substances is based on five schedules according to the potential for abuse and dependence, and on the existence of legitimate medical uses. The Attorney General must base scheduling on evidence of health effects. The American Medical Association (AMA) does not believe that anabolic steroids should have been scheduled, since their effects on health remain to be proven.

> *[The] medical facts do not support the scheduling of anabolic steroids as a controlled substance. Anabolic steroids can be used safely under medical supervision ... have an accepted medical use ... [and] abuse has not been shown to lead to physical or psychological dependence. (Legislation to Amend, 1988)*

Moreover, the AMA argues that legislative scheduling undermines the regular scheduling process through DHHS and the Attorney General. The

AMA regards the scheduling of anabolic steroids by Congress as an unwarranted precedent.

The scheduling of anabolic steroids created stiffer penalties for their illegal use. For example, simple illegal possession of anabolic steroids without any federal or state drug conviction is punishable by up to 1 year in prison and/or a fine of $1,000 to $5,000. If there is an existing drug conviction, illegal possession will result in not less than 15 days and no more than 2 years and/or a fine of no less than $2,500, but not to exceed $10,000. However, the sentencing system imposed by the United States Sentencing Guidelines results in significantly lower penalties in practice. Finally, the scheduling of anabolic steroids cannot address the reduction of performance-enhancing drug (PED) use on the whole, since other PEDs such as creatine and pseudoephedrine hydrochloride are not controlled.

There has been no single federal agency or state authority with complete responsibility for controlling the abuse and trafficking of anabolic steroids. Since the onset of a nationwide anabolic steroid investigation in 1985, the FDA and the Department of Justice, through the DEA, have assumed a leadership role in coordinating federal investigations of anabolic steroid trafficking. A number of federal agencies participate in enforcing statutes and regulations to reduce illicit trafficking of anabolic steroids. In addition, individual states play a role in investigating anabolic steroid offenses.

In 1990, a federal interagency task force was formed to coordinate federal and state approaches to steroid drug trafficking. Among the task force's conclusions were the following:

- A single federal agency should serve as the lead agency and be vested with the primary responsibility and commensurate resources and investigative authorities.
- Any effort to interdict anabolic steroid trafficking must also include counterfeit steroids in view of their possible health effects.
- Involving other agencies will be necessary to effectively interdict the smuggling and counterfeiting of anabolic steroids.

The task force called for further epidemiologic and etiologic research on which to build a steroid prevention program. It suggested involving other federal agencies in both disseminating information about the harmful effects of steroids and effective programs to combat their use (USDHHS, 1991).

In late 1994, the DEA, Office of Diversion Control, sponsored a conference in Annapolis, Maryland, on the impact of national steroid control legislation in the United States. The conference was attended by representatives of law enforcement, the federal government, and the international scientific community. The purpose of the conference was to analyze the impact of the Anabolic Steroid Control Act of 1990 both from law enforcement and scientific standpoints and to examine what has been accomplished as a result of this legislation. The conference sought to evaluate the current situation with regard to steroid abuse and diversion.

The participants examined the impact of the Anabolic Steroid Control Act of 1990. Although experts presented evidence that the coordinated federal investigative effort had significantly affected the illicit anabolic steroid market by making the steroids harder and more expensive to obtain, the data showed that abuse of anabolic steroids continues to constitute a significant threat to the general public health and safety, especially in adolescents and young adults. It was determined that, while there have been notable accomplishments under this legislation, there are several serious obstacles to its effectiveness. One of these obstacles is that the current provisions of the Federal Sentencing Guidelines establish grossly inadequate sentencing standards for steroid traffickers. The guidelines do not reflect realistic dosages and treat a given quantity of steroids as significantly less dangerous than other Schedule III substances or even marijuana. This prevents convictions from acting as a deterrent to serious trafficking, since the guidelines will frequently result in a sentence involving little or no imprisonment.

Another obstacle is that steroids are not controlled in many key countries, nor are they controlled under international treaty. This has created a situation in which no matter how successful we are in dealing with domestic diversion of steroids from other uses (such as veterinary supplies), there is a constant supply of these drugs being smuggled into the United States from legal international sources (see the introduction). In order for the United States to make any further progress against the steroid abuse problem, the conference concluded that these obstacles must be removed (Haislip, 1995).

Between 1991 and 1994, over 185 anabolic steroid investigations of major drug dealers of steroids were initiated by the DEA. There were 283 arrests made and 6 million dosage units and $2.5 million in assets seized (Bahrke, 1994). Only large dealers are prosecuted because they are the only ones who will be punished under current Federal Sentencing Guidelines. The cost to prosecute is great, and small dealers only get a slap on the wrist or a short visit to a "country club" prison. The inadequacy of sentencing guidelines makes bringing steroid cases difficult, and juries are often sympathetic to defendants in cases that are prosecuted (Haislip, 1995). In addition, prosecution of anabolic steroid traffickers must compete with that of traffickers in other controlled substances for the limited resources of enforcement and customs agents (Bahrke, 1994). In addition, police officers themselves are often users of anabolic steroids (Swanson, Gaines, & Gore, 1991).

The Anabolic Steroid Control Act has had some deterrent effect on some low-level dealers who may have something to lose from having a criminal conviction on their records (Haislip, 1995). Also, it may be possible for investigators to prosecute traffickers for other federal and state violations, such as tax evasion, firearms, money laundering, food and drug labeling, customs, and postal violations. This would help bring the full force of the law to bear against defendants involved in anabolic steroid trafficking.

Sources of Steroids

Athletes obtain anabolic steroids from a variety of sources. Although athletes primarily obtain steroids in a vast multifaceted black market, prescribing physicians, pharmacists, and veterinarians provide a significant amount of the anabolic steroids used today (Yesalis & Bahrke, 1995). Steroids intended for animals end up in humans. Veterinary steroids may be bought illegally by claiming that the drugs are for farm animals (Stejskal, 1994).

Nonetheless, the black market dwarfs the amount of steroids prescribed by physicians (Haislip, 1995). Conservatively reported to be about $500 million per year, this black market is as heterogeneous in its makeup as it is substantial in its size (Kouri et al., 1994; Kazubski, 1991). Physicians, veterinarians, pharmaceutical industry employees, coaches, and athletic trainers are all among those who provide anabolic steroids to the athlete (Yesalis & Bahrke, 1995). Supplies of anabolic steroids may be diverted to illegal distributors, often health clubs, by employees of legitimate pharmaceutical corporations and veterinary drug houses within the United States (Yesalis & Bahrke, 1995). Diverted anabolic steroids are generally of safe pharmaceutical quality (Burge, 1995). The products of clandestine laboratories and some imported anabolic steroids are more likely to be unsafe or low quality (Haislip, 1993). There has been a shift from illegal diversion of steroids legally manufactured in the United States to a distribution network fed by steroids smuggled in from places such as Mexico, South America, Canada, Europe, and Russia (Haislip, 1995). Experts estimate that anywhere from 50 to 80% of steroids used today for nonmedical purposes are obtained illegally on the black market (Bahrke, Yesalis, & Wright, 1996). Steroids are not controlled in international commerce, and the use of regular and special international mail systems allows massive quantities to be smuggled into the United States quickly and cheaply (Haislip, 1995).

Although distributing steroids without a prescription is illegal in the United States, obtaining the drugs is easy because in many Latin American and Eastern European countries anabolic steroids are available over the counter (Stejskal, 1994). Mexican pharmacies have been a big source of steroids for weight-training gyms and health clubs in the United States (Yesalis & Bahrke, 1995). Steroids are available from mail-order sources and over the Internet. Readily available publications such as the *Underground Steroid Handbook* (*USH*) (Duchaine, 1990), as well as a number of sites on the Internet, carry many advertisements for imported and domestically produced illicit steroids.

The presence of such a large, multifaceted black market has created the potential for a significant public health problem. Black marketeers often have no incentive to look out for the athletes' interests and will sell them virtually anything. As a result, users frequently buy steroids unaware of the true nature and quality of the drugs they purchase (Bidwill & Katz, 1989). There are also many small-scale clandestine laboratories (Burge, 1994). The component chemicals are readily available and can be combined with minimal equipment and knowledge. The products are likely to be impure, nonsterile, or both, creating further health risks for the user.

Indirect Legal Consequences of Steroid Abuse: Criminal Behavior

Athletes—and others—take steroids in the belief that using steroids will result in better athletic performance, better muscular structure and appearance, or both. Like so many drugs and substances, though, anabolic steroids work on more than just one type of tissue. Some medical evidence—although nothing yet conclusive—points to the potential for significant psychotropic effects from long-term steroid use. It remains unclear whether the apparent psychotropic effects are caused by the steroids or whether long-term steroid abusers have a predisposition for mental instability (Pope & Katz, 1988). The violent behavior, discussed in the following paragraphs, can have tragic consequences, including death (Nack, Yaeger, & Teagan, 1998).

When a state charges an anabolic steroid abuser with a crime, the possible effect of anabolic steroids on the state of mind of the defendant may be an issue. Physiological and psychological side effects have long been associated with the use of anabolic steroids (Pope & Katz, 1988). However, recent research has begun to reveal that there may be psychiatric repercussions of steroid use far beyond the mere increase in aggressiveness commonly reported in the past (Pope et al., 1996). Some researchers believe that anabolic steroids, when used in large doses, may lead to a severe toxic psychosis (Pope & Katz, 1994). Moreover, athletes often engage in sophisticated regimens of steroid use, combining many different steroids as well as other drugs, such as marijuana, stimulants, and alcohol. The results of these varied combinations of drugs are unpredictable. The effect of stacking anabolic steroids on the user's mental status is undocumented, except for anecdotal accounts presented in lay books like the *Underground Steroid Handbook* and *Anabolic Reference Guide* (Phillips, 1991).

The ingestion of other substances that can affect behavior, as well as pre-existing psychopathology, can substantially cloud the legal issues involved in a particular case. Prosecutors can argue that the use of anabolic steroids had very little to do with the psychotic criminal behavior at issue. For example, individuals willing to take anabolic-androgenic steroids and other drugs of questionable origin, content, and purity, which have serious legal implications as well as health effects, differ from the general population on a wide variety of characteristics, including mental health (Pope & Katz, 1988; Nack, 1998). Thus it may not be the use of anabolic steroids alone that has contributed to their temporary psychotic state. Fifteen percent of Pope and Katz's subjects reported past alcohol abuse or dependence, and 32% reported other prior substance abuse or dependence, including use of cannabis (17%) and cocaine (12%) (Pope & Katz, 1988). We do not know the extent to which concurrent use of alcohol and other drugs caused the users' psychotic state. Nor do we know how much their pre-existing psychopathology or their family predisposition to mental illness may have contributed to their becoming psychotic while using anabolic steroids (Bahrke, Yesalis, & Wright, 1996). Subsequent studies have shown that weightlifters in general, whether steroid users or not, exhibit flamboyant features and severe personality pathology, such as histrionic, narcissistic, antisocial, and borderline features (Bidwill & Katz, 1989). Bodybuilders, another group associated with steroid abuse, seem more extreme (Nack, 1998). Severe personality pathology could predispose a person to having a psychosis (Perry, Andersen, & Yates, 1990).

Some attorneys have argued that any such steroid-induced psychosis eliminates, or alternatively mitigates, criminal responsibility (Bidwill & Katz, 1989). They have coined the term "roid rage" to refer to the altered sense of judgment and increased anger and aggression that may result from the use over time of large doses of anabolic steroids. Steroids can influence human behavior and have been proffered as the etiology of criminal behavior. At least one criminal defendant has used the defense of steroid-induced insanity successfully to eliminate criminal responsibility in one case (*State v. Williams*, 1986).

States differ on how they define insanity (Rosner, 1994). Among the various forms of the insanity defense, the most common is the M'Naghten Rule. As originally formulated, the 1843 case of Daniel M'Naghten culminated in the cognitive test for insanity, which would relieve a defendant of criminal blame if

> *at the time of the committing of the act, the party accused was labouring under such a defect of reason from disease of the mind, as not to know the nature and the quality of the act he was doing; or if he did know it, that he did not know what he was doing was wrong. (M'Naghten's Case, 1843)*

Under the M'Naghten Rule, a sane person is presumed to know the consequences of their actions. To be ruled insane, a defendant must prove that he or she was unable to distinguish right from wrong or understand the nature and consequences of his or her acts. The Model Penal Code, promulgated by the American Law Institute, suggested another test for legal insanity, which contains both cognitive and volitional prongs:

> *A person is not responsible for criminal conduct if at the time of such conduct as a result of mental disease or mental defect he lacks substantial capacity either to appreciate the criminality of his conduct or to conform his conduct to the requirements of law. (Model Penal Code, 1955)*

While the differences between these formulations may not be apparent on a casual reading, they have dramatic effects in court. The M'Naghten test requires that the defendant prove he did not know he was doing anything wrong. The American Law Institute test allows a defendant who knew he was doing wrong to satisfy his burden of proving his insanity if he can show he nevertheless lacked substantial capacity to behave properly.

The mental state potentially produced by steroid use may be sufficient to establish an insanity defense in a state that uses a test that is modeled on the American Law Institute's "substantial capacity" test—the most liberal of the various definitions of insanity (*State v. Williams*, 1986; Taylor, 1987). On the other hand, in a state that relies on the M'Naghten test, "roid rage" would not establish an insanity defense, because steroids do not prevent a defendant from understanding he is engaging in improper conduct, even though the steroids may make it impossible for the defendant to behave properly.

Short of claiming legal insanity, a criminal defendant may attempt to claim that his or her capacity for obeying the law was diminished by intoxication caused by steroid side effects. While this kind of defense does not prevent a conviction for violent conduct, it may significantly reduce the consequences of the conviction by reducing a charge from, for example, murder to voluntary or involuntary manslaughter. Until recently, very little information about the effects of anabolic steroids on the mind was available to the average user. Research completed 10 years ago revealed that steroid-induced psychosis may be a side effect of steroid use (Pope & Katz, 1988; Bidwill & Katz, 1989). However, there is disagreement as to the actual causal role played by anabolic steroids. Even today there is less than unanimity concerning the psychological effects of anabolic steroids (Bahrke, Yesalis, & Wright, 1996).

If it could be argued that most users of steroids presently are unclear about or unaware of the potential psychiatric problems that may accompany steroid use, the legal defense of involuntary intoxication may be a persuasive theory for avoiding criminal responsibility. Involuntary intoxication is a complete defense to a crime in a M'Naghten jurisdiction (Lafave & Scott, 1986). Furthermore, it is recognized as a defense in many states by statute (Ga. Code Ann., 1988; Colo. Rev. Stat., 1986; Model Penal Code, 1985). The defendant must prove (1) that the defendant was intoxicated, (2) that the intoxication was involuntarily created, and (3) that as a result of this involuntary intoxication the defendant's mental state met the jurisdiction's test for insanity.

The common law has recognized intoxication that results from alcohol or drugs as involuntary when any of four conditions was met: (1) the intoxication was coerced or the result of duress; (2) the intoxication was pathological; (3) the intoxication resulted from a substance taken pursuant to a physician's advice; or (4) the intoxication was the result of an innocent mistake by the accused as to the intoxicating nature of the substance ingested. For the court to render the intoxication involuntary, the defendant will have to show that the facts surrounding his affliction with the steroid-induced psychosis parallel one of these four scenarios. As users become educated to the drugs' potential for producing psychiatric repercussions, the utility of this defense will diminish.

Involuntary intoxication is an affirmative defense, which means that the defendant has the burden of going forward with evidence of intoxication and the burden of persuading the fact-finder that he or she satisfies the requirements for the defense. Through the testimony of experts, the defense has to prove that the resulting psychosis was intoxication, that the intoxication was involuntary, and that the defendant was legally insane at the time he or she committed the criminal act (Bidwill & Katz, 1989).

As for users who are knowledgeable about the potential of drugs to produce psychiatric symptoms, but choose to use them anyway, the insanity defense would not be available. The rule in the majority of jurisdictions is that insanity that would excuse the accused from criminal responsibility cannot be the result of alcohol or drug use. One article has concluded that steroid-induced psychosis—even if it satisfies the cognitive test of insanity—fails as a method of completely eliminating culpability under the insanity defense because it would be a temporary insanity created by the voluntary, excessive use of a drug (Bidwill & Katz, 1989).

However, because anabolic steroids are taken voluntarily and could induce changes in mental status, the defense of voluntary intoxication might be appropriate. An individual who acts without criminal intent or without exercising free will is not morally blameworthy. This defense would be available only to an individual charged with a specific-intent crime, such as first-degree murder on the basis of premeditation, attempted murder, assault with intent to kill, common law burglary (intent to engage in breaking and entering), and common law larceny (intentional taking and carrying away). Specific intent is, in general terms, some intent beyond the mere intent to perform the physical act required for the crime (Lafave & Scott, 1986). Evidence that the defendant had become intoxicated using anabolic steroids could be introduced to show that the intoxication rendered that person incapable of forming the specific intent constituting an element of the crime. This rule is well accepted in most American jurisdictions (Annotation, 1966).

For most crimes, the state must prove that the defendant *intended* to commit the crime with which he or she is charged. The requisite intent of the crime is known as the *mens rea* (Morissette, 1952). Defense counsel would introduce evidence of voluntary intoxication to show that the defendant was incapable of possessing the mens rea that is an indispensable element of the crime. If this effort is successful, a necessary element of proof has failed and the law considers that the crime was not committed.

However, voluntary intoxication will not shield a defendant from criminal responsibility in all circumstances. While some crimes, such as murder, require proof of a specific intent, other crimes, such as unintentional manslaughter, require only a showing of a *general* intent, or that the person merely intended to do the physical act that the crime proscribes. The proof of voluntarily incurred intoxication will negate only a *specific*-intent element of a crime. It will not negate the *general* intent component, as mere proof of the commission of the proscribed act, *actus reus*, will be sufficient to show that the accused possessed general intent, regardless of his or her intoxicated state. Thus the evidence could be used for mitigation of the criminal responsibility and moral blameworthiness, rather than for exculpation.

Once the defense introduces enough evidence of intoxication that the jury is left with a reasonable doubt as to whether the defendant was capable of forming the specific intent, the prosecution must overcome the evidence of intoxication to prove beyond a reasonable doubt that the defendant in fact formed the requisite intent (*Patterson v. New York*, 1977; *In re Winship*, 1970; *State v. Schulz*, 1981). The defendant's voluntary ingestion of the intoxicant is irrelevant.

Some prosecutors may argue that much of the psychological and behavioral effects of steroid intake may be placebo (Bjorkqvist, 1994). They may also point to studies that show that the anticipation of the aggressiveness related to steroid use may lead to actual violent acts and become, in effect, an excuse for aggression (Bahrke, Yesalis, & Wright, 1996). As Bahrke and colleagues point out, attempting to evaluate and summarize the psychological and behavioral effects associated with the use of anabolic steroids is complicated by several methodological shortcomings, including weak research design and methodology and inadequate instrumentation and measurement (Bahrke, Yesalis, & Wright, 1996). Therefore, issues involving the contribution of anabolic steroids substance abuse, pre-existing personality pathology, and psychosis to a defendant's violent behavior will still have to be resolved on a case by case basis.

The Proper Role of the Legal System Regarding Steroid Abuse

This entire discussion makes a very large assumption: that the legal system must have a significant—and perhaps the leading—role in controlling abuse of anabolic steroids. The fact of such a role seems fairly clear. As discussed above, statutes and regulations have dealt directly with anabolic steroids, and the courts have struggled with some of the indirect questions. Even questioning this assumption puts the cart before the horse, however. The initial question must be whether the legal system *should* have such a significant role.

Direct legal efforts to limit steroid abuse should remind us of two similar efforts; neither was arguably a success. The War on Drugs has not succeeded (Currie, 1993). Purer, cheaper cocaine and heroin is more available now than before the campaign that began in the 1970s (Musto, 1997; Ryan, 1998). Similarly, Prohibition had little effect on alcohol availability (Levine, 1985). Both the current War on Drugs and Prohibition did have significant unwanted side effects: violence related to drug and alcohol trafficking, undermined respect for the law, and prevention of effective public health and education efforts to reduce demand for the drugs at issue (Rumbarger, 1989; Levine, 1985).

These difficulties arguably stem from misdefinition of the entire problem. The legal system treats the "drug problem," including the "steroid problem," as a moral or criminal issue (Ryan, 1998; Bertram et al., 1996). In a sense, this is as it should be. We cannot expect the legal system to respond adequately to, say, a public health crisis, because it simply is not equipped to do so. Yet, as the remainder of the chapters in this book amply demonstrate, that is precisely what the "steroid problem" appears to be—an ethical and public health problem.

The legal system can effectively diminish demand for steroids only through punishment of users and traffickers. The legal system does not educate users on the long-term effects of anabolic steroid abuse, or of needle sharing, or anything else. It waves a finger under the nose of the user, in effect saying, "You should not do this because it is naughty." As Kevin Ryan notes, however,

> *The idea behind the punishment of [illicit drug] users is that severe punishment threatened will deter use in the first place, and severe punishment suffered will deter continued use. The mountain of research on the presumed deterrent effect of punishment, however, has been inconclusive, and when applied to drug use the logic of deterrence is dubious indeed. People use and quit based on a wide variety of motivations and forces. . . . [D]rug users are highly unlikely to quit due to hypothetical threats of punishment. Worse, serious threats may simply drive users underground and into more dangerous patterns of use (Ryan, 1998, p. 225).*

Some of those more dangerous patterns of use include using veterinary supplies and other unverifiable sources, experimentation with multiple compounds, and sharing and reuse of needles for injectables.

If we want to reduce abuse of anabolic steroids for reasons of public health—such as the potential adverse health effects—then we must concentrate our efforts on public health and educational interventions. If, on the other hand, our goal is to reduce abuse of anabolic steroids for moral and ethical reasons—such as preserving the "purity" of athletic competition—or as part of a broader criminalization of drugs, we are unlikely to do better than the War on Drugs or Prohibition by relying solely on the legal system. Just relying on the legal system to stem the tide will lead to the same result: abject failure and creation of a thriving black market.

Conclusion

In this complex field, several conclusions and avenues for future policy action seem warranted. First of all, drug testing is well established in the area of competitive athletics. Sport organizations have accepted that drug testing must be done, and the courts have upheld their right to perform mandatory testing (Jacobs & Samuels, 1995). Drug testing has withstood challenges on both federal and state constitutional grounds.

Second, we need to rethink the Anabolic Steroid Control Act of 1990, under which anabolic steroids became a Schedule III controlled substance. Clearly, the Act has not had a major impact on the availability and use of anabolic steroids in the United States. The domestic black market and the constant supply coming from abroad have overwhelmed any positive enforcement of the Act. The legal and practical obstacles to the enforcement of the Act have also made it very difficult to prosecute offenders or get convictions. At the same time, the legislation has constrained legitimate medical uses of these drugs by physicians, a significant negative consequence (Black, 1992).

The Act has had little impact on steroid use by high school students, one of the most threatening aspects of the problem. Since anabolic steroids are so easy to obtain, and use and distribution so difficult to prosecute, governmental and private efforts in this area need to shift emphasis to improved education of the public. Young people in particular must be much better educated about the serious health hazards that may accompany use of steroids and steroid substitutes. Conversely, the failure of Prohibition and the War on Drugs graphically demonstrates that simply criminalizing behavior won't control that behavior. A well-conceived and well-funded set of educational programs would be far more effective for this purpose than further legislation, criminalization, and added bureaucratic machinery.

References

Amateur Sports Act of 1978, Pub. L. No. 95-606, 92 Stat. 3045 (codified at 36 U.S.C. § 371 *et seq.*).

Anabolic Steroid Control Act of 1990, Title XIX of Pub. L. No. 101-647, 104 Stat. 4851 (codified at 21 U.S.C. § 333,[e]).

Anabolic steroids. (1989, September). State Legislation Report, American Medical Association.

Annotation, Modern Status of the Rules as to Voluntary Intoxication as Defense to Criminal Charge, 8 *A.L.R.3d* 1236, 1240 (1966).

Anti-Drug Abuse Act of 1988, Pub. L. No. 100-690, § 2403, 102 Stat. 4230 (codified at 21 U.S.C. § 333).

Bahrke, M.S. (1994). International conference on abuse and trafficking of anabolic steroids. *The International Journal of Drug Policy*, *5*(1), 23–26.

Bahrke, M.S., Yesalis, C.E., & Wright, J.E. (1990). Psychological and behavioural effects of endogenous testosterone levels and anabolic-androgenic steroids among males: A review. *Sports Medicine*, *10*, 303–337.

Bahrke, M.S., Yesalis, C.E., & Wright, J.E. (1996). Psychological and behavioural effects of endogenous testosterone and anabolic-androgenic steroids: An update. *Sports Medicine, 22,* 367–390.

Barnes v. International Amateur Athletic Federation, 862 F. Supp. 1537 (D.W. Va. 1993).

Bertram, E. (Ed.), Blachman, M.J., Sharpe, K., & Andreas, P. (1996). *Drug war politics: The price of denial.* Berkeley: University of California.

Bidwill, M.J., & Katz, D.L. (1989). Injecting new life into an old defense: Anabolic steroid-induced psychosis as a paradigm of involuntary intoxication. *University of Miami Entertainment & Sports Law Review, 7*(1), 19–21.

Bjorkqvist, K., Nygren, T., Bjorklund, A-C., & Bjorkqvist, S.E. (1994). Testosterone intake and aggressiveness: Real effect or anticipation. *Aggressive Behavior, 20*, 17–26.

Black, J.A. (1992). The Anabolic Steroids Control Act of 1990: A need for change. *Dickinson Law Review, 97*(1), 131.

Blowman, D.J. (1992). *Regulating roids. Controlled substance scheduling of anabolic-androgenic steroids from a policy-analytic perspective.* Unpublished master's thesis, Pennsylvania State University.

Buckley, W.E., Yesalis, C.E., Friedl, K.E., Anderson, W., Streit, A., & Wright, J. (1988). Estimated prevalence of anabolic steroid use among male high school seniors. *Journal of the American Medical Association, 260*, 3441–3445.

Burge, J. (1994). Legalize and regulate: A prescription for reforming anabolic steroid legislation. *Loyola (Los Angeles) Entertainment Law Journal, 15,* 33–60.

Burge, J. (1995). Reforming anabolic steroid legislation. *Drug Law Report, 3*(19), 217–228.

California Health & Safety Code § 11153.5 (West 1988 Supp.).

Chastonay, R.J., Chief, Prescription Drug Branch (1984, July 9). Class action against products on the market without approval containing DHEA. *Dl.C RX Drug Study Bulletin.*

Colorado Rev. Stat. § 18-1-804(3) (1986).

Colorado Rev. Stat. § 12-36-117(1)(v)-(w) (Supp. 1989).

Currie, E. (1993). *Reckoning: Drugs, the cities, and the American future.* New York: Hill & Wang.

Downes, S. (1998, November 29). Drug charges haunt Slaney. *The Times* (London).

Duchaine, D. (1990). *Underground steroid handbook.* Santa Monica, CA: OEM.

Federal Arbitration Act, 9 U.S.C. §§ 1-16 (1994).

Federal Food, Drug, and Cosmetic Act of 1938, 21 U.S.C. § 301 *et seq.* (1994).

Ford, J.B. (1984). Drugs, athletes and the NCAA: A proposed rule for mandatory drug testing in college athletics. *John Marshall Law Review, 18,* 205–236.

Georgia Code Ann. § 26-704 (Harrison 1988).

Gilbert, W. (1969, July 7). Drugs in sport: Part 3, High time to make some rules. *Sports Illustrated,* 30–35.

Gorman, R. (1995). The *Gilmer* decision and the private arbitration of public-law disputes. *University of Illinois Law Review, 1995*, 635–681.

Gormley, K. (1992). One hundred years of privacy. *Wisconsin Law Review, 1992,* 1336.

Graham v. Scissor-Tail, Inc., 171 Cal. Rptr. 604 (1981).

Haislip, G.R. (1994). *Conference report: International Conference on the Abuse and Trafficking of Anabolic Steroids.* Washington, DC: U.S. Drug Enforcement Administration, Office of Diversion Control.

Haislip, G.R. (1995). *Conference on the impact of national steroid control legislation in the United States.* U.S. Drug Enforcement Administration, Office of Diversion Control.

Hill v. National Collegiate Athletic Assn., 865 P.2d 633, 7 Cal.4th 1, 26 Cal. Rptr.2d 834 (1994).

Hooters of America v. Phillips, 1998 U.S. Dist. LEXIS 3962 (D.S.C. March 12, 1998).

In re Winship, 397 U.S. 358, 364 (1970).

Jacobs, J.B., & Samuels, B. (1995). The drug testing project in international sports: Dilemmas in an expanding regulatory regime. *Hastings International and Comparative Law Review, 18*, 557–589.

Jancin, B. (1989). Is athlete's steroid use a valid insanity defense? *Clinical Psychiatry News, 2,* 15.

Kazubski, D. (1991). Overview of the illicit steroid market. In *Conference report: Scientific and investigational aspects of anabolic steroid control* (pp. 20–22). U.S. Department of Justice, Drug Enforcement Administration.

Kouri, E., Pope, H., Katz, D., et al. (1994). Use of anabolic-androgenic steroids: We are talking prevalence rates [Letter to the editor]. *Journal of the American Medical Association, 271*, 347–348.

Lafave, W.R., & Israel, J.H. (1992). *Criminal procedure* (2d ed.). St. Paul: West.

Lafave, W.R., & Scott, A. (1986). *Criminal law* (2d ed.). St. Paul: West.

Legislation to amend the Controlled Substances Act (anabolic steroids): Hearing on H.R. 3216 before the Subcommittee on Crime of the Committee on the Judiciary, House of Representatives, 100th Cong., 2d Sess. (1988, July 27).

Levine, H.G. (1985). The birth of American alcohol control: Prohibition, the power elite, and the problem of lawlessness. *Contemporary Drug Problems, 12,* 63–115.

Locke, E., & Jennings, M. (1986). The constitutionality of student-athlete mandatory drug testing programs: The bounds of privacy. *University of Florida Law Review, 38*, 581–613.

Lord, C. (1998a, June 5). IOC finds flaws in one of Smith's lines of defence. *The Times* (London).

Lord, C. (1998b, October 16). Smith takes on issue of right to test. *The Times* (London).

Martin, G.A., Jr. (1989). Why not understand drug testing? *New England Law Review, 3,* 645–649.

Meloch, S.L. (1987). An analysis of public college athlete drug testing programs through the unconstitutional condition doctrine and the fourth amendment. *Southern California Law Review, 60,* 815–850.

M'Naghten's Case, 8 Eng. Rep. 718, 722 (H.L. 1843).

Model Penal Code, § 401.1(1) (Tent. Draft 4) (1955). St. Paul: American Law Institute.

Model Penal Code, § 2.08 (1985). St. Paul: American Law Institute.

Morissette v. United States, 342 U.S. 246, 252 (1952).

Musto, D. (1997). *The American disease: Origins of narcotic control.* New York: Oxford.

Nack, W., (1998). The muscle murders. *Sports Illustrated, 88*(20), 96–106.

National Treasury Employees' Union v. von Raab, 489 U.S. 656 (1989).

New Jersey v. T.L.O., 469 U.S. 325 (1985).

O'Halloran v. University of Washington, 679 F. Supp. 977 (W.D. Wash.), *rev'd on other grounds,* 856 F.2d 1375 (9th Cir. 1988).

Ohio Monthly Record, January 1988, at 861–862 (to be codified at § 4731-11-05 in the Ohio Admin. Code).

Patterson v. New York, 432 U.S. 197 (1977).

Perry, P.J., Andersen, K.H., & Yates, W.R. (1990). Illicit anabolic steroid use in athletes. *American Journal of Sports Medicine, 18,* 422–428.

Phillips, W. (1991). *Anabolic reference guide* (5th ed.). Golden, CO: Mile High.

Pope, H.G., & Katz, D.L. (1988). Affective and psychotic symptoms associated with anabolic steroid use. *American Journal of Psychiatry, 145,* 487–490.

Pope, H.G., & Katz, D.L. (1994). Psychiatric and medical effects of anabolic-androgenic steroid use. *Archives of General Psychiatry, 51,* 375–382.

Pope, H.G., et al. (1996). Anabolic-androgenic steroid use among 133 prisoners. *Comprehensive Psychiatry, 37,* 322–327.

Preliminary draft. (1996). *The Medical Letter, 38,* 91.

Proper and improper use of drugs by athletes: Hearings before the Senate Subcommittee to Investigate Juvenile Delinquency, 93d Cong., 1st Sess. (1973, June 18, July 12–13). USY4.J89/2:D84/5.

Reynolds v. International Amateur Athletic Federation, 23 F.3d 1110, 1114 (6th Cir.), *cert. denied,* 115 S. Ct. 423 (1994).

Rosenberg v. Merrill Lynch, 976 F. Supp. 681 (D. Mass. 1998), *appeal pending.*

Rosner, R. (1994). *Principles and practice of forensic psychiatry.* New York: Chapman & Hall.

Rumbarger, J.J. (1989). *Profits, power, and prohibition: Alcohol reform and the industrializing of America, 1800–1930.* Albany, NY: State University of New York Press.

Ryan, K.F. (1998). Clinging to failure: The rise and continued life of U.S. drug policy. *Law & Society Review, 32*(1), 221–242.

Scanlan, J.A., Jr. (1987). Playing the drug-testing game: College athletes, regulatory institutions, and the structure of constitutional argument. *Indiana Law Journal, 62*, 863–983.

Schaill v. Tippecanoe County School Corporation, 679 F. Supp. 833 (N.D. Ind. 1988), *aff'd,* 864 F.2d 1309 (7th Cir. 1988).

Skinner v. Railway Labor Executives' Assn., 489 U.S. 602, 613–614 (1989).

State v. Schulz, 307 N.W.2d 151, 156, 102 Wis.2d 423, 429–430 (1981)

State v. Williams, No. C-5630/5631/5634 (Cir. Ct. St. Mary's Cty., Md., filed April 3, 1986).

Stejskal, G. (1994). They shoot horses, don't they? Anabolic steroids and their challenge to law enforcement. *FBI Law Enforcement Bulletin, 63,* 1–6.

Swanson, C., Gaines, L., & Gore, B. (1991, August). Abuse of anabolic steroids. *FBI Law Enforcement Bulletin,* 19–23.

Taylor, W.N. (1991). *Macho medicine: A history of the anabolic steroid epidemic.* Jefferson, NC: McFarland.

Taylor, W.N. (1987). Synthetic anabolic-androgenic steroids: A plea for controlled substance status. *The Physician and Sportsmedicine, 15*(5), 145.

Title XIX, Anabolic Steroid Control Act of 1990, 136 Cong. Rec., Senate p 18301.

Turner P. (1987). Clinical pharmacology in criminal cases: Discussion paper. *Journal of the Royal Society of Medicine*, 80.

U.S. Constitution. Amendment IV.

U.S. Department of Health and Human Services, Public Health Service. (1991, January). *Report of interagency task force on anabolic steroids.* Author.

Vernonia Schl. Dist. No. 47J v. Acton, 115 S.C. 2386 (1995).

Yesalis, C.E., & Bahrke, M.S. (1995). Anabolic-androgenic steroids: Current issues. *Sports Medicine, 19*, 326–340.

Yesalis, C.E., Barsukiewicz, C., Kopstein, A., & Bahrke, M. (1997). Trends in anabolic-androgenic steroid use among adolescents. *Archives of Pediatric and Adolescent Medicine, 151,* 1197–1206.

Yesalis, C.E., Kennedy, N.J., Kopstein, A.N., & Bahrke, M.S. (1993). Anabolic-androgenic steroid use in the United States. *Journal of the American Medical Association, 270*, 1217–1221.

PART III

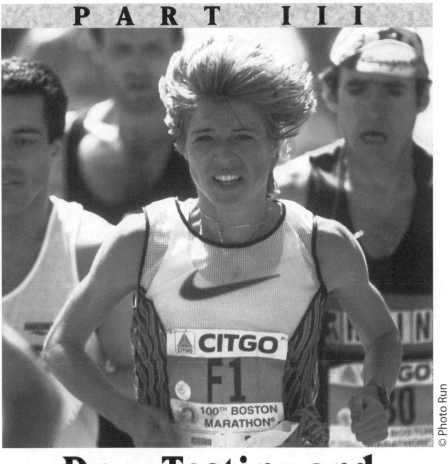

© Photo Run

Drug Testing and Societal Alternatives

The first two chapters of part III discuss drug testing in sport. Although testing involves a number of drugs besides anabolic steroids, significant attention is given to this topic because testing represents one of the primary strategies currently employed to combat drug use in sport. Politicians, fans, sport officials, the media, and even some athletes often appear to view drug testing as a "magic bullet" for this problem. Consequently, a critical analysis of the evolution, strengths, and frailties of drug testing is important.

Chapter 12 examines the drug-testing issue from a political angle. It includes a candid discussion of the problems inherent in the current drug-testing system, such as secrecy, pharmacological warfare, loopholes, outlaw laboratories, false positives, and roadblocks to enforcement.

Chapter 13, on the other hand, looks at the scientific aspects of drug testing. Following a short history of drug testing, the chapter focuses on the metabolism of anabolic steroids, the technology involved in testing, the philosophy of testing, the costs of testing, and the circumventing of positive test results. The author also discusses the use of other substances to enhance performance, and future directions in drug testing.

To provide closure to this text but impetus for change, the authors consider societal alternatives to anabolic steroid use. In **chapter 14,** they point out that identifying potential solutions is easy but agreeing on a proper course of action and successfully completing it are difficult. They propose four alternatives for dealing with the use of anabolic steroids and other performance-enhancing drugs.

It is the hope of the contributors that the reader will find this book to be not only a comprehensive resource on anabolic steroids but also a catalyst for individual and societal change.

CHAPTER

12

Evolution and Politics of Drug Testing

Jim Ferstle

***O** what a tangled web we weave,*
When first we practise to deceive!

Sir Walter Scott
Marmion, 1808

***L**ess is more . . .*
Ah, but a man's reach should exceed his grasp,
Or what's a heaven for?

Robert Browning
"Andrea del Sarto," 1855

Historians may come to view 1998 as a defining moment in the story of drugs in sport. After nearly forty years of grappling with what to do about athletes who attempt to aid their performances through drug use, in 1998 sport administrators and the public were dragged through a stream of sport doping scandals. These well-publicized events exposed the pervasive use of drugs by athletes and the inability of the testing systems to deal with the problem.

This chapter will attempt to provide some insight into the drug-testing system. It begins with a brief chronology of the extraordinary events of 1998–1999, then continues with the origins of drug testing and the politics that affect the scientific process of examining body fluids for the presence of prohibited substances. It deals primarily with the Olympic drug-testing system because the information on professional and collegiate sports is minimal and insufficient for any kind of analysis. Because the chapter deals with areas where the Olympic system may need improvement, the temptation is to brand it a failure. Nothing could be further from the truth. Victory and defeat are easy to measure in an athletic event, but are not quite as easy to determine in an area as complex as sport drug testing.

The Year of Scandals

The scandals began in January when a Chinese swimmer was stopped during a routine customs check in Australia and vials of human growth hormone (hGH) were discovered in her luggage. Although hGH was banned, athletes couldn't be sanctioned for its use because there was no test to detect it. In Europe, documents uncovered by German cancer researcher Werner Franke exposed GDR State Plan 14.25, a state-supported sport doping program run by the German Democratic Republic for more than twenty years.

With the full backing of the GDR government, sport officials administered drugs to athletes, checked their urines to ensure they did not flunk drug tests, and developed new drugs to aid athletes and avoid detection. Stasi (GDR secret police) files uncovered by Franke also indicated that GDR sport officials used their positions within sporting federations to keep either one step ahead of the testing system or to subvert the system by tampering with athletes' urine samples. Further evidence of systematic doping was uncovered during the 1998 Tour de France cycling race. French customs officers seized a car filled with banned drugs that was owned by Festina, the top-ranked cycling team in the world. Subsequent investigation revealed that cycling teams had doping programs, monitored by team doctors and partly financed through riders' winnings. As with the drugs found with the Chinese swimmer, those the cyclists were using, hGH and erythropoietin (EPO), were banned, but no reliable tests had been implemented to detect them. Other drugs, such as perfluorocarbon (PFC), were experimental and not even on the market. These cases provided clear illustration that athletes were ahead of the testers.

Also in 1998 an Associated Press reporter noted a bottle of androstenedione in the locker of home-run king Mark McGwire. McGwire admitted he used the "supplement," as did a lot of other major league baseball players. Androstenedione is banned by the IOC, the National Football League (NFL), and the National Collegiate Athletic Association (NCAA), but not by Major League Baseball. It is not regulated in the United States and is sold over the counter as a supplement. An act of Congress in 1994 provided this loophole by preventing the Federal Drug Administration from regulating substances unless proof of harm had been established. The ensuing public debate about the use of "andro" illustrated the lack of harmonization in the rules of the sport governing bodies. It also revealed a public ambivalence about the use of banned substances by professional athletes and the divided feelings of many about what should or should not be allowed.

On September 21, 1998, world record–setting sprinter and 1988 Olympic gold medalist Florence Griffith Joyner died in her sleep of what was later diagnosed as suffocation brought on by an epileptic seizure. She was 38. Instead of eulogizing a champion taken too soon, the media coverage of Flo Jo, as she was nicknamed, concentrated on one question: was it possible that use of performance-enhancing drugs contributed to her death? This public debate demonstrated that the drug-testing system also could not provide conclusive evidence that someone did *not* use drugs. Thus, any athletes whose appearance underwent dramatic change or who suddenly improved their performances were not lauded for their accomplishments. Instead they were suspected of drug use, and the testing system could not substantiate their innocence.

In the wake of the Tour de France scandal, the International Olympic Committee (IOC) called an emergency meeting of its executive committee to address the "doping crisis." Committees were formed to study the problem and propose solutions at an IOC doping congress to be held in February of 1999. The IOC also decided to lobby Major League Baseball to put androstenedione on its banned list. In addition, the IOC proposed getting the United Nations involved in some way with their self-proclaimed "War on Drugs." The IOC began developing proposals to raise the money necessary to fund these efforts. But, by the end of 1999, it was still not clear whether this war would be fought with rhetoric or with a serious, well-funded, comprehensive effort.

All Talk, No Action

The history of drug testing is full of rhetoric but short on well-funded and well-planned action. Sporting federations have always reacted to drug crises rather than attempting to anticipate problems or become proactive in their war on drugs. Having existed for only about thirty years, sport drug testing is not yet a mature industry, and its growing pains have been very public. To those administering elite sports, drug testing has often been seen as a necessary evil—something they have to do but often lack the commitment to do well. Sport administrators may see drug testing as former American football coach Woody Hayes saw the forward pass: "Three things can happen," said Hayes, "and two of them are bad." Drug testing may catch no one, which means your system is an exercise in futility. You may catch some of those who abuse drugs, which often leads to media characterizations of a sport tainted by drug use. Or you can attempt to deter athletes from taking drugs by implementing an expensive, effective, comprehensive testing program.

Although sport officials will often privately admit that drug use among athletes is high, relatively few athletes are ever caught. The perception, therefore, is that "only the stupid" flunk drug tests, and that the truly smart athletes know how to beat the system. Why test then? First, athletes who die during a competition threaten the health of the sport. Sport is promoted as a healthy activity, not a haven for those with a "win at all costs" mentality. Second, competition is based on the notion of the "level playing field," where every athlete has a chance to emerge victorious. Drug use can alter that perception by providing some with an unfair advantage. In political terms, sport administrators have little choice. To preserve the image of their sports, they must test for drug use.

By the time the IOC convened its anti-doping conference in February of 1999 in Lausanne, it was facing another crisis, the so-called Olympic bribery scandal. News reports had revealed details of corruption in the Olympic bid process for the 2002 Winter Olympics in Salt Lake City. Further investigation demonstrated that as a USOC report by former U.S. congressman, George Mitchell stated, a climate of corruption had been fostered within the IOC bidding process so that attempts were made by bidding cities to influence selection by "buying" IOC votes. The scandal threatened IOC sponsorship and overshadowed the doping conference. Instead of getting agreement on a plan to fight doping, the result of the Lausanne meeting was a declaration of the IOC's intent to continue the fight against doping, contribute $25 million to that cause, and to support the establishment of an "independent" World Anti-Doping Agency (WADA).

Because the IOC had proposed that IOC president Juan Antonio Samaranch and the head of its medical commission, Prince Alexandre de

Merode, lead this agency, most questioned its independence. European Union leaders also were concerned about potential loopholes in the declaration, which called for uniform bans for drug offenses except for "exceptional circumstances." The definition of exceptional circumstances was too broad for the EU leaders, who stated that a wealthy professional athlete could claim such circumstances because in some European countries there had been rulings that some drug penalties were too stiff as they deprived a professional athlete of the ability to earn a living.

Debate continued about formation of WADA throughout 1999. As the year 2000 approached, the IOC promised that an agency would be up and running by January 1, 2000, but nothing about leadership, budget, governing structure, or location of the agency had been made public as of September 1999. In addition, despite promising research on developing a test for synthetic Human Growth Hormone (rhGH), de Merode publicly stated that he doubted a test would be ready for the Sydney Olympics in 2000. Instead of immediately increasing the funding ($1 million) it had provided for the initial research into an rhGH test, the IOC waited until August of 1999 to announce it would provide $2 million for studies to validate the tests, although the GH-2000 study group had asked for $5 million in March to fund the project. There were similar stories about the development of a test for erythropoietin (EPO), where research funding was given to a California scientist by the USOC, but the funding stopped before work on a functional test could be completed.

The Testing Crisis

In addition to the fact that there were no tests for two banned substances, EPO and hGH, the IOC labs came under attack during 1999 for tests it currently used to detect use of testosterone and the anabolic steroid, nandrolone. Attorneys for Mary Decker Slaney filed suit in April of 1999 against the International Amateur Athletic Federation (IAAF) and the USOC charging, among other things, that the T/E ratio test used to screen for use of testosterone was an invalid test for females. The suit had the support of the U.S. Track & Field federation (USATF), which also cleared Slaney and a male sprinter, Dennis Mitchell, of doping offenses for alleged use of testosterone. The sport's international governing body, the IAAF, found both guilty of doping and banned each for 2 years. Several British sprinters, including 1992 Olympic 100 m champion Linford Christie, were accused of using nandrolone, but were found not guilty by their national federation, U.K. Athletics. The IAAF was reviewing those cases as this book went to press.

The athletes alleged that the IOC tests used on them did not differentiate between substances produced "naturally" within their bodies and substances used for doping. The U.K. Sports Council set up a scientific panel to investigate the claims that "false positive" tests for nandrolone could be legitimate. Attorneys for the athletes were poised to challenge any action taken by the IAAF. Scientists maintained that the test for nandrolone was sound and enforceable and noted that a new method that measured the carbon isotope ratio for endogenous and exogenous testosterone was being perfected for use in cases involving the hormone. The net result of the IOC scandal, inaction on testing procedures, and the questions over steroid testing was a decline in confidence in the drug testing system, especially among athletes. British distance runner Paula Radcliffe went so far as to begin soliciting volunteers who would undergo blood tests, which they would make public, in an attempt to demonstrate to the world that they were drug free and not using EPO.

Another British distance runner, Jon Brown, openly accused other distance runners of enhancing their performances by using EPO. Craig Masback, chairman of USATF, said that only an anti-doping agency free from any control by the sport federations or the IOC could be trusted to conduct an effective anti-doping program. Through it all the one constant of the anti-doping movement seemed to be that it is scandal driven and slow moving. It was started due to scandals surrounding the deaths of athletes and only seems to respond to new scandals. The more frequently the scandals erupt, the more the system is forced to change.

History of Drug Testing

For nearly a century, sport administrators have tapped the expertise of lab scientists in order to discover if athletes (or animal trainers) have attempted to enhance performance through the use of banned substances (Catlin, 1987). A far cry from the advanced testing machinery in use today, the first "doping" tests were probably done on saliva. Concerned about drugged horses, the Austrian Jockey Club brought a Russian chemist to Vienna in 1910 to see if he could detect the presence of alkaloids in the saliva of race horses. Austrian professor Dr. Sigmund Frankel later developed a similar saliva test, and 218 such exams were conducted on horses between 1910 and 1911 (IOC, 1973).

Testing of human urine did not begin until the 1950s, when the Italian soccer and cycling federations requested that the FMSI (Italian Medical Sports Federation) lab in Florence test soccer players and cyclists for stimulants. After the 1960 Summer Olympics in Rome, CONI (the Italian National Olympic Committee) joined forces with FMSI to set up a second drug-testing lab in Rome (Gasbarrone & Rosati, 1988).

At various times during the 1950s, sports medicine groups met in Austria and Germany to hold symposiums or inquiries into the problem, and in 1959, the International Sports Medicine Congresses focused on the issue at their meeting in Paris. Dr. Manfred Donike, director of the Institute for Biochemistry lab in Cologne, speaking at an International Athletic Foundation (IAF)–sponsored conference on doping in sports in 1987, traced the beginnings of "modern" drug testing: "Starting about 1960, the modern techniques of analytical chemistry, especially chromatography, provided the possibility to detect more and more dope agents or their metabolites in biological fluids, preferentially in urine" (Donike, de Merode, Beckett, & Dugal, 1988, p. 53).

In 1959, the Association Nationale d'Education Physique formed a doping commission in France. In 1962, FMSI organized a doping inquiry and the IOC passed a resolution condemning doping. On September 30, 1962, the Austrian government, through the federal ministry of education, set up a doping commission. These organizations passed their own regulations, including sanctions against those found guilty of doping offenses (*Investigative Hearings,* 1973).

In January 1963, at a meeting in Strasbourg, France, the Council of Europe defined doping as follows:

> *The administering or use of substances in any form alien to the body or of physiological substances in abnormal amounts and with abnormal methods by healthy persons with the exclusive aim of attaining an artificial and unfair increase of performance in competition. Furthermore, various psychological measures to increase performance in sports must be regarded as doping. (IOC, 1973)*

All the organizations involved in the issue struggled with the dual problem of defining doping and establishing what constituted proof of a doping offense. These issues continue to be debated up to the present. Some substances are banned before a test can be developed to test for them. This undermines the credibility of the system and causes some to recommend that substances not be banned unless tests exist to detect them. (A seemingly ludicrous debate occurred during the 1992 Summer Olympics in Barcelona, according to Professor Arnold Beckett, a founding member of the IOC Medical Commission. When tests done on the athletes revealed that they were most likely using sodium bicarbonate to "buffer" their systems, a move was made to ban it. Beckett then asked, "What are you going to do, ban cake? It's ludicrous, you can't test for it" [Beckett, 1993].)

Thus, during the early 1960s, considerable time was spent drafting the original language on the doping regulations in an attempt to find something that was acceptable to everyone. One concern was the difficulty of discriminating between doping and legitimate medical treatment with a substance that could improve performance; so in November 1963 in

Madrid, the European Doping Colloquium passed an amendment to the original doping definition to address this problem:

> *Where treatment with medicine must be undergone, which as a result of its nature or dosage is capable of raising physical capability above the normal level, such treatment must be considered as doping and shall rule out eligibility for competition. (IOC, 1973)*

To further define what constituted an offense, the group included with this amendment the first "official" list of banned substances. Instead of today's list, which includes over 100 substances, this first official list of banned substances consisted of broad categories of banned drugs, including narcotics; amine stimulants; alkaloids, such as strychnine and ephedrine; and all analeptic agents, respiratory tonics, and certain hormones (IOC, 1973). While tests for most of the substances were available, testing for the "hormones" was not. Scientifically, the process was "toothless," but was developed on the premise that banning these substances would have a deterrent effect on athletes. Many would not know that there was no test, and others would feel ethically bound to obey the rules.

By November 1964, the first known government-sponsored, antidoping legislation was proposed by members of the French Senate. The law forbade the misuse of pharmacological substances for doping, and it levied fines, disqualifications, and jail sentences of up to 1 year for the offenders. The law was passed, went into effect in 1965, and was followed that same year by a similar antidoping act passed in Belgium (IOC, 1973). All these proposals, position statements, definitions, and pieces of legislation were difficult to implement, however, because of various legal entanglements. The measures conflicted with other laws or international agreements or were difficult to enforce because of the lack of clear guidelines or regulations.

Even agreement regarding what substances should be on the banned list was difficult to achieve. Into this breach stepped the IOC, which had established its medical commission in 1961 under the leadership of Sir Arthur Porritt. The committee had done little, however, until 1967 when Prince Alexandre de Merode of Belgium, a former cyclist who had become aware of the doping problem in his sport, began to work to set up laboratories and a testing protocol for use at the Games.

Currently, nearly two dozen labs around the world are granted the IOC "seal of approval" as IOC-accredited drug-testing centers. Getting the labs involved brought scientists into the program whose reputations and lab income could benefit or be damaged by the success or failure of the

Olympic drug-testing program. A cursory certification process evolved. At first, certification meant merely being a testing lab set up at or near the site of the next Olympics. Donike became the major player in this process, as his was the first "full-service" testing lab, which was set up for the Summer Olympics in 1972. From the early minimal standards, this certification process evolved into a formal set of criteria set up by the IOC Medical Commission. The IOC's accreditation process has been monitored and administered entirely by the IOC Medical Commission. Plans are to expand that and require all IOC labs to pass a separate outside accrediting process, as well as the IOC's internal monitoring.

The Roots of Modern Drug Testing

Most medical research is targeted toward disease and disease prevention, not research on determining what an individual has ingested to improve his or her performance. Thus an entire industry had to be developed around the need to be able to identify substances in an athlete's urine. For some of the labs, sport drug testing can bring in as much as a million dollars a year. The type of testing done at these labs is quite specific and challenging. While other labs testing for drugs often specialize in certain categories or specific types of testing, Olympic labs have to test for a broad range of drugs in several different categories.

As the testing system becomes more adept at identifying and sanctioning athletes for specific drugs, more substances are discovered by the so-called doping gurus for use in aiding performance. And, as the use of drugs has increased, so have their effects on the outcome of sporting events. Many athletes have become human guinea pigs, experimenting with all sorts of substances in an attempt to enhance their athletic prowess. Some of these experiments have resulted in death ("Death of Birgit Dressel," 1988).

Motivation for Testing

It is the fear of athletes dying that spawned the IOC drug-testing process. Professor Beckett has said:

> *There is really no such thing as a level playing field. That is an admirable concept, but not within the bounds of reality. All we can really do by testing is to prevent athletes or unscrupulous individuals from doing damage to themselves through the use or misuse of certain substances. That is really what the drug testing system is designed to do. (1994)*

Others disagree. Dr. Don Catlin, head of the IOC-accredited lab in Los Angeles, says that it is part of the duty of the testing process to ensure fair competition, to protect honest athletes from those who attempt to gain an advantage by any means possible.

The major concern, however, remains that abuse of performance-enhancing substances by highly motivated, elite athletes or their coaches and trainers can have tragic consequences. In 1960, for example, a Danish cyclist died during the Olympics in Rome. His death was linked to the use of amphetamines. That same year, the death of track athlete Dick Howard was attributed to the use of "pep pills" (Wadler & Hainline, 1989). In the summer of 1967, British cyclist Tommy Simpson died during the Tour de France; amphetamines were found in his pockets and in his body. Governments and sport bodies reacted to the mounting pressure created by media reports of these incidents by passing legislation and instituting drug-testing programs (Donohoe & Johnson, 1986). By the end of 1967, the IOC had set up their medical commission, drafted rules prohibiting doping, and begun randomly testing athletes during both the 1968 Winter and Summer Games.

The IAAF also formed a subcommittee on doping under its medical commission and pioneered the process of accrediting drug-testing labs. In 1978, the IAAF Medical Commission Subcommission drafted a paper titled "Standardization of Analytical Procedures and Quality Tests for Doping Control Laboratories" (Donike et al., 1988). These standards were adopted for use in lab accreditation at the IAAF Medical Commission's annual meeting in March 1979 in Berlin and at the IAAF Council in April 1979 in Dakar, Senegal. In 1980, the medical commission of the IOC drafted its own requirements for accreditation. Labs passing this test are required to be reaccredited every two years. Used loosely at first, this method of certifying labs was begun in earnest in 1985 (Donike, 1988).

Out-of-Competition Testing

In 1985, the Sports Council of England provided financial assistance for a pilot program of out-of-season testing of British athletes eligible for international selection. The British Amateur Athletic Board (BAAB) began a program of random, out-of-competition testing in 1986 (Bottomley, 1988). Around the same time, Norway and Sweden also developed out-of-competition testing programs and began to coordinate efforts between the athletic governing bodies and their federal governments in an attempt to control the importation of banned substances (Norman, 1988). Customs officials in Norway confiscated 200,000 tablets in 1986, 5,000 of which were identified as narcotics and 20,000 as anabolic steroids (Norman, 1988). The directors of IOC labs, such as Cowan and Donike, repeatedly told sport authorities that merely testing during competition would not adequately address the problem of increasing drug use in sports.

Some countries resisted establishing more stringent testing programs, however, noting that their athletes would be put at a disadvantage if the testing program in their country was tougher than in the rest of the world. At a 1995 USOC executive board meeting, during a "town hall" session on drug testing, Brian Derwin, a former weightlifter and a member of the USOC board of directors said: "We can get our house in order, but there's a penalty to be paid for that if we go overseas and get beat. Internationally, we're getting our brains beat out. It's obvious when people at the venues are going around selling drugs that we're getting beaten up" (Longman, 1995).

De Merode and others on the IOC Medical Commission struggled to establish uniformity in a system rife with national and international differences. At the World Conference on Anti-Doping in Sport in June 1988, de Merode said: "It is totally unacceptable that in one country you can take this drug and in another country you cannot" (Boswell, 1988). "We need common legislation. The premises of doping control have been laid. . . . There is a lack of harmonization between sports federations and politicians" (Stuart, 1988).

Merely legislating against doping won't work for everyone, however. This was illustrated by the comments of another delegate to that conference, Dr. Eduardo de Rose of Brazil. When asked if Norway's approach would work in his country, de Rose said: "We will not use legislation because we are not used to following legislation. We have a law against everything and we do everything" (Hynes, 1988).

Challenge Testing

Because the sporting "superpowers" had the most at stake and the least amount of trust of each other's integrity, an attempt was made to try and deal with the major powers first, in hopes that others would follow their example. Officials of the United States Olympic Committee (USOC) and the then Soviet Union began work to establish a cooperative drug-testing program between the two countries in 1988. The program would have enabled testers from each country to "challenge test" each other. A pact was signed in 1989. Others were invited to join in the coalition, but the response was lukewarm at best. Canada, Italy, Czechoslovakia, and what was then West Germany joined the superpowers in a meeting in Moscow in October 1989, but East Germany and other nations did not. Representatives from U.S. and Soviet labs visited each other's labs and exchanged information in an attempt to achieve a standard of operation in their testing systems ("Doping Tests," 1989; Warshaw, 1989).

Another problem, acknowledged by IOC lab directors, was that, due to the different economic and political conditions in various countries, the capabilities of various labs within the IOC system varied. Well-funded labs in Cologne or Los Angeles, for example, have more resources than a lab in Czechoslovakia or Moscow (Catlin, 1991). Thus, it was suggested that a two-track accreditation system be implemented within the IOC, where one standard is applied to the established labs and another standard to those who do not have the resources. The concept was considered, but never implemented.

To bolster the notion of challenge testing, the United States Track & Field federation (USATF) proposed to the IAAF that an international system of challenge testing be tried, where each nation would choose a number of athletes from another country who would be subject to an unannounced test (Chriss, 1990). The idea was an adjunct to the joint monitoring program between the two Olympic sport superpowers. At the time of the breakup of the former Soviet Union, however, neither the U.S./USSR challenge testing program nor the USATF program had been implemented.

Even if the countries participated in testing programs, the further challenge is to get all the sporting federations within a country to comply. For example, at the 1995 USOC "town hall" meeting on drugs, it was noted that only 8 of the 41 sporting federations within the USOC conducted out-of-competition testing.

According to Catlin, out-of-competition testing is not enough; there must be no-notice or "surprise" out-of-competition testing. If the athlete knows the test is coming, he or she can use several methods to attempt to beat it. Catlin also emphasized that to truly monitor athletes, each athlete should be tested several times during the year to establish a baseline or "profile" data (Longman, 1995). Others, such as Donike, have pushed the concept of profiling for years. Mary Wayte, a former Olympic swimmer who was a member of the USOC's athletes advisory council, spoke for many athletes when she said that they would be receptive to the idea of submitting to four to eight tests a year to establish these profiles (Longman, 1995). For whatever reason, these suggestions have fallen on deaf ears, as nothing has been done by any of the sport governing bodies to implement them.

Enforcing the Rules

Two incidents illustrate the difficulty of enforcing out-of-competition testing rules. In 1996, Klaus Wengborski, an IAAF tester, was sent by the IAAF to test a group of Greek athletes. When he attempted to get them to provide urine samples, however, he was physically restrained by a Greek coach. The athletes fled, a protest was filed, and an inquest held by the IAAF. The result of this incident was that the coach was fined and banned, but none of the athletes were punished. Kenyan Olympic and world cross country champion John Ngugi had his ban for refusing an unannounced test commuted when protests were filed against the way the test was conducted by IAAF tester John Wetton.

For testers to be able to perform surprise tests, sport governing bodies must know where athletes are at all times. Michelle Smith de Bruin, Irish triple gold medal winning swimmer, was warned in 1997 when she missed an out-of-competition test because of failure to inform her federation of her movements. In 1998, the IAAF invoked a provision of their rules to deny prize money to two Kenyan athletes who had not had the required two out-of-competition tests during the past 12 months. To ensure that athletes are not avoiding testers, sport federations have begun writing in their rules that athletes who fail to keep the federation informed of their movements and miss tests could be subject to the same sanctions as those who flunk a test.

Challenges and Limitations in Drug Testing

Many factors, ranging from funding to technological considerations, influence testing.

Lack of Funding

Funding is a barrier for many sport federations. By 1998, out-of-competition testing cost from $500 to over $1,000 per test (Ferstle, Sept. 1997). The main reason for the high cost is the necessity of sending the testers where the athletes are. This and other factors led many sport administrators to view drug testing as a lost cause, something that keeps generating problems but few solutions. In 1991, Ollan Cassell, the former executive director of USA Track & Field, voiced concern:

> *Of all the things in our sport that I have to deal with, the thing that scares me the most is drugs. . . . Our (testing) system is one of the best in the world. We want fair competition. . . . [But] we don't have a test for testosterone, for EPO [erythropoietin] or blood doping, or hGH. . . . [The testing system] is something we're still wrestling with. We still don't have all the answers. (Cassell, 1991)*

In 1995, Dr. Ralph Hale, a USOC vice president, said, "Our anti-doping campaign, I'm afraid, has been a failure to this point. Many countries have lost confidence in our anti-doping effort. I'm not sure we're doing the right job" (Longman, 1995).

At the time this chapter is being written, seven years after Cassell's comments, the IOC still does not have tests for EPO, blood doping, or hGH, and its test for determining testosterone and nandrolone use is under attack (Patrick, 1997). While the problem of how to detect use of endogenous substances is a vexing one, one stark fact remains: sport federations do not fund the necessary research or provide the technology necessary to develop solutions to these problems.

Scope of Drugs Being Tested

When the technology is there, there are often problems using it or enforcing the rules once a "positive" finding is made. The IOC attempted to sanction several Russian athletes at the 1996 Olympics in Atlanta for using Bromantan, but the athletes' bans were overturned by the IOC's court of arbitration because the substance was not on the banned list. IAAF Medical Commission chairman and IOC member Arne Ljungqvist said that the ruling was a clear message to the IOC that the clause about related substances, used in several instances on the IOC banned list, does not allow the IOC to sanction an athlete. The substance must be listed by name on the list before an athlete can be banned for using it (Ferstle, Sept. 1997).

Another troubling scenario arose in the winter of 1996 when Kenyan world champion and world-record holder Daniel Komen tested above the allowed limit for caffeine. Komen was subsequently cleared of the offense, but not before several questions arose as to the validity of the caffeine test. As with testosterone, it appears that some athletes excrete more than a normal amount of caffeine (Ferstle, Sept. 1997). Some research has also been done that appears to indicate that caffeine above the IOC threshold (12 ng/dl) is actually a hindrance to performance, while levels below the IOC threshold can enhance one's endurance (Anderson, 1996). Thus, it would appear that the IOC list may be too broad or that what is on it has not been fully researched. However, when IOC President Juan Antonio Samaranch suggested in the summer of 1998 that the list needed to be pared, the subsequent firestorm of protest took that proposal off the table.

The previous year at the 1997 American College of Sports Medicine's annual meeting, Dr. Gary Wadler had attempted to form an ACSM working group to study the drug-testing process. Wadler noted that the IOC list needed paring. Having drugs on the list that cannot be tested for is counterproductive, he said, because it merely becomes an advertisement to athletes that this is a drug you can take and not have to worry about being caught (Wadler, 1997). If new methods need to be developed, the funding should be found to develop them quickly and with proper scientific scrutiny. But in many ways development of new doping methods often appears to be ahead of testing. For example, because of fears of AIDS transmission, scientists have been working on "recycling" blood and "manufacturing synthetic blood" ("Surgeons Cut Out the Need," 1997). Research is even being conducted on producing blood that is a cross between human blood and that of aquatic mammals and appears to have a protein that allows for more efficient use of oxygen. In 1998, one of these substances, PFC, was allegedly being used by cyclists as a substitute for blood doping, or EPO.

Barriers to Blood-Testing

Dr. Bo Berglund and the researchers at the Karolinska Institute in Sweden attempted to develop a test for blood doping in 1988. The first blood tests specifically designed to detect blood "boosting" were performed at the world cross-country skiing championships in 1988 (Videman, 1989), but the tests could detect "boosting" only if a person was using someone else's blood. Despite this, by 1991 the IOC Medical Commission recommended that blood tests be used at the Olympics, possibly starting with the Winter Games in 1994. The announcement was met with considerable resistance. Significant legal and cultural issues appeared to be barriers to implementing a blood test (Wilson, 1991). For example, legal experts advised the IOC that if an athlete's health was damaged by a mistake during collection of the blood, the organization could be sued. Others noted that some cultures did not allow drawing of blood.

By 1996 the experiment with blood testing appeared to have been abandoned. Wilfried Meert, director of the Ivo van Dame Grand Prix Athletics meet in Belgium, one of the Golden Four meets that did blood testing for two years, said:

> *We stopped the blood tests because there didn't seem any point in continuing. We expected the international federation to introduce a new rule that allowed blood testing, that our tests would be a first step. But this never happened. And the IAAF's own experts kept telling us that urine samples give just as good results. In the end it was very expensive, and we agreed that it is the sort of initiative that ought to come out of the international federation, not from individual meeting organisers (Downes, 1997).*

The IAAF Medical Commission chairman, Arne Ljungqvist, noted in 1997 that urine testing was superior to blood testing for detecting banned substances (Ferstle, March 1997). An IAAF experiment of using blood testing at the Golden Four track meets in Europe reinforced the conclusion that blood testing was not the wave of the future (Downes, 1997). By the end of 1998, however, blood tests gained credit from an Australian study that concluded that they would be the best way to detect the use of hGH and EPO. The GH 2000 project was also concluding its research into a blood test for hGH. Prior to this time, the only places where blood testing had been accepted was in the "protection" of athletes from the health risks of potential congestive heart failure.

Worried about the rumors of EPO use by endurance athletes, both the cycling and cross-country skiing federations imposed limits on the hematocrits of participants (Martin, 1997). The skiers set their limits at a hematocrit of 18.5 g/dl for men and 16.5 g/dl for women, while the bikers drafted a 50% rule. Any cyclist whose hematocrit was over 50% would be suspended, have his or her license to race revoked, and be subject to further testing to be readmitted to competition. While no skiers failed the test, several cyclists, including Italian star Claudio Chiappucci, were suspended by the International Cycling Union (UCI) during the spring of 1997 (Reuters, 1997).

The skiers' and cyclists' proactive approach to the rumor of EPO abuse contrasted with IOC nonaction when a situation developed prior to the 1992 Winter Olympics in France. When a Russian biathlete was hospitalized, rumors spread that his illness was due to blood doping. Donike wrote a letter to the IOC requesting the medical records of the athlete and stating that the IOC Medical Commission should investigate the matter (Donike, 1992). No probe was allowed, however, and the athlete returned for the 1994 Winter Olympics and won a gold medal.

Thus, although individual sport federations have moved to blood testing, the IOC has steadfastly resisted doing any form of blood tests. Despite repeated statements by de Merode that tests for EPO and hGH would be ready for the 2000 Olympics in Sydney, the reality is that 2000 has come and might go without such measures. By late 1999, even de Merode had changed his tune, now stating that the tests would not be ready in time. For the 1998 Winter Olympics in Nagano it was announced that the blood testing that had been applauded when used by cyclists and cross-country skiers would not be carried out. Only when Norwegian cross-country skiers, such as multigold medalist Bjorn Dahlie, threatened to boycott the Games if blood testing was not done, was some blood testing allowed.

Researchers for the GH 2000 program, the only research project funded by the IOC (the IOC contributed $1 million, the European Union $1 million), were also developing blood tests for detecting hGH. The question remains whether or not the IOC and other federations will be able to overcome the resistance to use such tests. De Merode said in the fall of 1998 that if a blood test was developed that could detect these substances, the IOC Medical Commission would approve it. It would then be passed on to the IOC legal department, where the final determination of whether or not to implement the test would be made prior to sending the measure before the IOC's executive committee.

Causes for Criticism of Drug Testing

Lack of funding and the inability to develop effective means of testing are not the only problems that plague the system. The cloak of secrecy that surrounds all testing and the fact that sport governing bodies still control nearly every aspect of the testing process have caused some to question the credibility of the system's enforcement process.

When East German swimmer Jorg Hoffmann admitted on German radio that he took anabolic steroids, Australian swimming coach Don Talbot was livid. Australian Kieren Perkins had been defeated by Hoffmann in the 1991 World Championships in a race where both swimmers broke the world record. To Talbot, Hoffmann's admission was yet another blemish on the credibility of the testing system, and he urged swimming's governing body, FINA, to release the results of drug tests to avoid suspicions of a cover-up ("Australian Chief Enraged," 1997).

I believe great efforts are made to cover-up positive tests.... It's like the ostrich putting its head in the sand as far as our leaders in the sport are concerned. They don't want to do anything. While I don't have proof, that's my gut feeling. It may well be that the people who are cheating are ahead of what FINA is testing for. But the very fact that FINA won't publish things ... makes you suspicious that something is wrong and that they won't release the results because something is being covered up (Talbot to Agence France-Presse, October 12, 1997).

Questionable Labs

Numerous athletes, coaches, and officials have charged that drug-testing rules are sometimes selectively enforced. Others contend that the system is easy to circumvent because there is no random testing and the sample collection process is easy to subvert. The economic disparity between nations often means that frequent out-of-competition testing may happen in one country, while another has little or no surprise testing. This often leads international federations to resist strict testing programs. The Dubin Inquiry report (see pp. 365–366) blasted the IOC's accreditation process because the people who do the accrediting are also directors of some of the labs being accredited.

The IOC's attempts to maintain the infallibility of its testing process received a blistering grilling during the Jessica Foschi case. In 1996, Foschi, a U.S. swimmer, provided a urine sample that contained metabolites of an anabolic steroid, mesterolone. Foschi's defense was that her urine had been sabotaged and that the drug was given to her without her knowledge by someone intent on ruining her career. During testimony, lawyers for the Foschis focused on the IOC's contention that mistakes are not made in IOC labs, that no "false positives" are produced by IOC testing.

> *For example, assume an extremely accurate laboratory that errs and declares a false positive once every one million tests for a banned substance. Testing for all of the IOC banned substances and their metabolites involves searching for over 100 drugs and over 400 metabolites. Using 500 tests for simplicity, that means the laboratory conducts a total of one million tests on every 2,000 urine samples. Accordingly, an error rate of one in one million tests yields one false positive in every 2,000 drug free urine samples tested. Assume that for every 2,000 drug free urine samples there are 40 (2%) urine samples with banned substances or their metabolites and the laboratory cautiously declares only 80% positive. That yields 32 positive tests of urine samples with banned substances. Given those numbers, for every 2,040 urine samples examined, 33 urine samples will be declared positive, and one out of 33, or 3%, will be false positive, despite the error rate of only one in a million. Even an error rate of one in ten million yields one false positive every 20,400 urine samples, and Dr. Catlin conducts tests on 15,000 urine samples each year. Assuming that Dr. Catlin's laboratory has examined 120,000 drug free urine samples over the past 12 years, conducting 500 tests for banned substances and metabolites per sample, Dr. Catlin's lab would have conducted sixty million tests without a single mistake. (Foschi v. FINA, 1996)*

The Foschi lawyers also suggested that the IOC had a financial motive for their claim that they do not make mistakes.

> *Dr. Catlin testified that he has tremendous incentive to cover-up a false positive. If it were ever to become known that he had a false positive, he says his lab, which generates over a million dollars per year from urine testing for sport organizations, "would be out of business in a flash" (Foschi, 1996).*

The Foschi lawyers' math is flawed in that it makes presumptions based on an open system where all the results of every test are known. As stated before, drug-testing results are not open to independent scrutiny or analysis, thus "false positive" tests would never become public. There is no accounting of the number of tests that have to be thrown out or not acted upon because laboratory directors may believe they are false positives.

According to IOC protocol, a second, confirmatory test must be done on each positive A-sample before the result is reported. Again, there is no record of how many false positives make it to this stage of the process but are never acted upon because they are discovered by this "fail safe" mechanism. So, while it is in the best interest of a defendant arguing a case against the system to make these arguments, the data to prove or disprove them are not available. A further safeguard built into the IOC system is that any analytical positive result must be reported to the IOC Medical Commission for analysis before action is taken against the individual producing the sample. So, there is, in effect, another stage where any errors in the process can be detected. While this does not mean that a false positive could not slip through the system, there are measures in place to prevent it from happening (Kammerer, 1997).

A Questionable System

Still, the system is solely administered by IOC personnel, which opens it to criticism that it is not subject to independent scrutiny. In a 1991 speech, Robert Armstrong, Chief Counsel to Canadian Justice Minister Charles Dubin, addressed these concerns:

While the concept of a universal standard for laboratory accreditation is to be applauded, the present system of accreditation is, in my view, subject to a serious problem of conflict of interest. The problem arises because some of the members of the IOC subcommission who determine which laboratories will be accredited and which laboratories will have their accreditation revoked also operate their own laboratories, which are accredited by the IOC. They have the ability to create a monopoly and an unfair price system....

To use a phrase from English common law, it is important not only that justice be done, but that justice appear to be done. Unless an athlete has full right of appeal, including the right and ability to challenge the scientific validity of the drug test, he or she will be denied a full right of review of any positive test. Chief Justice Dubin therefore recommended "that the grounds of appeal against a positive doping control test result be expanded to include challenges to the scientific validity of the test." *(Armstrong, 1991, pp. 24–25)*

Catlin, head of the IOC-accredited lab in Los Angeles, disputed the Canadians' conclusions (Catlin, 1991). He said that the Dubin Inquiry considered only limited testimony, mainly confined to the Canadian system, and that it is unfair to brand the entire IOC system as deficient based on this examination. He said he believes that the IOC system does allow for adequate review of tests. It is not a perfect system, he acknowledged, but it is the best that has yet been developed. To look merely at alleged shortcomings ignores the development of a sophisticated analytical system that must operate in a worldwide arena that is not immune from politics.

Dr. Robert Voy, former director of sports medicine for the USOC, agrees. He doesn't criticize the scientists who operate the labs, but rather the sport administrators who are charged with imposing sanctions based on the test results. He addressed this in his book *Drugs, Sport, and Politics:*

Allowing national governing bodies, international federations, and national Olympic Committees such as the United States Olympic Committee to govern the testing process to ensure fair play in sport is terribly ineffective. In a sense, it is like having the fox guard the henhouse.

There is simply too much money involved in international sports today. One needs to understand that the officials in charge of operating sport at the amateur level need world-class performances to keep their businesses rolling forward. . . . The athletes and officials realize this, so they're willing to do whatever it takes to win. And sometimes that means turning their backs on the drug problem. (Voy & Deeter, 1991, p. 101)

Irish cyclist-turned-journalist Paul Kimmage, in *A Rough Ride: An Insight Into Pro Cycling,* has been equally blunt in his criticism of the cycling sport authorities and their attitudes regarding enforcement of drug-testing rules (1990).

The men in power want a solution all right, but a painless one. . . . The grapevine is a dreadfully frustrating source of knowledge. Facts are often distorted, but there is no smoke without fire. I've heard stories of corruption that would make you ill. Of race organizers giving the green light to champions to take anything they want. Of urine samples that never reach laboratories. The temptation by those on the make is to cover up and not own up. But by not owning up we will continue to suck in the innocents and spit out the victims. (Kimmage, 1990, pp. 185–186)

Former French Open champion Yannick Noah openly questioned the tennis testing program's effectiveness. He said that testing was only done for public relations, not to catch cheaters. "I don't think they are going to find anything," he said. "They don't really want to. If they wanted to discover something they would test every week." ("Wimbledon-Drugs," 1990).

Still the IOC system is considered the most comprehensive of its kind in the world. It is, in effect, the industry standard (Dubin, 1990). The IOC Medical Commission has encouraged the sport governing bodies, under the umbrella of the IOC, to standardize the list of banned substances. It has supported economically and educationally the development of drug-testing labs at various Olympic venues, such as Montreal, Calgary, and Los Angeles (Hatton & Catlin, 1987). The IOC has tried, thus far unsuccessfully, to "harmonize" the drug-testing rules and procedures. Cultural, legal, and societal pressures have resulted in some federations having stricter doping legislation than others. Despite these shortcomings, the Olympic system is far ahead of that in the professional sports.

Possible Solutions Outside the IOC

American professional and collegiate sports have opted for something of a compromise, attempting to address the issue of drug use by athletes with testing programs structured to catch the obvious offenders, provide them with an opportunity for "rehabilitation," and shelter the sport from the stigma of harboring "cheaters." There are few public pronouncements about athletes who flunk drug tests. First-time offenders can be held out of games, often under the guise of an injury, and told to "clean up." After their period of rehabilitation, they can return to the game, subject only to a more strict monitoring program that involves more frequent testing. How effective this system is in minimizing drug use is unknown, as only chronic abusers are identified and the number of athletes who are truly rehabilitated is a secret. As the case of NFL lineman

Lyle Alzado illustrated, professional athletes can freely use drugs throughout their careers without fear of detection. When he was diagnosed with brain cancer, Alzado went public about his longtime use of performance-enhancing drugs and how he easily avoided detection because of the ineffectiveness of the NFL's drug-testing system.

None of the systems are open to public scrutiny, but the Olympic system has attracted the most attention due to the dire consequences of any offense and the recent litigation of disputed test results. Those who flunk drug tests in Olympic sports are publicly identified, banned from their respective sports, and lose the contracts they may have had with sponsors. While no professional "star" performer has ever been "busted" for use of performance-enhancing drugs during the "prime" of his or her career, Olympic athletes, such as 100 m champion Ben Johnson, have. For some this amounts to evidence of a double standard (Starkman, 1997).

Caught up in this system are the scientists. The laboratory scientists involved in the drug-testing system do not wage "war"; they merely analyze urine samples, and all indications are that they do that well. The cracks in the system form when the scientists are not given enough funding to properly research the tests they perform. Thus, even when a "positive" lab sample is produced, sport administrators have trouble enforcing their rules because lawyers can exploit loopholes in the system created by inadequate research. In other instances, lawyers will challenge rules that are written in such a way that enforcement is nearly impossible.

Sport administrators, fearful of the damage done to the sport's image and athletes' health through drug use, have declared that the drug-testing process should be confidential. Only when details emerged from many controversial cases, such as those involving track stars Harry "Butch" Reynolds and Mary Decker Slaney, and the Stasi files, have the legal and financial shortcomings of the testing system been exposed to the general public. What has emerged is a picture of a process conducted under the veil of confidentiality where little is truly confidential. Millions of dollars are at stake in the form of damaged reputations and lost income, but less is spent on the science than on lavish parties thrown by the sport officials in charge of administering the system (Ferstle, Sept. 1997). Although the process has actually accomplished a great deal in a short time, it is remembered more for its failures than its successes.

The failures have caused critics of the system, such as University of Texas professor John Hoberman, to predict that eventually there will be no drug testing. Sports stars will compete wearing the logos of performance-enhancing products, and the IOC will have a new sponsor category to sell (Patrick, May 1998). Others, such as U.S. Swim Coaches Association president John Leonard, say that they will fight for reform in the process.

Athletes' Rights in Drug Testing

The Olympic testing system is more extensive than that used by professional sports largely because the unions have been able to limit the scope of the testing program and what substances are banned. Professional athletes' rights are more pervasive. In the Olympic system, athletes have no union and few rights. Perhaps because of the difficulties faced by those attempting to enforce drug-testing rules, much of the legislation governing sanctions appears to conflict with common judicial practice. Once an athlete faces charges of providing a positive test, for example, the legal concept of "innocent until proven guilty" is thrown out the window. Lawyers in the Foschi case and later those representing U.S. 400 m intermediate hurdler Stephon Flenoy pointed out that governing bodies cannot "enforce an absolute liability rule: strict liability with no possibility of the athlete to defend" (Foschi, 1996).

The identification of a banned substance or its metabolite in an athlete's urine shall constitute an offense. From that rule, some members of FINA have tried to argue not only that the proof of a positive test and minimal chain of custody evidence satisfies FINA's burden to establish prima facie offense, but also that no defense to the report of a positive test will be permitted. Basic principles of fundamental fairness, due process, and natural justice require that members of a community not be punished through the application of rules that are contrary to the general understanding of the community. As the AAA [American Arbitration Association] panel held in this case, such rules are inconsistent with the basic concepts of United States justice. However, these are not concepts that are limited to the United States; they are concepts accepted in civilized nations around the world. (Foschi, 1996)

When challenged in court or before independent arbitration panels, the sport governing bodies have ultimately lost in attempting to enforce such draconian measures.

The IOC, fearful of the court costs associated with legal battles over their drug rules, had athletes competing in the 1996 Olympics sign a waiver committing them to resolving disputes through arbitration rather than in court. Arbitration of cases at the Olympics is handled quickly, in contrast to how disputed tests are handled by individual federations. There athletes have to first exhaust all appeals within their countries' federations and with the international governing body before there is the option of a hearing before an arbitration panel or some outside agency. By that time, however, they will have already served nearly all or a significant part of whatever sanction they face. This makes the concept of "speedy justice" something of a farce.

1984: The L.A. Cover-Up

Mistakes do happen in the system. Athletes can be subject to sanctions when the test results may be flawed. But, more often than not, when the testing system fails, it results in potentially guilty athletes escaping. Rumors of these failures generally emerge as tales of "cover-ups" of "positive tests." Not all of these tales are merely rumor. In sworn testimony given during the doping case of U.S. discus thrower Ben Plucknett in 1981, Arnold Beckett (of the IOC Medical Commission) acknowledged that some of the urine samples at the 1976 Winter Olympics had been tampered with. In a later interview Beckett revealed that the Soviets had "infiltrated" the lab and managed to get access to urine samples (Beckett, 1994). Testing had to be halted at those Games because of the incident (*Plucknett v. TAC/USA,* 1982).

The official report of the IOC issued after the 1984 Olympics in Los Angeles and a scientific paper published by Dr. Catlin and his associates at the UCLA lab that did the testing also yielded some discrepancies (Catlin, Kammerer, Hatton, et al., 1987; Dubin, 1990; Los Angeles Olympic Organizing Committee, 1985; Wadler & Hainline, 1989). When asked about the fact that the number of positives announced and the number reported in Catlin's paper did not match, Prince de Merode told a newspaper reporter in February 1988 that the IOC had waited until a medical commission meeting in November 1988 in Mexico to make public the other positive results (de Merode, 1988).

The only action taken at that meeting, however, was to ratify the results of a few positive tests that had not been formally announced during the Games. Several other positive tests remained, however. Dr. Voy, for one, wondered what happened. "The numbers don't add up," he said (Voy, unpublished interview, 1988).

In August of 1994, the answer became public. A letter signed by de Merode, Beckett, Dr. Robert Dugal, and Donike declared that the code necessary to identify an athlete's urine sample had been removed from de Merode's room and destroyed. The medical commission members said they had decided not to reveal this fact because nothing could be done to rectify the situation and going public with their concerns might only damage the testing system (Donike, unpublished letter, 1985). Several positive samples had been detected by the UCLA lab, but nothing could be done because the code documents, which had been stored in a safe in de Merode's room at the Biltmore Hotel, were removed by Los Angeles Olympic Organizing Committee (LAOOC) personnel ("Testing the Testors," 1994).

De Merode, when asked about the incident by reporters, said that the LAOOC's Dr. Tony Daly had initially told him the documents had been sent to Lausanne. When de Merode said he would get on a plane and retrieve them, Daly admitted the documents had been destroyed (Wilson, Sept. 1994). After this incident, said Beckett, steps were taken to make sure that the process could not be subverted in such a way again (Beckett, unpublished interview, 1994). The shredding in L.A., coupled with the fact that it remained a poorly kept "secret" for ten years, only increased the suspicion among many that positive test results had been "covered up" in the past and would be in the future.

These were not the only times the testing system was questioned. In the minutes of the IOC Medical Commission meetings in Los Angeles, de Merode was asked about the rumors of cover-ups of positive tests at the Moscow Olympics in 1980. De Merode responded that the problem in Moscow was the inability to detect all substances because of the use of an ineffective screening test that had been implemented for those Games (Minutes of IOC Medical Commission Meeting, 1984). Arnold Beckett, who helped set up the Moscow testing, acknowledged that political disputes had resulted in a less than adequate preparation and implementation of testing for the Moscow Games (Beckett, unpublished interview, 1994).

More Secrets

A previously secret doctoral study done in Germany by Johann Zimmermann revealed that analysis of the leftover samples from the Moscow Games in Donike's Cologne lab revealed potential use of testosterone. In 140 samples taken from female athletes, 10 had T/E (testosterone-to-epitestosterone) ratios above the IOC set limit of 6:1 and another 11 were above 5.3:1. Analysis of the 424 male samples indicated that 9 had T/E ratios above 6:1, and another 9 were above 5.3:1. Zimmermann's data also showed how the T/E ratios dropped dramatically from 1980 to 1983 when formal testing began using the T/E ratio to sanction athletes. In 1980, for example, 29 out of 342 samples tested were above 6:1, and another 34 were between 5.3:1 and 6:1. By 1983, out of 843 samples tested, only 7 were above 6:1, while 7 more were between 5.3:1 and 6:1 (Zimmermann, 1986).

The analysis of the samples by Dr. Donike fueled rumors that many positive tests had been covered up in Moscow. In Helsinki in 1983 at the IAAF World Track-and-Field Championships, Dr. Donike admitted in testimony before the Dubin Inquiry that some of the A-samples appeared to have excess levels of testosterone. On review, however, the medical panel decided not to test the B-samples. When an athlete provides a urine sample for testing, the sample is poured from the bottle in which it was collected into an A-sample bottle and a B-sample bottle. The A-sample is opened and tested at the lab. The B-sample is not tested unless a banned substance is found in the A-sample. The athlete has the right to be present when the B-sample is opened and tested. This system was created to help protect against tampering or sabotage of an athlete's specimen (Buffrey & Parrish, 1989).

If there is evidence of tampering, or if the seals on the bottles have been accidentally broken prior to testing, most organizations' drug-testing rules mandate that the test results are invalid and cannot be used to sanction an athlete. Examination of the previously secret files of the GDR sport system revealed that GDR officials conspired to protect their athletes from testing positive by substituting for "dirty" urine samples, destroying samples, and pretesting athletes prior to every competition (Berendonk & Franke, 1997). Because the process was not open to independent scrutiny, officials with access to it could subvert it, and the perception was created that some samples could be treated differently than others (Buffrey & Parrish, 1989).

For example, in 1988 10 athletes were banned from the Summer Olympics in Seoul for flunking drug tests. Dr. Jongsei Park, the director of the drug-testing lab in Seoul, told a reporter for the *New York Times* that "as many as 20 other athletes tested positive and were not disqualified" (Janofsky & Alfano, 1988). However, Park denied that there was any cover-up of positive tests when he was asked about the story at an IAF conference in Monte Carlo in 1989. He noted that four of the positive tests were cases in which HCG was detected in the urine samples, and four others were positive tests for marijuana, a substance not banned by the IOC. At least two of the urines containing HCG were from pregnant women, Park said (Park, 1989).

The IOC provided a summary of the drug testing at Seoul, listing four categories:

- The 10 positive tests
- 6 cases discussed and determined as not positive
- 3 IOC "control" samples—samples with known quantities of banned substances sent to the lab to test the lab's ability to make the proper analysis
- 15 samples that were studied "upon the request of the IOC Medical Commission" for "additional scientific research" (IOC, 1989)

Dr. Arne Ljungqvist, head of the IAAF Medical Commission and a member of the IOC Medical Commission, disputed the use of the term "positive" in the Seoul cases:

"It is completely wrong to refer to those cases as positive. The result of an analysis is not like a sheet of paper which says positive, but an analytical data which requires a specialist evaluation. In most cases, it's quite clear that a sample contains a banned substance and in other cases it's not." said Ljungqvist.

"But there are cases which are difficult to decide upon and require careful study. Some of those cases may then be judged as not positive and will therefore not be reported. This is, in all probability, what happened in some cases in Seoul like it happened in any other major competition." ("IOC-Drugs," 1988)

At the IAF-sponsored conference on drugs in sport in Monte Carlo in 1989, Ljungqvist and Beckett were grilled by the media regarding the issue of cover-ups. They steadfastly denied that there had ever been a cover-up of positive drug-test results. When asked if the drug-test records—test results with ID numbers attached, no identifying names—would ever be made public to squash the speculation and put an end to the rumors, both replied that they didn't believe that was possible (Beckett & Ljungqvist, 1989). Officials in charge of drug testing appear to believe that a closed system is necessary, that confidentiality can be protected only in a closed system. But little really remains totally confidential in Olympic sports, and when information "leaks," it is rarely flattering to the system.

In 1992, further evidence that targeting of athletes was not limited to the Olympics emerged. Near the opening of the Barcelona Olympics, two British weightlifters were sent home because tests they had taken prior to the Games revealed the presence of clenbuterol. While clenbuterol was not listed by name on the IOC list of banned substances, the IOC Medical Commission had been concerned about its use by athletes, and had recommended adding it to the list. Not all athletes or federations had been informed of this change, however. But, at the same time, Donike notified the German athletics federation by fax of the presence of clenbuterol in the urine of several female German sprinters, among them Katrin Krabbe.

Krabbe and her teammate Grit Breuer had been the subject of a controversy earlier in the year because the sample process for an out-of-competition test appeared to have been manipulated to subvert the system. The three urine samples that were taken from Krabbe, Breuer, and their teammate, who were training in South Africa, were all from the same person. The analysis of the samples appeared to indicate that the athletes could have used "artificial bladders" to store "clean" urine. These condomlike bladders would be inserted into the athlete's vagina and voided when the athlete was called to fill a sample bottle.

The suspension levied against the three athletes was overturned by the German courts because of rule irregularities. Thus, it appeared that the trio was being targeted by Donike for evidence of a violation. The fax revealed that several tests done on the trio were done by Donike's lab. Some revealed the use of clenbuterol; others were clean. But in all the tests, the code had been broken and the identity of the athletes was known to the lab. This practice demonstrated that confidentiality was not universally maintained within the system.

At the 1996 Games in Atlanta, the IOC system suffered another blow. It was revealed that tests done on the high resolution mass spectrometer (HRMS), a more expensive but more "sensitive" testing machine being used for the first time at these Games, had found traces of banned substances (Downes, 1997). However, instead of using the test results to impose sanctions, de Merode declared that they would be used only for "further study." Prior to the Games, the HRMS machine had been touted as a new weapon against drug abuse because it could theoretically detect more minute quantities of banned substances. After the Games were over, de Merode said that legal constraints prevented use of any of the data to sanction an athlete. At the very least, this incident was a public relations blunder. At worst, it was more fodder for those who claimed that the system is unnecessarily secretive and subject to abuse.

When you add to this the case of a Cuban judo participant who was merely given a warning despite the discovery of a banned diuretic in her urine, and the overturning of IOC sanctions for several Soviet athletes who tested positive for Bromantan, the testing at the Atlanta Games was considered by many to be a fiasco (Wadler, unpublished interview, 1997). Catlin was called in to operate the HRMS machines because the Atlanta lab, which received its certification only a month prior to the opening of the Games, did not have the necessary experience using the equipment. In Atlanta, Catlin tested the urine samples on regular mass spec equipment, the HRMS, and a carbon isotope spectrometer, which is being used to develop a more reliable test for the illegal use of testosterone (Catlin, unpublished interview, 1997).

According to Catlin, the steroid testing done in Atlanta was the most extensive of any Games. Yet the lingering impression after the Games, when only a couple of athletes had been banned and "positive" tests discovered on the HRMS machines were used only "for further study" ("Das Erbe," 1996), was that the system lacked credibility. Again, charges of "cover-up" were made, as few details were made public about potentially positive tests. This inability of the system to be open to independent scrutiny provides the most ammunition to its critics. As long as there is secrecy, the system will remain an easy target for those who want to use this issue as a club.

Testing Issues in Pro and U.S. Collegiate Sports

Drug use in the NFL was brought into the open in Dr. Arnold Mandell's 1976 book on the San Diego Chargers, *The Nightmare Season*. Major league baseball players' use of pep pills was exposed by well-publicized Pittsburgh grand jury findings in 1985 (Donohoe & Johnson, 1986) and by Jim Bouton's (1970) book, *Ball Four*. The NCAA was rocked by the drug-related death of a Clemson University athlete and by the prosecution of several coaches who were distributing drugs to student-athletes (Keisser, 1991).

The NFL had begun testing its players for drugs in training camps in 1982 (Demak & Kirshenbaum, 1990) but didn't test for anabolic steroids until 1987 (Forbes, 1989). By 1990 that program had expanded to include some random testing every 6 weeks. Currently players can be tested as many as 9 times during the year in a random selection process that is administered by Dr. John Lombardo (Wadler, 1997). NFL players are also tested during the off-season, but as in all the pro sports, the scope of the program is balanced against "individual rights" as defined by agreements between the league and players' unions.

In 1986 the NCAA began to develop a drug-testing program. This program is tightly controlled by the NCAA, and at first it included only limited testing at or before major bowl games or championships. It has since expanded to include some random testing of athletes and is bolstered by separate testing programs conducted by the universities (Yesalis, personal communication, 1991).

The Men's International Professional Tennis Council agreed in November 1985 that tennis players would submit to urinalysis at two of the five major tournaments. This initial testing was only for "social drugs," such as amphetamines and cocaine ("Drug Tests Sought," 1987). The program was later expanded in some situations to include anabolic steroids, and the players who competed in the 1988 Olympics were subject to IOC testing (Wadler & Hainline, 1989).

American professional sports have testing programs that are not remotely comparable to those conducted by Olympic sport federations. Major League Baseball and the NBA still have only very limited testing. Basketball and baseball are only concerned with recreational drugs, while the NFL does test for anabolic steroids (Wadler & Hainline, 1989). Their programs are based on a concept of rehabilitating offenders rather than sanctioning them after a first offense. By not imposing immediate sanctions, these programs have had better luck in maintaining the confidentiality of the process.

The disparity between professional sports and the Olympic sports became clear in 1998 when McGwire's use of androstenedione was reported during "Big Mac's" quest to set a new major league home run record. Randy Barnes, 1996 Olympic shot put champion, had been suspended earlier in the year for using the same substance. Obviously the rules were not the same for all athletes. What was even clearer was that stars are treated differently than other players. While it was known, prior to the McGwire revelations, that other players in the major leagues used andro, the story did not become front page news until it involved Big Mac. Also, in April two minor league ballplayers were suspended for use of anabolic steroids. Tests had been done on them, the league said at the time, because of suspicion of drug use by younger players (*USA Today*, 1998). This unequal treatment provoked less debate, however, than the impact these revelations had on kids who now saw their role models, famous athletes, condoning the use of performance-enhancing drugs.

Why should a professional baseball player be allowed to use a substance that an Olympic athlete cannot? In reality this disparity had always existed, but had not been brought into such a clear view. Professional sports do treat drug use differently, and, depending on your point of view, professional sport organizations are either getting away with it or are merely facing the fact that drug use in society is rampant and that athletes are not immune. The pro sport rules appear to be based on the premise that as long as the drugs don't harm or kill you, you can take them.

Politics and Pharmacological Warfare

As stated earlier, the testing system's major weakness is that it mixes politics with pharmacology. The governing bodies need absolute proof of guilt, and often the science necessary to provide that proof is not available, either because of inadequate funding or because those attempting to subvert the system have found yet another way to beat it. With the adverse publicity each positive drug test generates, governing bodies have little incentive to catch people. Doriane Lambelet Coleman, an attorney and a nationally ranked 800 m runner who was instrumental in drafting comprehensive legislation for USATF's out-of-competition testing program and revamping USATF's current rules in 1989, provided a revealing commentary on the rules that governed the drug-testing appeals process in track and field.

"It appeared that whoever drafted these rules was either not very bright or that they wanted people to get off," said Coleman (1989) about the old rules. "The way the legislation was drafted, there were plenty of loopholes." Several cases in the United States illustrated some of the loopholes to which Coleman referred. These cases prompted her and others to seek changes in the drug-testing appeals process after athletes successfully challenged lab results.

Dubin Commission lawyer, Robert Armstrong, further criticized the IOC's inaction at the International Symposium on Sport and Law in Monte Carlo in 1991:

> *The IOC and its Medical Commission have known for years that testing for anabolic steroids at the time of competition was a virtual waste of time in terms of providing effective deterrent for their use during training periods.... There had been a failure of leadership among our sporting governing organizations, both at the national and international level. If you examine the Dubin Report carefully, I think you will agree that our sport leaders have let us down. If you are going to lead, you must lead from the head of the line. You must be out front. You cannot lead by reacting after the fact. (Armstrong, 1991, pp. 19–20)*

De Merode and Hans Skaset, the president of Norway's Confederation of Sport, pointed out at the World Conference on Anti-Doping in Sport in 1988 that leadership in an international arena is not easy to achieve. Implementing an international plan involves negotiating with leaders of sometimes hostile nations to accomplish an often not-so-common goal. As Skaset pointed out:

> *You have all sorts of mistrust mixed in with this; you have the East-West dimension.... If we could have something like an INF treaty between the Soviet Union, the German Democratic Republic and the United States, then they would have to patrol each other.... (Hynes, 1988)*

De Merode added:

> *It's absolutely necessary to do it, to have random tests during competition, but through training as well. It's the next step we have to pass, but it's only possible if the concept is acceptable to everybody.... You cannot tell an international federation you cannot do this. We can only tell them of the problem. ("Down on Dope," 1988)*

The Opposition

The drug testers don't operate in a vacuum. In addition to dealing with the politicians and legislators, they have to fight a pharmacological war with athletes and their advisers, who are constantly attempting to stay one step ahead of the labs. Charlie Francis, Ben Johnson's coach from 1981 until 1988, was nicknamed by some of his peers "Charlie the chemist"—not because he had a degree in biochemistry but because he knew about drugs and the drug-testing system (Denton, 1989).

When he was coaching and after Johnson was caught, Francis was kept up to date on the latest in sports pharmacology by a wide array of individuals operating in and behind the scenes in track and field. From undetectable anabolic steroids to masking agents, Francis heard stories about all forms of substances athletes were taking in an attempt to beat the drug-testing system. When the testing for anabolic steroids became more sophisticated, the athletes turned to dihydrotestosterone, then clenbuterol, a supposed steroid substitute. Sydnocarb, a stimulant that was at one time unavailable to lab testers and, therefore, undetectable, was used until the labs caught up. There were rumors of a substance called lipoplex that is supposed to metabolize the metabolites of a steroid so that its by-products will not be recognized on a drug screen as those of a banned substance (Francis, 1991). Athletes were also taking gonadotropin-releasing hormones in an attempt to balance their endocrine profiles; as a result, their profiles looked normal and the athletes could not be sanctioned by any new test that used these profiles. Since then, testosterone precursors, such as DHEA, and another allegedly anabolic product, IGF-1 (insulinlike growth factor), have become the "hot" products pushed by the ergogenic gurus.

Dr. Mauro DiPasquale discussed this in the newsletter *Drugs in Sports*:

> *In the past few years there has been such an emphasis on the use of anabolic steroids that few people, other than the athletes themselves, have noticed the quiet revolution that has been occurring. While athletes are still using anabolic steroids (there has been little decrease in the use of anabolic steroids by the more pharmacologically sophisticated athletes), most are making extensive use of other compounds for the purposes of enhancing their performance, with or without the concomitant use of anabolic steroids.*

These compounds are used as ergogenic aids, masking agents to conceal the use of anabolic steroids, and therapeutic agents to deal with the side effects of anabolic steroid use. Many of these compounds are either not detectable or are not tested for, further increasing the incentive for their use. (DiPasquale, 1991, p. 2)

How a government-sponsored doping program operated was revealed in the GDR documents. Not only did GDR labs monitor the athletes to make sure they would not fail drug tests, but GDR pharmaceutical companies were also engaged to develop drugs that could be used to beat the drug tests. The GDR labs developed a special anabolic steroid, Turinabol, and a synthetic epitestosterone, which was used to prevent GDR athletes from showing up on a urine test with a T/E ratio above 6:1.

Each of these forms of subterfuge may fail if the lab knows what to look for, which is one reason why IOC lab directors are so concerned about secrecy, and why those attempting to beat the system are constantly scouring the medical journals to uncover those secrets.

Does masking work or is this merely the case of an enterprising individual attempting to take advantage of a new niche in the marketplace? In the mid-1980s, athletes used probenecid to block the excretion of banned substances (Catlin & Hatton, 1991). They diluted their urine, used catheters, and hid bags of "clean" urine on or in their bodies in an attempt to beat the system. In the 1990s, athletes are resorting to polypharmacy—use of a wide variety of substances—to beat the system (DiPasquale, 1991). The mystery remains: How much of this pharmacological competition is fact and how much is fiction?

Sports Illustrated reported in the spring of 1997 that athletes were consulting chemists to make designer steroids, drugs altered in chemical structure to mask their presence in the urine (Yaeger & Bamberger, 1997). Catlin maintains that such a practice, while theoretically possible, would be ultimately detected by IOC labs. "If it's a steroid, then I believe we could find it," said Catlin (Catlin, 1997). The trouble is that by the time the IOC labs find the substance, do the testing necessary to make sure they can reliably detect it, and put it on the banned list, the athletes have moved on to another substance that may provide the same ergogenic effect. In 1998, charges were made that cyclists were using perfluorocarbon (PFC), a blood substitute that could improve oxygen carrying capacity. It was also revealed that two German distance runners used HES, a blood plasma expander. Neither were banned at the time, but both may have aided performance.

The fact remains that there are substances that are difficult, if not impossible, to detect. Stories circulated in 1996 of a stimulant that was being used widely by athletes. The substance had been given to subjects, who were then tested in an IOC lab. The drug could not be found (Kammerer, 1996).

The Courts

By the 1990s, as Olympic sports became more openly professional, drug cases began to be litigated because the stakes for the athletes were so high. Clauses in sponsorship agreements called for the termination of any sponsorship if an athlete was convicted of a drug offense. In some cases, the clauses also allowed a company to recoup fees paid to that athlete if the athlete was found guilty of a doping offense. Until 1995, only three cases, the 1987 suspension of Swiss distance runner Sandra Gasser, the 1988 positive test of U.S. swimmer Angel Meyers (Martino), and the 1990 case of 400 m world-record holder Harry "Butch" Reynolds, had gone to court to challenge the results of drug tests.

Testimony by Dr. David Black (1991) in the Reynolds case created enough doubt about the validity of the test results in the minds of a U.S. federal arbitrator and a three-member USATF panel that they ruled in favor of Reynolds. Dr. Black's review of the test done in an IOC-accredited lab in Paris raised several questions about the accuracy and interpretation of Reynolds's test data. Doubts were also raised about the "chain of custody" when a lawyer for Reynolds demonstrated that the seal on the "envopak" that contains the urine sample could be "picked" with a dental pick.

This flaw in the chain of custody did not prove that Reynolds's sample had been tampered with, but it created doubt about the system that is supposed to ensure against tampering. Each sample is collected in a beaker that is selected by the athlete. After the athlete has been observed urinating into the beaker, the urine is poured into two bottles (these are the A and B samples). The bottles are marked with a code number, sealed, and sent to the lab in an envopak that is also sealed with a tab that has a coded number on it. Any serious breach of this chain-of-custody process can be grounds for invalidating the analytical results of the tests on the bottles' contents.

Although scientific issues were involved in the disposition of the Reynolds case, the main issues on which the case turned were procedural (i.e., problems in the chain of custody) (TAC Doping Control Review Board, 1991, p. 7). Such is also the case in the other way in which athletes have successfully overturned analytically positive tests: through the appeals process of a sport's governing body.

In 1987, U.S. discus thrower John Powell was informed that a sample he allegedly provided after the USATF championships had tested positive for nandrolone. Powell appealed, stating that USATF could not prove that the sample was his because of irregularities in the collection and labeling process (Almond, 1990). A key piece of evidence in Powell's appeal was the fact that the documents accompanying his sample rendered the test invalid, according to the members of the appeals panel. Others pointed out that the mislabeling could have easily been intentional and should not have invalidated the test (USOC, 1987). As a result of this case, USATF rules were changed so that a labeling error would not automatically invalidate a positive result (Coleman, 1989). Other USATF cases also resulted in a new USATF rule regarding testosterone.

In 1989, shot-putter August Wolf and pole vaulter Billy Olsen were informed that samples they provided at the USATF indoor championships had higher than the allowed limit for testosterone. Both appealed and presented witnesses challenging the validity of the testosterone test. Their appeals were successful and neither was disciplined (TAC, 1989).

Subsequently a rule was passed at the 1989 USATF convention stating that a T/E ratio of over 6:1 would be considered a positive result, and the onus was on the athlete to prove that his or her ratio was not the result of drug use (TAC, 1990). This doctrine of guilty until proven innocent has held up, even though challenged by Reynolds and Barnes. Both contended that USATF's rules violated the U.S. constitution, which ensures that a person is considered innocent until proven guilty. The burden is usually on the prosecutor to prove that the accused is guilty, rather than on the accused to demonstrate that the charges are false (TAC Doping Control Review Board, 1991). Reynolds won his appeal in the United States; Barnes did not.

The U.S. judicial philosophy of innocent until proven guilty contributed to Reynolds's winning his USATF appeal but may not be upheld in Europe, where the philosophy is "guilty until proven innocent," as the Sandra Gasser case illustrated. Gasser was also found innocent by her federation, but she lost her case in the British courts, which ruled that she failed to prove her innocence (*Gasser v. Stinson,* 1988).

This legal confusion amply illustrates some of the difficulties encountered by sport administrators and athletes who are forced to litigate what appears to be an analytically positive drug test.

The case of Diane Modahl, however, challenged the system on a more important arena, that of science. Modahl's urine sample, analyzed in the IAAF-accredited lab at Lisbon, contained what appeared to be a T/E level of 42:1, well over the limit of 6:1. A study done at Donike's lab in Cologne, however, revealed that errors in sample handling could account for abnormal T/E ratios (Donike, Geyer, Gotzmann, & Mareck-Engelke, 1995). Further study by scientists in Manchester, England, also revealed that the handling of Modahl's sample may have produced the positive test.

Because the sample had been left on a dock, exposed to sweltering temperatures and possible degradation, any results gained from it became suspect. The Manchester researchers revealed that urine exposed to heat could degrade. This degradation could result in the multiplication of testosterone and the degradation of epitestosterone, thus resulting in the huge ratio (Webb, 1996). Modahl won her case and is now seeking damages against the British Athletics Federation.

Modahl's case was not the only one where athletes have created doubt in the minds of appeal panels regarding an analytically positive drug test. Basketball player Stacey Augmon and hockey player Corey Millen were able to convince the USOC that their elevated testosterone levels were not the result of doping. Millen played for the U.S. Olympic hockey team in 1984 and 1988, and Augmon played basketball for the 1988 U.S. team. Millen was banned by the International Ice Hockey Federation in 1989 because of his over-the-limit testosterone ("Millen Barred," 1989), but Augmon successfully appealed his over-the-limit testosterone test results before an IOC medical panel at the 1988 Summer Olympics in Seoul (Almond, 1990). Both argued that their bodies produced naturally high levels of testosterone that caused their ratios to be outside the 6:1 IOC limit. The ice hockey federation, however, refused to accept Millen's defense.

Research done in Scandinavia has, in fact, indicated that there are a significant number of individuals similar to Millen and Augmon, called outliers by the scientists. Using results from a year's tests (8,946) on Swedish athletes, 27 were found to have "natural" high T/E ratios above 6:1 that were not the result of drug use (Garle, 1996). Further research done by Donike's lab and labs in several other European nations revealed that T/E ratios might also be affected by intake of alcohol, birth control pills, or female menstrual cycles (Donike, Geyer, Gotzmann, & Mareck-Engelke, 1996).

In the spring of 1997, two more T/E ratio cases raised more questions about the applicability of the test. American track stars Mary Decker Slaney and Sandra Farmer Patrick provided urine samples that tested above the 6:1 ratio at the 1996 U.S. Olympic track-and-field trials. Coleman, working for one of the athletes, challenged the finding on the basis of research done in Donike's Cologne lab that showed T/E ratios could be affected by alcohol consumption and a woman's menstrual cycle. These revelations further undermined the IOC's tests for testosterone (Longman, 1997; Ferstle, May 1997).

While these tests were highly publicized, insiders say that female athletes with T/E ratios between 6:1 and 10:1 have successfully appealed their cases and not been sanctioned (Muscle Media 2000, May 1997). One male bodybuilder with a 10:1 T/E ratio also had his ban overturned by using a test touted by the British IOC-accredited lab. The procedure involved giving the athlete ketoconazole, a substance that lowers natural production of testosterone. If the athlete's testosterone levels go down, he or she is innocent of doping. If the levels stay elevated, the athlete is guilty because the excreted testosterone could be coming only from an artificial source (Wadler, 1997).

The confusion over guilt or innocence that surrounds the T/E ratio test has allowed athletes to create doubt about the validity of the test for testosterone and opened a rather large loophole in the testing system. Donike advocated backing up positive results through the use of endocrine profiles, such as the one used in the Johnson case in Seoul to refute Johnson's contention that his drinks were spiked ("Update," 1989). Catlin has also developed a carbon isotope test that is being touted as a definitive answer to the problem of determining whether or not a T/E ratio higher than 6:1 is due to doping (Goodbody & Powell, *London Times,* May 20, 1997).

The endocrine profile has been controversial within the drug-testing community for the same reason that other natural substances cause problems—there is a lack of controlled scientific studies to determine normal and abnormal levels of the substances being identified and measured. Advised of the use of profiles, however, athletes have begun using substances such as gonadotropin-releasing hormones to give themselves "normal" profiles. If the carbon isotope test can pass scientific scrutiny, however, it may provide a partial answer for the T/E situation. The trouble with the test is that it can detect only synthetic testosterone; thus if an athlete dopes with DHEA or other testosterone precursors or stimulators, the ratio method would still have to be used to catch them (Ferstle, Sept. 1997). IOC lab directors maintain that they can detect use of these precursors in both regular mass spectrometry testing and with the high resolution carbon isotope method (Ayotte, 1999). The research on these methods is minimal, however, so their validity will ultimately be tested in court rather than in the lab.

The dispositions of the testosterone cases illustrate the difficulty that scientists and governing bodies have with substances that are naturally produced. Testosterone, hGH, and erythropoietin are banned substances that the human body produces naturally. Comprehensive studies of what constitutes normal levels of these substances have not yet been conducted (Catlin & Hatton, 1991). The studies by IOC labs have been primarily on athletes; only in recent years have these labs started to test other populations to validate or alter the 6:1 ratio that they currently use as the guideline for determining an analytically positive test for doping using testosterone. The NCAA considered raising the ratio above 6:1 in 1990 and the IOC considered lowering the ratio to 4:1 (Ferstle, 1991). When the Decker Slaney and Farmer Patrick cases were made public, the USOC put together a five-member panel that was designed to review each T/E case before any action would be taken.

"The scientific basis for the testosterone test is sound," said Dr. Catlin. "The problem develops in that it does not produce a positive test, but a finding that must be investigated. You cannot determine whether a violation has occurred from just one test, you have to examine the data from a series of tests." (Ferstle, Sept. 1997)

As a result, T/E cases often take months to years to be resolved. The basis of the decision often shifts from examination of a lab analysis to a subjective decision based on the accumulated evidence. Meanwhile an athlete is usually suspended from competition or has to sue to win the right to compete. There is no speedy justice in a T/E case, leaving some sport officials to suggest that action on T/E tests be suspended until swift, reliable testing can be done to determine the guilt or innocence of an athlete accused of taking testosterone.

Sometimes substances that are not banned show up in a urine screen as a banned drug. In 1995, for example, a U.S. woman tested positive for amphetamines. The positive test, however, was caused by taking Deprenyl, a drug used for treating Parkinson's disease and that was widely touted among heath gurus as an antioxidant (Austad, 1997). The athlete was not banned, but was forced to miss important competitions while appealing the test result.

Rogue Labs

The sport drug-testing labs face "competition" from commercial labs that protect athletes from being caught. The IOC lab directors call them "outlaw laboratories." These labs will test the urine of anyone who pays the fee (Catlin & Moses, 1989). The testing is done anonymously, and no sanctions are imposed. Athletes use the services, for example, to determine their T/E ratios so they can stay just under the detection limit of the IOC tests. A more serious example of this behavior has been the revelation in the Soviet and German press of the pretesting of Olympic athletes by labs in those countries to make sure athletes attending international competitions were clean (Harvey, 1990; Starcevic, 1990).

In 1984 the USOC allowed U.S. athletes to anonymously send urine samples to the UCLA lab for testing. USOC officials said that the program was designed to allow the UCLA lab to gain experience handling and analyzing drug samples but later admitted that the program was a mistake and that athletes used the program to learn about their clearance times (Patrick, 1989; Puffer, 1988). Craig Kammerer, who was the assistant director of the lab in 1984, said that the USOC did not give the same explanation to lab staff as to the public:

We were told that positive results from the tests at the Olympic trials would be grounds for keeping people off the team. And some people did lose their place on the Olympic team in 1984, but we saw more than the number who weren't allowed to compete. (Kammerer, 1991)

In response to the actions of the "rogue labs," de Merode announced in May 1988 the promulgation of a code of ethics for IOC-accredited labs. The code forbids IOC labs from doing testing for individuals ("Labs Under IOC Gun," 1988). This has not stopped athletes from seeking such assistance. IOC lab directors are called regularly by individuals seeking testing. Some non-IOC labs openly offer the service. Augie Wolf was actively soliciting business for one such lab in 1990, sending a prospectus offering anonymous testing at a lab in northern California (Moses, 1989).

Beating the System

Athletes will try almost anything to beat the system. They will consult with so-called steroid gurus for ways to beat the tests or for access to the latest undetectable substances. They will have a teammate or friend urinate for them and switch samples. They will be tipped off as to when the tests will be conducted so they will be "clean" (Bedell, 1991). They will inject epitestosterone to foil the tests that measure the T/E ratio. Or they will use vinegar, salt, bleach, WD-40 lubricant, hydrogen peroxide, or ammonia in an attempt to produce a negative sample (Bedell, 1991). Catheters and condoms have also been used to substitute or store urine, which is then emptied into the collection bottle at the appropriate time.

And, if all this fails, athletes will use more extreme measures. One American athlete "accidentally" dropped his B-sample bottle in an attempt to void his positive test. When the bottle didn't break, he picked it up and threw it, smashing the bottle and voiding the test. He could not be suspended for a failed drug test nor banned for smashing the bottle because the rules at the time did not cover such an offense (Ferstle, 1991).

Quality Control

Lab work that is not up to IOC standards can also produce false positives, as was illustrated by the following three cases. In 1989, Norwegian javelin thrower Trine (Solberg) Hattestad was convicted by her federation and the IAAF of flunking a drug test at the European Cup meet in Brussels. The IAAF later reversed the conviction and decertified the lab that did the test. Hattestad sued the Norwegian federation and was awarded a $50,000 judgment ("Solberg Wins Damages," 1990).

In early 1991, the female member of a Soviet pairs team was also accused of producing a positive test. The result was leaked after an A-sample tested in an uncertified lab in Sofia, Bulgaria, was deemed to be positive for excessive testosterone. The B-sample analysis done in Cologne was negative. The skating federation was reprimanded and told not to use noncertified labs for its testing (Zanca, 1991).

The conviction of a Yugoslavian long jumper at the 1990 European championships was also recently overturned by the IAAF ("Bilac Back," 1991). These cases illustrate that quality control is a major issue in drug testing. The competence of a lab can often determine whether an athlete is judged guilty or innocent. Since 1988, the IOC has worked hard to improve the accreditation process. It has made great strides in improving lab standards, but one criticism still applies. Unlike other lab accreditation programs, the IOC's is administered by member labs, not an outside accrediting body.

Sabotage

The element of sabotage has been raised in defense of U.S. Olympic hopeful swimmer Jessica Foschi. Prior to the 1996 Olympic trials, Foschi's urine sample contained mesterolone, an anabolic steroid. She maintained her innocence and scoured the test data for a reason to explain how the banned substance got into her body. Her only conclusion was sabotage, backed in part by the absence of an altered steroid profile and the large quantity of the drug found in her system. Foschi successfully fought the ban within the U.S. Swimming Federation, but was banned by FINA, the international swimming governing body, which maintained that athletes are responsible for whatever they ingest. The rules cannot be altered to include provisions for sabotage, they claimed. Foschi appealed her ban to the international court of arbitration, which ruled in her favor in the summer of 1997, awarding her slightly more than $10,000 in damages.

The Foschi case and that of American 400 m hurdler Stephon Flenoy raised the question of athletes' rights in the drug-testing process. Flenoy was suspended prior to being given an adequate hearing, said his lawyer Ed Williams. A U.S. district court arbitrator ruled in Flenoy's favor in the summer of 1997, voiding Flenoy's suspension and allowing him to compete in the USATF championship meet.

Whenever stiff penalties are proposed, they are often opposed by those citing legal objections. For example, several individuals challenged the NCAA's drug-testing programs on the grounds that they violated individuals' rights in the United States (Almond, 1989; "Court Backs NCAA's Drug Tests," 1988; "Update," 1989; Wong, 1988). In August of 1997, the IAAF voted to reduce its four-year ban for drug use to a two-year ban. The reason for this "climb down" was that courts in several countries had ruled that a four-year ban was too harsh and a "restraint of trade."

Many of the same arguments were made when individuals proposed out-of-competition, random testing of athletes in Olympic or professional sports. A strong players' union combined with NFL management's lack of enthusiasm for a strong drug-testing program hindered the development of any comprehensive attack against drug use in the NFL. Some players have even charged that NFL team personnel often openly subvert the process, as an unnamed NFL player told *Sports Illustrated:*

> *The problem is enforcement. Some clubs have a guy who enforces the testing. Our guy is like one of the boys. He sits by the weight room eating a sandwich. Say it's your turn to be tested. You say, "Pete, my urine's a little weak today, let me come back tomorrow," or you get the trainer to piss in the bottle for you and give Pete that one. It's a joke. (Wulf, 1991, p. 10)*

In the Olympic sports, the collection process presents a different hurdle to the effectiveness of drug testing. The collection of a urine sample from an athlete is an important first step in the drug-testing chain of custody. Almost universally, however, this process is operated by volunteers. Some may be well-trained medical professionals, others high school students. This reliance on volunteer help and the design of the collection process can create problems. In the celebrated first case of alleged doping involving Randy Barnes, testimony revealed what some consider a huge flaw in the collection process. According to documents and transcripts of Barnes's hearing before the Athletics Congress (TAC) (1990), the individual who served as the crew chief at the meet in Malmo, Sweden, where Barnes allegedly tested positive for methyltestosterone, (a) failed to list the envopak number for Barnes's sample on Barnes's form, and (b) possessed all the tools necessary to substitute another sample for the one Barnes had given and avoid detection of such a switch.

According to Alvin Chriss, who was special assistant to the executive director of USATF and involved in drafting USATF's current drug-testing legislation:

> *One guy had control of everything. Whether or not I have a doubt that this man and his wife did in fact attempt to subvert the process, which I do not believe they did, the IAAF should not be allowed to defend the sloppiness of a procedure that allows this kind of work to pass muster. (Chriss, 1991)*

As noted in the Powell case described earlier, mistakes in the process can invalidate a positive lab result and undermine the credibility of the system. Training for the volunteers who often play key roles in the collection process is often minimal, and there is no formal review of the process. Similar concerns were raised in the Michelle Smith de Bruin case when data showed that the sample tested on-site had a significantly different specific gravity than when it was tested in the lab. The key to the case seemed to be proving who tampered with the sample.

All these systemic problems underscore the need for more funds and independent scrutiny, but nobody is rushing to provide funding for the system. In effect, the sport governing bodies fund this "cottage industry" of sport dope testing through testing; only recently have the NCAA and IOC provided any research money independent of the testing funding. Money does not come in the form of grants for scientific research on drugs in sport, only in the form of fees for analyzing samples. The drug-testing system, therefore, is monetarily driven by testing.

This emphasis on testing has its roots in the belief of many sport administrators that merely the threat of testing would deter athletes from using drugs. These administrators ignored the advice of many of the emerging pioneers in the field of sport drug testing, such as Brooks and Beckett of London, Donike, and Dugal from Montreal, by adopting a minimalist approach to drug testing. They funded tests only during competitions and announced the testing in advance (Dubin, 1990).

Almost from the beginning, therefore, a gap existed between what many scientists advised and what sport authorities were willing to fund or enforce. The lack of early action to prevent the proliferation of drugs may well have been a costly mistake. Most observers agree that the best chance the governing bodies had to gain control of the problem came in the early 1970s when congressional hearings were held. The testimony fell largely on deaf ears, however, and drug use has continued to increase since then. Proponents of the IOC system note that all these problems are merely "growing pains" of a largely effective and comprehensive testing program. IOC officials constantly proclaim that they are winning the "war against drugs" and that the IOC system is the best in the world. In 1996, the IOC contributed $1 million to research for a project dubbed GH 2000. The research, commissioned for several labs in the IOC system, is designed to find effective tests for hGH and other endogenous substances. The project was undermined somewhat, however, when the promised delivery of the excess urine samples from the Atlanta Olympics to the labs doing research was never executed (Downes, 1997). Scientists within and outside the IOC system also maintain that $1 million is a paltry amount to spend on drug-testing research. The wife of an IOC lab director (Cowan) works for a major pharmaceutical company and notes that her company will routinely spend $10 million on developing a single drug. Cowan also noted that a single lab in Japan that tests race horses will perform the same number of tests in a year that are done in the entire IOC system during that same time.

Drug Testing and the Media

From 1968 to 1988, sport drug testing developed from a cottage industry to an amorphous, semiregulated business largely out of the public view. Then Ben Johnson tested positive, and drug use and drug testing became front-page news in almost every media outlet in the world. The Dubin Inquiry grabbed the world's attention. Since Johnson was caught in Seoul, hardly a week goes by without some mention of drugs in sports, and in 1998 the seemingly endless drug scandals increased public awareness of the proliferation of drug use in sports. Until Johnson was caught, the media often ignored the issue, looked the other way, or merely believed drug stories were bad copy. The following excerpt from a column written by Alan Greenberg (1991) of the *Hartford Courant* is typical of many reporters' treatment of the issue:

> *I was covering the Los Angeles Raiders when Alzado, who had played previously with the Denver Broncos and Cleveland Browns, joined [the team] in 1982. He had acne on his back and upper arms, classic signs of steroid use. And his moods? One minute, he was the greatest guy in the world; the next minute, he was an erupting volcano for seemingly no reason.*
>
> *In 1984, I was talking to one of his teammates across the Raiders' dressing room, when Alzado, with no provocation, picked up his gray metal stool and threw it in my direction, shouting something about "reporters in the locker room." Shaken, I asked several players who knew him best what was bugging him. They said Alzado had probably just had a steroid injection and to stay out of his way. Good advice.*

A more sobering analysis was delivered by Greenberg's colleague Jerry Trecker (1991) of the *Hartford Courant:*

A sports machine capable of pretending that it doesn't debase the nation's educational system with its flaunting of academic standards, is equally adept at convincing itself that drug use really isn't that widespread. A sports media that pretends to birddog its subject by analyzing every play of a Super Bowl or an NCAA basketball final is also good at imagining that an occasional "expose" discharges the responsibility to truly profile the athletes it glorifies. And fans who may care more about the money they bet on a game than the way their favorites win are unlikely to insist upon high standards in the locker room.

With the revelations from the Dubin hearings, GDR files, and disputed test results, the media has become more aware of the strengths and weaknesses of the drug testing system. While pro sports are generally not exposed to much scrutiny in this area, Olympic sports have been frequently attacked for the perceived flaws in the testing system. Some members of the media have even attempted to expose the double standard that exists. *Toronto Star* reporter Randy Starkman (1997), for example, recently noted the "hypocrisy" of the uneven scrutiny between professional and Olympic hockey players.

When the worlds of NHL players and Olympic athletes collided for the first time in Nagano in 1998, one thing that became more striking than ever was the difference in the levels of scrutiny each is under when it comes to drug testing.

Just think about it for a moment: Canadian Olympians—the freestyle skiers, figure skaters, biathletes or bobsledders—are subject to year-round, random drug testing throughout their careers. NHL players who became Olympians were subjected to the same level of testing for a period of less than three months. Does society care less if an NHL star uses steroids to strengthen himself than if a bobsledder does?

The hypocrisy of the issue really becomes clear when you consider that the 60-plus NHL candidates who represented Canada in hockey at the 1998 Nagano Olympics provided urine samples for confidential testing. Even if a player were loaded up on steroids, testosterone, or amphetamines, there were to have been no sanctions. League officials say the testing was done for educational purposes, because of all the innocuous substances, such as cough medicines, on the IOC list. If one of the other Canadian Olympians had been caught taking something, he or she would have been booted off the team. They didn't get the benefit of these "educational" tests.

The revelation, in the summer of 1998, of McGwire's use of androstenedione, seemed to confirm the lack of concern about drug use in professional sports. While many commentators contrasted the treatment of Barnes and McGwire, others said, in effect, what's the big deal? Baseball doesn't ban it. McGwire didn't break any rules. McGwire even criticized the Olympic testing system, scoffing that it tests for cold medicine. Still, it was clear that by 1998 the media had become more educated about the issues of drug use in sports. It was no longer our little secret, but a well-established fact that drug use was widespread. Concern over the use of substances such as creatine, which was not banned, focused attention on what public policy should be on the issue. Far from having a consensus, however, there seemed to be more debate than agreement over what the world's athletes should or shouldn't be allowed to use.

Conclusion

The concept of analyzing an athlete's urine for the presence of prohibited substances seems simple. Just put the fluids into the machine and wait for the results. But, like everything else, what seems simple has a way of becoming complex. Machines fail. They are designed and operated by humans. Humans make mistakes. A mistake in a drug test can cost an athlete a medal or a career. Thus, much of the debate surrounding drug testing concerns ways to avoid those mistakes. Catch the cheaters, but don't ban an innocent man or woman.

This aversion to accusing the innocent is the rationale sport administrators cite when explaining the cloak of secrecy in drug testing. Test results are supposed to be private until a final determination is made on the guilt or innocence of the athlete. But there are leaks, rumors, and accusations of cover-ups that a system draped in confidentiality is ill equipped to deal with effectively.

Thus a process based on science becomes embroiled in human emotion. As Cassell (1991) told a meeting of race directors, drug testing is one of the most emotional issues an athlete, coach, or sport administrator encounters because the stakes are so high.

Testing is complex because the research in the field is so new and limited to only a very select group of labs. Thus the seemingly simple question of whether or not an athlete is truly guilty of using a banned substance is often obscured by conflicting testimony, testimony that is often slanted for political or economic gain.

Although drug testing is offered as the solution to the problem of drug use by athletes, the system's effectiveness is directly related to the competence and integrity of those who operate it. Because of the high stakes involved, that competence and integrity will always be challenged. The key to evaluating the system's effectiveness, therefore, is how well its operators maintain their high standards in the face of the constant barrage of criticism directed at their operations.

In its infancy, drug testing was established as a deterrent to athletes using drugs. As the testing system enters adulthood, the burdens on it have increased. Now, it is supposed to be a world-wide police agency, ferreting out cheaters and ensuring a "level playing field"—and do this with only a meager budget.

It is easier to find flaws in such an operation than to understand how far the system has grown in the past 30 years. With all its imperfections, it has accomplished a great deal. With proper funding, it could have accomplished a great deal more. Like an adult, it is entering what could potentially be its most productive years. With all the publicity directed toward this system since the Seoul Olympics, the time appears to be right for the full maturation of the system. From the publicity and outcry about drug abuse during 1998, there appears to be momentum to devote significant funds to the war on drugs. It remains to be seen if the funding will match the rhetoric and if a truly independent system that recognizes and protects athletes' rights will develop.

References

Almond, E. (1989, Sept. 8). Colorado case fuels drug-testing furor. *Los Angeles Times.*

Almond, E. (1990, June 12). U.S. track group's drug enforcement in question. *Los Angeles Times.*

Anderson, O. (1995, January/February). More buzz about "Joe". *Running Research News.*

Armstrong, R. (1991, February 1). *The lessons learned from Canada's Dubin Inquiry.* Speech delivered at the International Symposium on Sport and Law, Monte Carlo.

The Athletics Congress (TAC). (1989). *Decisions of hearing panels in cases of Augie Wolf and Billy Olsen.* (Available from The Athletics Congress, P.O. Box 120, Indianapolis, IN 46206)

The Athletics Congress. (1990, December 20). *Official transcript of hearings: Application of Randy Barnes.* (Available from The Athletics Congress, P.O. Box 120, Indianapolis, IN 46206)

The Athletics Congress Doping Control Review Board. (1991, October 4). *Decision of DCRB in the case of Harry L. Reynolds.* (Available from The Athletics Congress, P.O. Box 120, Indianapolis, IN 46206)

Austad, S.N. (1997). *Why we age: What science is discovering about the body's journey through life.* New York: Wiley.

Australian chief outraged by Hoffmann drug admission. (1997, October 12). Agence France-Presse.

Ayotte (1999, May 13). E-mail correspondence.

Beckett (1993). Interview by author. Hilton Head, SC.

Beckett, A.H. (1994). Phone interview by author.

Beckett, A.H. (1997). Phone interview by author.

Beckett, A.H., & Ljungqvist, A. (1989, June 5-7). Interview by author conducted at Second International Athletic Foundation World Symposium on Doping in Sport, Monte Carlo.

Bedell, D. (1991, April 17). Athletes use a variety of methods to overcome drug tests. *Dallas Morning News.*

Berendonk, B., & Franke, W.W. (1997). Hormonal doping and androgenization of athletes: A secret program of the German Democratic Republic government. *Clinical Chemistry, 43,* 1262–1279.

Bilac back in business. (1991, July). *Track & Field News,* 50.

Black, D. (1991). Phone interview by author.

Boswell, R. (1988, June 27). World conference attacks illicit drugs. *Ottawa Citizen.*

Bottomley, M. (1988). Report. In P. Bellotti, G. Benzi, & A. Ljungqvist (Eds.), *International Athletic Foundation World Symposium on Doping in Sport: Official proceedings* (pp. 209-211). Monte Carlo, Monaco: International Athletic Foundation.

Bouton, J. (1970/1990). *Ball four.* New York: Macmillan.

Buffrey, S., & Parrish, W. (1989, August 2). World body ignored positive drug tests and Doc rips "rescue." *Toronto Sun.*

Cassell, O. (1991, November 16). Speech delivered at Road Race Management Conference, Washington, DC.

Catlin, D.H. (1987). Detection of drug use by athletes. In R. Strauss (Ed.), *Drugs and performance in sports* (pp. 103-121). Philadelphia: Saunders.

Catlin, D.H. (1991). Phone interview by author.

Catlin, D.H. (1997). Phone interview by author.

Catlin, D.H., & Hatton, C.K. (1991). Use and abuse of anabolic and other drugs for athletic enhancement. *Advances in Internal Medicine, 36,* 399–424.

Catlin, D.H., Kammerer, R.C., Hatton, C.K., et al. (1987). Analytical chemistry at the Games of the XXIIIrd Olympiad in Los Angeles, 1984. *Clinical Chemistry, 33,* 319–327.

Catlin, D.H., & Moses, E. (1989). Interviews by author.

Chriss, A. (1990). Phone interview by author.

Chriss, A. (1991). Phone interview by author.

Coleman, D. Lambelet (1989). Phone interviews by author.

Court backs NCAA's drug tests. (1988, February 26). *St. Paul Pioneer Press.*

Das Erbe von Atlanta: Vier Vertusche Dopingfålle. (1996, November 19). *Süddeutsche Zeilung.*

The death of Birgit Dressel. (1988, February/March). *Athletics,* 6–10.

Demak, R., & Kirshenbaum, J. (1990, January). The NFL fails its drug test. *Sports Illustrated.*

de Merode, A. (1988, February 19). Unpublished telephone interview by author conducted during Winter Olympics. Calgary.

Denton, H. (1989, March 5). Charlie Francis: The doctor is in. *Washington Post.*

DiPasquale, M. (1991). Polypharmacy: Anabolic steroids and beyond. *Drugs in Sports, 1*(1), 2–3.

Donike, M. (1992). Letter to IOC Executive Board.

Donike, M., de Merode, A., Beckett, A., & Dugal, R. (1985). Letter regarding 1984 Olympic testing subversion.

Donike, M., Geyer, H., Gotzmann, A., et al. (1988). Dope analysis. In P. Bellotti, G. Benzi, & A. Ljungqvist (Eds.), *International Athletic Foundation World Symposium on Doping in Sport: Official proceedings* (pp. 53–80). Monte Carlo, Monaco: International Athletic Foundation.

Donike, M., Geyer, H., Gotzmann, & Mareck-Engelke, U. (Eds.). (1995). *Proceedings of the 12th Cologne Workshop on Dope Analysis.* Cologne: Sport & Buch Strauss.

Donohoe, T., & Johnson, N. (1986). *Foul play.* Oxford, England: Blackwell.

Doping tests. (1989, December 13). Associated Press Wire Service.

Down on dope. (1988, June 27). *Toronto Sun,* p. 80.

Downes, S. (1997, May 27). Reuters.

Drug tests sought. (1987, June 12). *Toronto Sun.*

Dubin, C.L. (1990). *Commission of inquiry into the use of drugs and banned practices intended to increase athletic performance.* Ottawa, ON: Canadian Government Publishing Centre.

Ferstle, J. (1991, August 18). U.S. authorities might have key player in drug network. *St. Paul Pioneer Press.*

Ferstle, J. (1997, April). EPO testing provides glimpse of possible new drug testing protocols: Blood testing remains controversial. *Road Race Management.*

Ferstle, J. (1997, May 18). *Sunday Times* (London).

Ferstle, J. (1997, September). A brief chat with Arne Ljungqvist. *Runner's World Daily* [Online serial].

Forbes, G. (1989, September 1). Steroids losers: Daringly foolish to try. *USA Today.*

Foschi, J. (September 27, 1996). Brief filed by Williams & Connolly law firm for the Court of Arbitration for Sport: Jessica K. Foschi v. Federation Internationale de Natation Amateur.

Francis, C. (1991). Phone interview by author.

Garle, M., Ocka, R., Palonek, E., & Björkhem, I. (1996). Increased urinary testosterone/epitestosterone ratios found in Swedish athletes in connection with a national control program. Evaluation of 28 cases. *Journal of Chromatography Biomedical Applications, 686,* 55–59.

Gasbarrone, E., & Roasti, F. (1988). Report. In P. Bellotti, G. Benzi, & A. Ljungqvist (Eds.), *International Athletic Foundation World Symposium on Doping in Sport:*

Official proceedings (pp. 222–224). Monte Carlo, Monaco: International Athletic Foundation.

Gasser v. Stinson (and another). (1988, June 15). Lexis Nexis case summary of decision.

Greenberg, A. (1991, June 29). Alzado has a serious message to kids about steroids—Don't use 'em. *Hartford Courant.*

Harvey, R. (1990, December 3). Magazine says East Germans used steroids. *Los Angeles Times.*

Hatton, C.K., & Catlin, D.H. (1987). Detection of androgenic anabolic steroids in urine. *Clinics in Laboratory Medicine, 7,* 655–668.

Hynes, M. (1988, June 28). Controls sought for drugs. *Globe and Mail.*

Hynes, M. (1988, June 29). Norway cracks down on steroids. *Globe and Mail.*

International Olympic Committee. (1989). *Analytical results of A-samples at the games of the XXIVth Olympiad in Seoul, 1988.* (Available from IOC, Chateau Vidy, CH-1007, Lausanne, Switzerland)

Investigative hearings on the proper and improper use of drugs by athletes: Hearings before the Committee on the Judiciary, U.S. Senate. 93rd Cong., 1st Sess. (1973, June 18, July 12 & 13) (testimony of International Olympic Committee).

IOC-drugs. (1988, November 17). Associated Press Wire Service.

Janofsky, M., & Alfano, P. (1988, November 17). System accused of failing test posed by drugs. *New York Times,* pp. 1, 45.

Kammerer, C. (1991). Phone interview by author.

Kammerer, C. (1996). Phone interview by author.

Kammerer, C. (1997). Phone interview by author.

Keisser, B. (1991, July 16). We need to pass Alzado's painful lesson on to the kids. Knight-Ridder News Service.

Kimmage, P. (1990). *A rough ride: An insight into pro cycling.* London: Stanley Paul.

Labs under IOC gun. (1988, May 5). *Toronto Sun.*

Longman, J. (1995, April 9). USOC experts call drug testing a failure. *New York Times.*

Longman, J. (1997, May 15). Slaney angry over duration of drug study. *New York Times.*

Los Angeles Olympic Organizing Committee. (1985). *Official report of the games of the XXIIIrd Olympiad, Los Angeles, 1984* (2 vols.). Los Angeles: Author.

Mandell, A.J. (1976). *The nightmare season.* New York: Random House.

Martin, D. (1997, January–February). Blood testing for professional cyclists: What's a fair hematocrit limit? *Sportscience* [Online serial].

Millen barred but U.S. plans to file appeal. (1989, April 22). *St. Paul Pioneer Press.*

Minutes of IOC Medical Commission meeting. (1984).

Moses, E. (1989). Phone interview by author.

National Athletics Board of Review of The Athletics Congress. (1990, July 16). *Decision of the NABR panel on the case of Charles R. DeBus* (SP No. 1-07-07/1989).

Norman, N. (1988). Report. In P. Bellotti, G. Benzi, & A. Ljungqvist (Eds.), *International Athletic Foundation World Symposium on Doping in Sport: Official proceedings* (pp. 211-213). Monte Carlo, Monaco: International Athletic Foundation.

Park, J. (1989, June 5–7). *Review of the Seoul Laboratory activities—Seoul Olympic Games 1988.* Paper presented at the Second International Athletic Foundation World Symposium on Doping in Sport, Monte Carlo, Monaco.

Patrick, D. (1989, June 20). Doctor's account confirms rumors. *USA Today.*

Patrick, D. (1997, May 23). Olympians come under fire. *USA Today,* p. 3.

Plucknett v. TAC/USA. U.S. District Court for the Northern District of California, Palo Alto (Document No. C820545MHP) (1982, April 24).

Puffer, J. (1988, May). Interview by author conducted at American College of Sports Medicine annual meeting, Dallas.

Reuters Information Service, (1997, May 8).

Solberg wins damages. (1990, October 11). *Athletics Today,* p. 4.

Starcevic, N. (1990, December 3). Doping—East Germany. Associated Press Wire Service.

Starkman, R. (1997, October 4). NHL Olympians get break on drug testing. *Toronto Sun.*

Stuart, H. (1988, June 27). Down on dope. *Toronto Sun.*

Surgeons cut out need for blood transfusions. (1997, October 12). *Sunday Times* (London).

"Testing the testors," (1994). BBC *On the Line.*

Trecker, J. (1991, July 16). Sports continue without real concern for drug abuse. *Hartford Courant.*

United States Olympic Committee. (1987). Unpublished letters from George Miller and Ollan Cassell. (USOC address: 1750 E. Boulder St., Colorado Springs, CO 80909)

Update: Drug testing out. (1989, August 23). *USA Today.*

Videman, T. (1989, June 5–7). Speech delivered at Second International Athletic Foundation World Symposium on Doping in Sport, Monte Carlo, Monaco.

Voy, R. (1988). Phone interview by author.

Voy, R., & Deeter, K.D. (1991). *Drugs, sport, and politics: The inside story about drug use in sport and its political cover-up, with a prescription for reform.* Champaign, IL: Leisure Press.

Wadler, G.I., & Hainline, B. (1989). *Drugs and the athlete.* Philadelphia: Davis.

Wadler, G.I. (1997, May). Interview by author at ACSM Meeting in Denver.

Warshaw, A. (1989, October 12). Doping. Associated Press Wire Service.

Webb, J. (1996, March 23). A sporting chance. *New Scientist, pp. 25–27.*

Wilson, S. (1991, April 16). IOC meetings. Associated Press Sportswire.

Wilson, (1994, September). AP Sportswire.

Wimbledon-Drugs. (1990, June 24). Associated Press Wire Service.

Wong, G. (1988). *Essentials of amateur sports law.* Dover: Auburn House.

Wulf, S. (Ed.). (1991, July 22). Scorecard: Eye openers. *Sports Illustrated,* 10.

Yaeger, D., & Bamberger, M. (1997, April 14). Over the edge: Aware that drug testing is a sham, athletes seem to rely more than ever on banned performance enhancers. *Sports Illustrated.*

Zanca, S. (1991, February 12). Figure skating—drugs. Associated Press Wire Service.

Zimmermann, J. (1986). Untersuchung zum Nachweis von exogenen gaben von Testosteron. Unpublished doctoral thesis.

CHAPTER

13

Drug Testing and Anabolic Steroids

R. Craig Kammerer, PhD

Athletes should be freed from the use of clay and mud and other irksome medicines.

Gymnastikos, 200 A.D.

Our anti-doping campaign, I'm afraid, has been a failure to this point. Many countries have lost confidence in our anti-doping effort. I'm not sure we're doing the right job.

"U.S.O.C. Experts Call Drug Testing a Failure"
New York Times, Sunday, April 9, 1995, S-11.

A small part of this work has appeared elsewhere (Kammerer, 1998a,b).

This chapter's topic is testing methods for anabolic steroids and related compounds. Following a short history of drug testing, the chapter will focus on metabolism, the technology involved in testing, the philosophy of testing, the costs of testing, and the circumventing of positive test results. The last part of the chapter discusses the use of other substances for their anabolic effects and future directions in steroid testing.

Drug testing of humans began on a limited scale in the late 1950s when, after several European cycle races, evidence of drug use was observed. In the 1960 Rome Olympic Games, a cyclist died after apparent amphetamine use. In 1965, Beckett, Tucker, and Moffat (1967), who had developed procedures capable of detecting a number of different stimulants, tested participants in the Tour of Britain cycling races. In the 1967 Tour de France, another cyclist died, with amphetamines found both on his person and in his body. Since Professor Beckett was a member of the newly formed International Olympic Committee (IOC) Medical Commission, his procedures were employed on an experimental basis in the 1968 Olympic Games. No testing for anabolic steroids was performed at this time due to the lack of assay procedures. The first "formal" testing for nonsteroidal drugs occurred at the 1972 Munich Olympic Games (Donike & Stratmann, 1974), though there still was no official testing for steroids. The development of complex radioimmunoassay (RIA) screening procedures (Brooks, Jeremiah, Webb, & Wheeler, 1979) as well as analytical advances in gas chromatography–mass spectrometry (GC-MS) techniques led to the introduction of tests for anabolic steroids at the 1976 Montreal Olympic Games (Bertrand, Masse, & Dugal, 1978). However, only 275 of the 1,800 total samples could be analyzed for steroids due to the complexity of these procedures, and eight positive cases were reported publicly.

During both the 1976 Montreal Olympics and the 1980 Moscow Olympics, RIA screening procedures (Brooks, Firth, & Sumner, 1975; Rogozkin, Morozov, & Tchaikovsky, 1979) were used to analyze samples for the presence of anabolic steroids, and GC-MS analysis was used to confirm positive screening results. Because of the inherent lack of specificity in RIA screening assays for many of the steroid metabolites, whose detection is necessary to infer the presence of anabolic steroids, and because endogenous testosterone was added to the list of banned drugs, GC-MS was adopted at the 1984 Olympic Games as both the screening and confirmatory method of analysis of anabolic steroids (Catlin, Kammerer, Hatton, Sekera, & Merdink, 1987). The method of determining whether or not the testosterone was from illegal supplementation by the athlete was developed by Donike, Barwald, Kosterman, Schänzer, & Zimmermann, (1983), based upon an earlier study (Baba et al., 1980). The test consists of measuring both testosterone (T) and its epimeric form (a geometric isomer called epitestosterone) (E) in the same sample. Since E is not converted to testosterone and the normal ratio of the quantity of T to the quantity of E is in a ratio of approximately 1:1 (hereinafter called T/E) for both males and females, administration of testosterone raises this ratio. Initially, a ratio of over 6:1 was considered evidence of having administered testosterone, but as natural exceptions to this threshold of guilt (discussed later) have appeared, the "rules" now are more like over 6:1 suspicious and over 10:1 guilty. Further refinement in these guidelines may be forthcoming.

Drug testing at the 1988 Olympics was summarized by Chung et al. (1990) and Park and colleagues (1990), but in terms of testing procedures for steroids, these articles provided little significant new information. In the 1992 Barcelona Olympic Games, the laboratory reported the detection of several banned drugs in the participating athletes: three cases of stimulant medications, two clenbuterol positives, and three T/E ratios over 6:1 (between 6:1 and 10:1) (Segura et al., 1995). The samples containing the stimulant drugs and clenbuterol were formally reported for punitive action, while the three T/E ratios were referred for further study without action against the athletes.

Since the publication of the first edition of this book, progress has been made in study of the metabolism (chemical changes imparted to a drug after ingestion but before excretion) of some of the lesser-known anabolic steroids (Bowers, 1996; Deboer, Dejong, Maes, & Van Rossum, 1992; Geyer, Schänzer, Schindler, & Donike, 1996; Goudreault & Masse, 1991; Kim, Suh, Ryu, Chung, & Park 1996; Schänzer, 1996b). For a good up-to-date summary of steroid use in sport, see chapters 2 and 3.

Blood or Urine Testing?

Although a few athletic federations utilize limited blood testing outside Olympic competition, and some experimental blood testing was performed at the Lillihammer Olympic Games, urine is usually the only permitted testing fluid in most testing programs, and thus metabolites (final excretion products) are the molecules that must be detected to prove an athlete's anabolic steroid use. There are several reasons for limiting testing to the urine matrix. First, athletes (and most athletic federations) feel that taking a blood sample is an unnecessary trauma to the athlete. Second, giving a urine sample does not involve needles or any invasive procedure, the use of which introduces the variables of technique of the staff, possible transmission of disease, and legal and religious considerations. The possibility of using blood for drug testing is not a new idea (Donike, 1976), and in recent years has again become of interest because of the probable addition of more natural endogenous compounds (such as human growth hormone; see later in the chapter) to the banned list. However, the litigious nature of society today (Jacobs & Samuels, 1995) will probably preclude any blood-based drug testing on a wide scale. An extremely valuable application of the use of blood as the drug-testing matrix has recently been shown (de la Torre, Segura, & Polettini, 1995; de la Torre, Segura, Polettini, & Montagna, 1995), with the report that intact testosterone esters have been found in the blood of people who have taken testosterone (usually supplied as an ester of some type in pharmaceutical preparations). Since testosterone esters are *not* found naturally, and are *not* excreted into the urine, the detection of an intact ester proves unequivocally that synthetic testosterone was consumed, which could not have been proven in this manner by a urine test. Thus, the use of blood testing for the verification of testosterone abuse removes any doubt of exogenous supplementation in such a case. Theoretically, however, the use of testosterone skin patches/gels/creams would still circumvent this test, as intact esters either would not be used or esters would not survive the passage through the skin to the bloodstream intact. Also of interest is the work that has been published on the detection of various hormones in blood after testosterone administration (e.g., LH, FSH, 17-hydroxyprogesterone, testosterone, etc.) as well as the use of the ketoconazole suppression test, all of which are being investigated to verify the recent abuse of testosterone (see Carlström et al., 1992; Cowan, Kicman, Walker, & Wheeler, 1991; Kicman et al., 1990; Oftebro, Jensen, Mowinckel, & Norli, 1994; Palonek, Gottlieb, Garle, Björkhem, & Carlstroem, 1995).

A review of the metabolism and detection of anabolic steroids in human urine has appeared, containing significant new data (Schänzer, 1996b). It is important to remember that a significant number of anabolic steroids are excreted into human urine primarily or exclusively as metabolites (structures chemically different than the original drug, formed in the body before excretion into the urine); so it is often not relevant to look for the actual steroid in urine. Frequently, detection time of the parent drug is short, whereas detection time of the appropriate metabolites is much longer. Therefore, for drug-testing purposes and for verification of abuse of an anabolic steroid, monitoring the presence of metabolites is often indicated because the parent drug may not be found. That is, testing for the presence of an anabolic steroid can be formidable or impossible without availability of the metabolite standards or metabolic information in the testing laboratory. Although many of the authentic anabolic steroid metabolite standards have been made (Sanaullah & Bowers, 1996; Schänzer & Donike, 1993; Schänzer, Horning, & Donike, 1995; Schänzer, 1996b), the quantities available are extremely limited and are available primarily to IOC testing laboratories and not to private, clinical, or hospital laboratories. Thus, even though considerable published information now exists, many of the reference chemicals are still not *readily* available. Since many of the drugs are not on the U.S. market, urine from excretion studies is often difficult to obtain for corroborating a positive test result. As an example of this testing situation in the United States, an accreditation program was begun by the American Association for Clinical Chemistry and the College of American Pathologists to identify capable athletic drug-testing (ADT) laboratories. Of the 35 initially interested laboratories, only 6 lasted through the accreditation process. Additionally, 3 of these 6 laboratories had direct IOC experience or accreditation already, and only a shortened list of anabolic steroids was included in the testing process (e.g., many of the world's anabolic steroids were not part of this ADT program).

Structures, Chemistry, and Metabolism

The significant anabolic steroids reported in the literature are listed in tables 13.1 to 13.3. Table 13.1 lists the anabolic steroids on the U.S. market (generic and black markets included), table 13.2 the more common non-U.S. anabolic steroids, and table 13.3 the uncommon non-U.S. anabolic steroids. Each table is organized as follows: chemical name or names; molecular formula; Chemical Abstracts Service (CAS) registry number, which uniquely identifies that substance; Negwer number (referring to a standard reference compendium on drugs: Negwer [1987]); and synonyms (drug company and trade names).

Some anabolic steroids are sold as many different ester derivatives (particularly nortestosterone and testosterone; table 13.1). Therefore, the actual number of marketed anabolic steroids is quite large when these different esters are included in the list, even though in the human body all of these different esters of a specific anabolic steroid are converted to the same parent drug. Thus, for example, all esters of nortestosterone form only nortestosterone metabolites, which are excreted in the urine; so that for testing purposes, all the different esters of nortestosterone yield the same group of metabolites in the urine.

Anabolic steroids are a class of chemical compounds consisting structurally of four rings (three 6-membered and one 5-membered) fused together into a carbon atom skeleton. These compounds confer anabolic activity to a living organism—that is, the ability to promote the utilization of nutrients. Drug company chemists originally synthesized anabolic steroids as analogues of the natural androgenic steroid testosterone (see chapter 1).

Often during these synthetic development programs the chemical substitution process involved adding of an alkyl substituent to the 17 position of the anabolic steroid four-ring system; the primary goals were to enhance the anabolic and decrease the androgenic activity of the new drug with the hope that the presence of a 17α-alkyl-substituent would decrease the metabolic degradation of the drug by the liver.

Table 13.1 Anabolic Steroids—U.S. Drugs

Names	Formula	CAS	Negwer	Synonyms
1. Dianabol a. 17β-Hydroxy-17α-methyl-androsta-1, 4-dien-3-one b. 1-Dehydro-17α-methyltestosterone	$C_{20}H_{28}O_2$	72-63-9	5907	BA 17309; NSC 42722; TMV 17; Methandienone
2. Fluoxymesterone a. 11β, 17β-Dihydroxy-9α-Fluoro-17α-methylandrost-4-en-3-one b. 9α-Fluoro-11β-hydroxy-17α-methyltestosterone	$C_{20}H_{29}FO_3$	76-43-7	5917	U. 6040; NSC 12165; Halotestin
3. Metandren a. 17β-Hydroxy-17α-methylandrosten-3-one b. 17α-Methyl-testosterone	$C_{20}H_{30}O_2$	58-18-4	5944	NSC 9701; Numan; Oreton-M
4. Nortestosterone a. 17β-Hydroxy-estr-4-en-3-one b. 19-Nortestosterone	$C_{18}H_{26}O_2$	434-22-0	4988	SG 4341; Nandrolone

5. Oxandrolone 17β-Hydroxy-17α-methyl-2-oxa-5α-androstan-3-one	$C_{19}H_{30}O_3$	53-39-4	5497	Sc 11585; NSC 67068; Anavar; 8075 C.B.
6. Oxymetholone a. 17β-Hydroxy-2-[Hydroxymethylene]-17α-methyl-5α-androstan-3-one b. 2-[Hydroxymethylene]-17α-methyldihydrotestosterone	$C_{21}H_{32}O_3$	434-07-1	6370	NSC 26198; C.I. 406; RS 992
7. Stanozolol 17β-Hydroxy-17α-methyl-5α-androstano [3, 2-c]-Pyrazole	$C_{21}H_{32}N_2O$	10418-03-8	6359	WIN 14833; NSC 43193; Stromba; Winstrol
8. Testosterone 17β-Hydroxyandrost-4-en-3-one	$C_{19}H_{28}O_2$	58-22-0	5458	

CAS = Chemical Abstracts Service.

Table 13.2 Anabolic Steroids—Common Non-U.S. Drugs

Names	Formula	CAS	Negwer	Synonyms
1. Clostebol	$C_{19}H_{27}ClO_2$	A. 1093-58-9	5429	4-Chlorotestosterone
4-Chloro-17β-hydroxy-androst-4-ene-3-one	$C_{21}H_{29}ClO_3$	B. 855-19-6	6301	Acetate; Steranabol
	$C_{22}H_{31}ClO_3$	C. 2162-44-9	6702	Propionate; Yonchlon
	$C_{25}H_{37}ClO_3$	D. 32361-10-7	7345	Caproate: Macrobin-Depot
2. Drostanolone				
a. 2α-Methyldihydrotestosterone;	$C_{20}H_{32}O_2$	A. 58-19-5	5971	Methalone (Syntex)
b. 17β-Hydroxy-2α-methyl-5α-androstan-3-one	$C_{23}H_{36}O_3$	B. 521-12-0	7014 12198	Propionate; Lilly 32379; RS 877; NSC
3. Ethylestrenol	$C_{20}H_{32}O$	965-90-2	5967	Org 483; Orgabolin; Maxibolin
a. 19-Nor-17α-pregn-4-ene-17β-ol;				
b. 17α-Ethylestr-4-ene-17β-ol				
4. Mesterolone	$C_{20}H_{32}O_2$	1424-00-6	5970	SH 60723; NSC 75054; Testiwop
17β-Hydroxy-1α-methyl-5α-androstan-3-one				
5. Methenolone	$C_{22}H_{32}O_3$	A. 434-05-9	6727	Acetate; SH 567; NSC 74226; SQ 16496
17β-Hydroxy-1-methyl-5α-androst-1-ene-3-one	$C_{27}H_{42}O_3$	B. 303-42-4	7600	Enanthate; SH 601; SQ 16374; NSC 64967; Primobolan

6. Norethandrolone a. 17α-Ethyl-19-nortestosterone b. 17α-Ethyl-17β-hydroxyestr-4-ene-3-one	$C_{20}H_{30}O_2$	52-78-8	5948	Nilevar; Ethylnortestosterone
7. Oral-Turinabol a. 4-Chloro-17β-hydroxy-17α-methyl-1, 4-androstadien-3-one b. 4-Chloro-1-dehydro-17α-methyltestosterone	$C_{20}H_{27}ClO_2$	2446-23-3	5850	Chlorodianabol; Chlorodehydromethyltestosterone
8. Oxymesterone a. 4-Hydroxy-17α-methyltestosterone b. 4, 17β-Dihydroxy-17α-methylandrost-4-en-3-one	$C_{20}H_{30}O_3$	145-12-0	5950	Balnimax; Theranabol; SKF 7304; Oranabol
9. Stenbolone 17β-Hydroxy-2-methyl-5α-androst-1-en-3-one	$C_{20}H_{30}O_2$ $C_{22}H_{32}O_3$	A. 5197-58-0 B. 1242-56-4	5943 6728	 Acetate; RS 2106; S.3760; Anatrofin

CAS = Chemical Abstracts Service.

Table 13.3 Anabolic Steroids—Uncommon Non-U.S. Drugs

Names	Formula	CAS	Negwer	Synonyms
1. Androisoxazole	$C_{21}H_{31}NO_2$	360-66-7	6349	AIZ, Neoponden
a. 17α-Methyl-5α-androstano [3, 2-c] isoxazol-17β-ol				
b. 17β-Hydroxy-17α- methyl-5α-androstano [3, 2-c]-isoxazole				
2. Allyltrenbolone	$C_{21}H_{26}O_2$	850-52-2	6209	RH or RU 2267; A 35957; DRC 6246
a. 17α-Allyl-17β-Hydroxyestra-4, 9, 11-trien-3-one				
b. 17α-Allyl-17β-Hydroxy-19-norandrosta-4, 9, 11-trien-3-one				
3. Bolandiol	$C_{24}H_{32}O_2$	1986-53-4	7209	SC 7525; Anabiol; Dipropionate
Estr-4-ene-3β, 17β-diol				
4. Bolasterone	$C_{21}H_{32}O_2$	1605-89-6	6365	U.19763; NSC 66233; Myagen
a. 7α, 17α-Dimethyltestosterone				
b. 17β-Hydroxy-7α, 17α-dimethylandrost-4-en-3-one				
5. Bolazine	$C_{40}H_{64}N_2O_2$	A. 4267-81-6	8169	
17β-Hydroxy-2α-methyl-5α-androstan-3-one-azine	$C_{52}H_{84}N_2O_4$	B. No number	8321	Capronate
6. Boldenone	$C_{19}H_{26}O_2$	A. 846-48-0	5423	1-Dehydrotestosterone
17β-Hydroxyandrosta-1, 4-dien-3-one	$C_{30}H_{44}O_3$	B. 13103-34-9	7884	Undecylenate; Ba 29038; Equipoise; Boldene

7. Bolenol a. 19-Nor-17α-pregn-5-en-17β-ol b. 17α-Ethylestr-5-en-17β-ol	$C_{20}H_{32}O$	16915-78-9	5968	Organon compound
8. Bolmantalate a. 19-Nortestosterone-1-adamantane carboxylate b. 17β-Hydroxyestr-4-en-3-one-1-adamantanecarboxylate	$C_{29}H_{40}O_3$	1491-81-2	7799	Lilly 38851
9. Calusterone 7β, 17α-Dimethyl-17β-hydroxyandrost-4-ene-3-one	$C_{21}H_{32}O_2$	17021-26-0	6366	U-22550; Methosarb
10. Chlordrolone a. 4-Chloro-17α-methyl-19-nortestosterone b. 4-Chloro-17β-hydroxy-17α-methylestr-4-en-3-one	$C_{19}H_{27}ClO_2$	3415-90-5	5430	SKF 6612
11. Chloroxydienone a. 4-Chloro-1-dehydro-11β-hydroxy-17α-methyltestosterone b. 4-Chloro-11β, 17β-dihydroxy-17α-methyl-1, 4-androstadien-3-one	$C_{20}H_{27}ClO_3$	2614-57-5	5851	
12. Chloroxymesterone a. 4-Chloro-11β-hydroxy-17α-methyltestosterone b. 4-Chloro-11β, 17β-dihydroxy-17α-methylandrost-4-en-3-one	$C_{20}H_{29}ClO_3$	10392-52-6	5915	

(continued)

Table 13.3 *(continued)*

Names	Formula	CAS	Negwer	Synonyms
13. Dihydrotestosterone				
17β-Hydroxy-5α-androstan-3-one	$C_{19}H_{30}O_2$	521-18-6	5496	DHT, Stanolone, Anaprotin
-propionate	$C_{22}H_{34}O_3$	855-22-1	6746	
-valerate	$C_{24}H_{38}O_3$	26271-72-7	7216	
-benzoate	$C_{26}H_{34}O_3$	1057-07-4	7444	
-enanthate	$C_{26}H_{42}O_3$	33776-88-4	7491	
14. Enestebol 4, 17β-Dihydroxy-17α-methylandrosta-1, 4-dien-3-one	$C_{20}H_{28}O_3$	2320-86-7	5908	
15. Formebolone a. 11α-17β-Dihydroxy-17α-methyl-3-oxo-androsta-1, 4-diene-2-carboxaldehyde b. 2-Formyl-11α, 17β-dihydroxy-17α-methylandrosta-1, 4-diene-3-one	$C_{21}H_{28}O_4$	2454-11-7	6293	Hubernol; Esiclene; Formyldienolone
16. Furazabol a. 17α-Methyl-5α-androstano [2, 3-c] furazan-17β-ol b. 17α-Methyl-5α-androstano [2, 3-c] [1, 2, 5] oxadiazol-17β-ol	$C_{20}H_{30}N_2O_2$	1239-29-8	5938	DH 245; Androfurazanol
17. Mebolazine a. 17β-Hydroxy-2α-17α-dimethyl-5α-androstan-3-one-azine b. 2α, 17α-Dimethyl-5α-androstan-17β-ol-3-one-azine	$C_{42}H_{68}N_2O_2$	3625-07-8	8217	Dimethazine; Roxilon

18. Metribolone 17β-Hydroxy-17α-methylestra-4, 9, 11-trien-3-one	$C_{19}H_{24}O_2$	965-93-5	5380	R 1881; RU 1881; methyltrienolone
19. Mestanolone 17β-Hydroxy-17α-methyl-5α-androstan-3-one	$C_{20}H_{32}O_2$	521-11-9	5972	Androstalone
20. Methandriol				
17α-Methylandrost-5-ene-3β, 17β-diol	$C_{20}H_{32}O_2$	521-10-8	5969	Methylandrostenediol
-diacetate	$C_{24}H_{36}O_6$	2061-86-1	No #	
-dipropionate	$C_{26}H_{40}O_4$	3593-85-9	7487	Probolin, Anabolin
-propionate	$C_{23}H_{36}O_3$	60883-73-0	7013	Protobolin
-bisenanthoylacetate	$C_{38}H_{60}O_6$	No number	8144	Notandron-depot
21. Mibolerone 17β-Hydroxy-7α, 17α-dimethylestr-4-ene-3-one	$C_{20}H_{30}O_2$	3704-09-4	5946	U.10997; CDB 904; CHEQUE
22. Norbolethone a. 13-Ethyl-17β-hydroxy-18, 19-dinor-17α-pregn-4-en-3-one b. 13, 17α-Diethyl-17β-hydroxygon-4-en-3-one	$C_{21}H_{32}O_2$	797-58-0	6367	Wy 3475; Genabol
23. Norclostebol				
a. 4-Chloro-19-nortestosterone	$C_{18}H_{25}ClO_2$	13583-21-6	4956	SKF6611; Lentabol; Cp-73;
b. 4-Chloro-17β-hydroxyestr-4-ene-3-one	$C_{20}H_{27}ClO_3$	1164-99-4	5852	Anabol 4-19; acetate
24. Normethandrolone a. 17α-Methyl-19-nortestosterone b. 17β-Hydroxy-17α-methylestr-4-ene-3-one	$C_{19}H_{28}O_2$	514-61-4	5460	P-6051; NSC 10039; Organon; methylnortestosterone

(continued)

Table 13.3 *(continued)*

Names	Formula	CAS	Negwer	Synonyms
25. Oxabolone 4-Hydroxy-19-nortestosterone	$C_{26}H_{38}O_4$	1254-35-9	7478	Cipionate; F.I.5852; Steranabol Depot
26. Penmesterol 17α-Methyltestosterone-3-cyclopentyl-enolether	$C_{25}H_{38}O_2$	67-81-2	7349	R.P. 12222; Pandocrine
27. Roxibolone 2-Carboxy-11β, 17β-dihydroxy-17α-methylandrost-1, 4-dien-3-one	$C_{21}H_{28}O_5$ $C_{31}H_{48}O_5$ $C_{33}H_{52}O_5$	60023-92-9 60023-91-8 No number	6295 7931 8006	BR 906 Decylester; BR 917 Dodecylester
28. Silandrone 17-β-(Trimethylsilyoxy)-androst-4-ene-3-one	$C_{22}H_{36}O_2Si$	5055-42-5	6760	SC 16148; NSC 95147
29. Thiomesterone 1α-7α-Bis (acetylthio)-17β-hydroxy-17α-methylandrost-4-ene-3-one	$C_{24}H_{34}O_4S_2$	2205-73-4	7196	Embadol; Sta 307; Protabol; E Merck; Germany
30. Tibolone 17α-Ethynyl-17β-Hydroxy-7α-methylestr-5 (10)-en-3-one	$C_{21}H_{28}O_2$	5630-53-5	6286	Org OD14; Livial
31. Trenbolone 17β-Hydroxyestra-4, 9, 11-trien-3-one	$C_{18}H_{22}O_2$ $C_{20}H_{24}O_3$	10161-33-8 10161-34-9	4876 5769	R 2580; Hexabolan; Parabolan Ru 1697; Finaplix; Acetate
32. Trestolone 17β-Hydroxy-7α-methylestr-4-ene-3-one	$C_{21}H_{30}O_3$	6157-87-5	6338	U.15614; CDB 903; NSC 6994; Acetate

CAS = Chemical Abstracts Service.

Regardless of the resultant total biological activity, the toxicity of the new anabolic steroid was often higher than that of testosterone. As measured by in vitro lab assays, these resultant 17α-alkyl-substituted anabolic steroids had higher anabolic activity, equal or lower androgenic activity, but higher toxicity than the corresponding unsubstituted anabolic steroids. These conclusions have been shown to not always be accurate when measured by newer in vitro assays.

The metabolism of anabolic steroids varies considerably from drug to drug and cannot be consistently predicted in terms of the major excretion products in humans (Schänzer, 1996b). Until quite recently, the published literature contained little of this metabolic information for many of the anabolic steroids. A summary of the human metabolism of most types of anabolic steroids is presented in table 13.4. The primary urinary metabolites are those present in the largest concentrations or for the longest time after ingestion of that anabolic steroid. Therefore, for valid and effective testing, these metabolites (or excretion products) must be detected in order to prove ingestion of a specific anabolic drug.

Technology of Anabolic Steroid Testing

Originally, anabolic steroid testing was based upon RIA, a procedure utilizing the principle of antibody response to a specific steroid with a radioactive tracer present. Brooks, Firth, and Sumner (1975) and Brooks et al. (1979) developed several antibodies directed toward 19-nortestosterone analogues, norethandrolone analogues, and 17α-substituted anabolic steroid analogues. These antibodies had broad specificity ranges and were combined into two RIA kits for testing for anabolic steroids. Several steroids were detected with very low sensitivity, including stanozolol and methenolone. Also, testosterone and epitestosterone were not quantitated reliably by these procedures, so tests for these substances in urine would require two additional RIA assays (Bilek, Hämpl, Putz, & Starka, 1987). Additional antibodies developed by other groups for anabolic steroids did not vastly improve the RIA assays for several reasons (Hämpl, Picha, Chundela, & Starka, 1978, 1979; Hämpl, Putz, Protiva, Filip, & Starka, 1982; Hämpl & Starka, 1979). Analysis of a chemical with an RIA method proves to be nonspecific, in that a wide range of molecules with some structural similarities to the original drug react with the antibody and show a positive result. Because of the general response with this type of test, results from an RIA alone would never be accepted as proof that a specific drug entity is present, without any doubt. Due to this inherent lack of specificity of RIA as a technique, the only accepted method of analysis for confirmation and proof of a positive drug-screening test is gas chromatography–mass spectrometry (GC-MS).

Table 13.4 Primary Human Urinary Metabolites of Some Anabolic Steroids

Anabolic steroid	Metabolites	Reference
Bolasterone	a. 7α, 17α-Dimethyl-5β-androstane-3α, 17β-diol b. 7α, 17α-Dimethyl-5β-androstane-3α, 17α-diol	Schänzer, 1996b
Boldenone	a. Boldenone b. 3α-Hydroxyl-5α-androsten-17-one c. 3-Keto-5α-androsten-17β-ol	Cartoni et al., 1985 Schänzer & Donike, 1992 Schänzer et al., 1995a
Calusterone	a. 7β, 17α-Dimethyl-5β-androstane-3α, 17β-diol b. 7β, 17α-Dimethyl-5α-androstane-3α, 17β-diol	Schänzer, 1996b
Chloro-dianabol	a. 6β-Hydroxy-chlorodianabol b. 6β, 12-Dihydroxychlorodianabol c. 6β, 16β-Dihydroxy-chlorodianabol d. 3α, 6β, 17β-Trihydroxychlorodianabol	Dürbeck et al., 1983 Schänzer, Horning, & Donike, 1995 Schänzer, Horning, et al., 1996
Clostebol	a. 4-Chloro-17-keto-androst-4-ene-3α-ol b. 4-Chloro-3α, 16β-dihydroxy-5-androstan-17-one c. 4-Chloro-17-keto-5α-androstan-3α-ol d. 4-Chloro-17-keto-5β-androstan-3α-ol	Dörner et al., 1963 Schänzer, Horning, et al., 1996
Dianabol	a. 17-Epi Dianabol b. 6β-Hydroxy Dianabol	Dürbeck & Büker, 1980 Schänzer et al., 1991 Schänzer, Delahaut, et al., 1996
Dihydrotes-tosterone	a. Androsterone b. Epiandrosterone c. 5α-Androstane-3α, 17β-diol d. 5α-Androstane-3β, 17β-diol	Geyer, Schänzer, Schindler, & Donike, 1996
Drostanolone	a. Drostanolone b. 2α-Methyl-3α-hydroxy-5α-androstan-17-one c. 2α-Methyl-5α-androstan-3α, 17β-diol	Chung et al., 1990 DeBoer et al., 1992
Ethylestrenol	19-Nor-5ξ, 17α-pregnane-3ξ, 17β, 21-triol	Björkhem et al., 1982

Anabolic steroid	Metabolites	Reference
Fluoxymesterone	a. 9α-Fluoro-17α-methyl-4-androsten-3α,6β,11β,17β-tetraol b. 9α-Fluoro-17α-methyl-6β,11β,17β-trihydroxy-4-androsten-3-one (6β-hydroxyfluoxymesterone) c. 9α-Fluoro-17α-methyl-5β-androstan-3α,11β,17β-triol	Kammerer et al., 1990 Schänzer, Horning, et al. 1996
Formebolone	2-Hydroxymethyl-11α, 17β-dihydroxy-17α-methyl-androstan-1, 4-diene-3-one	Chung et al., 1990 Masse et al., 1991
Furazabol	a. Furazabol b. 16-Hydroxy-furazabol	Gradeen et al., 1990 Kim et al., 1996
Mestanolone	17α-Methyl-5α-androstane-3α, 17β-diol	Masse et al., 1991 Schänzer, 1996b
Mesterolone	a. Mesterolone b. 1α-Methyl-17-keto-5α-androstan-3α-ol	Huck & Egg, 1972 DeBoer et al., 1992
Metandren	a. 5α-Androstan-17α-methyl-3α, 17β-diol b. 5β-Androstan-17α-methyl-3α, 17β-diol	Quincey & Gray, 1967
Methandriol	17α-Methyl-5β-androstane-3α, 17β-diol	Schänzer, 1996b
Methenolone	a. Methenolone b. 3α-Hydroxy-1-methylene-5α-androstan-17-one	Björkhem & Ek, 1983
Mibolerone	a. Tetrahydromibolerone b. 7α, 17α-Dimethyl-5β-estrane-3α, 17β-diol	Bowers, 1996
Nandrolone	a. 19-Norandrosterone b. 19-Noretiocholanolone c. 19-Norepiandrosterone	Masse et al., 1985
Norclostebol	a. 4-Chloro-3α-hydroxy-estra-4-ene-17-one b. 4-Chloro-3α-hydroxy-5β-estrane-17-one c. 4-Chloro-3α-hydroxy-5α-estrane-17-one d. 4-Chloro-3α, 16β-dihydroxy-5-androstane-17-one	Schänzer, 1996b
Norethandrolone	19-Nor-5ξ,17α-pregnane-3ξ, 17β, 21-triol	Ward et al., 1977

(continued)

Table 13.4 *(continued)*

Anabolic steroid	Metabolites	Reference
Oxandrolone	a. Oxandrolone b. 17-Epi oxandrolone	Masse, Hongang, et al., 1989
Oxymesterone	Oxymesterone	Schänzer, 1996b
Oxymetholone	a. 17α-Methyl-5α-androstan-3α, 17β-diol b. Other proposed structures	Bi et al., 1992a, b
Stanozolol	a. 3'-Hydroxy stanozolol b. 4β-Hydroxy stanozolol c. 16β-Hydroxy stanozolol d. Stanozolol e. 4β, 16β-Dihydroxy stanozolol	Schänzer et al., 1990 Schänzer, Delahaut, et al., 1996
Stenbolone	a. Stenbolone b. 3α-Hydroxy-2α-methyl-5α-androst-1-ene-17-one c. 16ξ-Hydroxy-stenbolone	Goudreault et al., 1991 Masse et al., 1992
Testosterone	See articles.	Baba et al., 1980 Donike et al., 1983
Trenbolone	17-Epitrenbolone	Uralets et al., 1996

In the future, other analytical technique combinations will be utilized, because of the need to employ such analyses to detect and confirm the presence of some of the newer, larger, and less stable hormone drugs being abused. These newer mass spectrometric techniques would include those with gentler sample introduction methods (liquid chromatography instead of gas chromatography), softer ionization techniques (time of flight, electrospray and ionspray interfaces), and more sensitive or more specific detection methods (isotope ratio MS, high-resolution MS, and MS-MS techniques). Some combination of techniques, which still employ mass spectroscopy, will undoubtedly be used to retain certainty about any reported positive analysis.

Gas Chromatography—Mass Spectrometry

During gas chromatographic analysis, a solvent extract of a urine sample is injected into a long column that interacts with the various components of the sample, retarding some components more than others. The time that a substance takes to pass through a particular column under a specified set of conditions is peculiar to that substance and thus helps identify it. A mass spectrometer attached to the end of that GC column detects substances passed into it by bombarding the molecules with a beam of electrons that fragments the molecules into ionic pieces; these data constitute an ion fragment fingerprint of that particular substance. That spectrum (collection) of fragment ions, along with the retention time (time spent in the GC column before detection), constitutes information unique for each substance; thus, identification without any doubt is confirmed when these data are the same as that collected when the authentic reference substance or sample from an excretion study is analyzed under the same conditions.

Liquid Chromatography—Mass Spectrometry (LC-MS)

LC-MS is, in principle, similar to gas chromatography–mass spectrometry, except the sample is passed through the separation column in the liquid state, rather than in the gas phase, and the inert carrier medium, which moves the sample through the separation column, is a liquid, instead of a gas.

The LC-MS technique is rapidly entering the drug-testing laboratory because of several advantages over the traditional GC-MS techniques. An LC analysis usually proceeds at room temperature, along with movement of larger hormone drugs through the separation column, whereas GC analysis requires the drug or hormone to be heated, vaporized into the gaseous state, in order to move through the separation column. Recent research (Barron, Barbosa, Pascual, & Segura, 1996) has reduced or eliminated some of the other disadvantages of LC-MS analysis, which were poor sensitivity and low sample volume capacity before service and maintenance of the instrument was required. Thus, in the future, LC-MS will become a technique of increasingly major importance in the drug-testing laboratory because of its ability to confirm the presence of most drugs, including the unstable, polar, and large-molecular-weight natural hormones (hGH, EPO, etc.).

High-Resolution Mass Spectrometry (HRMS)

Until recently HRMS would not have been an advantage in drug testing because sensitivity would have been sacrificed for specificity. In addition, the instruments have been extremely expensive (approximately $500,000 or more per instrument). However, costs of these instruments, like LC-MS instrumentation, have been declining recently, so that these instruments may soon be within the budgets of major laboratories. Because of the improvement in several different electronic and instrumental aspects of HRMS analysis, the technique now possesses increased sensitivity for some drugs. However, background signal (also called experimental noise) is also increased with increased sensitivity, such that the technique may not be of greater value for all substances, since endogenous interferences (background signal) vary with the metabolite being analyzed (Schänzer, Delahaut, et al., 1996; Schänzer, Horning, et al., 1996; Thieme, Grosse, & Mueller, 1996). HRMS analysis was introduced in the testing program of the 1996 Summer Olympic Games in Atlanta, but the "positives" found with the technique were not formally reported, presumably due to the potential legal problems. Namely, how are negative results obtained with the "old, proven" method judged vis-à-vis positive results obtained with the "new" HRMS method? In other words, a database of results must be collected, particularly comparing the two methods on the same samples, in order to validate a result with the "new" HRMS machine. Only after sufficient results are published, addressing detection limits, any false negative and positive issues, and statistics showing the validity of results, will the technique be acceptable both scientifically and legally.

Isotope Ratio Mass Spectrometry (IRMS)

The relatively new technique of isotope ratio mass spectrometry is being proposed for verification of testosterone positives that could be explained by means other than drug taking. It is based on the simple fact that the percentage of carbon 13 (a naturally occurring, stable, nonradioactive isotope of carbon of approximately 1.1% natural abundance) found in endogenous testosterone, which is made in the body from dietary components whose carbon sources are plants and animals, is different than the percentage of carbon 13 present in the synthetic testosterone found in a drug preparation. IRMS analysis can determine the percent carbon 13 to percent carbon 12 (% ^{13}C:^{12}C) ratio in the sample (note that normally ^{12}C is approx. 98.9% of the carbon and ^{13}C approx. 1.1%), and thus whether it came from a synthetic drug or from diet (Aguilera et al., 1996a,b). Even though anabolic steroids are an old class of drugs (Hoberman & Yesalis, 1995), with the ban on athletic use of testosterone occurring in 1983, it has been reported quite recently that several different situations (see later discussion) will raise the T/E ratio into the "illegal" >6:1 range, without the athlete ever having taken testosterone! If enough data are published verifying the veracity of IRMS and establishing that it can corroborate whether an athlete has taken testosterone, then the technique will be used, despite its expense, time, and special equipment needs. It should be emphasized here that an IRMS is used only for isotope ratio analyses in T/E drug cases, cannot be used for other routine assays (such as steroid screening or confirmation tests), and still costs over $100,000 per instrument. IRMS can be of great value in resolving the "problems" associated with the documented increase in T/E ratios after alcohol use (Falk, Palonek, & Björkhem, 1988; Karila, Kosunen, Leinonen, Tachtelae, & Seppaelae, 1996), a fluctuation in the ratio in women apparently caused by many factors (Engelke, Geyer, & Donike, 1995; Engelke, Flenker, & Donike, 1996), some experimental conditions during sample preparation and their effects on the results (Geyer, Schänzer, Mareck-Engelke, & Donike, 1996), possible use of DHEA (Haning et al., 1991; Haning et al., 1993), or even simultaneous use of both testosterone and epitestosterone (Dehennin, 1994). However, because of both the complexity of and possible sex differences in metabolism of DHEA (Haning et al., 1991; Haning et al., 1993), it is not clear that IRMS can distinguish between the use of pharmaceutical and "dietary" DHEA. In other words, use of DHEA, which may convert in some small degree to testosterone, may not contribute enough "synthetic testosterone" to the ^{13}C:^{12}C ratio to weight the result in favor of suspicion of synthetic supplementation rather than "normal fluctuation." Nonetheless, use of the IRMS instrument will increase dramatically in the future, after the verification test for testosterone abuse is validated. However, it will add considerable costs to the operation of the laboratories, since this instrument will still be useful only in the small numbers of samples in which a "testosterone problem" is present.

Philosophy of Anabolic Steroid Testing

In the past, testing for anabolic steroids was simple, in terms of what constitutes a positive and what does not. The presence of any amount of an anabolic steroid scientifically documented as real, and shown to be significantly above background (signal level attributable to instrument noise) was considered doping. This was because no known anabolic steroid was found in the body naturally. With the addition of the endogenous anabolic steroid, testosterone, to the control list in 1983, and the many other conditions subsequently found to interfere with testing for anabolic steroid (see discussions above and below), criteria for what constitutes a drug positive today are exceedingly complex because of the increasingly lengthy list of conditions under which a "false positive" result may occur. These false positive possibilities include consumption of meat from animals treated with anabolic steroids (Hemmersbach et al., 1995), "normal" production of nandrolone metabolites after use of contraceptive medication or in pregnancy (Reznick et al., 1987), endogenous production of "boldenone" metabolites without drug use (Schänzer, Geyer, et al., 1995), "illegal" T/E ratios after alcohol use (Karila et al., 1996), or improper storage/enzyme treatment of the urine specimen (Geyer, Schänzer, Mareck-Engelke, et.al., 1996).

Levels of commonly found agents (testosterone, caffeine) are purposefully set high in laboratories to protect innocent athletes from being falsely accused of drug abuse. Because of this philosophy, some positives will not be reported in order to avoid any chance of a false positive result. Thus, some abuse will not be deterred by testing, particularly for those substances for which only very high drug levels constitute a positive result (e.g., testosterone and caffeine). If the IRMS test is validated (discussed above), then much of the abuse of testosterone now apparent because of the current high guilt threshold will become less possible. It is still not clear how effective IRMS will be in detecting those athletes who carefully use testosterone while keeping their T/E ratios below 6:1.

Despite the frequent requests for information on detectability of anabolic steroids, there are no absolute guidelines an athlete can use and no definable time period in which an athlete can cease drug use in order to escape a positive test result. This is because there are too many inherent variables that can profoundly affect the drug elimination/excretion process. These variables (figure 13.1) can affect a test result quantitatively in different directions, indicating why it is impossible to define reliable detection guidelines for anabolic steroids.

Figure 13.2 lists ways an athlete can theoretically avoid a positive anabolic steroid test result while taking the drugs. Although any drug that dilutes or inhibits the excretion of anabolic steroids into urine is now banned, new designer inhibitors and other possible options will be available. As athletes learn of new options, testing will be circumvented. Laboratories will become aware of these new drugs and processes and will take appropriate countermeasures, and the vicious cycle will continue.

- Urine output/volume for that athlete
- Urine pH (acidity or alkalinity, usually affected by diet)
- Urine volume used by laboratory to test for AS
- Dosage of AS taken, when last taken, and formulation used (e.g., oral)
- Acute or chronic use of AS
- Other AS taken simultaneously
- The AS being detected: some AS are easier to detect at lower levels than others
- Lab variabilities
  - Tuning of mass spectrometer affects sensitivity of tests
  - Cleaning of mass spectrometer source affects sensitivity
  - Meticulousness in sample clean-up, handling, and derivatization affects sensitivity
- Agents present, promoting-inhibiting excretion of AS
- Drug metabolism inhibitors/promoters taken concurrently with AS, for example, barbiturates, alcohol, nicotine, some anti-ulcer medications (H_2 receptor antagonists), and others
- Metabolic activity of individual athlete (such as genetic variations)
- Fat content of athlete
- Athlete's diet during testing/competition
- Recent trauma/shock to athlete

Figure 13.1 Variables influencing the concentration or detectability of anabolic steroids (AS) in urine.

- The user can dilute the urine (e.g., by using diuretics, which is now illegal).
- The user can prevent AS excretion into urine (e.g., by using probenecid, which is now illegal).
- The user can mask/interfere with peak detection by coelution of an interfering substance on the gas chromatograph–mass spectrometer system.
- The user can cease dosing in time for AS levels to drop too low to detect.
- The user can take testosterone but keep the level low enough that the ratio to epitestosterone stays below 6:1.
- The user can take epitestosterone so that the testosterone-to-epitestosterone ratio stays below 6:1; this is illegal, and the user could be convicted of illegal testosterone levels by means other than the testosterone-to-epitestosterone ratio.
- The user can take birth control pills in an attempt to "hide" the use of nandrolone; this is illegal, and the user will be convicted of nandrolone use anyway (see Masse, Ayotte, & Dugal, 1989).

Figure 13.2 Theoretical ways to prevent a positive test for anabolic steroids (AS).

Costs of Anabolic Steroid Testing

Many factors enter into the high cost of testing for anabolic steroids. Acquisition, maintenance, and use of GC-MS systems, and the hiring, training, and retention of qualified people to conduct anabolic steroid testing by GC-MS analysis, constitute much of the cost. Expensive high-purity reagents and careful, meticulous, reliable lab work are also required, the latter possible only with extensive training of lab personnel. With the addition of HRMS and IRMS testing methods as discussed above, the costs are much higher. HRMS machines could be used to test for any drug but cost about $300,000 each; although IRMS instruments are cheaper (about $100,000 each), they may be used only for T/E analyses. Addition of both types of instruments increases the lab operation costs substantially. Additional expensive MS techniques will likely be needed in the near future (LC-MS-MS, time of flight/laser desorption mass spectroscopy, etc.) to be used for the analysis of the several natural polypeptide drugs currently being abused (see later discussion), which shall greatly increase the costs of operating a testing program, as some of these instruments currently cost about $200,000 each. Recent LC-MS-MS benchtop instruments (Stevenson, 1998) have come down in price significantly, so it is possible that even high-resolution and time of flight/laser desorption instruments may dramatically drop in price in the near future. These "new" techniques will be discussed further in future editions when they are in common use.

Even with contracts guaranteeing a large volume of testing, in 1999 a charge of $100 or more per anabolic steroid analysis was usual. There is considerable expense in the intensive, laborious efforts for confirmation of screening positives, relative to the initial screening. Should the number of screening positives become very high, the laboratory becomes overwhelmed with GC-MS/LC-MS confirmation work, slowing other work as well as the output of screening results on other samples.

Thus, the costs of testing for anabolic steroids and hormones are not likely to decline much in the future, because of the introduction of more expensive, high-resolution, isotope equipment needed both for testing for the polypeptide hormones and for increased sensitivity. Improvements in testing procedures and the introduction of cheaper and faster screening procedures are not likely to offset these additional expenses.

In addition, in order to corroborate a T/E positive (Garle, Ocka, Palonek, & Björkhem, 1996; Kicman et al., 1990; Palonek et al., 1995; Raynaud et al., 1992; Raynaud et al., 1993; Dehennin & Matsumoto, 1993), the chronic use of other anabolic steroids in the recent past (Oftebro, 1992; Norli et al., 1995), or the use of dihydrotestosterone (DHT) (Southan et al., 1992; Kicman, Coutts, Walker, & Cowan, 1995; Kicman et al., 1997; Donike et al., 1995; Geyer, Schänzer, Schindler, et al., 1996), steroid profiling analysis data are being analyzed more frequently. Basically, more data are being analyzed in order to evaluate the effects of exogenous anabolic steroids on endogenous steroids, both relative to one another and in absolute amounts. This work entails considerable data analysis and validation of the amounts of each endogenous steroid via comparison with authentic reference standards after use of the appropriate internal and external standards. First, collection of all the appropriate peak area data and verification of the identity of those peaks by comparison of the retention time (time spent in the analysis column after injection of the sample up to the detection time) with that of authentic standard steroids is needed. Then calculation of the quantities present is made by comparison of the peak response with that obtained from authentic standards, which then allows calculation of the amount of the relevant steroids present in the sample. The dilution of urine, genetics, sex, disease conditions present, legal drugs taken, and other criteria all may have an effect on the results, so that steroid profile analysis is not an exact science! However, regardless of the results, the need for additional evaluation of more data than was routinely obtained in the past will increase the time needed to process samples, as well as the costs to do so.

Circumventing Positive Test Results

It is possible but unlikely that an athlete can prevent a positive anabolic steroid test result by using a substance containing appropriate interfering or masking ion fragments. This is because laboratories use both the gas chromatographic retention time (RT) and the mass spectrometric fragment ions for declaring a positive, and the chances of an interfering substance possessing both the same RT and ion spectrum as the drug are extremely low.

An athlete is considered guilty of using testosterone if the T/E ratio exceeds 6:1, although in actual practice many organizations will not pursue a "positive" below 9:1 or 10:1 because a finite though still low number of cases of T/E ratios over 6:1 have been shown not to result from testosterone abuse (Oftebro, 1992; Raynaud et al., 1992; Raynaud et al., 1993; Garle et al., 1996; Karila et al., 1996). Simultaneous consumption of epitestosterone and testosterone to keep the ratio of the two substances close to the "normal" ratio of 1:1 should not prevent the identification of exogenous testosterone use (Dehennin, 1994) because the laboratories can calculate the ratios of testosterone, as well as the ratios of epitestosterone, to other endogenous steroids measured during the drug-screening process. These resulting ratios will then change and will be interpreted as atypical by scientists evaluating the data (Dehennin & Matsumoto, 1993; Dehennin, 1994; Norli et al., 1995; Palonek et al., 1995; Geyer, Schänzer, Mareck-Engelke, et al., 1996). Laboratories have indeed set reference range values for many endogenous steroid levels and ratios (Donike et al., 1995), but the published data to date are rare. In other words, reference range values will be arbitrary until data are published that address the natural variation in the levels of epitestosterone and many other natural hormones—that is, how they normally vary with age, sex, weight, diet, female hormonal fluctuation, use of legal dietary supplementation or birth control or other legal medication, and so on! This fact implies considerable legal problems whenever such a positive drug case is made public.

To my knowledge, there have been no reported positive cases of testosterone due to the use of both epitestosterone and testosterone. This may be due to the astute use of both testosterone and epitestosterone so that urinary levels are not high enough to be conclusive, or due to the anticipated legal issues involved in proving such dual usage. The use of moderate amounts of both testosterone and epitestosterone will not only prevent the T/E ratio from exceeding 6:1 but also will not raise the ratios relative to other endogenous steroids sufficiently to be conclusive. This situation is analogous to the use of moderate amounts of testosterone, which raises the T/E ratio but not over 6:1. Thus, some positive results may not be reported because of the obvious need to protect individuals whose T/E ratios or ratios of testosterone and epitestosterone to other endogenous steroids vary due to "natural" reasons and not to drug use. In either case, use of both testosterone and epitestosterone constitutes a problem in anabolic steroid testing because they are both endogenous substances and thus illegal levels must be shown to be due to the illegal use of those substances and not to normal variations in natural hormones (Dehennin, 1994).

Even the published scientific data on the validity of the 6:1 T/E ratio as a means to substantiate testosterone abuse are still relatively sparse. This situation confers advantages to the abusers and their lawyers, because the independent, peer-reviewed data for the test are not available in quantity sufficient to withstand legal challenge. In other words, there is no specific source in which one may find substantial data on the relationship of T/E ratios to sex, age, diet, and common drugs taken (cold medications, alcohol, nicotine-tobacco use, caffeine, H_2-receptor antagonists [used for ulcer treatment], birth control pills, etc.). Data should also be available for the time of the menstrual cycle, bacteria count in the sample, pH of the sample, and any use of other common, permitted drugs. The data should be on a sufficiently large sample for each category of functional variable (>10,000) so that there is no chance that a false positive would occur in the population of athletes that normally attend a summer Olympics (usually approx. 10,000+). In other words, control of any natural substance requires the establishment of the "normal" endogenous level in the population and subsequent statistical determination of what is "abnormal" or abuse. Although some of these data exist, the quantity is relatively small, and therein lies the legal problem. A recent paper summarizes the testosterone testing "problems" and suggests some possible solutions, which are discussed elsewhere (Catlin, Hatton, & Starcevic, 1997).

A strongly rumored method for abusing testosterone is use of the available skin patches (gels) for the application of controlled-release testosterone. A controlled-release preparation delivers the drug into the body on a more consistent, even basis over time, rather than as the larger, more sudden dose that occurs soon after parenteral administration. Controlled release means a relatively even dosing over a longer time period—usually 8 to 12 hours—resulting in a lower peak plasma level than a regular dose, but a level that varies less and lasts longer. Thus, relative to parenteral administration, the use of a sustained-release testosterone preparation will yield a more stable blood level of drug with fewer high fluctuations in drug level, thereby making drug use "safer" than parenteral administration, and with less chance of exceeding the 6:1 T/E ratio (Meikle et al., 1992, 1996). The fact that an IOC laboratory has recently published a preliminary method to detect the use of a testosterone skin patch application strongly suggests that such testosterone use is common (Brisson et al., 1997). Furthermore, skin (particularly scrotal skin) contains high levels of reductase activity, so that applied testosterone is relatively quickly converted to dihydrotestosterone (DHT). Thus, DHT levels could be raised by either use of a testosterone skin patch or actual consumption of DHT. A number of Chinese female swimmers were found positive for DHT (Donike et al., 1995; Geyer, Schänzer, Schindler, et al., 1996) at the World Swimming Championships in 1994. Their positives were determined by careful comparison of the amount found in the samples with the amounts of several other endogenous steroids (steroid profile analysis), and reported in the world press (Southan et al., 1992; Kicman et al., 1995; Donike et al., 1995; Coutts et al., 1997). It was clear that those athletes thought that DHT would not be found during testing. However, once again, relatively arbitrary limits were used to determine guilt. In other words, the data base of reference values for the determination of normal versus supplemented levels was not substantial.

Illegal use of testosterone by female athletes is more difficult to prove than in male athletes because absolute levels are much lower in females and because both the levels of testosterone and epitestosterone and the T/E ratios fluctuate greatly (Karila et al., 1996; Engelke et al., 1995; Engelke et al., 1996). In addition, there may be a hormonal cycle–dependent T/E ratio fluctuation (Engelke et al., 1995), and a relatively large increase in T/E ratio after alcohol consumption (Falk et al., 1988; Karila et al., 1996).

Therefore, if the dose of testosterone is carefully chosen and/or combined with sustained release dosing, significant amounts of drug may be used during training and continuing relatively close to competition time, with a very low risk of reaching an illegal T/E ratio or drug positive. The ratio of T/E was chosen such that some drug abuse would be tolerated in order to protect all innocent athletes who may have a naturally higher T/E ratio.

If future experiments prove that the use of IRMS analysis does indeed distinguish between endogenous and exogenous testosterone, or if collection of competition blood specimens is allowed such that the nonendogenous intact testosterone esters may be found when testosterone has been taken, then the labs will have fewer problems in proving testosterone abuse.

Use of Other Substances

Many other substances have become popular for either their purported anabolic effects or their effects on endogenous anabolic substances, including the following:

- Zeranol
- clenbuterol
- Deprenyl
- orotic acid
- polypeptide hormones
- cafedrine
- Bromantan

- creatine
- bicarbonate
- Mesocarb/Sydnocarb

Zeranol is a nonsteroid but is a potent anabolic agent commonly used to fatten cattle (Roche & Davis, 1972). The USOC has banned Zeranol because of its anabolic activity. When an athlete consumes beef that contains Zeranol, low levels of the drug can be detected. Also, because Zeranol has no structural similarity to any other anabolic steroid and is not chemically a steroid, the legal issues of a positive case are unclear.

Clenbuterol, a B^2-receptor agonist commonly used to treat asthma in Europe (but not approved for medical use in the United States as of this writing), has been shown in animal studies to increase skeletal muscle mass and reduce body fat (Maltin et al., 1987; Satchell, 1996). Widespread abuse of this drug by athletes, including reported positives in the 1992 Barcelona Olympic Games (Segura et al., 1995) has kept it on most lists of banned drugs. A mass spectroscopic method for the detection of clenbuterol and analogues, which also can be used as a confirmation assay, has appeared recently (Doerge et al., 1995). The laboratories can detect use of the drug, but since it is used at very low dosage, and during training prior to competition, it is not known whether use has been totally deterred.

Deprenyl, a monoamine oxidase (MAO) inhibitor that was approved for use in the United States for Parkinson's disease in 1990, is probably used by athletes for its stimulation effects because there is no evidence of direct anabolic activity. However, this drug is converted to methamphetamine and amphetamine in humans by metabolism, so that any athlete taking this drug will undoubtedly be convicted of methamphetamine/amphetamine use (Heinonen, 1994). Thus, athletes must be careful when taking drugs that are presumed to be allowed, since the drugs may be metabolized to a banned substance.

Orotic acid is a naturally occurring vitamin (not a steroid) that possesses both anabolic and uricosuric properties. Testing for it is not currently available since "normal" levels are undetermined. Only rumor has indicated use of this "vitamin-drug." Since there are no data on its "normal" levels or the potency of its effects, the size of any problem is not known.

Several polypeptide hormones, including human growth hormone (hGH), human chorionic gonadotropin (HCG), gonadotropin-releasing hormone (GnRH), insulin, and erythropoietin (EPO) are very likely being abused in competition. The polypeptide hormones are abused for reasons other than the difficulty of confirming positive screening tests, as discussed later. Human growth hormone, GnRH, and HCG all have anabolic effects in their own rights or stimulate the release of testosterone or other natural anabolic agents (Bradley & Sodeman, 1990; Papadakis et al., 1996; Conn & Crowley, 1994; Laidler et al., 1995). EPO increases the production of red blood cells, increasing the body's oxygen-carrying capacity (Casoni et al., 1993). It was widely rumored that EPO was abused at the 1996 Atlanta Olympic Games because no confirmatory lab test was available to enforce the ban or confirm any potential reported positives (Bamberger & Yaeger, 1997).

Testing for the many polypeptide hormones is difficult because the confirmatory assays for these compounds by MS are not currently developed and validated and thus not available to laboratories yet (for hGH, see Kabouris, Platen, & Donike, 1996; for HCG, see Laidler et al., 1995; Liu & Bowers, 1995, 1996; Stenman, Kallio, Korhonen, & Alfthan, 1997; for EPO, see Wide, Bengtsson, Berglund, & Ekblom, 1995; Ekblom, 1996). Besides the fact that the presence of polypeptide hormones is difficult to confirm by a specific assay, these compounds are naturally present in all healthy people. Thus, doping control programs must establish what levels of polypeptide hormones are abnormal or indicative of abuse and what levels are normal. A considerable database is needed to confirm what concentration range for each of these natural components is normal and what variations occur for a variety of "natural" causes. Otherwise, testing programs are going to face considerable legal problems not unlike what is happening today with T/E positive cases. The problem with epitestosterone and its potential use started in 1983 with the ban on exogenous testosterone usage, and the problem still exists today: namely, what constitutes "normal" levels and what constitutes "illegal" levels, given the natural fluctuations that may occur in different individuals. Endogenous HCG levels are minute, at best, in men or are often undetectable but not in certain cases of malignancy. Levels of HCG are higher in women; shortly after conception, the levels become huge because this compound is a placental hormone and is the basis of a commonly used pregnancy test. Consequently, an athlete accused of HCG abuse can counter with contentions of illness or pregnancy. No one knows whether these "reasonable" excuses will work for an athlete who has abused these drugs.

Athletes take many other endogenous natural agents for a variety of effects, such as release of endogenous growth hormone, enhanced fat burning, and enhanced normal testosterone levels and synthesis (Conn & Crowley, 1994; Laidler et al., 1995). It is important that the athlete take due care in using new or experimental drugs or dosages that significantly exceed therapeutic levels. Although no scientific proof has appeared, deaths presumably due to the abuse of erythropoietin emphasize this point (Leith, 1991).

Testing for the many other products is a difficult issue. Designer steroids can be and are being made (Bamberger & Yaeger, 1997; Franke & Berendonk, 1997), which may lead to long-term drug abuse without detection. In addition, when such a drug is initially found, the agent must be banned by the various sport federations, the athletes and members must be apprised of such bans, and relevant sanctions must be listed so that all athletes, coaches, trainers, physicians, and other appropriate people are notified. The IOC, sport federations, and World Court of Arbitration for Sport usually require evidence that the prohibition of use of an agent is indicated (i.e., that it enhances performance) before issuing the ban (e.g., positives for the use of Bromantan in the 1996 Olympic Games were disallowed). However, the recent IOC ban on the use of THC (cannabinoids) suggest that performance enhancement is not a condition for banning the use of an agent. Most would agree that, in the majority of instances, THC use would not enhance performance.

Assays for Zeranol already exist, and testing for it is relatively trivial, involving only collection of the appropriate retention times and mass fragment data for GC-MS confirmatory analysis. Athletes use clenbuterol at very low doses (typically, 20 to 120 μg per day), so that levels are low in the urine and development of confirmatory tests requires high sensitivity. The half-life of clenbuterol in humans is approximately 34 hours; so the time required to remove more than 95% of the drug in the body after the last dose is 5 half-lives or about 7 days. Testing for Deprenyl is an easy task, but because a large fraction of the dose is converted into methamphetamine and amphetamine before excretion (Heinonen, 1994), tests for the latter two drugs (already on all banned lists) are already in place.

Not only the use of new drugs but also new applications for old drugs may occur, and evidently both occurred in recent international sporting events. Cafedrine is an old drug, a chemical linkage of ephedrine and theophylline, and is used after anesthesia to help wake a patient. It is a potent stimulant, which is *not* a simple mixture of ephedrine and theophylline (a stimulant related to caffeine) and thus would not yield a positive test for either drug (although theophylline, often used in the treatment of asthma, is not banned at this time). However, no metabolism data for cafedrine exists in the published literature, so that its use would be difficult to detect unless a laboratory knew what to look for by doing an excretion study and the corresponding metabolic identifications. Although not named specifically on any banned list to date, this drug is chemically related to a banned drug (ephedrine), and thus would be banned theoretically by the phrase "and related compounds." However, the 1996 Bromantan fiasco might suggest that the phrase "and related compounds" can no longer be effectively used.

A previously unknown drug, Bromantan, was found in five athletes in the 1996 Atlanta Olympic Games, but the positive cases were disallowed by the World Court of Arbitration for Sport because the drug was too new; namely, insufficient data, scientific knowledge, and research literature were available to enforce the recent ban. In other words, sufficient scientific knowledge must be readily available in the world's literature to justify consideration of a ban, and such a consideration must then be sent to the various athletic federations, who must approve the addition of such an agent to the banned lists. A computer search of the world's literature in July 1996 revealed that Bromantan was developed in Russia for thermoprotective and stimulant effects and was reportedly to be used in army troops. The only articles found in the Russian language described the compound as a psychostimulant. Its chemical structure was unlike any other known drug (even though one might construe it to be a distant cousin of amantadine, an antiviral drug currently on the market). There was no known metabolic information available in the public scientific literature from 1967 through July 1996. Rumors had been circulating that there was a new drug, which had been abused in the 1992 Barcelona Olympic Games. Thus, the IOC laboratories began to look in competition samples for a new unknown peak during screening, which was identified by mass spectrometry as Bromantan before the 1996 Olympic Games.

Creatine supplementation is claimed to be widespread and to positively affect performance (Volek & Kraemer, 1996). Creatine is a simple nitrogenous compound that is found in most meat and fish at about 0.5% by weight. In addition, it is also made in the body. It appears to help maintain the high-energy usage during strenuous exercise and is involved in energy output and maintenance in muscle tissue. Potential control of use or abuse is fraught with difficulties because of the variations in endogenous levels. In other words, there would have to be substantial data proving "normal" fluctuations of levels with exercise levels, age, sex, diet, and weight before any test could ever prove what constitutes an "illegal" level. Creatine does not currently appear on any banned list and may be used without any risk of penalty as of this date.

Sodium bicarbonate has been used for enhancing training and prolonging exercise levels (Webster, Webster, Crawford, & Gladden, 1993). The mechanism of action is presumably the neutralization of excess lactate that increases in muscle tissue as exercise and strenuous activity is continued. There is little hope of ever controlling bicarbonate abuse, in that large amounts exist in both the diet as well as in the body. In addition, there would be no easy way to isolate bicarbonate for a specific analysis from the myriad of other inorganic ions and species naturally present in the body.

Sydnocarb (Mesocarb) is a polar derivative of amphetamine and classed as a psychostimulant (Breidbach, Sigmund, & Donike, 1995). Its use could confer an advantage in those sports where short-term stimulation confers an advantage. Because of its polar structure as well as its instability under some conditions of laboratory analysis, Mesocarb is poorly detected by some screening procedures. Recent papers demonstrate how to detect the drug by standard methods, in order to enforce a ban on its use by athletes (Thieme, Grosse, Lang, & Mueller, 1995; DeBoer, Ooijen, & Maes, 1995).

Future Directions in Anabolic Steroid Testing

New developments in drug testing may make this process cheaper, faster, and more reliable. On the other hand, it's also likely that new drugs will be developed that escape detection in current test procedures. Conversely, the introduction of (1) high-resolution MS-MS analysis; (2) LC-MS-MS assays for unstable compounds and polypeptide hormones; and (3) isotope ratio combustion MS analysis for use in the T/E assay will make the testing process more expensive, slower, and more difficult. These latter instruments and associated assays are considerably more complicated, and will require more staff, further training, and greatly increased overhead costs in such a testing laboratory.

- Development of specific sensitive immunoassays, based on antibodies raised against relevant anabolic steroid metabolites, may make screening tests much more reliable than current RIA methodology. The downside is that development and validation of such tests will be very difficult, time consuming, and expensive. Estimates range to $250,000 or more *per steroid* for development costs for a validated immunoassay
- Confirmation assays are under development for HCG, GnRH, hGH, EPO, and other abusable natural products. The IOC has budgeted some funds for a research project to develop a definitive test for hGH. In addition, there have been preliminary reports that a test for EPO is nearing completion. Some federations have been using the hemocrit as an indicator of EPO abuse; for example, above a certain value, the athlete is simply prohibited from competing, without any punitive action taken. Using an indirect test such as the hemocrit for "proof" of drug use would not appear to be legally sound, at least in the United States. Although the mass spectrometric technology clearly exists for the assay and detection of these products today, there is another major component to the valid detection of abuse of these products. Namely, the aforementioned problem of what levels constitute abuse and what levels simply reflect "normal" fluctuation of compounds that are present in all athletes. That is, each of these substances naturally varies in amount as normal physiological processes occur in the human body, and both genetic background and various diseases also affect levels of these natural hormones. Thus, the moral, legal, and ethical issues of calling a drug test positive for any of these agents are extremely complex, and not ease to define. Under current guidelines, MS should be used for all confirmatory procedures, but only RIA methods currently are readily available for these peptide hormones.
- New anabolic steroids may be synthesized that will initially escape detection by testing laboratories. Design of such drugs by someone who knows the screening ion programs currently used for anabolic steroids testing may produce drugs that do not yield the common screening ion

fragments and thus will escape detection until the information becomes available to the laboratories.

• Some athletic federations may allow blood samples to be used for testing purposes. Although in some cases, blood (plasma) may contain higher concentrations of a drug than does urine, only limited amounts of blood may be taken (10–20 ml), while much larger amounts of urine are more easily obtainable. Thus, any potential benefit of blood as the testing matrix may be minimal. When esters of testosterone are abused, they cannot be detected intact in urine but can in plasma, which will constitute proof of testosterone abuse. This is important, because testosterone esters are not endogenous (produced in the body), so that detection of an intact testosterone ester constitutes proof of exogenous testosterone supplementation. Thus, the controversy over the use of the T/E ratio will be avoided and the interpretation of the test result will become obvious (the first scientific proof that this technique is feasible has appeared: de la Torre, Segura, & Polettini, 1995; de la Torre, Segura, Polettini, & Montagna, 1995). However, the general use of blood is still tentative at best, because all international athletic federations must still approve blood as a testing matrix.

• Hair analysis may be used. The hair of a drug user does contain many of the drugs taken by that individual, and analysis of older sections of the hair can reliably indicate chronic use. Since limited excretion data of anabolic steroids into human hair has been reported, more research is needed to determine if anabolic steroids are excreted into human hair to confirm the plausibility and the clinical relevance of using human hair samples for anabolic steroid testing. Recent reviews of clinical analysis of hair samples (Deng, Kurosu, & Pounder, 1999; Gleixner & Meyer, 1997) show that testosterone may be found in human hair, and stanozolol has recently been found in the hair of rats treated with stanozolol (Hold et al., 1996). Thus, additional research is needed to validate what steroids and related drugs are excreted into hair, as well as whether hair is a valid sample for athletic drug-testing programs. If this testing of hair works, athletes will probably shave their heads, which will mean further testing to validate the use of other body hair for analysis.

Testing for anabolic steroids is complex, expensive, and technically very difficult. An intimate marriage of medicine, pharmacology, analytical chemistry, endocrinology, and clinical chemistry is necessary for building an effective anabolic steroid-testing laboratory that produces no false positive and minimal false negative results.

The average clinical laboratory is not capable of carrying out effective and comprehensive anabolic steroid testing because it does not have the necessary expertise and information available, unless extraordinary effort, expense, and collaboration with an already experienced laboratory is part of the program. Testing, even at IOC laboratories, is not foolproof, in that false negatives do occur for a variety of reasons (see figures 13.1 and 13.2). In addition, control of the endogenous anabolic steroid testosterone is difficult and only somewhat effective because protecting all innocent athletes from being falsely accused is a legitimate goal. Because of genetic variations and other induced variations in testosterone levels (Cowan, Kicman, Walker, & Wheeler, 1991; Engelke et al., 1995; Engelke et al., 1996; Karila et al., 1996), laboratories must set a sufficiently high threshold in defining the illegal level of testosterone; so it is likely that some abusers of testosterone will not be caught. Drug testing, in order to become more effective as a deterrent as well as to enhance health and promote fairness in competition, has to become much more widespread, and must include unannounced (out of competition) testing with more unvarying enforcement of sanctions. Some officials have gone so far as to say that only out-of-competition blood testing will make it possible for the testing process to "clean up" sport. Certainly, much more uniform, strict laboratory standards of testing for anabolic steroids are needed. If athletes knew that no one would escape detection for drug abuse and that all competitors would face the same uniformly enforced sanctions for use of drugs, most abuse would cease. Athletes are still afraid of being at a disadvantage by not using certain performance-enhancing agents, because they believe that a majority of their competitors (in certain sports) do use performance-enhancing agents.

Sanctions against athletes must be much more fairly and uniformly applied. This does not mean that an athlete must be punished in all cases in which his or her sample shows the presence of a drug, as other circumstances may affect whether or not true drug abuse has occurred. Such circumstances must always be based on scientific facts or uncertainty, and not on politics, quotas, or other irrelevant criteria. Besides the actual test results, scientific facts that should decide a testing positive include, but are not limited to, any evidence of sabotage; fluctuation of T/E levels, as happens due to female hormonal cycle variance (Engelke et al., 1995; Engelke, et al., 1996); genetics; evidence of endocrine disease; sample history; conditions during preparation for testing; and chain of custody. In addition, any positive case showing very low levels of drug coupled with a normal steroid profile, which indicates no chronic use, should not be called positive, since it has been shown that nandrolone metabolites may be generated from the use of some birth control medications (Reznick et al., 1987), that boldenone and metabolites have been found in totally naive people who have never taken boldenone or any steroid (Schänzer, Geyer, et al., 1995), and that several anabolic steroid metabolites have been found in people who have consumed animals that were treated with the steroids as fattening agents during the raising of the animal (Debruyckere, deSagher, & Peteghem, 1992, 1995; Kicman et al., 1994; Hemmersbach et al., 1995). In addition, pretest consumption of alcohol, incorrect storage of the urine sample, or use of certain specific deconjugation enzymes in sample preparation (Geyer, Schänzer, Mareck-Engelke, et al., 1996) can artificially raise a T/E ratio and create a false positive testosterone sample. It should always be borne in mind that a publicly announced drug testing positive most probably will ruin the athlete's career, often forever, so that when there is *any* doubt about a result for any reason whatsoever, a drug testing positive should be considered negative! On the other hand, society has become skeptical about the relative value of drug-testing programs. The titles of recent articles both in academic journals ("Performance-Enhancing Drugs, Fair Competition, and Olympic Sport," *Journal of the American Medical Association*: Catlin & Murray, 1996) and in the popular media ("Doped to Perfection," *Newsweek:* Cowley & Brant, 1996; "Bigger, Stronger, Faster," *Sports Illustrated:* Bamberger & Yaeger, 1997) certainly reflect considerable skepticism.

To predict the future of drug-testing programs for anabolic steroids and related hormones, one would really need a crystal ball. However, it is very likely that the present situation will persist. The monetary implications and political overtones of a drug positive found in an elite or famous athlete are too great to predict anything other than controversy and protracted legal challenges for most drug-testing programs. Unannounced out-of-competition testing may improve any drug-control program's effectiveness, but universal application of such an approach will be difficult to implement worldwide.

Recent publication (Franke & Berendonk, 1997) of the secret, extensive hormonal doping program used on athletes in the GDR (German Democratic Republic) emphasizes that testing is not yet good enough nor is it a really effective deterrent; yet it has enhanced fair competition in certain sports because without testing, drug use would certainly be much greater. In the future, testing can be a more effective deterrent to drug abuse. This will happen only if considerably more money, research, cooperation, and planning are forthcoming; if increased out-of-competition testing is introduced; and if, at the same time, the incentives for drug abuse decrease.

References

Aguilera, R., Becchi, M., Grenot, C., Casabianca, H., Hatton, C.K., Catlin, D.H., Starcevic, B., & Pope, H.G. (1996a). Improved method of detection of testosterone abuse by gas chromatography/combustion/isotope ratio mass spectrometry analysis of urinary steroids. *Journal of Mass Spectrometry, 31*, 169–176.

Aguilera, R., Becchi, M., Grenot, C., Casabianca, H., & Hatton, C.K. (1996b). Detection of testosterone misuse: Comparison of two chromatographic sample preparation methods for gas chromatographic-combustion/isotope ratio mass spectrometric analysis. *Journal of Chromatography Biomedical Applications, 687*(1), 53–54.

Baba, S., Shinohara, Y., & Kasuya, Y. (1980). Differentiation between endogenous and exogenous testosterone in human plasma and urine after oral administration of deuterium-labeled testosterone by mass fragmentography. *Journal of Clinical Endocrinology and Metabolism, 50*, 889–894.

Bamberger, M., & Yaeger, D. (1997, April 14). Bigger, stronger, faster. *Sports Illustrated,* pp. 62–70.

Barron, D., Barbosa, J., Pascual, J.A., & Segura, J. (1996). Direct determination of anabolic steroids in human urine by on-line solid-phase extraction/liquid chromatography/mass spectrometry. *Journal of Mass Spectrometry, 31,* 309–319.

Beckett, A.H., Tucker, G.T., & Moffat, A.C. (1967). Routine detection and identification in urine of stimulants and other drugs, some of which may be used to modify performance in sport. *Journal of Pharmacy and Pharmacology, 19,* 273–294.

Bertrand, M., Masse, R., & Dugal, R. (1978). GC-MS: Approach for the detection and characterization of anabolic steroids and their metabolites in biological fluids at major international sporting events. *Farmaceutische Tijdschrift Voor Belgie, 55*(3), 85–101.

Bhasin, S., Storer, T.W., Berman, N., Callegari, C., Clevenger, B., Phillips, J., Bunnell, N., Tricker, R., Shirazi, A., & Casaburi, R. (1996). The effects of supraphysiologic doses of testosterone on muscle size and strength in normal men. *New England Journal of Medicine, 335*(1), 1–7.

Bi, H., Masse, R., & Just, G. (1992). Studies on anabolic steroids 10. Synthesis and identification of acidic urinary metabolites of oxymetholone in man. *Steroids, 57,* 453–459.

Bilek, R., Hämpl, R., Putz, Z., & Starka, L. (1987). RIA of epitestosterone, methodology, thermodynamic aspects and applications. *Journal of Steroid Biochemistry, 28*, 723–729.

Björkhem, I., & Ek, H. (1983). Detection and quantitation of 3α-hydroxy-1-methylene-5α-androstan-17-one, the major urinary metabolite of methenolone acetate (Primobolan) by isotope dilution-mass spectrometry. *Journal of Steroid Biochemistry, 18*, 481–487.

Björkhem, I., Ek, H., & Lantto, O. (1982). Assay of ethylestrenol in urine by isotope dilution-mass spectrometry. *Journal of Chromatography, 232,* 154–159.

Bowers, L.D. (1996). Metabolic pattern of mibolerone. In M. Donike (Ed.), *Proceedings of the 13th Cologne Workshop on Dope Analysis* (pp. 81–82). Cologne: Sport & Buch Strauss.

Bradley, C.A., & Sodeman, T.M. (1990). Human growth hormone: Its use and abuse. *Clinics in Laboratory Medicine, 10*, 473–477.

Breidbach, A., Sigmund, G., & Donike, M. (1995). Combination of screening procedures—Mesocarb detection as an example. In M. Donike, H. Geyer, A. Gotzmann, & U. Mareck-Engelke (Eds.), *Proceedings of the 12th Cologne Workshop on Dope Analysis* (pp. 301–304). Cologne: Sport & Buch Strauss.

Brisson, G.R., Sainz, A.G., Ayotte, C., Gareau, R., Senecal, L., & Castillo, M.J. (1997). Influence of a transscrotal testosterone propionate administration on the serum level of selected hormones of the hypophyso-gonadal axis. *Journal of Steroid Biochemistry and Molecular Biology, 62*(1), 65–71.

Brooks, R.V., Firth, R.G., & Sumner, N.A. (1975). Detection of anabolic steroids by radioimmunoassay. *British Journal of Sports Medicine, 9,* 89–92.

Brooks, R.V., Jeremiah, G., Webb, W.A., & Wheeler, M. (1979). Detection of anabolic administration to athletes. *Journal of Steroid Biochemistry, 11,* 913–917.

Carlström, K., Palonek, E., Garle, M., Oftebro, H., Stanghelle, J., & Björkhem, I. (1992). Detection of testosterone administration by increased ratio between serum concentrations of testosterone and 17 α-hydroxyprogesterone. *Clinical Chemistry, 36,* 1779–1784.

Cartoni, G.P., Giarrusso, A., Ciardi, M., & Rosati, F. (1985). Capillary gas chromatography and mass spectrometry detection of anabolic steroids II. *Journal of High Resolution Chromatography and Chromatographic Communications, 8,* 539–543.

Casoni, I., Ricci, G., Ballarin, E., Borsetto, C., Grazzi, G., Guglielmini, C., Manfredini, F., Mazzoni, G., Patracchini, M., Vitali, E.D.P., Rigolin, F., Bartalotta, S., Franze, G.P., Masotti, M., & Conconi, F. (1993). Hematological indices of erythropoietin administration. *International Journal of Sports Medicine, 14,* 307–311.

Catlin, D.H., Hatton, C.K., & Starcevic, S.H. (1997). Issues in detecting abuse of xenobiotic anabolic steroids and testosterone by analysis of athletes' urine. *Clinical Chemistry, 43*, 1280–1288.

Catlin, D.H., Kammerer, R.C., Hatton, C.K., Sekera, M.H., & Merdink, J.L. (1987). Analytical chemistry at the games of the XXIIIrd Olympiad in Los Angeles, 1984. *Clinical Chemistry, 33*, 319–327.

Catlin, D.H., & Murray, T.H. (1996). Performance-enhancing drugs, fair competition, and Olympic sport. *Journal of the American Medical Association, 276,* 231–237.

Chung, B.C., Choo, H.Y.P., Kim, J.W., Eom, K.D., Kwon, O.S., Suh, J., Yang, J.S., & Park, J.S. (1990). Analysis of anabolic steroids using GC/MS with selected ion monitoring. *Journal of Analytical Toxicology, 14,* 91–95.

Conn, P.M., & Crowley, W.F. (1994). Gonadotropin-releasing hormone and its analogs. *Annual Reviews of Medicine, 45,* 391–405.

Coutts, S.B., Kicman, A.T., Hurst, D.T., & Cowan, D.A. (1997). Intramuscular administration of 5α-dihydrotestosterone heptanoate: Changes in urinary hormone profile. *Clinical Chemistry, 43*, 2091–2098.

Cowan, D.A., Kicman, A.T., Walker, C.J., & Wheeler, M.J. (1991). Effect of administration of human chorionic gonadotrophin on criteria used to assess testosterone administration in athletes. *Journal of Endocrinology, 131,* 147–154.

Cowley G., & Brant, M. (1996, July 22). Can cheaters be stopped? Doped to perfection. *Newsweek*, pp. 31–34.

DeBoer, D., Dejong, E.G., Maes, R.A.A., & Van Rossum, J. (1992). The methyl-5α-dihydrotestosterones mesterolone and drostanolone: Gas chromatographic/mass spectrometric characterization of the urinary metabolites. *Journal of Steroid Biochemistry and Molecular Biology, 42,* 411–419.

DeBoer, D., Ooijen, R.D.V., & Maes, R.A.A. (1995). Thermostable derivatives of mesocarb and its p-hydroxy-metabolite. In M. Donike, H. Geyer, A. Gotzmann, & U. Mareck-Engelke (Eds.), *Proceedings of the 12th Cologne Workshop on Dope Analysis* (pp. 305–316). Cologne: Sport & Buch Strauss.

Debruyckere, G., deSagher, R., & Peteghem, C.V. (1992). Clostebol positive urine after consumption of contaminated meat. *Clinical Chemistry, 38,* 1869–1873.

Debruyckere, G., deSagher, R., & Peteghem, C.V. (1995). Detection of interferences in urinary anabolic steroid analysis. In M. Donike, H. Geyer, A. Gotzmann, & U. Mareck-Engelke (Eds.), *Proceedings of the 12th Cologne Workshop on Dope Analysis* (pp. 173–184). Cologne: Sport & Buch Strauss.

Dehennin, L. (1994). Detection of simultaneous self-administration of testosterone and epitestosterone in healthy men. *Clinical Chemistry, 40,* 106–109.

Dehennin, L., & Matsumoto, A.M. (1993). Long-term administration of testosterone enanthate to normal men: Alterations of the urinary profile of androgen metabolites potentially useful for detection of testosterone misuse in sport. *Journal of Steroid Biochemistry and Molecular Biology, 44,* 179–189.

de la Torre, R., Segura, J., & Polettini, A. (1995). Detection of testosterone esters in human plasma by GC/MS and GC/MS/MS. In M. Donike, H. Geyer, A. Gotzmann, & U. Mareck-Engelke (Eds.), *Proceedings of the 12th Cologne Workshop on Dope Analysis* (pp. 59–80). Cologne: Sport & Buch Strauss.

de la Torre, R., Segura, J., Polettini, A., & Montagna, M. (1995). Detection of testosterone esters in human plasma. *Journal of Mass Spectrometry, 30,* 1393–1404.

Deng, X.S., Kurosu, A., & Pounder, D.J. (1999). Detection of anabolic steroids in head hair. *Journal of Forensic Science, 44,* 343–346.

Doerge, D.R., Bajic, S., Blankenship, L.R., Preece, S.W., & Churchwell, M.I. (1995). Determination of β-agonist residues in human plasma using liquid chromatography/atmospheric pressure chemical ionization mass spectrometry and tandem mass spectrometry. *Journal of Mass Spectrometry, 30,* 911–916.

Donike, M. (1976). The detection of doping agents in blood. *British Journal of Sports Medicine, 10*(3), 147–154.

Donike, M., Bärwald, K.R., Kostermann, K., Schänzer, W., & Zimmermann, J. (1983). The detection of exogenous testosterone. In H. Heck, W. Hollmann, H. Liesen, & R. Rost (Eds.), *Sport: Leistung und Gesundheit* (pp. 293–298). Cologne: Deutscher Arzte-Verlag.

Donike, M., & Stratmann, D. (1974). Temperature programmed gas-chromatographic analysis of nitrogen containing drugs. Reproducibility of retention times and sample sizes by automatic injection (II). The screening procedure for volatile drugs at the 20th Olympic Games, Munich, 1972. *Chromatographia, 7*(4), 182–189.

Donike, M., Ueki, M., Koroda, Y., Geyer, H., Nolteemsting, E., & Rauth, S. (1995). Detection of dihydrotestosterone (DHT) doping: Alterations in the steroid profile and reference ranges for DHT and its 5α-metabolites. *Journal of Sports Medicine and Physical Fitness, 35,* 235–250.

Dörner, G., Stahl, F., & Zabel, R. (1963). Various experiments on the metabolism of 4-chlorotestosterone and testosterone derivatives in man. *Endokrinologie, 45,* 121–128.

Dürbeck, H.W., & Büker, I. (1980). Studies on anabolic steroids. The mass spectra of 17α-methyl-17β-hydroxy-1, 4-androstadien-3-one (Dianabol) and its metabolites. *Biomedical Mass Spectrometry, 7,* 437–445.

Dürbeck, H.W., Büker, I., Scheulen, B., & Telin, B. (1983). Anabolic steroids II. 4-Chloro-methandienone (Oral-Turinabol) and its metabolites. *Journal of Chromatographic Science, 21,* 405–410.

Ekblom, B. (1996). Blood doping and erythropoietin. *American Journal of Sports Medicine, 24*(6), S40–S42.

Engelke, U.M., Flenker, U., & Donike, M. (1996). Stability of steroid profiles (5): The annual rhythm of urinary ratios and excretion rates of endogenous steroids in females and its menstrual dependency. In M. Donike, H. Geyer, A. Gotzmann, & U. Mareck-Engelke (Eds.), *Proceedings of the 13th Cologne Workshop on Dope Analysis* (pp. 177–190). Cologne: Sport & Buch Strauss.

Engelke, U.M., Geyer, H., & Donike, M. (1995). Stability of steroid profiles (4): Ratios and excretion rates of endogenous steroids in female urines collected four times over 24 hours. In M. Donike, H. Geyer, A. Gotzmann, & U. Mareck-Engelke (Eds.), *Proceedings of the 12th Cologne Workshop on Dope Analysis* (pp. 135–156). Cologne: Sport & Buch Strauss.

Falk,O., Palonek, E., & Björkhem, I. (1988). Effect of ethanol on the ratio between testosterone and epitestosterone in urine. *Clinical Chemistry, 32,* 1462–1464.

Franke, W.W., & Berendonk, B. (1997). Hormonal doping and androgenization of athletes: A secret program of the German Democratic Republic government. *Clinical Chemistry, 43,* 1262–1279.

Garle, M., Ocka, R., Palonek, E., & Björkhem, I. (1996). Increased urinary testosterone/epitestosterone ratios found in Swedish athletes in connection with a national control program. Evaluation of 28 cases. *Journal of Chromatography Biomedical Applications, 687*(1), 55–60.

Geyer, H., Schänzer, W., Schindler, U., & Donike, M. (1996). Changes of the urinary steroid profile after sublingual application of dihydrotestosterone (DHT). In M. Donike, H. Geyer, A. Gotzmann, & U. Mareck-Engelke (Eds.), *Proceedings of the 13th Cologne Workshop on Dope Analysis* (pp. 215–230). Cologne: Sport & Buch Strauss.

Geyer, H., Schänzer, W., Mareck-Engelke, U., & Donike, M. (1996). Factors influencing the steroid profile. In Donike, M., Geyer, H., Gotzmann, A. & Mareck-Engelke, U., eds., *Proceedings of the 13th Cologne Workshop on Dope Analysis,* pp. 95-114, Sport & Buch Strauss, Cologne.

Gleixner, A. & Meyer, H.H.D. (1997, December). Methods to detect anabolics in hair: Use for food hygiene and doping control. *American Laboratory,* pp. 44–47.

Goudreault, D., & Masse, R. (1991). Studies on anabolic steroids 6. Identification of urinary metabolites of stenbolone acetate (17β-acetoxy-2-methyl-5α-androst-1-en-3-one) in human by gas chromatography/mass spectrometry. *Journal of Steroid Biochemistry and Molecular Biology, 38,* 639–655.

Gradeen, C.Y., Chan, S.C., & Przybylski, P.S. (1990). Urinary excretion of furazabol metabolites. *Journal of Analytical Toxicology, 14,* 120–122.

Hämpl, R., Picha, J., Chundela, B., & Starka, L. (1978). Radioimmunoassay of 17α-alkylated anabolic steroids. *Journal of Clinical Chemistry and Clinical Biochemistry, 16,* 279–282.

Hämpl, R., & Starka, L. (1979). Practical aspects of screening of anabolic steroids in doping control with particular accent to nortestosterone radioimmunoassay using mixed antisera. *Journal of Steroid Biochemistry, 11,* 933–936.

Hämpl, R., Picha, J., Chundela, B., & Starka, L. (1979). Radioimmunoassay of nortestosterone and related steroids. *Journal of Clinical Chemistry and Clinical Biochemistry, 17,* 529–532.

Hämpl, R., Putz, Z., Protiva, J., Filip, T., & Starka, L. (1982). Radioimmunoassay of norandrosterone. *Radiochemistry and Radioanalytic Letters, 56*(5), 273–280.

Haning, R.V., Jr., Flood, C.A., Hackett, R.J., Loughlin, J.S., McClure, N., & Longcope, C. (1991). Metabolic clearance rate of dehydroepiandros-terone sulfate, its metabolism to testosterone, and its intrafollicular metabolism to dehydroepiandrosterone, androstenedione, testosterone, and dihydrotestosterone in vivo. *Journal of Clinical Endocrinology and Metabolism, 72,* 1088–1095.

Haning, R.V., Jr., Hackett, R.J., Flood, C.A., Loughlin, J.S., Zhao, Q.Y., & Longcope, C. (1993). Plasma dehydroepiandrosterone sulfate serves as a prehormone for 48% of follicular fluid testosterone during treatment with Mentropins. *Journal of Clinical Endocrinology and Metabolism, 76,* 1301–1307.

Heinonen, E.H. (1994). Pharmacokinetic aspects of l-deprenyl (selegiline) and its metabolites. *Clinical Pharmacology and Therapeutics, 56,* 742–749.

Hemmersbach, P., Tomten, S., Nilsson, S., Oftebro, H., Havrevoll, O., Oen, B., & Birkeland, K. (1995). Illegal use of anabolic agents in animal fattening—consequences for doping analysis. In M. Donike, H. Geyer, A. Gotzmann, & U. Mareck-Engelke (Eds.), *Proceedings of the 12th Cologne Workshop on Dope Analysis* (pp. 185–192). Cologne: Sport & Buch Strauss.

Hoberman, J.M., & Yesalis, C.E. (1995, February). The history of synthetic testosterone. *Scientific American,* pp. 60–65.

Hold, K.M., Wilkins, D.G., Crouch, D.J., Rollins, D.E., & Maes, R.A. (1996). Detection of stanozolol in hair by negative ion chemical ionization mass spectrometry. *Journal of Analytical Toxicology, 20*(10), 345–349.

Huck, H., & Egg, D. (1972). Gas chromatographic investigation of urinary metabolites during treatment with mesterolone. *Wiener Klinische Wochenschrift, 84*(7), 114–117.

Jacobs, J.B., & Samuels, B. (1995). The drug testing project in international sports: Dilemmas in an expanding regulatory regime. *Hastings International and Comparative Law Review, 18*, 557–589.

Kabouris, M., Platen, P., & Donike, M. (1996). Detection of human growth hormone in urine of athletes. In M. Donike, H. Geyer, A. Gotzmann, & U. Mareck-Engelke (Eds.), *Proceedings of the 13th Cologne Workshop on Dope Analysis* (pp. 313–324). Cologne: Sport & Buch Strauss.

Kammerer, R.C. (1998a, February 9). *Steroids, designer drugs, and detection problems.* Paper presented at American Academy of Forensic Sciences 50th Annual Meeting, Drugs and Athletes Workshop, San Francisco.

Kammerer, R.C. (1998b, April 24–25). *What is doping and how is it detected?* Paper presented at the Amateur Athletic Foundation, Doping in Elite Sport Conference, Los Angeles.

Kammerer, R.C., Merdink, J.L., Jagels, M., Catlin, D.H., & Hui, K.K. (1990). Testing for fluoxymesterone (Halotestin) administration to man: Identification of urinary metabolites by gas chromatography–mass spectrometry. *Journal of Steroid Biochemistry, 36*, 659–666.

Karila, T., Kosunen, V., Leinonen, A., Taehtelae, R., & Seppaelae, T. (1996). High doses of alcohol increase testosterone-to-epitestosterone ratio in females. *Journal of Chromatography Biomedical Applications, 687*(1), 109–116.

Kicman, A.T., Brooks, R.V., Collyer, S.C., Cowan, D.A., Nanjee, M.N., Southan, G.J., & Wheeler, M.J. (1990). Criteria to indicate testosterone administration. *British Journal of Sports Medicine 24,* 253–264.

Kicman, A.T., Coutts, S.B., Walker, C. J., & Cowan, D. A. (1995). Proposed confirmatory procedure for detecting 5α-dihydrotestosterone doping in male athletes. *Clinical Chemistry, 41,* 1617–1627.

Kicman, A.T., Cowan, D.A., Myhre, L., Nilsson, S., Oftebro, H., Havrevoll, O., Oen, B., & Birkeland, K. (1994). Effect on sports drug tests of ingesting meat from steroid (methenolone)-treated livestock. *Clinical Chemistry, 40,* 2084–2087.

Kicman, A.T., Miell, J.P., Teale, J.D., Powrie, J., Wood, P.J., Laidler, P., Milligan, P.J., & Cowan, D.A. (1997). Serum IGF-I and IGF binding proteins 2 and 3 as potential markers of doping with human GH. *Clinical Endocrinology, 47,* 43–50.

Kim, T., Suh, J.W., Ryu, J.C., Chung, B.C., & Park, J. (1996). Excretion study of furazabol, an anabolic steroid, in human urine. *Journal of Chromatography Biomedical Applications, 687*(1), 79–84.

Laidler, P., Cowan, D.A., Hider, R.C., Keane, A., & Kicman, A.T. (1995). Tryptic mapping of human chorionic gonadotropin by matrix-assisted laser desorption/ionization mass spectrometry. *Rapid Communications in Mass Spectrometry, 9,* 1021–1026.

Leith, W. (1991, July 14). Cyclists don't die like this. *Independent,* pp. 3–4.

Liu, C., & Bowers, L.D. (1995). Studies towards confirmation of HCG using HPLC/MS. In M. Donike, H. Geyer, A. Gotzmann, & U. Mareck-Engelke (Eds.), *Proceedings of the 12th Cologne Workshop on Dope Analysis* (pp. 235–242). Cologne: Sport & Buch Strauss.

Liu, C., & Bowers, L.D. (1996). Immunoaffinity trapping of urinary human chorionic gonadotropin and its high-performance liquid chromatographic-mass spectrometric confirmation. *Journal of Chromatography Biomedical Applications, 687*(1), 213–220.

Maltin, C., Delday, M., Hay, S., Smith, F., Lobley, G., & Reeds, P. (1987). The effect of the anabolic agent, clenbuterol, on the overloaded rat skeletal muscle. *Bioscience Reports, 7,* 143–148.

Masse, R., Laliberte, C., Tremblay, L., & Dugal, R. (1985). Gas chromatographic/ mass spectrometric analysis of 19-nortestosterone urinary metabolites in man. *Biomedical Mass Spectrometry, 12*(3), 115-121.

Masse, R., Ayotte, C., & Dugal, R. (1989). Studies on anabolic steroids I: Integrated methodological approach to the gas chromatographic mass spectrometric analysis of anabolic steroid metabolites in urine. *Journal of Chromatography, 489,* 23–50.

Masse, R., Honggang, B., Ayotte, C., & Dugal, R. (1989). Studies on anabolic steroids II: Gas chromatographic/mass spectrometric characterization of oxandrolone urinary metabolites in man. *Biomedical and Environmental Mass Spectrometry, 18,* 429–438.

Masse, R., Bi, H., & Du, P. (1991). Studies on anabolic steroids VII. Analysis of urinary metabolites of formebolone in man by gas chromatography–mass spectrometry. *Analytica Chimica Acta, 247,* 211–221.

Masse, R., & Goudreault, D. (1992). Studies on anabolic steroids XI. 18-hydroxylated metabolites of mesterolone, methenolone, and stenbolone: new steroids isolated from human urine. *Journal of Steroid Biochemistry & Molecular Biology, 43,* 399–410.

Meikle, A.W., Arver, S., Dobs, A.S., Sanders, S.W., Rajaram, L., & Mazar, N.A. (1996). Pharmacokinetics and metabolism of a permeation-enhanced testosterone transdermal system in hypogonadal men: Influence of application site—a clinical research center study. *Journal of Clinical Endocrinology and Metabolism, 81,* 1832–1840.

Meikle, A.W., Mazer, N.A., Moellmer, J.F., Stringham, J.D., Tolman, K.G., Sanders, S.W., & Cdell, W.D. (1992). Enhanced transdermal delivery of testosterone across nonscrotal skin produces physiological concentrations of testosterone and its metabolites in hypogonadal men. *Journal of Clinical Endocrinology and Metabolism, 74*, 623–628.

Negwer, M. (1987). *Organo-chemical drugs and their synonyms* (3 vols., 6th ed.). New York: VCH.

Norli, H., Esbensen, K., Westad, F., Birkeland, K.I., & Hemmersbach, P. (1995). Chemometric evaluation of urinary steroid profiles in doping control. *Journal of Steroid Biochemistry and Molecular Biology, 54*(1-2), 83–88.

Oftebro, H. (1992). Evaluating an abnormal urinary steroid profile. *Lancet, 359,* 941–942.

Oftebro, H., Jensen, J., Mowinckel, P., & Norli, H.R. (1994). Establishing a ketoconazole suppression test for verifying testosterone administration in the doping control of athletes. *Journal of Clinical Endocrinology and Metabolism, 78,* 973–977.

Palonek, E., Gottlieb, C., Garle, M., Björkhem, I., & Carlstroem, K. (1995). Serum and urinary markers of exogenous testosterone administration. *Journal of Steroid Biochemistry and Molecular Biology, 55*(1), 121–127.

Papadakis, M.A., Grady, D., Black, D., Tierney, M.J., Gooding, G.A.W., Schambelan, M., & Grunfeld, C. (1996). Growth hormone replacement in healthy older men improves body composition but not functional ability. *Annals of Internal Medicine, 124,* 708–716.

Park, J.S., Park, S., Lho, D.S., Choo, H.P., Chung, B., Yoon, C., Min, H., & Choi, M.J. (1990). Drug testing at the 10th Asian Games and 24th Seoul Olympic Games. *Journal of Analytical Toxicology, 14,* 66–72.

Quincey, R.V., & Gray, C.H. (1967). The metabolism of [1, 2^{-3}H] 17α-methyltestosterone in human subjects. *Journal of Endocrinology, 37,* 37–55.

Raynaud, E., Audran, M., Brun, J.F., Fedou, C., Chanal, J.L., & Orsetti, A. (1992). False-positive cases in detection of testosterone doping. *Lancet, 340,* 1468–1469.

Raynaud, E., Audran, M., Pages, J. Ch., Fedou, C., Brun, J.F., Chanal, J.L., & Orsetti, A. (1993). Determination of urinary testosterone and epitestosterone during pubertal development: A cross-sectional study in 141 normal male subjects. *Clinical Endocrinology, 38,* 353–359.

Reznik, Y., Herrou, M., Dehennin, L., Lemaire, M., & Leymarie, P. (1987). Rising plasma levels of 19-nortestosterone throughout pregnancy: Determination by radioimmunoassay and validation by gas chromatography-mass spectrometry. *Journal of Clinical Endocrinology and Metabolism, 64*, 1086–1088.

Roche, T., & Davis, W. (1972). Evaluating growth promoters for beef cattle. *Farm and Food Research, 7,* 146–148.

Rogozkin, V.A., Morozov, V.I., & Tchaikovsky, V.S. (1979). Rapid radioimmunoassay for anabolic steroids in urine. *Schweizerische Zeitschrift fur Sport Medizin, 27*(4), 169–173.

Sanaullah, & Bowers, L.D. (1996). Facile synthesis of [16,16,17-$^2H_3$]-testosterone,-epitestosterone and their glucuronides and sulfates. *Journal of Steroid Biochemistry and Molecular Biology, 58*(2), 225–234.

Satchell, M. (1996, March 18). Raising "boxcars" out in the barn. *U.S. News & World Report,* pp. 40–41.

Schänzer, W. (1996a). Metabolism of anabolic androgenic steroids. *Clinical Chemistry, 42,* 1001—1020.

Schänzer, W. (1996b). Metabolism of anabolic androgenic steroids. Clinical Chemistry, 42, 1001–1020.

Schänzer, W., Opfermann, G., & Donike, M. (1990). Metabolism of Stanozolol: Identification and synthesis of urinary metabolites. *Journal of Steroid Biochemistry, 36*(1-2), 153–174.

Schänzer, W., & Donike, M. (1992). Metabolism of boldenone in man: Gas chromatographic-mass spectrometric identification of urinary excreted metabolites and determination of excretion rates. *Biological Mass Spectrometry, 21,* 3–16.

Schänzer, W., & Donike, M. (1993). Metabolism of anabolic steroids in man: Synthesis and use of reference substances for identification of anabolic steroid metabolites. *Analytica Chimica Acta, 275,* 23–48.

Schänzer, W., Geyer, H., Gotzmann, A., Horning, S., Mareck-Engelke, U., Nitschke, R., Nolteemsting, E., & Donike, M. (1995). Endogenous production and excretion of boldenone (17β-hydroxyandrosta-1,4-dien-3-one), an androgenic anabolic steroid. In M. Donike, H. Geyer, A. Gotzmann, & U. Mareck-Engelke (Eds.), *Proceedings of the 12th Cologne Workshop on Dope Analysis* (pp. 211–212). Cologne: Sport & Buch Strauss.

Schänzer, W., Horning, S., & Donike, M. (1995). Metabolism of anabolic steroids in humans: Synthesis of 6β-hydroxy metabolites of 4-chloro-1, 2-dehydro-17α-methyltestosterone, fluoxymesterone, and metandienone. *Steroids, 60,* 353–366.

Schänzer, W., Horning, S., Opfermann, G., & Donike, M. (1996). GC/MS identification of long-term excreted metabolites of the anabolic steroid 4-chloro-1,2-dehydro-17α-methyltestosterone in human. *Journal of Steroid Biochemistry and Molecular Biology, 57*(5/6), 363–376.

Schänzer, W., Delahaut, P., Geyer, H., Machnik, M., & Horning, S. (1996). Long-term detection and identification of metandienone and stanazolol abuse in athletes by gas chromatography–high-resolution mass spectrometry. *Journal of Chromatography: Biomedical Applications, 687*(1), 93-108.

Segura, J., de la Torre, R., Pascual, J.A., Ventura, R., Farre, M., Ewin, R.R., & Cami, J. (1995). Antidoping control laboratory at the games of the XXV Olympiad Barcelona '92. In M. Donike, H. Geyer, A. Gotzmann, & U. Mareck-Engelke (Eds.), *Proceedings of the 12th Cologne Workshop on Dope Analysis* (pp. 413–430). Cologne: Sport & Buch Strauss.

Segura, J., Pascual, J.A., Ventura, R., Ustaran, J.I., Cuevas, A., & Gonzalez, R. (1993). International cooperation in analytical chemistry: Experience of antidoping control at the XI Pan American Games. *Clinical Chemistry, 39*, 836–845.

Southan, G.J., Brooks, R.V., Cowan, D.A., Kicman, A.T., Unnadkat, N., & Walker, C.J. (1992). Possible indices for the detection of the administration of dihydrotestosterone to athletes. *Journal of Steroid Biochemistry and Molecular Biology, 42*(1), 87–94.

Stenman, U.H., Kallio, L.U., Korhonen, J., & Alfthan, H. (1997). Immunoprocedures for detecting human chorionic gonadotropin: Clinical aspects and doping control. *Clinical Chemistry, 43*, 1293–1298.

Stevenson, R. (1998). New instruments draw attention at Pittcon® '98. *American Laboratory 30*(12), 56.

Thieme, D., Grosse, J., Lang, L., & Mueller, R.K. (1995). Detection of Mesocarb metabolite by LC-TS/MS. In M. Donike, H. Geyer, A. Gotzmann, & U. Mareck-Engelke (Eds.), *Proceedings of the 12th Cologne Workshop on Dope Analysis* (pp. 275–284). Cologne: Sport & Buch Strauss.

Thieme, D.J., Grosse, R., & Mueller, R.K. (1996). Application of high-resolution and tandem-MS to the identification of anabolic agents. In M. Donike, H. Geyer, A. Gotzmann, & U. Mareck-Engelke (Eds.), *Proceedings of the 13th Cologne Workshop on Dope Analysis* (pp. 285–297). Cologne: Sport & Buch Strauss.

Volek, J.S., & Kraemer, W.J. (1996). Creatine supplementation: Its effect on human muscular performance and body composition. *Journal of Strength and Conditioning Research, 10*(3), 200–210.

Ward, R.J., Lawson, A.M., & Schackleton, C.H.L. (1977). Metabolism of anabolic steroid drugs in man and the marmoset monkey. I. Nilevar and Orabolin. *Journal of Steroid Biochemistry, 8,* 1057–1063.

Webster, M.J., Webster, M.N., Crawford, R.E., & Gladden, L.B. (1993). Effect of sodium bicarbonate ingestion on exhaustive resistance exercise performance. *Medicine and Science in Sports and Exercise, 25*, 960–965.

Wide, L., Bengtsson, C., Berglund, B., & Ekblom, B. (1995). Detection in blood and urine of recombinant erythropoietin administered to healthy men. *Medicine and Science in Sports and Exercise, 27*, 1569–1576.

Yesalis, C.E., & Cowart, V.S. (1998). *The Steroids Game.* Champaign, IL: Human Kinetics.

CHAPTER

14

Societal Alternatives

Charles E. Yesalis, ScD; Michael S. Bahrke, PhD; and James E. Wright, PhD

Where large sums of money are concerned, it is advisable to trust nobody.

Agatha Christie

Portions of this chapter are reprinted from *The Physician and Sportsmedicine* 1990; see credits page for more information.

When the first edition of this book was published in 1993, this chapter opened with a quote from Robert Voy, MD (1991), former Chief Medical Officer of the U.S. Olympic Committee:

> *If we will have reached a point of no return with this win at all costs attitude, the gold medals won't shine as brightly, the flags won't wave as boldly, the torch will flicker dimly, and we will have lost one of the greatest treasures ever known.*

With this second edition, it appears that Dr. Voy's predictions have already come to pass. In 1998 alone, the public was bombarded with continual reports of drug scandals (Dickey, Helmstaedt, Nordland, & Hayden, 1999; "Drug Trial, Take II," 1998; "Snowboarder Loses Medal," 1998; "Drugs and Cycling," 1998; "Track Star Blazed Trail," 1998; see chapter 2), including the following:

1. Chinese swimmers being ejected from the World Championships in Australia after having tested positive for banned substances.
2. Former East German coaches and physicians tried for their roles in the systematic doping of East German athletes over three decades.
3. Canadian snowboarder Ross Rebagliati testing positive for marijuana after having won a gold medal at the Winter Olympics in Nagano, Japan.
4. Olympic gold medalist Michelle Smith de Bruin accused of "manipulating" her urine sample in an out-of-competition drug test.
5. Cyclists, coaches, physicians, and trainers participating in the Tour de France implicated in a widespread, systematic doping scheme.
6. Olympic champion Randy Barnes testing positive for androstenedione.
7. Home run king Mark McGwire admitting the use of androstenedione.
8. Olympic champion Florence Griffith Joyner dying at age 38. Rumors of prior performance-enhancing drug use that surrounded her victories at the Seoul Olympic Games are resurrected.
9. Uta Pippig, three-time winner of the Boston Marathon, testing positive for a high level of testosterone.
10. Australian Open champion Petr Korda testing positive for an anabolic steroid.

When discussing the problem of performance-enhancing drug use, it is important to remember that sport is a microcosm of our society and the problems in sport are not limited to drug use. During the 1980s, 57 of 106 universities in Division I-A were punished by the NCAA via sanctions, censure, or probation for rule violations (Leaderman, 1990). These offenses did not involve illicit drug use by athletes but rather the unethical behavior of coaches, athletic administrators, staff, and faculty, the very men and women who should be setting the example. More recently, collegiate athletes have been convicted of criminal offences related to sports gambling (Lassar, 1998; Saum, 1998). In addition, an NCAA survey of 2,000 Division I male football and basketball players found 72% had gambled in some form, and 25% reported gambling on collegiate sports; 4% bet on games in which they played (Saum, 1998; "Study: Gambling in NCAA Rampant," 1999). Among members of the International Olympic Committee, bribery, graft, and other corruption appear entrenched in the culture of the organization (Simson & Jennings, 1992; Swift, 1999). A common factor among all these scandals is money. In the 1990s there is no doubt sport has become a multinational industry of huge proportions. The IOC, NCAA, NFL, NBA, and MLB, among others, are all billion-dollar businesses ("A Survey of Sport," 1998; Hiestand, 1999).

A free society relies on the news media to inform the populace of the incidence and magnitude of social problems such as doping in sport. Even though the epidemic of drug use in sport has been common knowledge among insiders, the news media, especially in the United States, have not engaged in a widespread concerted effort to chronicle this issue (see chapter 2). Unfortunately the media, in particular television news, are often influenced by conflicts of interest within their parent companies between those reporting the news and those responsible for the broadcast of major sporting events. Few would argue that an in-depth expose of drug use, for example, in the NFL or the Olympics, would enhance the marketing of these highly lucrative sporting events.

Before any effort can be made to address the issue of doping in sport, it is critical that all of the stakeholders acknowledge that a problem exists. In this regard, we need to fully appreciate the high entertainment value placed on sport by society. Some go so far as to argue that sport is the opiate of the masses—a contention made earlier by Karl Marx regarding religion. If sport has become the opiate of the masses, then we must be prepared for the public to be indifferent to drug use in sport, at least at the elite level. Moreover, it could be argued that if substantial progress is made in the fight against epidemic doping, fans may express anger, rather than appreciation, toward those fighting drug use. Many people view competitive sports to escape from the problems of daily life and do not wish to be confronted with the moral and ethical aspects of doping. Besides, if antidoping efforts are successful, the once bigger-than-life idols could begin to appear all too human in stature and the eclipsing of records at national, Olympic, and world levels could become so rare that the fervor of fans would wane and the business of sports would suffer. Even high school sport appears to be expanding as a source of entertainment for adults, as shown by the increasing level of television coverage of high school football and basketball games. Consequently, it can be argued that the growth of the high school sport entertainment business is contributing to the increase in anabolic steroid use among adolescents during the 1990s (see chapter 3).

Sport has also been used by governments as a tool to control the masses or as justification for their social, political, and economic systems. "Bread and circuses" (panem et circenses) were used in this fashion by the emperors of Rome (Benario, 1983). Nazi Germany, the Soviet Union, East Germany, and Communist China all used sport for political advantage (Hoberman, 1984). Consequently, such governments, arguably, would be less than enthusiastic participants in the fight against doping or, for that matter, even in publicly acknowledging the existence of widespread doping. On the contrary, there is a reasonable amount of evidence that the governments of the Soviet Union, East Germany, and Communist China all played significant roles in the systematic doping of their athletes (see chapter 2).

With many societal problems, identifying potential solutions is easy, but agreeing on a proper course of action and successfully completing it are difficult. The following are our alternatives for dealing with the use of anabolic steroids and other performance-enhancing drugs: legalization, interdiction, education, and alteration of societal values and attitudes related to physical appearance and winning in sport.

Legalization: An End to Hypocrisy?

The legalization of illicit drugs has for some time been the subject of heated debate: comments range from "morally reprehensible" to "accepting reality." Legalization would reduce the law enforcement costs associated with illicit anabolic steroid use as well as the substantial cost of drug testing. Even some opponents of legalization must concede that such an action would lessen the level of hypocrisy in sport. It can be argued that society and sports federations have turned a blind eye or have subtly encouraged drug use in sport as long as the athletes have not been caught or spoken publicly about their use of anabolic steroids (Bamberger & Yaeger, 1997; Dubin, 1990; Lemonick, 1998; "Drugs and Cycling," 1998; "Longtime Drug Use," 1999; Voy, 1990; Yesalis & Friedl, 1988).

Legalization of anabolic steroid use in sport would involve two levels of authority. At one level, federal and state laws related to the possession, distribution, and prescription of anabolic steroids would have to be changed. If in the future anabolic steroids become an accepted means of contraception or as treatment for "andropause" (see chapter 1), it is difficult to understand how anabolic steroids could remain a Schedule III controlled substance. At the second level, bans on anabolic steroids now in place in virtually every sport would have to be rescinded. Legalization would bring cries that the traditional ideals of sport and competition were being further eroded. On the other hand, given the continued litany of drug and other sport scandals (see above) that have taken place in full public view, it is hard to imagine in this jaundiced age that many people believe that the so-called traditional ideals in elite sports even exist.

It has long been asserted that the legalization of anabolic steroids would force athletes to further expose themselves to possible physical harm or else to compete at a disadvantage (see introduction). Others have even questioned the basic premise that banning drugs in sport benefits the health of athletes and have argued that "the ban has in fact increased health risks by denying users access to medical advice and caused users to turn to high risk black market sources" (Black, 1996).

Further, legalization would allow athletes to use pharmaceutical grade steroids while being monitored by a physician. It can also be argued that the "danger" of steroid use is not, in itself, a realistic deterrent given the existing levels of tobacco, alcohol, and other illicit drug use.

In 1999 it seems that legalization of anabolic steroid use in sport is not acceptable. However, if the impotence of drug testing, now in full public view, persists for much longer, it is easy to imagine the IOC or other sport federations throwing up their hands in frustration and allowing the athlete with the best chemist to prevail.

Interdiction: A Question of Cost-Effectiveness

The U.S. federal government and all state governments currently have laws regarding the distribution, possession, or prescription of anabolic steroids (USDHHS, 1991). The Federal Food, Drug, and Cosmetic Act (FFDCA) was amended as part of the Anti-Drug Abuse Act of 1988 such that distribution of steroids or possession of steroids with intent to distribute without a valid prescription became a felony. This legislation not only increased the penalties for the illicit distribution of steroids but also facilitated prosecution under the FFDCA. In 1990 the Anabolic Steroids Control Act was signed into law by President Bush and added anabolic steroids to Schedule III of the Controlled Substances Act. This law institutes a regulatory and criminal enforcement system whereby the Drug Enforcement Administration (DEA) controls the manufacture, importation, exportation, distribution, and dispensing of anabolic steroids. However, the act did not provide extra resources to the DEA to shoulder the added responsibility.

Furthermore, as the use of anabolic steroids is increasingly criminalized, drug use will likely be driven further underground, and the source of the drugs will increasingly be clandestine laboratories, the products of which are of questionable quality. It also appears that in some areas criminalization has already altered the distribution network for anabolic steroids; athletes used to sell to other athletes, but sellers of street drugs are now becoming a major source (U.S. Department of Justice, 1994).

Even though the legal apparatus to control steroid trafficking exists, enforcement agents already are struggling to handle the problems of importation, distribution, sales, and use of other illicit drugs such as cocaine and heroin (U.S. Department of Justice, 1994). Based on what we know about the physical, psychological, or social effects of steroids, it is neither realistic nor prudent that enforcement efforts for steroids take precedent over those for more harmful drugs. On the other hand, this line of reasoning should not be used as a rationale for a lack of effective action against steroids. Nevertheless, the outlook that limited resources can be stretched to cover yet another class of drugs is not optimistic (U.S. Department of Justice, 1994), especially given the increase in recreational drug use among adolescents (Office of Applied Studies, 1999). The availability of anabolic steroids in this country suggests there is some reason to believe the United States may simply not have sufficient law enforcement personnel to deal with apprehending and punishing sellers of anabolic steroids and other performance-enhancing drugs.

Nonetheless, between February 1991 and February 1995, 355 anabolic steroid investigations were initiated by the DEA (Yesalis & Cowart, 1998). There have been more than 400 arrests, and more than 200 defendants have been convicted. However, because of the way criminal penalties were developed for steroid infractions, an individual brought to court on charges of distribution or selling must be a national-level dealer to receive more than a "slap on the wrist" and perhaps a short visit to a "country club" prison. For this reason, law enforcement agents often do not bother pursuing small cases because the costs of prosecution vastly outweigh any penalties that will be assessed.

Drug testing by sport federations is yet another form of interdiction. Such testing has been partially successful when directed at performance-enhancing drugs that, to be effective, must be in the body at the time of competition, such as stimulants and narcotics. As discussed in chapters 12 and 13, drug testing has been even less effective against anabolic steroids that are used during training or used to enhance an athlete's capacity to train. Testing can be circumvented by the steroid user in several ways. Generally, to avoid a positive test, athletes can determine when to discontinue use prior to a scheduled test, or, in the case of an unannounced test, they titrate their dose using transdermal patches or skin creams containing testosterone so as to remain below the maximum allowable level. Further confounding the testing are other drugs used by athletes, such as human growth hormone and erythropoietin, for which no effective tests currently exist (see chapter 13). Moreover, testing for anabolic steroids is expensive (approx. $120 per test), and although organizations like the IOC, NFL, or NCAA may be able to institute such procedures, the cost is prohibitive for the vast majority of secondary schools. Consequently, only a handful of secondary school systems test for anabolic steroids.

In summary, although interdiction through law enforcement and drug testing has intuitive appeal, its impact on the nonmedical use of anabolic steroids and other performance-enhancing drugs is open to debate. Since the flurry of legislative activity at the state and national levels regarding the control of the manufacture, distribution, prescription, and possession of steroids in the late 1980s and the early 1990s, use among adolescents has increased significantly (see chapter 3). As for the future of testing, it is difficult to be optimistic: over the past 30 years, drug users have consistently outplayed the drug testers. In addition, one can only speculate as to the future challenges to testing created by impending advances in genetic engineering. Will we be able to genetically enhance muscle mass, aerobic capacity, vision, and neurological response (Barton-Davis, Shoturma, Musaro, Rosenthal, & Sweeney, 1998)?

Education: Is Anybody Listening?

Since the 1980s, the U.S. Public Health Service, the U.S. Department of Education, as well as many state education departments, state and local medical societies, private foundations, and sport federations have been involved in prevention efforts related to steroid abuse. For the most part, these have centered on the development and distribution of educational materials and programs such as posters, videos, pamphlets, and workshops. For example, the Iowa High School Athletic Association has developed an educational booklet that provides information on the effects of steroid use, but also includes strength-enhancing alternatives to steroids and prevention ideas (Beste, 1991). The U.S. Department of Education and other sources have developed a variety of informational posters targeted at high school students to provide facts about steroids, their adverse effects, alternatives to their use, and their illegal status (American Academy of Orthopaedic Surgeons; U.S. Department of Health & Human Services [USDHHS], 1988). Video distributors now have a wide range of videotape programs available on steroid use prevention as well as bodybuilding techniques (William C. Brown Communications Inc., 1993). Educational consulting firms provide antisteroid training, program, and curriculum development to junior and senior high schools across the United States (Griffin & Svendsen, 1990; Harding Ringhofer, 1993). Major television networks have presented special programming targeted at adolescent audiences to relay the possible consequences of steroid use (*ABC Afterschool Special:* "Testing Dirty" and *CBS Schoolbreak Special:* "The Fourth Man"; Disney Educational Productions: "Benny and the Roids").

Health educators have made some inroads in changing several high-risk behaviors, such as high-fat diets, sedentary lifestyles, and smoking. Educators are well armed with vast quantities of scientific data regarding the deleterious nature of these activities. Furthermore, these are behaviors on which society has increasingly frowned. In sports, on the other hand, athletes who use anabolic steroids have enjoyed significant improvements in physical performance and appearance. Society is much less likely to shun these people. The adulation of fans, the media, and peers is a strong secondary reinforcement, as are financial, material, and sexual rewards.

Another fly in the education ointment is the possibility that anabolic steroids taken intermittently in low to moderate doses may have only a negligible impact on health, at least in the short term (see chapter 6). In 1989, several experts at the National Steroid Consensus Meeting concluded that according to the existing evidence, these drugs represent more of an ethical dilemma than a public health problem (Yesalis, Wright, & Lombardo, 1989). Although there is still little available evidence regarding the long-term health effects of anabolic steroids, many current or potential anabolic steroid users unfortunately mistake absence of evidence for evidence of absence. Even more frustrating is the fact that in two national studies, a substantial minority of the anabolic steroid users surveyed expressed no intention to stop using anabolic steroids if deleterious health effects were unequivocally established (Yesalis, Herrick, Buckley, Friedl, Brannon, & Wright, 1988; Yesalis, Streit, Vicary, Friedl, Brannon, & Buckley, 1989). Clearly, the paucity of scientific information has impeded the formulation of effective health education strategies. Far more than that, the unsubstantiated claims of dire health effects made by some in sports medicine and sensationalized by the news media have further eroded communication between athletes and doctors. However, even if long-term deleterious effects were well documented for anabolic steroids, our experience with teenagers and smoking suggests that substantial abuse would probably persist (Centers for Disease Control and Prevention, 1994; U.S. Department of Health and Human Services, 1989).

All of these problems and limitations in developing and disseminating effective prevention and intervention strategies could largely explain the significant increase in anabolic steroid use among adolescents since 1990 (see chapter 3).

Changing a behavior that has resulted in major benefits to the user, such as improved appearance and athletic performance, presents a monumental challenge. Traditional cognitive and affective education approaches to tobacco, alcohol, and drug abuse prevention have not been effective (Schaps, Bartolo, Moskowitz, Palley, & Churgin, 1981). In fact, there is evidence that providing a prevention program that uses "scare tactics" to dissuade adolescents from becoming involved with anabolic steroids may actually lead to increased usage, possibly because additional information stimulated curiosity (Goldberg, Bents, Bosworth, Trevisan, & Elliot, 1991). This observation helped lead to a prevention program (ATLAS, see chapter 4) focused, in part, on positive educational initiatives related to nutrition and strength training. The program also focused on increasing adolescents' awareness of the types of social pressures they are likely to encounter to use anabolic steroids, and attempts to "inoculate" them against these pressures. Adolescents are taught specific skills for effectively resisting both peer and media pressures to use anabolic steroids. Periodic monitoring and reporting of actual anabolic steroid use among adolescents was conducted in an effort to dispel misinformation concerning the widespread use of anabolic steroids among peers. Using peers as program leaders is an additional component. This program has been successful in significantly affecting attitudes and behaviors related to steroid use and remained effective over several years (Goldberg et al., 1996).

Unfortunately, the generalizability of the ATLAS program is open to question. The program focused on male high school football players and was not designed specifically to address anabolic steroid use among teenage girls, whose rate of steroid use, as we have stated, has doubled since 1990 (see chapter 3). In addition, the long-term effectiveness of this school-based program is still unknown and the program has yet to be replicated in other states. Moreover, there are two important and, as yet, unanswered questions regarding the ATLAS program. First, are school boards, in an age of constrained resources, willing to commit time and money to this relatively demanding program? Efficacy aside, it would be far easier and cheaper to continue to give only "lip service" to this problem and limit efforts to an occasional talk by the coach and the use of readily available educational videos and posters.

The second question is even more threatening to school officials. In an era when some believe that the "win at all costs" philosophy is gaining the upper hand, will some schools hesitate to unilaterally "disarm"? That is, will some schools hesitate to institute a program that could significantly reduce steroid use at the cost of conferring an advantage to an opponent who chooses to maintain a "see no evil" stance on the use of performance-enhancing drugs? This question is given some legitimacy by pervasive anecdotal accounts of high school coaches encouraging the use of, and in some instances selling, so-called supplements such as creatine, DHEA, and androstenedione to their athletes.

In summary, although educating athletes about the health risks and ethical issues associated with anabolic steroid use can help reduce use, this strategy is not a panacea.

Conclusion: Our Values Must Change

Compared with legalization, interdiction, and education, the influence of our social environment on anabolic steroid use receives far less attention. Yet in many ways the social environment exerts a more fundamental influence on drug use in sport than do the more superficial strategies to reduce use described earlier.

A number of performance-enhancing drugs, including anabolic steroids, are not euphorigenic, or mood altering, immediately following administration. Instead, the appetite for these drugs was created predominantly by our societal fixation on winning and physical appearance. An infant does not innately believe that a muscular physique is desirable—our society teaches this. Likewise, children play games for fun, but society preaches the importance of winning—seemingly, at an increasingly younger age.

Ours is a culture that thrives on competition, both in business and in sport. However, we long ago realized that competition of all types must exist within some boundaries. A primary goal of competition is to win or be the very best in any endeavor. Philosophically, many in our society appear to have taken a "bottom-line" attitude and consider winning the *only* truly worthwhile goal of competition. If we accept this philosophy, then it becomes easy to justify, or be led to the belief, that one should win at any cost. At that point doping becomes a very rational behavior, with the end (winning) justifying the means (use of anabolic steroids and other drugs).

This "win at any cost/winner take all" philosophy is not new. The winners in the ancient Greek Olympics were handsomely rewarded, and episodes of athletes cheating to obtain these financial rewards are well documented (Thompson, 1986a, 1986b; Young, 1985). Smith (1988) argued persuasively that the level of cheating in college athletics at the turn of the century exceeded what we see today. Even the legendary Knute Rockne was quoted as saying, "Show me a good and gracious loser and I'll show you a failure." Vince Lombardi went a step further with his philosophy that winning isn't everything—it's the only thing. Indeed episodes of cheating, including drug use, have been commonplace at the collegiate, professional, and Olympic levels over the past four decades (Dealy, 1990; Dickey et al., 1999; Dubin, 1990; Francis, 1990; Sperber, 1990; Swift, 1999; Telander, 1989; Voy, 1990). Moreover, because of reports in the news media as well as written and oral testimonials by athletes, adolescents are aware that anabolic steroids and other performance-enhancing drugs have played a part in the success of many so-called role-model athletes (Alzado, 1991; Bamberger & Yaeger, 1997; Dickey et al., 1999).

Our fixation on appearance, especially the muscularity of males, is also long lived. An entire generation of young men aspired to the physique of Charles Atlas, followed by yet another generation who marveled at the muscles of Mr. Universe, Steve Reeves, who played Hercules in several movies in the 1950s. Today's children look with envy at the physiques of Sylvester Stallone, Jean-Claude Van Damme, Wesley Snipes, Linda Hamilton, and other actors *and actresses* whose movie roles call for a muscular athletic build. In addition, a number of professional wrestlers such as Hulk Hogan and "Stone Cold" Steve Austin as well as some elite athletes like Mark McGwire are admired in part for their bigger-than-life muscularity. Anabolic steroid use among professional wrestlers, including Hulk Hogan, was given national attention during a steroid trafficking trial in 1991 (Demak, 1991). President Bush's appointment of Arnold Schwarzenegger, an individual who attained his prominence as a bodybuilder and movie star at least in part as a result of steroid use, as chair of the President's Council on Physical Fitness and Sports was yet another inappropriate message sent to our children. Such messages of material reward and fame as a result of drug-assisted muscularity and winning grossly overshadow posters on gym walls and videos that implore "Just Say No to Steroids."

Some might argue that our attitudes and values related to sports and appearance are too deeply entrenched to change. That may be so, in particular when it comes to elite sport—there is simply too much money involved. However, if we cannot control our competitive and narcissistic natures, we then must resign ourselves to anabolic steroid use, even among our children.

Society's current strategy for dealing with the use of anabolic steroids in sport is multifaceted and primarily involves interdiction and education. However, 10 years after our society was made aware that our children were using steroids, our efforts to deal with this problem have not been very successful. Since 1989 a number of national conferences on anabolic steroid use have been held, sponsored by either the U.S. federal government or sport and educational organizations. The purpose of these meetings was to gather and/or disseminate information or to achieve a consensus for action. At this point all these activities appear to have been a sincere effort to deal with the problem, but this strategy of attacking the symptoms while ignoring the social influence of drug use in sport is obviously ineffective. If we maintain our current course in the face of increased high levels of anabolic steroid use (or use of other performance-enhancing drugs), then we as sports medicine professionals, parents, teachers, and coaches are guilty of duplicity—acting for the sake of acting. We plan and attend workshops, distribute educational materials, lobby for the passage of laws, and seek the assistance of law enforcement. All these activities merely soothe our consciences in the face of our inability, or unwillingness, to deal with our addiction to sport and our fixations on winning and appearance.

References

Alzado, L. (1991, July 8). I'm sick and I'm scared. *Sports Illustrated*, 20–27.

American Academy of Orthopaedic Surgeons and the U.S. Department of Health and Human Services. *STEROIDS DON'T WORK OUT!* (a poster). Washington, DC: Center for Substance Abuse Prevention, Substance Abuse and Mental Health Services Administration.

Bamberger, M., & Yaeger, D. (1997, April 14). Over the edge. *Sports Illustrated*, 60–70.

Barton-Davis, E.R., Shoturma, D.I., Musaro, A., Rosenthal, N., & Sweeney, H.L. (1998). Viral mediated expression of insulin-like growth factor I blocks the aging-related loss of skeletal muscle function. *Proceedings of the National Academy of Sciences, 95,* 15603–15607.

Benario, H. (1983). Sport at Rome. *The Ancient World, 7,* 39.

Beste A. (1991). *Steroids: You make the choice*. N.p.: Iowa High School Athletic Association Printing Department.

Black, T. (1996). Does the ban on drugs in sport improve societal welfare? *International Review for Sociology of Sport, 31,* 367–380.

Centers for Disease Control and Prevention (1994). *Preventing tobacco use among young people: A report of the Surgeon General*. Atlanta: Author.

Dealy, F. (1990). *Win at any cost: The sell out of college athletics.* New York: Birch Lane Press Books.

Demak, R. (1991, July). The sham is a sham. *Sports Illustrated,* 8.

Dickey, C., Helmstaedt, K., Nordland, R., & Hayden, T. (1999, February 15). The real scandal. *Newsweek,* pp. 48–54.

Drug trial, take II. (1998, August 19). *USA Today,* p. 3C.

Drugs and cycling. (1998, September 29). *USA Today,* p. 1C.

Dubin, C. (1990). *Commission of inquiry into the use of drugs and banned practices intended to increase athletic performance* (Catalogue No. CP32-56/1990E, ISBN 0-660-13610-4). Ottawa, ON: Canadian Government Publishing Centre.

Francis, C. (1990). *Speed trap.* New York: St. Martin's Press.

Goldberg, L., Bents, R., Bosworth, E., Trevisan, L., & Elliot, D. (1991). Anabolic steroid education and adolescents: Do scare tactics work? *Pediatrics, 87,* 283–286.

Goldberg, L., Elliot D.L., Clarke G., MacKinnon, D., Zoref, L., Moe, E., Green, C., & Wolf, S. (1996). The Adolescents Training and Learning to Avoid Steroids (ATLAS) prevention program: Background and results of a model intervention. *Archives of Pediatrics and Adolescent Medicine, 150,* 713–721.

Griffin T., & Svendsen R. (1990). *Steroids and our students: A program development guide.* St. Paul: Health Promotion Resources and WBA Ruster Foundation.

Harding Ringhofer & Associates and Media One. (1993). *Students and steroids: The facts . . . straight up* (a steroid use prevention program for adolescents). Minnetonka, MN: Author.

Hiestand, M. (1999, January 12). The B word—billion—no longer out of bounds. *USA Today,* pp. 1–2a.

Hoberman, J. (1984). *Sport and political ideology.* Austin, TX: University of Texas Press.

Lassar, S. (1998, December 3). Four former Northwestern football players indicted on perjury charges related to sports gambling investigation (press release). U.S. Justice Department, U.S. Attorney, Northern District of Illinois.

Leaderman, D. (1990, January 3). 57 of 106 universities in NCAA's top unit punished in 1980s. *Chronicle of Higher Education,* p. A31.

Lemonick, M. (1998, August 10). Le Tour des Drugs. *Time,* p. 76.

Longtime drug use. (1999, January 28). *USA Today,* p. 3C.

Office of Applied Studies (1999). *National Household Survey on Drug Abuse: Main findings, 1997* (SMA # 99-3295). Rockville, MD: U.S. Department of Health and Human Services, Substance Abuse and Mental Health Services Administration.

Saum, B. (1998, November 10). Written testimony of Bill Saum, Director of Agent and Gambling Activities, National Collegiate Athletic Association, before the National Gambling Impact Study Commission, Las Vegas, Nevada.

Schaps, E., Bartolo, R., Moskowitz, J., Palley, C., & Churgin, S. (1981). Review of 127 drug abuse prevention program evaluations. *Journal of Drug Issues, 2,* 17–43.

Simson, V., & Jennings, A. (1992). *The lords of the rings: Power, money, and drugs in the modern Olympics.* London: Simon & Schuster.

Smith, R. (1988). *Sports and freedom: The rise of big-time college athletics.* New York: Oxford University Press.

Snowboarder loses medal after drug test. (1998, February 11). *USA Today,* p. 9E.

Sperber, M. (1990). *College sports inc.* New York: Holt.

Study: Gambling in NCAA rampant. (1999, January 12). *USA Today,* p. 3C.

A survey of sport: Not just a game. (1998). *Economist, 347,* 2–23.

Swift, E. (1999, February 1). Breaking point. *Sports Illustrated,* 34–35.

Telander, R. (1989). *The hundred yard lie.* New York: Simon & Schuster.

Thompson, J. (1986a). Historical errors about the ancient Olympic games. *Gamut, 17*(winter), 20–23.

Thompson, J. (1986b). The intrusion of corruption into athletics: An age-old problem. *Journal of General Education, 23,* 144–153.

Track star blazed trail. (1998, September 22). *USA Today,* pp. 1–2C.

U.S. Department of Health and Human Services, Department of Education. (1988). *Steroids: Playing with trouble* (a poster). Washington, DC: U.S. Government Printing Office, 1988-0-208-087.

U.S. Department of Health and Human Services. (1989, March). *Health United States: 1988* (DHHS Publication [PHS] 89-1232, U.S.). Hyattsville, MD: USDHHS, National Center for Health Statistics.

U.S. Department of Health and Human Services, Public Health Service. (1991, January). *Interagency Task Force on Anabolic Steroids.* Washington, DC: Author.

U.S. Department of Justice (1994). *Report of the International Conference on the Abuse and Trafficking of Anabolic Steroids.* Washington, DC: Drug Enforcement Administration.

Voy, R. (1990). *Drugs, sport, and politics.* Champaign, IL: Leisure Press.

Wm. C. Brown Communications. (1993). *1992–1993 Weight training fitness and conditioning catalog.* Dubuque, IA: Brown and Benchmark.

Yesalis, C., & Cowart, V. (1998). *The steroids game.* Champaign, IL: Human Kinetics.

Yesalis, C., & Friedl, K. (1988). Anabolic steroid use in amateur sports: An epidemiologic perspective. In R. Kretchmar (Ed.), *Proceedings of the US Olympic Academy XII* (pp. 83–89). Colorado Springs: U.S. Olympic Committee.

Yesalis, C.E., Herrick, R.T., Buckley, W.E., Friedl, K.E., Brannon, D., & Wright, J.E. (1988). Self-reported use of anabolic-androgenic steroids by elite power lifters. *The Physician and Sportsmedicine, 16,* 91–100.

Yesalis, C., Wright, J., & Lombardo, J. (1989, July 30–31). *Anabolic androgenic steroids: A synthesis of existing data and recommendations for future research.* Keynote research address, National Steroid Consensus Meeting, Los Angeles.

Yesalis, C., Streit, A., Vicary, J., Friedl, K., Brannon, D., & Buckley, W. (1989). Anabolic steroid use: Indications of habituation among adolescents. *Journal of Drug Education, 19,* 103–116.

Young, D. (1985). *The Olympic myth of Greek amateur athletics.* Chicago: Ares.

Index

The letters *f* and *t* after page numbers indicate figures and tables, respectively.

About the Editor

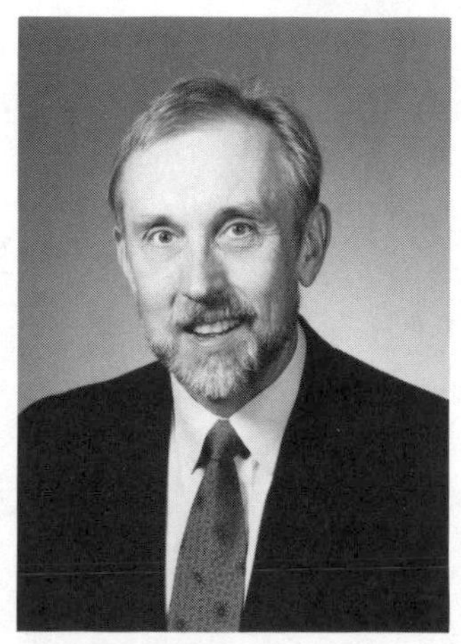

Renowned worldwide for research and teaching experience related to nonmedical use of steroids and other performance-enhancing drugs, Charles Yesalis, ScD, MPH, is currently professor of Health Policy and Administration and Exercise and Sport Science at The Pennsylvania State University.

Author or coauthor of more than 60 journal articles and a frequent presenter at international conferences throughout the United States, Canada, France, Sweden, and the Czech Republic, he has also edited or coauthored three books concerning steroid usage.

In addition to testifying before the U.S. Congress, he has acted as consultant for the U.S. Senate Judiciary Committee, Drug Enforcement Administration, NFL Players Association, Food and Drug Administration, Centers for Disease Control and Prevention, U.S. Olympic Committee, National College Athletic Association, and the National Strength and Conditioning Association.

Dr. Yesalis earned a master's degree in Public Health from the University of Michigan and a doctoral degree from Johns Hopkins School of Hygiene and Public Health.

In his leisure time he enjoys military history as well as racquetball, weightlifting, and running.

About the Contributors

Michael S. Bahrke received his MS in exercise physiology and his PhD in sport psychology from the University of Wisconsin–Madison. Dr. Bahrke has been an assistant professor at the University of Kansas, director of research for the U.S. Army Physical Fitness School, fitness area coordinator at the University of Wisconsin, and project director for a National Institute of Drug Abuse–funded anabolic steroids research grant in the School of Public Health, Division of Epidemiology and Biostatistics, at the University of Illinois in Chicago. He is currently an acquisitions editor in the Scientific, Technical, and Medical Division of Human Kinetics.

Kirk J. Brower received his BA in psychobiology from the University of California, Los Angeles, and his MD from the University of California, Irvine. After completing his residency in psychiatry at UCLA in 1985, Dr. Brower joined the faculty at the University of Michigan in Ann Arbor, where he is currently an associate professor of psychiatry. He is also executive director of the Chelsea Arbor Treatment Center, which is devoted to the treatment and research of substance abuse problems.

Stephen P. Courson attended the University of South Carolina, where he was a tri-captain of the football team in 1976. He was drafted by the Pittsburgh Steelers in 1977 and was a member of the 1978 and 1979 Super Bowl championship teams. Mr. Courson was one of the first players to openly acknowledge his steroid use and the predicament in sports while still an active player (he did so in *Sports Illustrated* in 1985). He is now involved with Charles Yesalis in research and lectures to high schools, colleges, and civic groups about performance-enhancing drug use in sport and society. He has released his own book dealing with drugs in sport (*False Glory,* Longmeadow Press, 1991).

Diane L. Elliot, MD, is professor of medicine and associate director of the Human Performance Laboratory in the Division of Health Promotion & Sports Medicine of the Department of Medicine at Oregon Health Sciences University. With her colleague, Linn Goldberg, MD, she developed and assessed the ATLAS (Adolescents Training and Learning to Avoid Steroids) program, a sport team–centered drug prevention and health promotion program for male adolescent athletes. Dr. Elliot currently is principal investigator for the newly implemented ATHENA (Athletes Targeting Healthy Exercise and Nutrition Alternatives) program for adolescent female athletes. She is a crew chief for the U.S. Olympic Committee's drug testing program. Dr. Elliot has many scientific publications and, with Dr. Goldberg, wrote the popular book *The Healing Power of Exercise.*

Jim Ferstle is a freelance writer who specializes in participatory sports, sports medicine, and education. Ferstle's award-winning reporting on drugs and sports has brought him notoriety as an expert in the field. His work has appeared in *Runner's World, The London Sunday Times, 60 Minutes,* the BBC's *Panorama,* and *St. Paul Pioneer Press.*

Karl E. Friedl, PhD, is the research manager for the Military Operational Medicine Research Program at the U.S. Army Medical Research and Materiel Command in Frederick, Maryland. Prior to this assignment, he conducted research in the Occupational Physiology Division of the U.S. Army Research Institute of Environmental Medicine in Natick, Massachusetts, where he specialized in physiological limits of prolonged, intensive military training. Previously, Lieutenant Colonel Friedl worked in the Department of Clinical Investigation at Madigan Army Medical Center in Tacoma, Washington, performing studies in endocrine physiology. He received his PhD in physiology in 1984 from the Institute of Environmental Stress at the University of California, Santa Barbara.

Linn Goldberg, MD, FACSM, received his medical degree with distinction from the George Washington University Medical School. Currently, he is professor of medicine, director of the Human Performance Laboratory and head of the Division of Health Promotion & Sports Medicine at the Oregon Health Sciences University. Dr. Goldberg is a fellow of the American College of Sports Medicine, an expert panelist for the U.S. Department of Education's Safe, Disciplined and Drug-Free Schools and serves as a crew chief for the U.S. Olympic Committee. He has served as a special consultant to the U.S. Department of Health and Human Services and delegate to the World Health Organization, regarding drug use in sport.

R. Craig Kammerer, PhD, is a senior research scientist, consultant, and medical writer in the pharmaceutical industry in New Jersey. Dr. Kammerer has been assistant professor of pharmacology (1978–1987) at the UCLA School of Medicine and was the founding associate director of the Paul Ziffren Olympic Analytical Lab (1982–1987). This first IOC-accredited lab in the United States performed drug testing for the 23rd Summer Olympics in Los Angeles in 1984.

Carol C. Kleinman, MD, JD, received her BA in political science from Northwestern University in Evanston, Illinois, and her JD, with honors, and her MD from George Washington University, Washington, D.C. After completing her residency in psychiatry at the University of Maryland in Baltimore in 1984, she worked as a staff psychiatrist and Director of Women's Forensic Programs, at Clifton T. Perkins Hospital Center in

Jessup, Maryland. She is a clinical assistant professor at the Uniformed Services University of the Health Sciences in Bethesda, Maryland. She is also a past president of the Washington Psychiatric Society. She is currently in the practice of general and forensic psychiatry in Chevy Chase, Maryland.

Charles D. Kochakian received his PhD in physiological chemistry in 1936 from the University of Rochester. A pioneer in the research of anabolic-androgenic steroids, Dr. Kochakian discovered the anabolic action of a male hormone extract on human urine, determined the sites of protein synthesis, and delineated the mechanism of action of testosterone on protein synthesis. He was a professor emeritus of the University of Alabama at Birmingham. Dr. Kochakian died February 12, 1999, at the age of 90.

Andrea N. Kopstein received her MPH in epidemiology from the University of Texas School of Public Health and her PhD in epidemiology from Johns Hopkins University. For more than 10 years, she was a project officer and statistician at the National Center for Health Statistics, part of the Centers for Disease Control and Prevention. She also spent 10 years as a project officer and statistician at the National Institute on Drug Abuse, part of the National Institutes of Health. Currently, Dr. Kopstein is a statistician with the Substance Abuse and Mental Health Services Administration where she works on the National Household Survey on Drug Abuse.

C.E. Petit, JD, earned his JD magna cum laude from the University of Illinois College of Law, where he was articles editor for the *University of Illinois Law Review.* He became interested in drug testing while studying for an AB in chemistry at Washington University (St. Louis), and became familiar with the legal intricacies of drug testing while serving as a commanding officer while handling the aftermath of twenty-odd positive drug tests, including two for steroid abuse. He is currently in private practice in Urbana, Illinois.

James E. Wright holds a bachelor's degree in biology from Farleigh Dickenson University and a doctoral degree in zoology from Mississippi State University. He has been an NIH postdoctoral fellow at the Institute of Environmental Stress, University of California, Santa Barbara. Dr. Wright served in the USMC and later in the U.S. Army. He was a research team leader and chief of the Muscle Strength Section at the U.S. Army Research Institute of Environmental Medicine (1977–1982). From 1985 to 1988 he was chief of the Exercise Science Branch at the U.S. Army Physical Fitness School and Liaison of the Office of the (Army) Surgeon General to that organization.